Liver Fibrosis: Pathophysiology, Diagnosis and Management

Liver Fibrosis: Pathophysiology, Diagnosis and Management

Edited by Finley Bush

hayle
medical

New York

Hayle Medical,
750 Third Avenue, 9th Floor,
New York, NY 10017, USA

Visit us on the World Wide Web at:
www.haylemedical.com

ISBN: 978-1-63241-910-1

Cataloging-in-Publication Data

Liver fibrosis : pathophysiology, diagnosis and management / edited by Finley Bush.
 p. cm.
Includes bibliographical references and index.
ISBN 978-1-63241-910-1
1. Liver--Fibrosis. 2. Liver--Fibrosis--Pathophysiology. 3. Liver--Fibrosis--Diagnosis.
4. Liver--Fibrosis--Treatment. 5. Liver--Diseases. I. Bush, Finley.
RC848.F53 L58 2020
616.362--dc23

Table of Contents

Preface

Liver fibrosis is a condition of the liver characterized by the excessive accumulation of extracellular matrix proteins such as collagen. Advanced liver fibrosis leads to cirrhosis of the liver. Cirrhosis leads to hepatocellular dysfunction and a high intrahepatic resistance to blood flow that results in hepatic insufficiency and portal hypertension. Liver biopsy is the standard procedure for diagnosing and assessing liver fibrosis. To determine the degree of liver damage, several scales such as Ishak fibrosis score (stages I–V) and METAVIR scoring system (stages I–IV) are used for the staging of liver fibrosis. Other evaluations such as platelet count, ascites, Bonacini cirrhosis discriminant score and spider angiomata can help to diagnose cirrhosis. Recent evidence points to the reversibility of liver fibrosis even in its advanced stages. Typically, this may happen with a cessation of liver injury, via the successful treatment of the underlying disease. For patients with cirrhosis, liver transplantation is currently the only curative strategy with improved quality of life and better chances of survival. A lot of research is being undertaken to develop non-invasive and reliable markers of liver fibrosis, and liver specific antifibrotic therapies. This book aims to shed light on some of the unexplored aspects of liver fibrosis and the recent researches in this pathological condition. The objective of this book is to give a general view of the different aspects of its pathophysiology, diagnosis and management. This book, with its detailed analyses and data, will prove immensely beneficial to professionals and students involved in hepatology at various levels.

The researches compiled throughout the book are authentic and of high quality, combining several disciplines and from very diverse regions from around the world. Drawing on the contributions of many researchers from diverse countries, the book's objective is to provide the readers with the latest achievements in the area of research. This book will surely be a source of knowledge to all interested and researching the field.

In the end, I would like to express my deep sense of gratitude to all the authors for meeting the set deadlines in completing and submitting their research chapters. I would also like to thank the publisher for the support offered to us throughout the course of the book. Finally, I extend my sincere thanks to my family for being a constant source of inspiration and encouragement.

Editor

TRPV4 Channel Inhibits TGF-β1-Induced Proliferation of Hepatic Stellate Cells

Yang Song[1,2,3], **Lei Zhan**[1,2], **Mingzhe Yu**[1,2], **Cheng Huang**[1,2], **Xiaoming Meng**[1,2], **Taotao Ma**[1,2], **Lei Zhang**[1,2], **Jun Li**[1,2]*

1 School of Pharmacy, Anhui Medical University, Hefei, China, **2** Institute for Liver Diseases of Anhui Medical University (AMU), Hefei, China, **3** The First Affiliated Hospital of Anhui Medical University, Hefei, China

Abstract

TRPV4, one of the TRP channels, is implicated in diverse physiological and pathological processes including cell proliferation. However, the role of TRPV4 in liver fibrosis is largely unknown. Here, we characterized the role of TRPV4 in regulating HSC-T6 cell proliferation. TRPV4 mRNA and protein were measured by RT-PCR and Western blot in patients and rat model of liver fibrosis in vivo and TGF-β1-activated HSC-T6 cells in vitro. Both mRNA and protein of TRPV4 were dramatically increased in liver fibrotic tissues of both patients and CCl_4-treated rats. Stimulation of HSC-T6 cells with TGF-β1 resulted in increase of TRPV4 mRNA and protein. However, TGF-β1-induced HSC-T6 cell proliferation was inhibited by Ruthenium Red (Ru) or synthetic siRNA targeting TRPV4, and this was accompanied by downregulation of myofibroblast markers including α-SMA and Col1α1. Moreover, our study revealed that miR-203 was downregulated in liver fibrotic tissues and TGF-β1-treated HSC-T6 cell. Bioinformatics analyses predict that TRPV4 is the potential target of miR-203. In addition, overexpression of miR-203 in TGF-β1-induced HSC significantly reduced TRPV4 expression, indicating TRPV4, which was regulated by miR-203, may function as a novel regulator to modulate TGF-β1-induced HSC-T6 proliferation.

Editor: Partha Mukhopadhyay, National Institutes of Health, United States of America

Funding: This project was supported by the National Science Foundation of China (NO 81072686, 81273526, 81202978) and publication fees were covered by NSFC (NO 81273526). The funder had no role in study design, data collection and analysis, decision to publish, or preparation of the manuscript.

Competing Interests: The authors have declared that no competing interests exist.

* Email: lj@ahmu.edu.cn

Introduction

Liver fibrosis is a medical problem worldwide with high morbidity and mortality, and endangers human health seriously [1]. Hepatic stellate cells (HSC) play an essential role in the development of liver fibrosis. For example, following fibrotic injury, HSC undergo transdifferentiation from quiescent vitamin-A-storing cells to an activated myofibroblastic phenotype identified by upregulation of α-smooth muscle actin (α-SMA) and type I collagen, thereby contributing to the progression of liver fibrosis [2,3]. However, the molecular mechanisms responsible for the proliferation and activation of HSC are still unclear. In the case of HSC, this proliferation and activation responses can be prevented by treatment with chemical inhibitors of ion channels [4,5]. But so far, the detailed mechanisms, by which ion channels regulate liver fibrosis, are complex and have not been fully elucidated.

Transient receptor potential vanilloid 4 (TRPV4) was firstly identified as a channel activated by hypotonicity-induced cell swelling, however, TRPV4 is also sensitive to a wide variety of physical and chemical stimuli [6]. Importantly, it is able to integrate different stimuli and confer many distinct cellular functions in various cell types throughout the body [7,8,9,10]. Here, we detected increased TRPV4 mRNA and protein level in the liver of rats subjected to liver injury. The blockade of TRPV4 with Ruthenium Red (Ru) or TRPV4-siRNA inhibited the proliferation of activated HSC-T6 cells and decreased α-SMA and Col1α1 expressions. Moreover, we explored the potential function of miR-203 in the regulation of TRPV4 in vitro. Our results suggested a pathological role of TRPV4 in the activation and proliferation of HSC, indicating that TRPV4 may be a potential therapeutic target in the treatment of liver fibrosis.

Materials and Methods

2.1 Materials and reagents

Non-tumorous portions of the liver were obtained from patients undergoing partial liver resection at the Department of Surgery, The First Hospital of Anhui Medical University. The degree of fibrosis was classified as normal liver and mild to moderate fibrosis according to the Liver Cancer Study Group of Japan. Written informed consent was obtained from all patients. The study was approved by the Ethical Committee of Anhui Medical University and followed the ethical guidelines of the Declaration of Helsinki.

CCl_4 was obtained from Shantou Xilong Chemistry Plant (Shantou, China). Dimethylsulfoxide (DMSO) were purchased from Sigma Inc. (St. Louis, MO, USA). Mouse monoclonal antibodies against α-SMA and β-actin were obtained from Boster (Wuhan, China). TRPV4 antibodies were purchased from Abcam (Cambridge, UK). TGF-β1 was purchased from Peprotech (New Jersey, USA). miR-203, TRPV4, α-SMA and Collagen I primers were produced from Shanghai Sangon Biological and Technological Company (Shanghai, China). Ruthenium Red was purchased from Sigma (Deisenhofen, Germany). DNA extraction kit was acquired from Axygen. Streptavidin peroxidase (SP) immunohistochemical kit was acquired from Zhongshan Biotechnology Corporation (Beijing, China). Secondary antibodies for goat anti-rabbit immunoglobulin (IgG) horse radish peroxidase (HRP), and goat anti-mouse IgG HRP were purchased from Santa Cruz Biotechnology (Santa Cruz, California, USA).

2.2 CCl$_4$ liver injury model

Liver fibrosis was generated by a 12-week treatment of adult male Sprague-Dawley (200–220 g) rats with CCl$_4$ (CCl$_4$/olive oil, 1:1 (vol/vol) per kg body weight by intraperitoneal injection twice weekly) as previously described [11]. Vehicle control animals were treated intraperitoneally with 1 ml/olive oil/kg body weight at the same time intervals. 24 h after the final CCl$_4$ injection, rats were sacrificed and liver tissues were harvested for the further analysis. Animals were provided by the Experimental Animal Center of Anhui Medical University. The animal experimental protocol was approved by the University Animal Care and Use Committee of Anhui Medical University.

2.3 Cell culture and cell treatment with TGF-β1

HSC-T6 cell line was obtained from Shanghai FuMeng Gene Bio-technology Co., LTD. (Shanghai, China). HSC-T6 cells were cultured in Dulbecco's modified Eagle's medium (DMEM, USA) supplemented with 10% fetal bovine serum, 100 U/ml penicillin and 100 mg/ml streptomycin in a humidified incubator at 37°C with 5% CO2. These cells were propagated for 48 h and serum-starved with 0.5% FBS for 24 h before adding 10 ng/ml Platelet-derived growth factor (PDGF-BB, peprotech, USA).

2.4 Cell transient transfection of miR-203 mimics and siTRPV4

HSC-T6 cells were cultured in serum-free DMEM for 12 h and then subjected to transfection with miR-203 mimics, (NS)-miRNA (GenaPharma, China) and Si-TRPV4, Si-control using Lipofectamine 2000 (Invitrogen, USA)according to the manufacturer's instruction. The culture medium was changed 6 h after transfection, and TGF-β1 (Peprotech, USA) was added at a concentration of 10 ng/ml. The sequences of oligonucleotides used are as follows:

miR-203 mimics: 5'-GUGAAAUGUUUAGGACCACUAG-3'
      5'-AGUGGUCCUAAACAUUUCACUU-3
NS-miRNA: 5'-UUCUCCGAACGUGUCACGUTT-3'
      5'-ACGUGACACGUUCGGAGAATT-3'
Si-TRPV4: 5'- CCGUGUCCUUCUACAUCAATT -3'
      5'- UUGAUGUAGAAGGACACGGTT -3'
si-control: 5'-UUCUCCGAACGUGUCACGUTT-3'
      5'-ACGUGACACGUUCGGAGAATT-3'

2.5 Ruthenium Red (Ru) treatment

Ru was dissolved in Dulbecco's modified Eagle's medium (DMEM, Gibco, USA) with 10% fetal bovine serum and used at a concentration of 1 uM. HSC-T6 cells were seeded overnight in culture dishes and treated with TGF-β1 plus Ru.

2.6 Semi-quantitativereversetranscription-polymerasechainreaction(RT-PCR)

Total RNA was extracted from rat liver tissues and HSC-T6 cells using TRIzol reagents (Invitrogen). The first-strand cDNA was synthesized from total RNA using Thermoscript RT-PCR System (Takara) according to the manufacturer's instructions. RT-PCR was carried out under standard protocol using the following primers: β-actin (forward: 5'-TGAGCTGCGTGTGGCCCCT-GAG-3'; reverse: 5'-GGGGCATCGGAA CCGCTCATTG-3'), TRPV4(forward: 5'-CGCCTCCGCAGGGATCGCTGGTC-3'; reverse: 5'-TGAGCTGGCTTAGGTGACTCCATGGGAGTG-3', α-SMA (forward: 5'-TGGCCACTGCTGCTTCCTCTTC-TT-3'; reverse: 5'-GGGGCCAGCTTCGTCAT ACTCCT-3'), Col1a1: (forward: 5'-TACAGCACGCTTGTGGATG-3'; reverse: 5'-TT GAGTTTGGGTTGTTGGTC-3'). PCR was performed at 94°C for 5 min, followed by 35 or 38 cycles of amplification at 94°C for 36 s, 52 or 60°C for 36 s and 72°C for 1 min by using ABI9700. The band intensities were measured by a densitometer and the results were normalized with β-actin. The results were repeated at least three times independently from three different pools of templates, while each pool of template was extracted from at least three ventricles.

2.7 Quantitative real-time PCR

Total RNA was extracted from the cultured cells using a RISO RNA Isolation Reagent (Biomics, USA). Expression of miR-203 was measured using an EzOmics miRNA qPCR Detection Primer Set (Biomics, USA) and EzOmics One-Step qPCR Kit (Biomics, USA) in PikoReal 96 real-time PCR system (Thermo Fisher Scientific, Finland).The fold-change for miR-203 relative to U6 was calculated using the 2- $\Delta\Delta$Ct method, where $\Delta\Delta$Ct = ΔCt BEL/5-FU-ΔCt BEL-7402 and ΔCt = Ct miR-203-Ct U6. PCR was performed in triplicate. Total RNA was isolated from the cultured cells using the TRIzol reagents (Invitrogen, USA), and the first strand cDNA was synthesized using a ThermoScript RT-PCR synthesis kit (Fermentas, USA) according to the manufacturer's instructions. Quantitative real-time PCR analyses for mRNA of TRPV4, α-SMA, β-actin were performed by using the QuantiFast SYBR Green RT-PCR kits (QIAGEN, Germany). The mRNA level of β-actin was measured as an internal control.

2.8 RNA interference (RNAi) analysis

RNAi experiments in HSC-T6 cells were performed by forward transfection in day 2 cultured HSC-T6 (2×10^5 cells per 200 mm^2 dish) using Lipofectamine RNAiMax (Invitrogen) according to the manufacturer's protocol. For TRPV4 immunoblotting, HSC-T6 cells were cultured in serum-free DMEM for 12 h and then subjected to reverse transfection with RNAiMax in Opti-MEM. Small interfering RNA (siRNA) oligonucleotides against TRPV4 genes or scrambled sequences were synthesized by the Shanghai GenePharma Corporation. The following siRNA sequences were used: si-TRPV4 (rat), 5'-CCCAGAGUAUGCACCAAUATT-3' (sense) and 5'-UAUUGGUGCAUACUCUGGGTT-3' (antisense); si-control with scrambled sequence (negative control siRNA having no perfect matches to known rat genes), 5'-UUCUCC-GAACGUGUCACGUTT-3' (sense) and 5'-ACGUGACAC-GUUCGGAGAATT-3' (antisense). Transfection was allowed to proceed for various times and cells were processed for different assays. The siRNA transfection efficiency of Lipofectamine RNAiMax in cells was determined by the BLOCK-iT Alexa Fluor Red Fluorescent Oligo protocol (Invitrogen).

2.9 MTT assay

Cellular proliferation was measured using MTT assay. 5×10^3 cells were seeded in 96-well plates and cultured with siRNA-TRPV4 at 37°C in a humid chamber with 5% CO2 for 2 days. 5 mg/ml MTT was then added to each well and incubated with cells at 37°C for 4 h. After removal of supernatant, 150 ul of DMSO were added to each well. The optical density (OD) was measured at 490 nm. The percentage of viability was calculated according to the following formula: viability $\% = T/C \times 100\%$, where T and C refer to the absorbance of transfection group and cell control, respectively.

2.10 Western blotting

Rat liver tissues and cells were lysed with lysis buffer. Whole-cell extracts were prepared, and protein concentration of samples was determined using a BCA protein assay kit (Boster, China). Whole-cell extracts (30 or 50 mg) were then fractionated by electrophoresis through an 10% sodium dodecyl sulfate-polyacrylamide gel electrophoresis (SDS-PAGE). Gels were run at a 120 V for 2 h before being transferred onto a PVDF membrane (Millipore Corp, Billerica, MA, USA). After blockade of nonspecific protein binding, nitrocellulose blots were incubated for 1 h with primary antibodies diluted in TBS/Tween20 (0.075%) containing 3% Marvel. Anti-TRPV4 (Cell Signaling, Beverly, MA, USA) was diluted 1:400, and rabbit monoclonal anti-α-SMA (Boster) was diluted 1:200. Rabbit monoclonal antibodies directed against TRPV4 (Abcam, Cambridge, UK) or β-actin (Santa Cruz Biotechnology, CA, USA) were used at 1:400. Following incubation with primary antibodies, blots were washed four times in TBS/Tween-20 before incubation for 1 h in goat anti-rabbit horseradish peroxidase conjugate antibody at 1:10000 dilution in TBS/Tween-20 containing 5% skim milk. After extensive washing in TBS/Tween-20, the blots were processed with distilled water for detection of antigen using the enhanced chemiluminescence system. Proteins were visualized with the ECL-chemiluminescent kit (ECL-plus, Thermo Scientific).

2.11 Immunohistochemistry

Liver tissues were fixed in 10% neutral buffered formalin solution, embedded in paraffin, and stained for routine histology. The sections were dewaxed in xylene and dehydrated in alcohol, antigen retrieval was achieved by microwaving in citric saline for 15 min. Thin sections were deparaffinized and treated with 0.3% hydrogen peroxide for 15 min to block endogenous peroxidase activity. The sections were further blocked by 2% bovine serum albumin followed by incubation with primary antibody against TRPV4 (1:400) for 16 h at 4°C. After rinsing, the sections were incubated with biotinylated secondary antibody for 60 min at room temperature. TRPV4 expression was visualized by 3,3'-diaminobenzidine tetrahydrochloride (DAB) staining. Slides were counterstained with hematoxylin before dehydration and mounting. TRPV4 positive areas within the fibrotic region were then observed. Quantitative analysis was calculated from five fields for each liver slice.

2.12 Luciferase reporter assays

Luciferase reporter assays were carried out in HSC. Briefly, HSC-T6 cells (5×104 cells/well) were cultured into 24-well plates and co-transfected with 200 ng DNA of TRPV4-UTR wt plasmid in the presence of 60 nmol of miR-203 mimics and NS-miR-203 (Gene Pharma, Shanghai, China), using 2.5 uL lipofectamine 2000 and 100 uL Opti-MEM (Invitrogen, USA). The cells were harvested and lysed 48 h after transfection and the luciferase activities were measured consecutively by the Dual-Luciferase Reporter 1000 Assay system (Promega, USA). Renilla luciferase activity was normalized to Firefly luciferase activity. All experiments were performed independently in triplicate.

2.13 Double Immunofluorescent Staining

For double immunofluorescent staining, sections were firstly blocked with 10% normal serum blocking solution in order to avoid unspecific staining. Then, the sections were incubated with rabbit polyclonal primary antibodies for TRPV4 (1:50; Abcam) and mouse monoclonal primary antibodies for α-SMA (1:100; Santa Cruz). Sections were incubated with both primary antibodies over-night at 4°C, followed by a mixture of anti-mouse FITC (1:200) and anti-rabbit TRITC (1:200) conjugated secondary antibodies for 2 h at room temperature. Then the stained sections were examined with a Leica sp5 laser confocal microscope (Germany).

2.14 Statistical analysis

Data are represented as mean ± SE. Statistical analysis was performed using ANOVA followed by Student's t-test. For changes in mRNA or protein levels, ratios of mRNA (relative expression) and protein (densitometric values) to respective housekeeping controls were compared. Significance was defined as $p < 0.05$.

Results

3.1 Upregulation of TRPV4 mRNA and protein in the liver tissues from liver fibrosis patients and CCl$_4$-treated rats

First, we investigated the expression of TRPV4 in the liver tissues from liver fibrosis patients. As shown in Fig. 1A, TRPV4 immunostaining signal was increased in the liver tissues from liver fibrosis patients compared to the normal liver. Additionally, the results of Immunofluorescence in human samples indicated that TRPV4(red) was highly expressed in α-SMA positive cells(green) in the fibrotic area, indicating HSC may be one of main cell types which express TRPV4 (Fig. 1B). Second, in order to identify the expression of TRPV4 in the liver tissues from CCl$_4$-treated rats, the severity of liver fibrosis was determined by hematoxylin and eosin (H&E) staining and Masson's trichrome staining. H&E and Masson's trichrome staining showed normal lobular architecture with central veins and radiating hepatic cords in the vehicle group (Fig. 1C). The CCl$_4$ treatment resulted in steatosis, inflammatory infiltration, and fibrosis in the main block of experiments of 12 weeks (Fig. 1C). Immunostaining from vehicle treated groups showed scarce α-SMA staining, whereas the liver tissues from CCl$_4$-treated rats were extensively stained (Fig. 1D). Moreover, compared with the vehicle-treated groups, both RT-PCR and western blot analysis demonstrated that expression of TRPV4 mRNA and protein extracted from rat liver were elevated in CCl$_4$-treated livers (Fig. 1E, F and G). Together, these data suggested that the TRPV4 was induced and may have certain functions in hepatic fibrosis.

3.2 Increasing expression of TRPV4 mRNA and protein during HSC activation

In chronic liver injury, quiescent HSCs change into proliferative myofibroblast-like cells, which is a main source of extracellular matrix. To validate the alteration of TRPV4 gene expression during HSC activation also occurs in vitro, we examined the expressions of TRPV4 mRNA and protein in cultured rat HSC-T6 cells. As illustrated in Fig. 2A and B, HSC-T6 cells was incubated with 10 ng/ml TGF-β1 for 24 h, both mRNA and protein levels of TRPV4 were elevated. Additionally, α- SMA and Col1α1 expressions were increased according to the progression of HSC-T6 cell activation (Fig. 2C) and significantly correlated with the level of TRPV4.

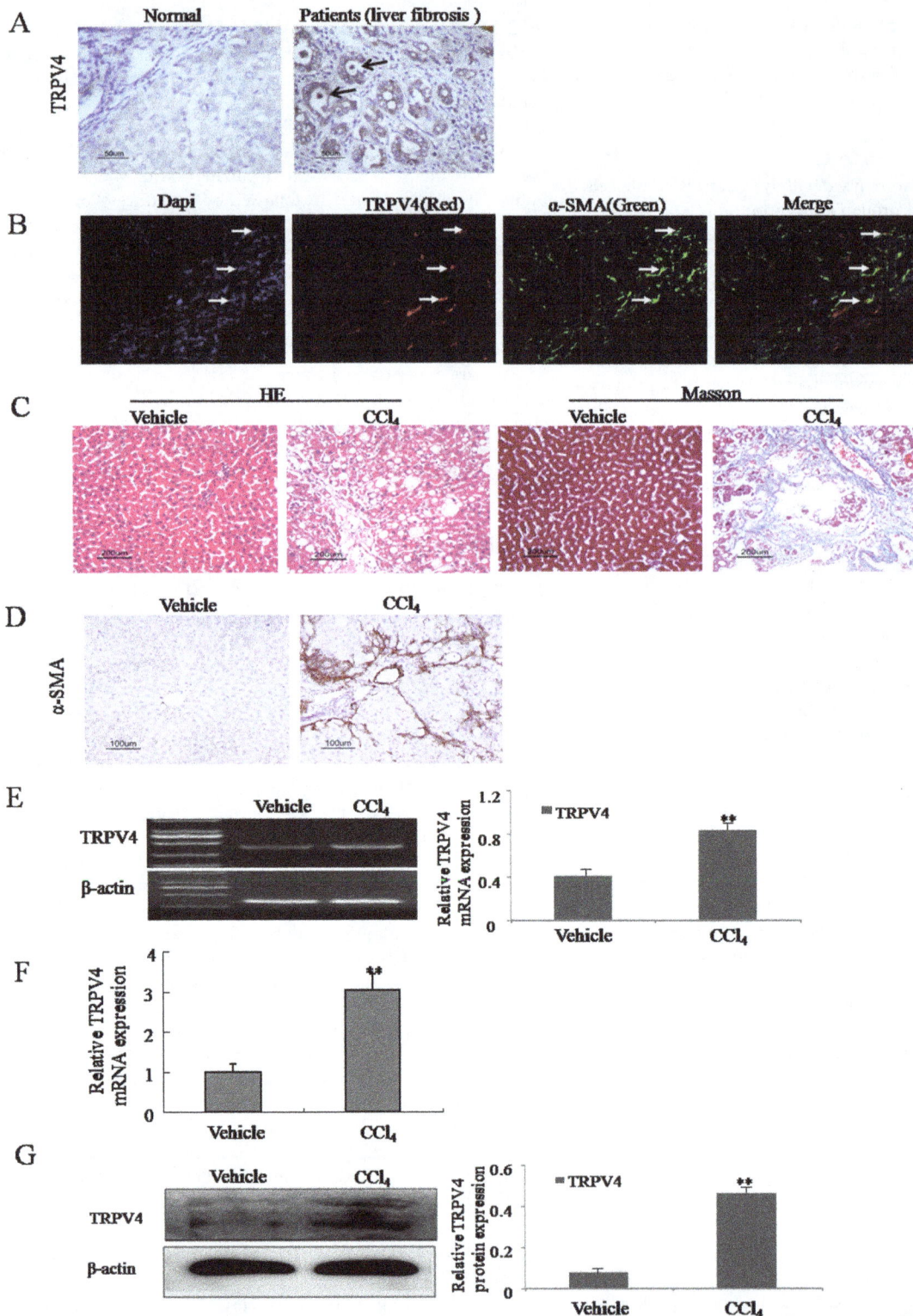

Figure 1. Upregulation of TRPV4 mRNA and protein in the liver tissues from liver fibrosis patients and CCl4-treated rats. A. The level of the TRPV4 was analyzed by immunohistochemistry in human normal liver and liver fibrosis patients. Representative views from each group are presented (original magnification, ×50). B. Liver tissues from liver fibrosis patients tissue were double stained with TRPV4 and α-SMA antibodies. Representative photomicrographs are shown (original magnification, ×40) in B. C. Pathology observation of the experimental rat liver sections stained with hematoxylin and eosin (H&E) staining and massion staining (×200). D. The level of the α-SMA was analyzed by immunohistochemistry in vehicle control livers and liver fibrotic tissue. Representative views from each group are presented (original magnification, ×50). E-F. Total RNAs were isolated from the livers of CCl4-treated rats or vehicle-treated groups. The expression of TRPV4 mRNA was assessed by RT-PCR(E) and realtime PCR(F). Representative images of three independent experiments are shown. *p<0.05, **p<0.01 vs. vehicle control. G. Whole-cell extracts were isolated from the liver tissues of CCl4-treated rats or vehicle-treated groups, and subjected to immunoblot for TRPV4 and β-actin control. Representative images of three independent experiments are shown. *p<0.05, **p<0.01 vs. vehicle control.

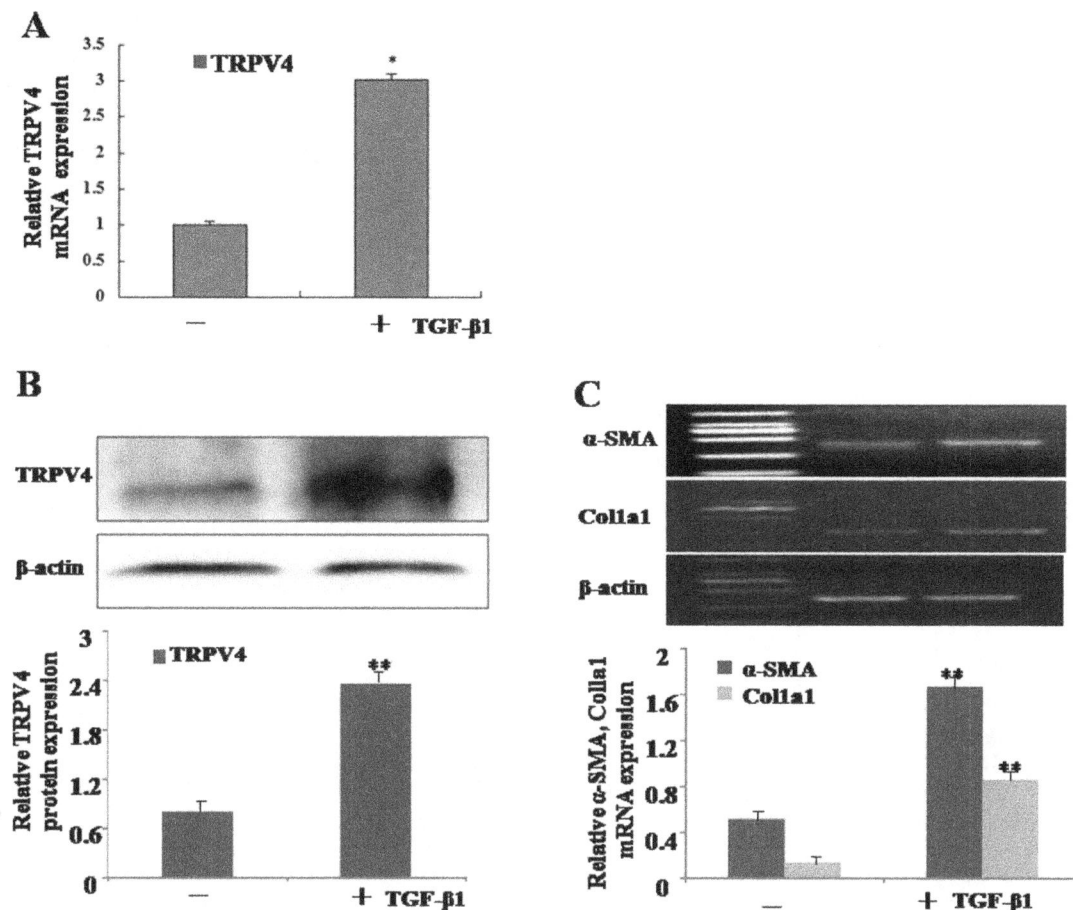

Figure 2. Increasing expression of TRPV4 mRNA and protein during HSC activation. A. Total RNAs were isolated from TGF-β1-treated HSC-T6 cells, and subjected to qRT-PCR analyses. Representative images of three independent experiments are shown. *p<0.05 vs. non-treated cells. B. Whole-cell extracts were isolated from TGF-β1-treated HSC-T6 cells, and subjected to Western blot analyses with TRPV4 and β-actin antibodies. Representative blots of three independent experiments are shown. **p<0.01 vs. non-treated cells. C. Total RNAs were isolated from TGF-β1 treated HSC-T6 cells at different time points. The expression of α-SMA and Col1a1 mRNA was assessed by RT-PCR. Representative images of three independent experiments are shown. **p<0.01 vs. non-treated cells.

3.3 Blockade of TRPV4 inhibited the proliferation and decreased α-SMA expression in activated HSC-T6 cells

To elucidate the functional role of TRPV4 during activation of HSC-T6 cells, Ruthenium Red (Ru), a common non-specific blocker of TRPV4 channel, was used to block this channel in TGF-β1-induced HSC-T6 cells. First, we tested the effect of Ru on the expression of TRPV4, as shown in Fig. 3A, Ru could inhibit the expression of TRPV4. Results of MTT assays demonstrated that Ru inhibited the proliferation of TGF-β1-treated HSC-T6 cells (Fig. 3B). To determine whether TRPV4 was capable of modulating α-SMA expression in vitro, we performed real time RT-PCR and Western blot assays on the liver tissues from CCl4-treated rats. The expression of α-SMA, an event associated with liver fibrosis, was suppressed in Ru-treated HSCs (Fig. 3C and D). To further establish the critical role of TRPV4 in the proliferation of activated HSC-T6 cells, siRNA specific for rat TRPV4 (TRPV4-siRNA) was used to knockdown the TRPV4 expression. As illustrated in Fig. 3E, MTT assay demonstrated that the viability of HSC-T6 cells was dramatically reduced after incubation with TGF-β1 and TRPV4-siRNA when compared to TGF-β1 and the scrambled-siRNA transfected cells. TGF-β1-activated HSC-T6 cells transfected with TRPV4-siRNA also expressed lower levels of α-SMA as compared to that transfected

with the scrambled-siRNA (Fig. 3F). These data suggested that the blockade of TRPV4 channel inhibited TGF-β1-induced HSC-T6 cell proliferation and decreased the production of α-SMA in activated HSC.

3.4 Overexpression of miR-203 inhibits TGF-β1-induced HSC proliferation

miR-203, a tumor suppressor microRNA, is often silenced in different malignancies, but the roles of miR-203 during liver fibrosis remain obscure at the present. To our surprise, miR-203 was downregulated in rat liver fibrotic tissues compared with the normal liver tissues by one-step quantitative RT-PCR (Fig. 4A). To investigate whether miR-203 has a role in TGF-β1 induced HSC activation, we firstly sought to determine whether TGF-β1 regulates miR-203 expression in activated HSC. In this experiment, we observed a remarkable declined of miR-203 in response to TGF-β1, in addition, as shown in Fig. 4B, the expression of miR-203 was suppressed by TGF-β1 in a dose-dependent manner (range from 5 to 10 ng/ml at 24 h). These findings convincingly indicated that miR-203 was down-regulated dose-dependently in TGF-β1-induced HSC. In order to investigate the roles of miR-203 in regulating TGF-β1-induced HSC proliferation, we tested the effect of miR-203 overexpression on the proliferation of TGF-

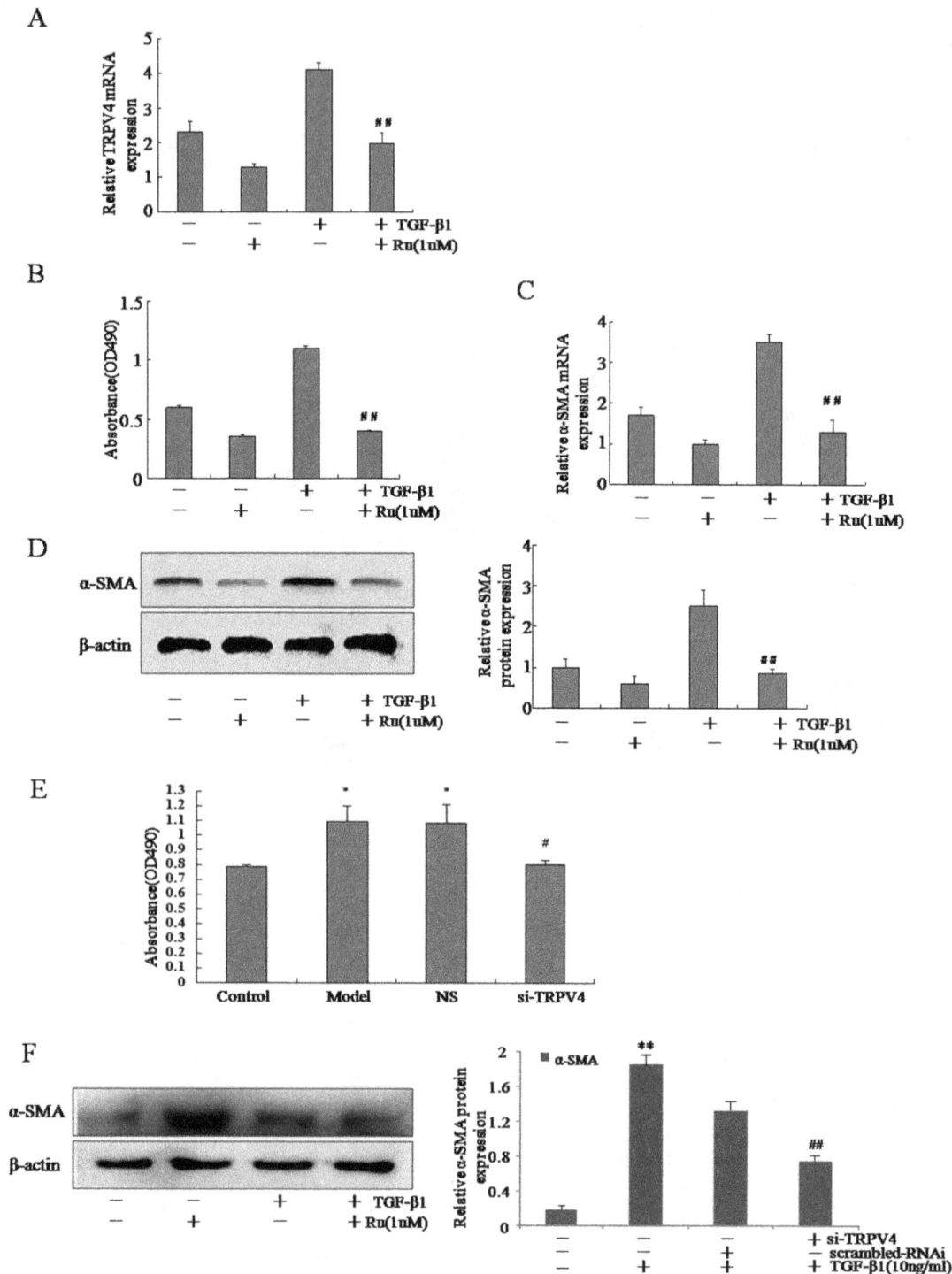

Figure 3. Blockade of TRPV4 inhibited the proliferation and decreased α-SMA expression in activated HSC-T6 cells. A. Total RNA extracts were made from HSC-T6 cells treated with or without TGF-β1 and Ru, and subjected to qRT-PCR analyses of TRPV4. Representative images of three independent experiments are shown. #p<0.05 vs. TGF-β1-treated cells. B. HSC-T6 cells were seeded in triplicate on day 0 and incubated in DMEM containing 10% fetal bovine serum or same media supplemented with Ru for further 24 h. Proliferation was measured by adding 5 mg/ml MTT reagent per well and incubating it for 4 h. #p<0.05 vs. TGF-β1-treated cells. C. Total RNA extracts were made from HSC-T6 cells treated with or without TGF-β1 and Ru, and subjected to qRT-PCR analyses of α-SMA. Representative images of three independent experiments are shown. #p<0.05 vs. TGF-β1-treated cells. D. Whole-cell protein extracts were made from HSC-T6 cells treated with or without TGF-β1 and Ru, and subjected to Western blot analyses of TRPV4. Representative images of three independent experiments are shown. ##p<0.01 vs. TGF-β1-treated cells. E. HSC-T6 cells were treated with TGF-β1 for 48 h, followed by transfection with TRPV4-siRNA for an additional 48 h, and cell viability was determined by MTT assay. Mean±SE of two HSC preparations in quadruplets is shown; *p<0.05 vs. non-treated cells, #p<0.05 vs. TGF-β1-treated cells. F. Whole cell extracts were isolated from TGF-β1-treated HSC-T6 cells with RNAi transfection, and subjected to Western blot analyses. Representative images of three independent experiments are shown. **p<0.01 vs. non-treated cells, ##p<0.01 vs. TGF-β1-treated cells.

β1 induced HSC. The cells transfection with miR-203 mimics significantly increased mature miR-203 expression (Fig. 4C). The MTT assay showed that introduction of miR-203 caused a significant inhibition of cell proliferation in TGF-β1-induced HSC (Fig. 4D). These results indicated that overexpression of miR-203 inhibited TGF-β1-induced HSC proliferation.

3.5 TRPV4 is a Target of MiR-203 in HSC

To determine the potential role of miR-203 in mediating TGF-β1-induced HSC proliferation, potential targets that are components of TGF-β1 signaling pathway were identified by using miRbase Targets, miRanda, and TargetScan 5.1. Among the candidate miR-203 targets, we paid more attention to TRPV4 (Fig. 5A). MiR-203 mimics was transfected into TGF-β1-treated HSC. Real-time PCR analysis revealed that TRPV4 expression was significantly lower in miR-203 transfected HSC compared with the NS-miRNA-transfected cells (Fig. 5B). To determine whether TRPV4 gene is a true directly target of miR-203, luciferase reporter vectors encoding a fragment of wild TRPV4 mRNA 3'-UTR, namely, TRPV4-wt was subcloned into a reporter vector downstream of the luciferase gene in HSC. Luciferase reporter assays showed that the relative luciferase activity of the reporter that contained wild-type 3'-UTR of TRPV4 mRNA was significantly decreased in miR-203-overexpressed cells compared to control cells (Fig. 5C). These results demonstrated that TRPV4 is likely a direct target of miR-203.

Discussion and Conclusion

Activation of HSC to a myofibroblast-like phenotype is the pivotal event in liver fibrogenesis [12,13]. HSC activation is characterized by enhanced cell proliferation and over-production of ECM. Recent studies indicated that ECM stiffening influenced the fibroblast differentiation to myofibroblasts, resulting in further increases in ECM deposition leading to the progression of the disease [14,15]. Therefore, inhibition of HSC activation/proliferation and blockage of ECM production are important strategies for therapeutic intervention. However, the molecular mechanisms for regulation of HSC activation/proliferation have not been well elucidated. Here, our study provided the initial evidence that, as the target of miR-203, TRPV4 is significantly increased in fibrotic rat livers and plays a critical role in controlling HSC activation.

TRPV4 cation channel, a member of the TRP vanilloid subfamily, is widely expressed in a broad range of tissues [16,17]. Subsequent studies have shown that TRPV4 channels possess multiple activation and regulatory sites that allow them to integrate distinct physical and chemical stimuli from the environment, offering a wide range of possible physiological roles, such as cell proliferation, survival, differentiation, migration, adhesion [18,19,20,21]. It is reported that TRPV4 regulates cardiac fibroblast differentiation to myofibroblasts by integrating signals from TGF-β1 [22,23]. And an exciting possibility raised by Arniges opens up in which TRPV4 could become a translational target in cystic fibrosis [24]. In the present study, we found that

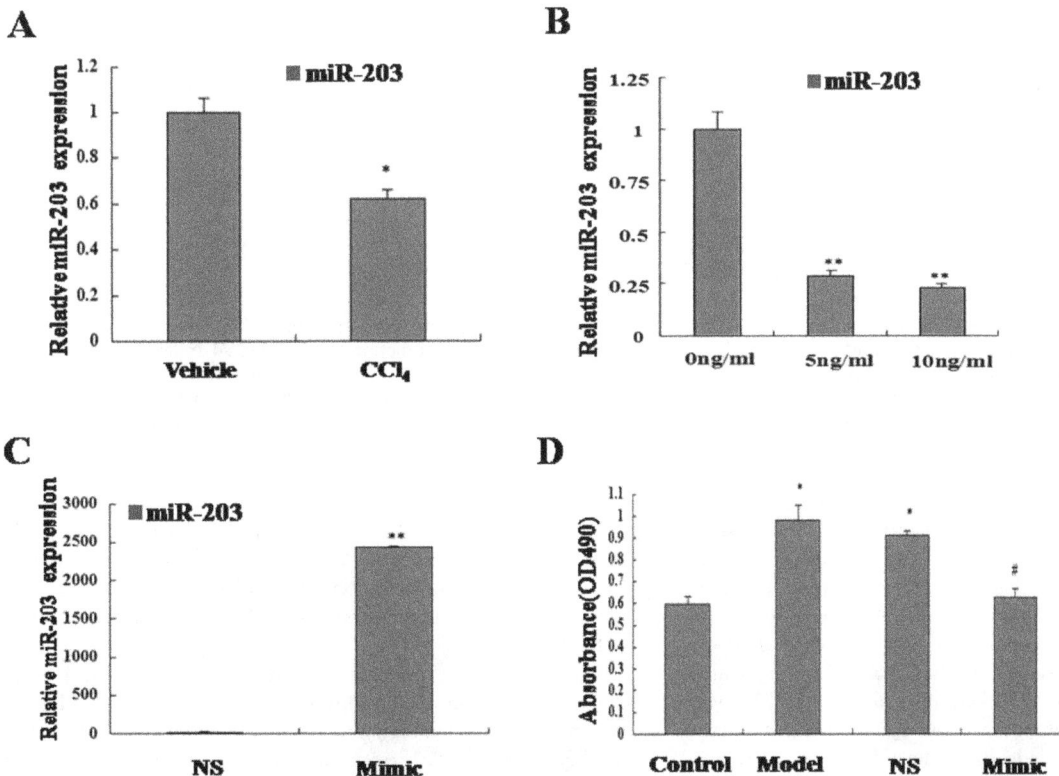

Figure 4. Overexpression of miR-203 inhibited of TGF-β1-induced HSC proliferation. A. Downregulation of miR-203 expression in liver fibrotic tissues compared with vehicle-treated groups. The miR-203 expression was analyzed by one-step quantitative real-time PCR. *P<0.05 vs vehicle control. B. Downregulation of miR-203expression in response to TGF-β1 (0, 5, 10 ng/ml) for 24 h. The miR-203 expression was analyzed by one-step quantitative real-time PCR. **P<0.01 vs non-treated cells. C. Upregulation of miR-203 expression in transfected HSC. The miR-203 expression of HSC was analyzed by one-step quantitative real-time PCR. **P<0.01 vs NS-miRNA. D. MiR-203 overexpression significantly inhibited proliferation of TGF-β1-induced HSC. The role of miR-203 in regulating TGF-β1-treated HSC proliferation was tested by MTT assay. The data represent the mean±SD of three different experiments. *P<0.05 vs control(non-treated cells), #P<0.05 vs NS-miRNA.

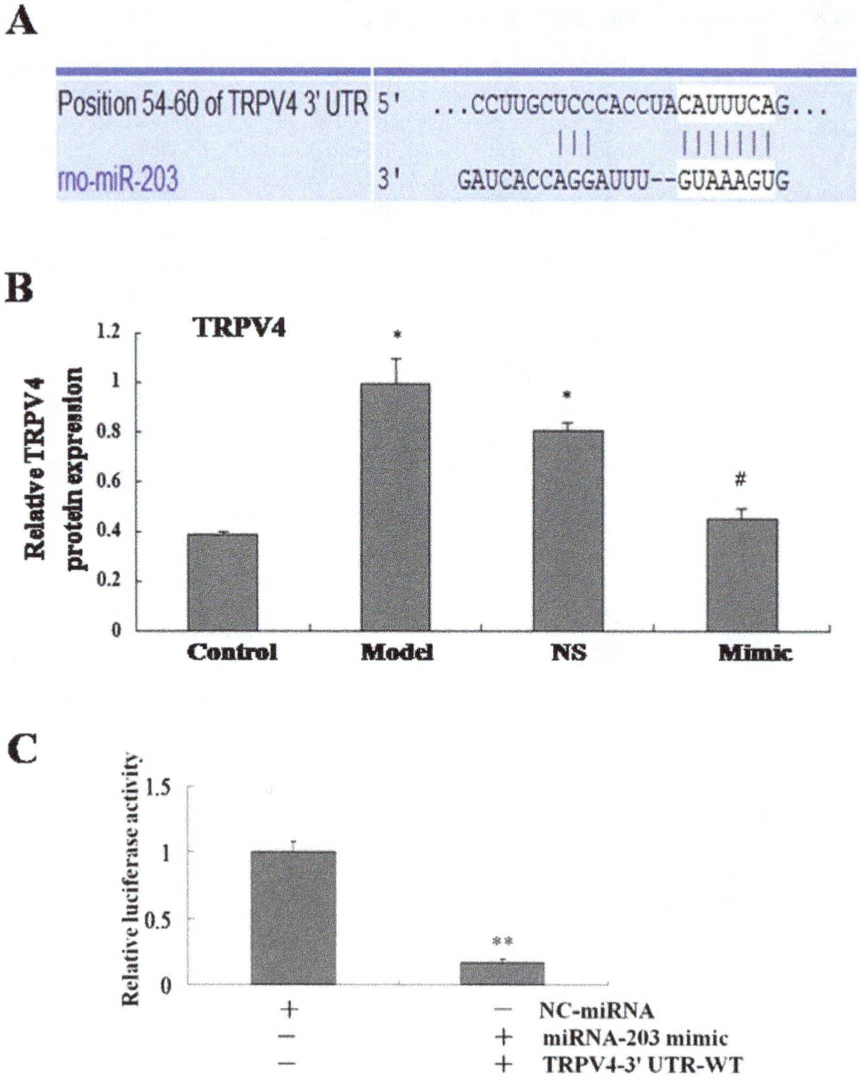

A

Position 54-60 of TRPV4 3' UTR	5'	...CCUUGCUCCCACCUACAUUUCAG...
		¦¦¦ ¦¦¦¦¦¦¦
rno-miR-203	3'	GAUCACCAGGAUUU--GUAAAGUG

B

C

Figure 5. TRPV4 is a target of miR-203 in HSC. A. The region of the rat TRPV4 mRNA 3′UTR predicted to be targeted by miR-203. Three different bioinformatics approaches (miRbase, miRANDA, and Targetscan 5.1) were used for the target prediction. B. The TRPV4 mRNA expression was analyzed by real-time PCR. The results are expressed as relative expression against control expression. *P<0.05 vs control(non-treated cells), #P<0.05 vs model(TGF-β1-treated cells).C. Dual-luciferase reporter assays of TRPV4 in HSC-T6 cells. Reporter construct containing wt TRPV4 3′-UTR was cotransfected with miR-203 mimics or NC-miRNA. Relative luciferase activity was normalized to firefly luciferase. Data are representative of at least three separate experiments. *P<0.05, **P<0.01vs. NC-miRNA.

TRPV4 channel was dramatically increased in the liver tissues from patients with liver fibrosis and CCl₄-treated rats in vivo and its expression was strongly correlated the HSC activation identified by the induction of α-SMA and Col1α1. And we found that TRPV4 is increased in HSC-T6 cells is response to TGF-β1 stimulation. These results suggested that TRPV4, in activated HSCs and in fibrotic livers, was likely upregulated. TRPV4 was associated with cell proliferation in various cell types. Accordingly, blockade of TRPV4 channels leads to the inhibition of proliferation in different cell types. In the present study, exposure of activated HSC-T6 cells to Ruthenium Red (Ru), dramatically decreased the cell viability. Additionally, knockdown of TRPV4 with siRNA strongly inhibited the proliferation of activated HSC-T6 cells. Moreover, induction of collagen and α-SMA is considered as a marker of HSC activation and liver fibrosis. Expression level of Col1α1 and α-SMA were upregulated in activated HSC-T6 cells and CCl₄-treated liver. In current study,

results indicated that the blockade of TRPV4 with Ru or siRNA down-regulated the expressions of Col1α1 and α-SMA in activated HSC-T6 cells. In combination with MTT results, we suggested that TRPV4 may be required for HSC activation and proliferation.

microRNAs are a group of small non-coding RNA, which can regulate expression of hundreds of target genes and thereby influencing various biologic processes such as cellular proliferation and differentiation [25]. Accumulating studies have demonstrated that miRNAs played important roles in regulating HSC functions such as cell proliferation, differentiation, and apoptosis [26,27,28]. For an instance, miR-146a inhibits TGF-β1-induced HSC differentiation, at least in part, via decreasing the expression of SMAD4 [27]. Recently the microarray analysis revealed that the expression of miR-203 was significantly downregulated in chronic liver disease and HCC [29,30]. It has also been shown that miR-203 could up-regulate NO expression in female rat MCCs via

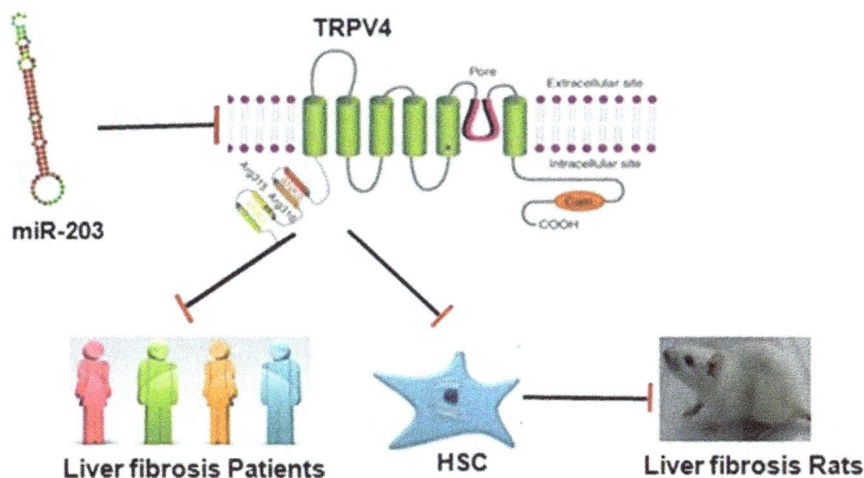

Figure 6. Overview of TRPV4 on liver fibrosis.

targeting TRPV4 [31]. The present study was destined to determine whether miR-203 could play a functional role in regulating HSC proliferation in response to TGF-β1 stimulation. In our study, miR-203 expression was downregulated dose-dependently in response to TGF-β1, MTT assay showed that transfection of miR-203 mimics led to a significant inhibition of cell proliferation in TGF-β1-treated HSC. Moreover, our experiments demonstrated that miR-203 overexpression resulted in significantly decreased TRPV4 expression, suggesting the inhibitory role of miR-203 in liver fibrosis may be correlated to function of TRPV4.

In summary, our findings in the present study suggested that TRPV4 may play a pivotal role during hepatic stellate cell activation. The blockade of TRPV4 channels offset TGF-β1-induced HSC-T6 cell proliferation, indicating the potential of TRPV4 as a therapeutic target for liver fibrosis. Moreover, it appeared that the expression of TRPV4 was directly regulated by miR-203 in TGF-β1-induced HSC (As shown in Fig. 6). To our knowledge, this is the first report focusing on the role of TRPV4 in liver fibrosis. This study gave us novel insights into the potential roles of TRPV4 channels in HSC activation, further functional analysis to determine the precise role of TRPV4 in HSC bioactivity could provide a novel therapeutic approach for treating hepatic fibrosis.

Author Contributions

Conceived and designed the experiments: YS CH X-MM L. Zhang JL. Performed the experiments: YS L. Zhan. Analyzed the data: YS M-ZY T-TM. Contributed reagents/materials/analysis tools: YS L. Zhan M-ZY. Contributed to the writing of the manuscript: YS JL.

References

1. Hernandez-Gea V, Friedman SL (2011) Pathogenesis of liver fibrosis. Annu Rev Pathol 6: 425–456.
2. Friedman SL (2008) Mechanisms of hepatic fibrogenesis. Gastroenterology 134: 1655–1669.
3. Lee UE, Friedman SL (2011) Mechanisms of hepatic fibrogenesis. Best Pract Res Clin Gastroenterol 25: 195–206.
4. Fang L, Zhan S, Huang C, Cheng X, Lv X, et al. (2013) TRPM7 channel regulates PDGF-BB-induced proliferation of hepatic stellate cells via PI3K and ERK pathways. Toxicol Appl Pharmacol 272: 713–725.
5. Liu H, Li J, Huang Y, Huang C (2012) Inhibition of transient receptor potential melastain 7 channel increases HSCs apoptosis induced by TRAIL. Life Sci 90: 612–618.
6. Nilius B (2007) TRP channels in disease. Biochim Biophys Acta 1772: 805–812.
7. Chun JN, Lim JM, Kang Y, Kim EH, Shin YC, et al. (2013) A network perspective on unraveling the role of TRP channels in biology and disease. Pflugers Arch.
8. Patel A, Sharif-Naeini R, Folgering JR, Bichet D, Duprat F, et al. (2010) Canonical TRP channels and mechanotransduction: from physiology to disease states. Pflugers Arch 460: 571–581.
9. Clark K, Middelbeek J, van Leeuwen FN (2008) Interplay between TRP channels and the cytoskeleton in health and disease. Eur J Cell Biol 87: 631–640.
10. Jordt SE, Ehrlich BE (2007) TRP channels in disease. Subcell Biochem 45: 253–271.
11. Lafyatis R (2006) Targeting fibrosis in systemic sclerosis. Endocr Metab Immune Disord Drug Targets 6: 395–400.
12. Friedman SL (1993) Seminars in medicine of the Beth Israel Hospital, Boston. The cellular basis of hepatic fibrosis. Mechanisms and treatment strategies. N Engl J Med 328: 1828–1835.
13. Friedman SL (2008) Hepatic fibrosis — overview. Toxicology 254: 120–129.
14. Troeger JS, Mederacke I, Gwak GY, Dapito DH, Mu X, et al. (2012) Deactivation of hepatic stellate cells during liver fibrosis resolution in mice. Gastroenterology 143: 1073–1083 e1022.
15. Jiao J, Friedman SL, Aloman C (2009) Hepatic fibrosis. Curr Opin Gastroenterol 25: 223–229.
16. Watanabe H, Vriens J, Prenen J, Droogmans G, Voets T, et al. (2003) Anandamide and arachidonic acid use epoxyeicosatrienoic acids to activate TRPV4 channels. Nature 424: 434–438.
17. Everaerts W, Nilius B, Owsianik G (2010) The vanilloid transient receptor potential channel TRPV4: from structure to disease. Prog Biophys Mol Biol 103: 2–17.
18. Fiorio Pla A, Ong HL, Cheng KT, Brossa A, Bussolati B, et al. (2012) TRPV4 mediates tumor-derived endothelial cell migration via arachidonic acid-activated actin remodeling. Oncogene 31: 200–212.
19. Troidl C, Troidl K, Schierling W, Cai WJ, Nef H, et al. (2009) Trpv4 induces collateral vessel growth during regeneration of the arterial circulation. J Cell Mol Med 13: 2613–2621.
20. Hatano N, Suzuki H, Itoh Y, Muraki K (2013) TRPV4 partially participates in proliferation of human brain capillary endothelial cells. Life Sci 92: 317–324.
21. Zaninetti R, Fornarelli A, Ciarletta M, Lim D, Caldarelli A, et al. (2011) Activation of TRPV4 channels reduces migration of immortalized neuroendocrine cells. J Neurochem 116: 606–615.
22. Adapala RK, Thoppil RJ, Luther DJ, Paruchuri S, Meszaros JG, et al. (2013) TRPV4 channels mediate cardiac fibroblast differentiation by integrating mechanical and soluble signals. J Mol Cell Cardiol 54: 45–52.
23. Thodeti CK, Paruchuri S, Meszaros JG (2013) A TRP to cardiac fibroblast differentiation. Channels (Austin) 7: 211–214.
24. Arniges M, Vazquez E, Fernandez-Fernandez JM, Valverde MA (2004) Swelling-activated Ca2+ entry via TRPV4 channel is defective in cystic fibrosis airway epithelia. J Biol Chem 279: 54062–54068.

25. Ambros V (2001) microRNAs: tiny regulators with great potential. Cell 107: 823–826.

26. Sun X, He Y, Huang C, Ma TT, Li J (2013) The epigenetic feedback loop between DNA methylation and microRNAs in fibrotic disease with an emphasis on DNA methyltransferases. Cell Signal 25: 1870–1876.

27. He Y, Huang C, Sun X, Long XR, Lv XW, et al. (2012) MicroRNA-146a modulates TGF-beta1-induced hepatic stellate cell proliferation by targeting SMAD4. Cell Signal 24: 1923–1930.

28. He Y, Huang C, Zhang SP, Sun X, Long XR, et al. (2012) The potential of microRNAs in liver fibrosis. Cell Signal 24: 2268–2272.

29. Pogribny IP, Starlard-Davenport A, Tryndyak VP, Han T, Ross SA, et al. (2010) Difference in expression of hepatic microRNAs miR-29c, miR-34a, miR-155, and miR-200b is associated with strain-specific susceptibility to dietary nonalcoholic steatohepatitis in mice. Lab Invest 90: 1437–1446.

30. Furuta M, Kozaki KI, Tanaka S, Arii S, Imoto I, et al. (2010) miR-124 and miR-203 are epigenetically silenced tumor-suppressive microRNAs in hepatocellular carcinoma. Carcinogenesis 31: 766–776.

31. Hu F, Zhu W, Wang L (2012) MicroRNA-203 up-regulates nitric oxide expression in temporomandibular joint chondrocytes via targeting TRPV4. Arch Oral Biol.

2

Col1A1 Production and Apoptotic Resistance in TGF-β1-Induced Epithelial-to-Mesenchymal Transition-Like Phenotype of 603B Cells

Jun Liu, Alex N. Eischeid, Xian-Ming Chen*

Department of Medical Microbiology and Immunology, Creighton University School of Medicine, Omaha, Nebraska, United States of America

Abstract

Recent studies have suggested that proliferating cholangiocytes have an important role in the induction of fibrosis, either directly via epithelial-to-mesenchymal transition (EMT), or indirectly via activation of other liver cell types. Transforming growth factor beta 1 (TGF-β1), a critical fibrotic cytokine for hepatic fibrosis, is a potent EMT inducer. This study aimed to clarify the potential contributions of TGF-β1-induced EMT-like cholangiocyte phenotype to collagen production and cell survival of cholangiocytes *in vitro*. Mouse cholangiocytes (603B cells) were treated with TGF-β1 and EMT-like phenotype alterations were monitored by morphological changes and expression of EMT-associated genes. Alterations in Col1A1 gene, Col1A1-associated miR-29s, and pro-apoptotic genes were measured in TGF-β1-treated 603B cells. Snail1 knockdown was achieved using shRNA to evaluate the contribution of EMT-associated changes to Col1A1 production and cell survival. We found TGF-β1 treatment induced partial EMT-like phenotype transition in 603B cells in a Snail1-dependent manner. TGF-β1 also stimulated collagen α1(I) expression in 603B cells. However, this induction was not parallel to the EMT-like alterations and independent of Snail1 or miR-29 expression. Cells undergoing EMT-like changes showed a modest down-regulation of multiple pro-apoptotic genes and displayed resistance to TNF-α-induced apoptosis. TGF-β1-induced apoptosis resistance was attenuated in Snail1 knockdown 603B cells. TGF-β1-induced Col1A1 production seems to be independent of EMT-like transition and miR-29 expression. Nevertheless, TGF-β1-induced EMT may contribute to the increased survival capacity of cholangiocytes via modulating the expression of pro-apoptotic genes.

Editor: Srinivasa M. Srinivasula, IISER-TVM, India

Funding: This study was supported by the Nebraska Tobacco Settlement Biomedical Research Program (LB506, LB692 and LB595) (to X-MC). The funders had no role in study design, data collection and analysis, decision to publish, or preparation of the manuscript.

Competing Interests: The authors have declared that no competing interests exist.

* E-mail: xianmingchen@creighton.edu

Introduction

Liver fibrosis results from the accumulation of interstitial or "scar" extracellular matrix (ECM) after either acute or chronic liver injury. The advanced stage of hepatic fibrosis is liver cirrhosis, which gradually destroys the hepatic architecture and causes significant deaths worldwide. Mechanistic studies have been focused on hepatic stellate cells (HSCs), as these cells can undergo "activation" into proliferative and fibrogenic myofibroblast-like cells during liver injury [1,2]. Other live cell types may also play an important role in the pathogenesis of liver fibrosis [3]. Pathologically, ECM proteins are predominantly deposited around the portal region during development of hepatic fibrosis [4]. Cholangiocytes, epithelial cells lining the biliary tree, become aberrantly accumulated in the portal region and form clustered bile ducts during hepatic fibrosis [5]. Such reaction reflects a dysregulated balance between cell growth and cell death, referred as "ductular reaction" [6]. Recent studies demonstrate that cholangiocytes display features of epithelial-to-mesenchymal transition (EMT) during hepatic fibrosis [4,7–9]. EMT describes the molecular reprogramming and phenotypic changes involved in the conversion of polarized immotile epithelial cells to motile mesenchymal cells [10]. This process allows the remodeling of tissues during embryonic development and is recently implicated in tumor progression and development of fibrosis [11,12]. Pathophysiologically, cholangiocytes with mesenchymal features may contribute to the generation of fibroblast-like cells to facilitate collagen production and promote the "ductular reaction" at the portal region during hepatic fibrosis [13,14].

Transforming growth factor beta (TGF-β) is the prototype of most powerful EMT inducer in many epithelial tissues [15]. Interestingly, TGF-β1 is a critical fibrotic cytokine which plays an important role in the initiation and progression of liver fibrosis [16]. TGF-β1 has been demonstrated to induce collagen production as well as EMT-associated changes in several liver cell types, including cholangiocytes *in vitro* and *in vivo* [8,17–19]. Uncovering unique EMT-associated molecular events in cholangiocytes in response to TGF-β1 may identify valuable targets for anti-fibrotic therapies. Nevertheless, it's not clear whether TGF-β1-induced collagen production in cholangiocytes depends on the occurrence of EMT. Whether TGF-β1 promotes "ductular reaction" through induction of cholangiocyte EMT is also still obscure.

EMT can be viewed as a manifestation of extreme epithelial cell plasticity, characterized by loss of polarity, loss of epithelial markers, cytoskeletal reorganization, and transition to a spindle-shaped morphology concomitant with acquisition of mesenchymal markers [10]. Loss of epithelial adhesion does not necessarily lead to full transition to a mesenchymal phenotype [20]. EMT in response to TGF-β1 is mediated by the activation of a variety of downstream mediators of TGF-β1 signaling, including Smads and Snails [15]. Recent studies indicate that epithelial cells undergoing EMT also display distinct expression profile of microRNAs (miRNAs), a class of small regulatory RNAs which suppress gene expression at post-transcriptional level by base pairing with the 3′ untranslated regions (UTRs) of mRNAs [21]. Given the importance of miRNAs in gene regulation, they may play a pathogenic role in the many aspects of EMT, such as collagen production. Indeed, miR-29s have been demonstrated to directly target 3′UTRs of collagen mRNAs and downregulation of miR-29 family has been shown to correlate with the development of fibrosis in several tissues [22–24]. Although the detailed mechanisms for miR-29 downregulation during fibrosis remain to be elucidated, TGF-β1 decreases the transcription of this miRNA family in myofibroblasts *in vitro* [24]. In addition, EMT is well established to be associated with death resistance [10]. The main inducers of EMT can also promote apoptosis, suggesting that EMT could potentially serve as a pathway for escape from cell death depending on the particular cytokine milieu [25,26]. It has recently been found that Snail1 directly regulates the expression of apoptosis genes [27], suggesting that down-regulation pro-apoptotic gene by EMT-associated transcriptional factor may contribute to the development of ductular reaction during fibrosis.

Using a non-tumorigenic mouse 603B cholangiocyte cell line, in this study, we investigated the development of EMT induced by TGF-β1, its relationship to collagen production and finally its involvement with the acquisition of apoptotic resistance in cholangiocytes *in vitro*. The data we report here show that TGF-β1 induces EMT-like phenotypic alterations and promotes collagen α1(I) (Col1A1) production in 603B cells. However, TGF-β1-induced Col1A1 production is independent of EMT-like alterations and miR-29 expression. Moreover, TGF-β1-induced EMT may contribute to the increased survival capacity of cholangiocytes via modulating the expression of pro-apoptotic genes.

Materials and Methods

Cell Culture and TGF-β1 Treatment

A non-tumorigenic mouse cholangiocyte cell line 603B, was maintained in Dulbecco's modified Eagle's medium (Gibco) with 10% fetal bovine serum (Invitrogen). These cells were developed by transfection with the SV40 T antigen and they display typical morphology of well-differentiated cholangiocytes, express biliary epithelial cell markers consistent with biliary function and with the tight junctions between cells as previously documented [28]. 603B cells were seeded at 5% confluence and, 18 h later, were moved to a medium with 5% fetal bovine serum. TGF-β1 (R&D System) was added to a finial concentration of 3 ng/mL. Medium was changed every other day.

Establishment of Cells Stably Expressing Snail1 shRNA

Cells were transfected with control shRNA or shRNA against murine Snail1 (Origene) with lipofectamin2000. Transfection efficiency was 40% with this method. Forty-eight hours post-transfection, cells were selected with puromycin (1 μg/mL) for 3 weeks. Drug-resistant clones were isolated, expanded and confirmed by PCR and Western blot. All experiments were conducted using pools of colonies to avoid a clonal bias.

Quantitative Reverse-transcription PCR (qRT-PCR)

Total RNA was extracted from 603B cells with TRIzol (Invitrogen). qRT-PCR was performed with ABI-Prism 7900HT (Applied Biosystems) with the SYBR Green polymerase chain reaction master mix (Applied Biosystems). The PCR primers used were as follows: mouse E-cadherin, forward (5′-GGATAGA-GAAGCCATTGCCAAGTA-3′) and reverse (5′-TCAAA-GACCGGCTGGGTAAA-3′); α-smooth muscle actin (α-SMA), forward (5′-ATCATCACCAACTGGGACGAC-3′) and reverse (5′-TTTCTCCCGGTTGGCCTTAG-3′); Fibronectin1 (Fn-1), forward (5′-TGACACTTATGAGCGCCCTAAAGA-3′) and reverse (5′-TCATGGCAGGGATTTGCAAT-3′); Col1A1, forward (5′-GGGTCTAGACATGTTCAGCTTTGTG-3′) and reverse (5′-ACCCTTAGGCCATTGTGTATGC-3′); Bcl-2-associated X protein (Bax), forward (5′-CAGGATGCGTCCACCAAGAA-3′) and reverse (5′-GCAAAGTGAAAGAGGGCAACCA-3′); BH3 interacting domain death agonist (Bid), forward (5′-ACAGC-TAGCCGCACAGTTCAT-3′) and reverse (5′-CAG-CATGGCGTTGTCGTTCT-3′); Bcl-2-like protein 11 (Bim), forward (5′-AACCGCAAGCTTCCATACGA-3′) and reverse (5′-TCTTCAGCCTCGGGGTAATC-3′); phosphatase and tensin homolog (Pten), forward (5′-GCGTGCAGATAATGACAAG-GAGTA-3′) and reverse (5′-CCTCTGGATTT-GATGGCTCCTCTA-3′); p53 up-regulated modulator of apoptosis (Puma), forward (5′-CCCAGAAATGGAGCC-CAACT-3′) and reverse (5′-CCAGTATGCTACATGGTGCA-GAA-3′); beta-actin, forward (5′-TGGTGGGAATGGGTCA-GAA-3′) and reverse (5′-TCTCCATGTCGTCCCAGTTG-3′); Snail1, forward (5′-TAGGTCGCTCTGGCCAACAT-3′) and reverse (5′-TAGGGCTGCTGGAAGGTGAA-3′). Data analysis was performed with ABI-Prism 7900HT SDS2.0 software (Applied Biosystems). Experiments were performed in triplicate and the values were normalized to beta-actin. The cycle threshold (Ct) values were analyzed using the comparative Ct (ΔΔCt) method and the amount of target was obtained by normalizing to the endogenous reference (beta-actin) and relative to the control (non-treated cells).

For analysis of miR-29, total RNA was isolated from cells with the TRIzol reagent (Invitrogen). An amount of 0.05 μg total RNAs was reverse-transcribed by using the Taqman MicroRNA Reverse Transcription Kit (Applied Biosystems). Specific primers and probes for mature miR-29 a/b/c and snRNA RNU6B were obtained from Applied Biosystems. All reactions were run in triplicate. The amount of miR-29a/b/c was obtained by normalizing to snRNA RNU6B and relative to the control (untreated cells). Comparative qRT-PCR was performed in triplicate using Taqman Universal PCR Master Mix (Applied Biosystems) on the Applied Biosystems 7500 FAST real-time PCR System. Relative expression was calculated by using the comparative CT method.

Western Blot

Whole cell lysates were obtained with the M-PER Mammalian Protein Extraction reagent (Pierce) plus protease inhibitors (1 mmol/L phenylmethanesulfonylfluoride, 10 μg/mL leupeptin, and 2 μg/mL pepstatin). Antibodies to actin, caspase-3, E-cadherin (Sigma-Aldrich), N-cadherin (Cell Signaling), fibroblast-specific protein-1 (FSP-1), vimentin and Col1A1 (Abcam) were used.

Luciferase Reporter Constructs and Luciferase Assay

A 280 bp fragment from Col1A1 3′UTR containing three potential miR-29 binding sites was cloned into the multiple-cloning site of the pMIR-REPORT Luciferase vector (Ambion).

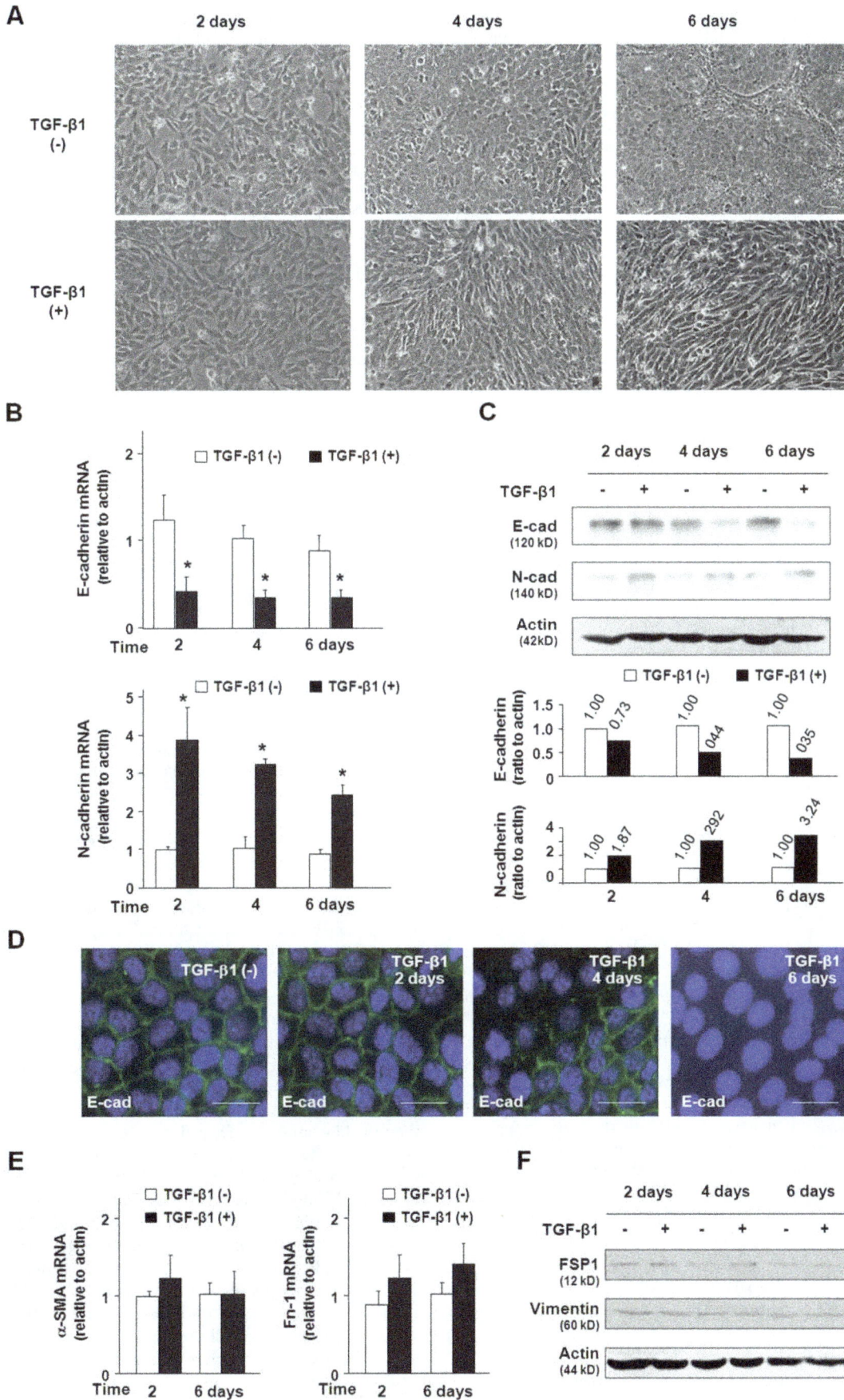

A

B

C

D

E

F

Figure 1. TGF-β1 induces EMT-associated changes in 603B cells. (A) Morphological alterations of 603B cells induced by TGF-β1 (3 ng/ml) at indicated time points. Upper panel are representative phase images showing the 603B cells cultured in the absence of TGF-β1 and lower panel shows the 603B cells stimulated with TGF-β1. After TGF-β1 exposure, 603B cells gradually assumed a spindle-like shape. (B) Alterations of E-cadherin and N-cadherin mRNA expression in 603B cells after exposure to TGF-β1 for various periods of time as assessed by qRT-PCR. TGF-β1 treatment induced steady down-regulation of E-cadherin and up-regulation of N-cadherin. The qRT-PCR results shown represent an average of three independent experiments. (C) Cellular levels of E-cadherin and N-cadherin proteins in TGF-β1-treated 603B cells as determined by Western blot. Consistent with qRT-PCR analysis, TGF-β1 induced down-regulation of E-cadherin and up-regulation of N-cadherin, respectively. Representative blots from three independent experiments are shown and actin was blotted to ensure equal loading. Densitometric levels of E-cadherin and N-cadherin signals were quantified and expressed as the ratio to actin. (D) Decreased cell membrane distribution of E-cadherin protein in 603B cells in respond to TGF-β1 stimulation as assessed by immunofluorescent staining. E-cadherin was stained green and DAPI stained nuclei blue. (E) α-SMA and Fn-1 mRNA expression levels were determined by qRT-PCR and (F) FSP-1 and vimentin protein expression levels were determined by Western blot. No significant change of these genes was detected. Values are means ± SE. *$p<0.05$ compared to non-TGF-β1-treated cells; E-cad = E-cadherin; N-cad = N-cadherin. Bar = 10 μM.

The empty pMIR-REPORT vector was used as a control. We then transfected cultured cells with each reporter construct. Luciferase activity was measured 24 h later and normalized to the control β-galactosidase level.

Cell Death and Propidium Iodide (PI) Staining Assay

For trypan blue staining, 5000 cells were plated in each well of a 6-well cluster dish and TGF-β1 was added at indicated time points. Medium was then removed; TNF-α (100 ng/ml) and SC-514 (50 nM) were added to induce apoptosis for 24 h. Floating cells were collected by centrifuge at 200 g for 5 min. The attached cells were trypsinized and combined with floating cells for staining. The numbers of dead and viable cells were counted under the microscope. For PI staining, 5000 cells were plated in 6 cm dishes and treated as described above. Cells were washed with phosphate buffered saline (PBS) and then fixed for 15 min with 4% formaldehyde in PBS. Cells were then washed with PBS and stained with PI for 5 min. Dye was removed, cell monolayers were washed with PBS, and apoptosis was assessed under the fluorescence microscope.

Immunofluorescence (IF) Staining

The 603B cells for immunofluorescence staining of E-cadherin and Col1A1 were plated in 8-well culture slides and treated in the same method as above described. Cells were washed with PBS three times and fixed with 4% paraformaldehyde in PBS for 10 min at room temperature and permeabilized in 0.5% Triton X-100/PBS for 5 min at room temperature. After washing with PBS for 5 min (three times), cells were incubated with blocking buffer (Cell Signaling IF protocol) containing 5% serum (from same species as secondary antibody) for 1 h at room temperature, and then incubated with the specific primary antibodies. The following primary antibodies were used for immunostaining: rat anti-E-cadherin (clone ECCD-2) (Sigma-Aldrich), and rabbit anti-procollagen/type I collagen (Chemicon, Temecula, CA). Alexa fluor-488 conjugated secondary antibodies were used. Cells were co-stained with 4',6-diamidino-2-phenylindole (DAPI), to visualize the nuclei. Stained cells were mounted with fluorescent mounting medium (Dako Cytomation), and assessed by a conventional fluorescent microscopy (Olympus BX51/DP71). The exposure time for FITC and DAPI signals was 2 seconds and 0.08 seconds, respectively.

The Enzyme Poly (ADP-ribose) Polymerase (PARP) Cleavage Assay for Assessing Apoptosis by Flow Cytometry

The PARP cleavage was determined using FITC-conjugated anti-PARP (85-kDa fragment) antibody (Abcam) to quantify apoptotic cells, as previously reported [29]. Cells were fixed with 0.01% formaldehyde for 15 min, and were then incubated with

200 μl of permeabilizing solution (0.5% BSA, 0.02% NaN3, and 0.5% Tween 20, in PBS) for 30 min at 37°C. After permeabilization, cells were stained with the anti-PARP antibody conjugated with FITC for 1 h. Cells were washed with PBS and analyzed by flow cytometry [29].

Data Analysis

All values are given as mean ± SE. Means of groups were compared with the Student's t test (unpaired) or ANOVA test when appropriate. p values <0.05 were considered statistically significant.

Results

TGF-β1 Induces EMT-like Phenotypic Changes in 603B Cells

Murine immortalized 603B cholangiocytes were seeded at low density and cultured in the medium with or without TGF-β1 (3 ng/ml) for up to 6 days. In the absence of TGF-β1, 603B cells maintained epithelial morphology during the culture period. In the presence of TGF-β1, the cells gradually displayed morphological appearances of mesenchymal cells and after 6 days of TGF-β1 treatment, the majority of cells became spindle-shaped (Fig. 1A). These morphological features suggested that TGF-β1 may induce EMT-like phenotypic changes in 603B cells.

EMT is characterized by loss of epithelial cell polarity, loss of cell-cell contacts, and acquisition of mesenchymal markers and phenotypic traits that include increased cell motility. E-cadherin is universally expressed by epithelial cells and plays essential roles to form the tight junctions between epithelial cells. Loss of E-cadherin expression is a marker for the occurrence of EMT. We found that after 2 days of TGF-β1 treatment, E-cadherin mRNA levels were steadily decreased in 603B cells as compared with the controls (p<0.05, Fig. 1B). TGF-β1 treatment did not significantly affect actin mRNA level during the culture (data not shown) and thus, it was used as the internal control to normalize the qRT-PCR data. Western blot analysis revealed a similar but delayed decrease in E-cadherin protein level in TGF-β1-treated cells, comparing with mRNA changes. Specifically, TGF-β1 treatment for 4 days only induced a modest decrease of E-cadherin protein in 603B cells, and a dramatic decrease of E-cadherin protein was detected 6 days after TGF-β1 stimulation (Fig. 1C). Decreased expression of E-cadherin in TGF-β1-treated 603B cells was further confirmed by immunofluorescent staining. As shown in Fig. 1D, whereas cells cultured in the absence of TGF-β1 predominantly expressed E-cadherin on the cell membrane, cells in the presence of TGF-β1 gradually lost E-cadherin expression. In contrast, TGF-β1-treated cells showed an increased expression of N-cadherin, a mesenchymal marker upregulated during EMT [20]. Expression of N-cadherin at both the message and protein levels

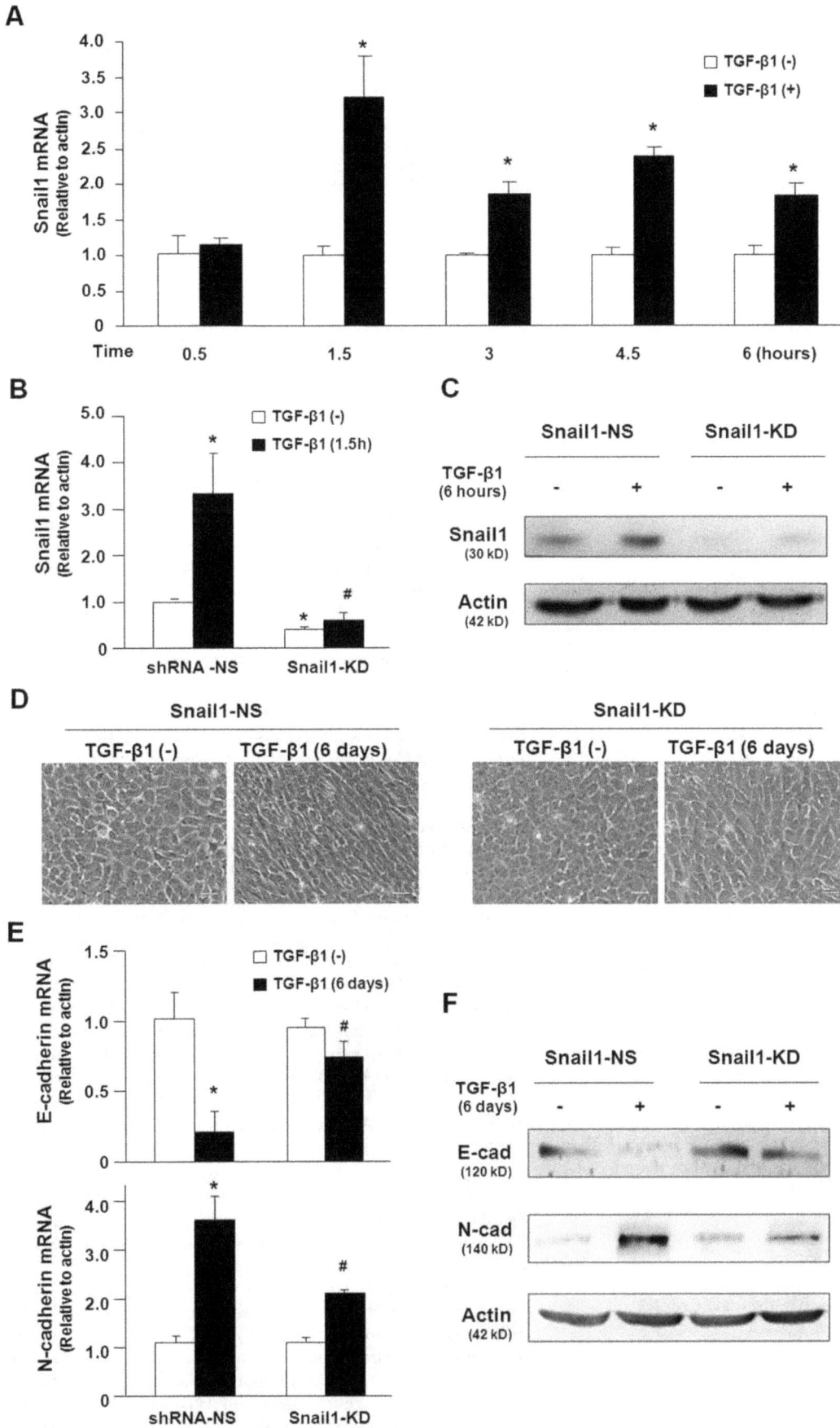

A

B

C

D

E

F

Figure 2. Snail1 knockdown attenuates TGF-β1-induced EMT-associated changes in 603B cells. (A) qRT-PCR revealed the rapid up-regulation of Snail1 mRNA levels in 603B cells after TGF-β1 (3 ng/ml) treatment. Data represent an average of three independent experiments. (B) Snail1 shRNA but not control shRNA abolished the upregulation of Snail1 mRNA levels by TGF-β1 in 603B cells. Cells stably expressing the Snail1 shRNA or control shRNA were exposed to TGF-β1 (3 ng/ml) for 1.5 h and expression of Snail1 mRNA levels were determined by qRT-PCR. (C) Snail1 shRNA decreases Snail1 protein expression in 603B cells. Cells stably expressing the Snail1 shRNA or control shRNA were exposed to TGF-β1 (3 ng/ml) for 6 h and expression of Snail1 protein levels were determined by Western blot. (D) Morphological changes of 603B cells stably expressing control shRNA or Snail1 shRNA after TGF-β1 (3 ng/ml) treatment for 6 days. (E) and (F) Effects of Snail1 knockdown on E-cadherin and N-cadherin expression in 603B cells following TGF-β1 treatment. Cells stably expressing the control shRNA or Snail1 shRNA were treated with TGF-β1 (3 g/ml) for 6 days and expression of E-cadherin and N-cadherin were determined by qRT-PCR (E) and Western blot (F), respectively. Values are means ± SE. *$p<0.05$ compared to non-TGF-β1-treated cells; #$p<0.05$ compared to cells expressing the shRNA-NS after TGF-β1 treatment; E-cad = E-cadherin; N-cad = N-cadherin; shRNA-NS = non specific shRNA control; Snail1-KD = snail shRNA knockdown. Bar = 10 μM.

was increased in cells in response to TGF-β1 treatment as assessed by qRT-PCR (Fig. 1*B*) and Western blot (Fig. 1*C*). In addition, cells undergoing EMT frequently express higher levels of α-SMA, Fn-1, FSP-1 and vimentin [20]. Nevertheless, no changes in α-SMA and Fn-1 mRNA levels were detected in cells following TGF-β1 treatment by real-time PCR (Fig. 1*E*). TGF-β1 stimulation failed to induce the expression of FSP-1 and vimentin at the protein levels (Fig. 1*F*). These data together suggested that TGF-β1 alone may only induce a partial EMT in 603B cells.

Snail1 is Required for TGF-β1-induced EMT-like Changes in 603B Cells

Snail1 is an important downstream effector of TGF-β1 signaling to induce EMT in various cells and functions as a transcriptional suppressor of E-cadherin [20]. We examined whether TGF-β1 influences Snail1 expression in 603B cells. Consistent with data from previous reports [27,17], we found that Snail1 mRNA levels were rapidly increased after TGF-β1 stimulation (Fig. 2*A*) and remained a modest increase (1.3–1.5 folds) at 2, 4 and 6 days after treatment, indicating that the induction of Snail1 may be an early event of TGF-β1-induced EMT-like changes.

To elucidate whether up-regulation of Snail1 contributed to the EMT-like changes, stable Snail1 knockdown in 603B cells was achieved by a specific shRNA to Snail1. As expected, Snail1 shRNA significantly reduced the basal Snail1 mRNA (Fig. 2*B*) and protein (Fig. 2*C*) levels, compared with the control shRNA. Moreover, TGF-β1-induced up-regulation of Snail1 was abolished in cells stably expressing Snail1 shRNA (Fig. 2*B* and 2*C*). We then cultured these cells in the absence or presence of TGF-β1 for 6 days and examined the morphological changes and expression patterns of E-cadherin and N-cadherin. As shown in Fig. 2*D*, Snail1 knockdown attenuated TGF-β1-induced EMT-like morphological alterations. Snail1 knockdown did not significantly change the basal expression of E-cadherin and N-cadherin at both the message and protein levels (Fig. 2*E* and 2*F*). However, TGF-β1-induced downregulation of E-cadherin was significantly impaired in the Snail1 knockdown cells. Moreover, Snail1 knockdown attenuated the upregulation of N-cadherin mRNA induced by TGF-β1 (Fig. 2*E*). Western blot analysis showed that Snail1 knockdown blocked TGF-β1-induced downregulation of E-cadherin and upregulation of N-cadherin in 603B cells (Fig. 2*F*). Taken together, these results clearly indicate that Snail1 was induced by TGF-β1 in 603B cells and this induction was required for TGF-β1-induced EMT-like changes.

Snail1 is Dispensable for TGF-β1-induced Col1A1 Expression in 603B Cells

It has been proposed previously that epithelial cells undergoing EMT may be an important source of ECM protein-producing cells during tissue fibrosis. Therefore, we examined whether TGF-β1 could induce the expression of Col1A1, a gene encoding collagen α1(I) which is predominantly accumulated in the portal

region during liver fibrosis. Col1A1 mRNA levels were increased 1 day after TGF-β1 exposure but decreased to the basal level at 2 days after TGF-β1 stimulation (Fig. 3*A*). Immunofluorescent staining and Western blot showed similar but delayed changes in Col1A1 protein levels in TGF-β1-treated cells (Fig. 3*B* and 3*E*). To test the role for snail1 in TGF-β1-induced up-regulation of Col1A1, we evaluated the Col1A1 mRNA levels in Snail1 knockdown 603B cells cultured in the absence or presence of TGF-β1 for 24 h (for Col1A1 mRNA) and 48 h (for Col1A1 protein). As shown in Fig. 3*D* and 3*F*, Snail1 knockdown neither affected the basal level of Col1A1 nor prevented TGF-β1-induced Col1A1 expression in 603B cells. These data suggested that although Col1A1 expression is upregulated by TGF-β1 signaling in cultured 603B cells, production of Col1A1 may be transient and not dependent on snail1-associated EMT-like phenotypic alterations.

miR-29s are not Involved in TGF-β1-induced Col1A1 Expression in 603B Cells

Col1A1 is a target for miR-29 [24]. It has recently been shown that decreased miR-29 expression results in the excessive production of Col1A1 in cardiac fibrosis and liver fibrosis patients [23,24]. To explore the potential involvement of miR-29 in TGF-β1-induced Col1A1 upregulation in 603B cells, we generated a luciferase vector which contains a 280-bp fragment of Col1A1 3′UTR with three conserved seed sequences for miR-29 targeting (Fig. 4*A*), conserved for miR-29a, -29b, and -29c [24]. As shown in Fig. 4*B*, the luciferase activity in 603B cells transfected with this construct was much lower than that in cells transfected with the empty control plasmid, suggesting repression of Col1A1 translation by endogenous miR-29s. Nevertheless, qRT-PCR analysis showed no significant change for the expression of miR-29 family members after TGF-β1 exposure (Fig. 4*C*). Thus, although Col1A1 is a target for miR-29, miR-29-mediated posttranscriptional mechanisms may not be involved in TGF-β1-induced Col1A1 expression in 603B cells.

TGF-β1 Induces Apoptotic Resistance in 603B Cells in a Snail1-dependent Manner

Cholangiocytes are aberrantly accumulated during liver fibrosis, suggesting the impaired balance between cell growth and cell death. Interestingly, during the liver development, high level TGF-β1 favors the accumulation of ductular-like cells [30]. We then evaluated whether TGF-β1 treatment promotes 603B cells survival *in vitro*. Cells were treated with TNF-α plus the NF-κB inhibitor SC-514 for 24 h. This treatment resulted in substantial cells death in 603B cells (Fig. 5*A* and 5*B*). PI staining revealed apoptotic nuclear fragmentation in a considerable portion of these cells after TNF-α and SC-514 treatment, suggesting occurrence of apoptosis (Fig. 5*A*). Pre-treatment with TGF-β1 for 5 days exerted a significant protective effect against TNF-α/SC-514-induced cell death (Fig. 5*A* and 5*B*). Consistent with these data, PARP cleavage

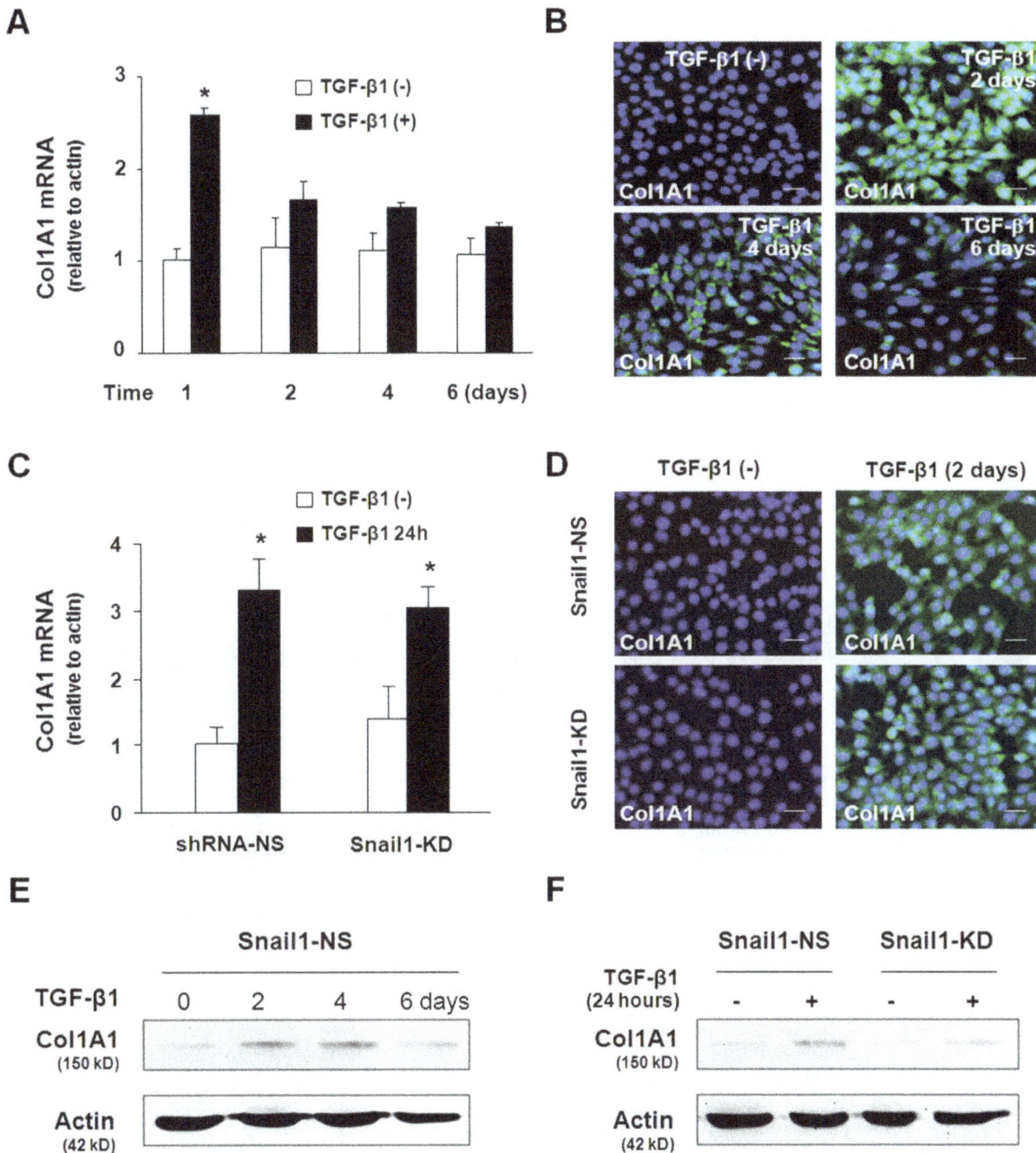

Figure 3. TGF-β1-induced Col1A1 expression is independent of Snail1 up-regulation. TGF-β1 (3 ng/ml) treatment transiently increased Col1A1 mRNA and protein in 603B cells, as determined by qRT-PCR (A and C), immunofluorescent staining (B and D) and Western blot (E and F). Snail1 knockdown did not affect TGF-β1-induced up-regulation of Col1A1 in 603B cells (C–F). Cells stably expressing the Snail1 shRNA or control shRNA were exposed to TGF-β1 (3 ng/ml) for 24 h (for qRT-PCR of Col1A1 in C) and for 2 days (for Conl1A1 protein staining in D and Western blot in E and F). The qRT-PCR results shown represent an average of three independent experiments. Values are means ± SE. *$p < 0.05$ compared to non-TGF-β1-treated cells; shRNA-NS = non specific shRNA control; Snail1-KD = snail shRNA knockdown; Bar = 10 μM.

assay by FACS showed that TGF-β1 pretreatment decreased apoptotic cell death induced by TNF-α/SC-514 treatment in 603B cells (Fig. 5C). To further demonstrate the nature of TNF-α/SC-514-induced cells death, we evaluated the caspase-3 activation by Western blot. Without TNF-α/SC-514 stimulation, 603B cells predominantly expressed the uncleaved procaspase-3. Addition of TNF-α plus SC-514 switched inactive procaspase-3 into active (cleaved) caspase-3, substantiating the induction of apoptosis

(Fig. 5D). 603B cells after 5 days of TGF-β1 exposure showed no significant difference in the expression level of inactive procaspase-3 as compared to non-treated cells. However, TNF-α/SC-514 induced caspase-3 cleavage was significantly attenuated (Fig. 5D). Interestingly, pre-treatment with TGF-β1 for 1 day failed to prevent TNF-α/SC-514 induced caspase-3 activation (Fig. 5D), suggesting the acquisition of apoptotic resistance by TGF-β1 might be a relatively late event.

A

B

C

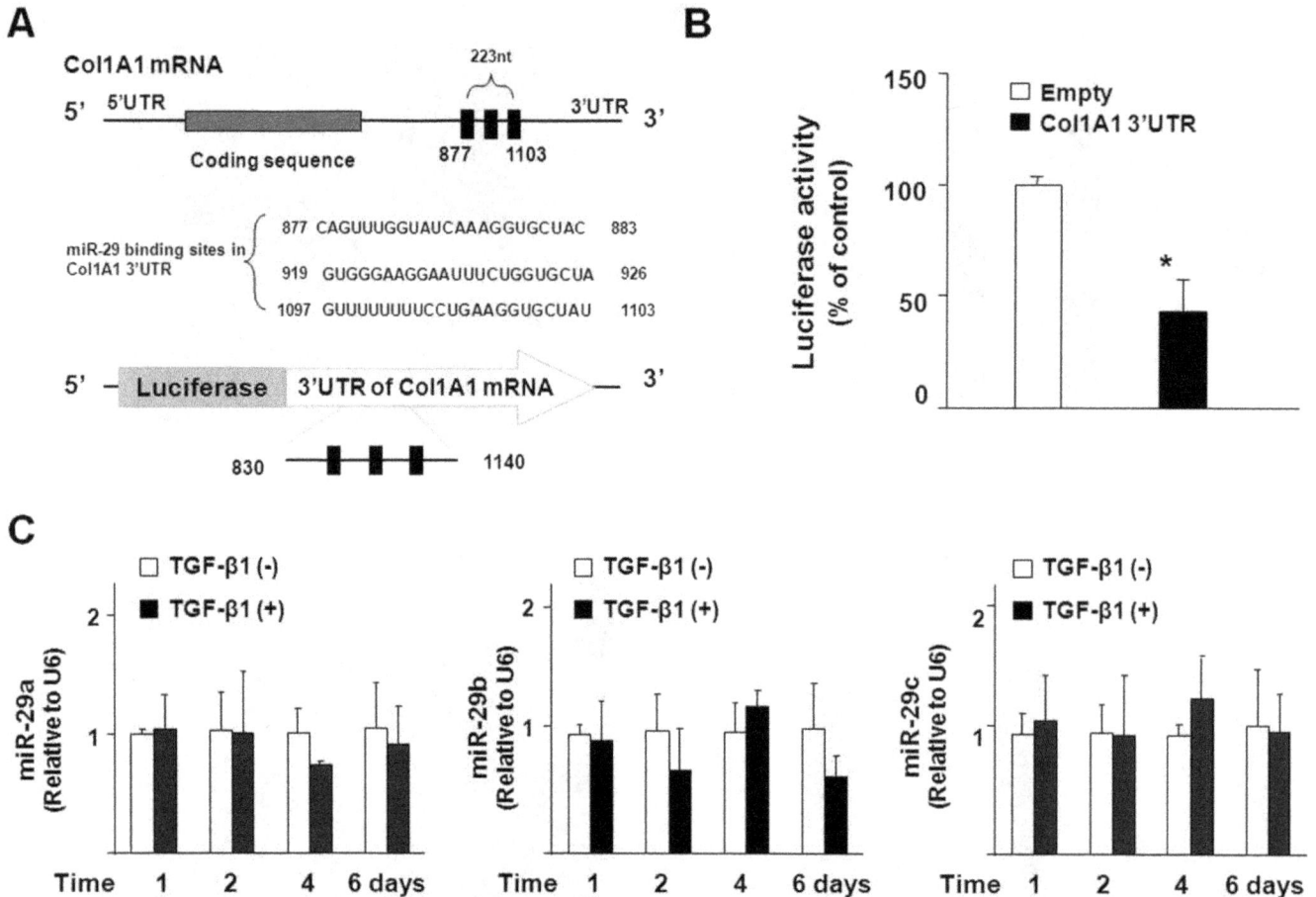

Figure 4. TGF-β1-induced Col1A1 expression is independent of miR-29 downregulation. (A) The schematic of Col1A1 mRNA showed three potential binding sites in its 3'UTR for miR-29 targeting. (B) Col1A1 3'UTR fragments containing miR-29 potential binding sites results in translational suppression in 603B cells as assessed by luciferase reporter assay. The Col1A1 3'UTR sequence covering the potential binding sites for miR-29 was inserted into the pMIR-REPORT luciferase plasmid. The empty pMIR-REPORT luciferase plasmid was used as the control. 603B cells were transfected with the constructs and luciferase analysis was performed 48 h later. Values are means ± SE. *$p<0.05$ compared to cells transfected with the empty pMIR-REPORT luciferase vector. (C) qRT-PCR analysis revealed no significant down-regulation of miR-29 family members in 603B cells following TGF-β1 treatment for up to 6 days. Data represent an average of three independent experiments.

To explore the underlying mechanisms, we measured associated caspase-3 activation in snail1 knockdown 603B cells. Cells stably expressing control shRNA or Snail1 shRNA were treated with TGF-β1 for 5 days and then exposed to TNF-α plus SC-514 for 24 h. Western blot analysis showed that TGF-β1 treatment significantly decreased caspase-3 activation in cells transfected with the control shRNA. In contrast, the suppressive effect of TGF-β1 treatment on TNF-α/SC-514 induced caspase-3 activation was attenuated in the snail1 knockdown cells (Fig. 5E), suggesting that Snail1 might contribute to TGF-β1-induced apoptotic resistance in 603B cells.

Snail1 functions as a transcriptional factor to suppress the expression of multiple genes, including several pro-apoptotic genes, Bax, Bid, Bim, Pten and Puma [27,31–33]. We found that the mRNA levels of these genes were steadily down-regulated in cells 4 days and 6 days after TGF-β1 treatment (Fig. 6A). Snail1 knockdown attenuated or even reversed TGF-β1 suppressive effects on some of these genes. Specially, Snail1 knockdown increased the basal expression of Bim in 603B cells, which was further induced by TGF-β1 treatment. Although Snail1 knockdown did not enhance basal Bid and Puma expression, downregulation of their expression induced by TGF-β1 was attenuated in

the Snail1 knockdown cells (Fig. 6B). No significant impact on expression of Bax and Pten was detected in the Snail1 knockdown cells. These data suggest that Snail1 may be a key mediator for TGF-β1 pathway to modulate cell survival by regulating pro-apoptotic genes.

Discussion

Whether cholangiocytes can transdifferentiate into myofibroblast-like cells via EMT to promote liver fibrosis development is still under debate [34]. Cholangiocytes display morphological features of EMT during hepatic fibrosis [4,7–9]. However, recent data from cell fate mapping experiments suggested that there were no FSP1 or α-SMA positive cells derived from cholangiocytes during murine liver fibrosis, suggesting that cholangiocytes might not be a key origin of myofibroblast during liver fibrosis [35–37]. In this study, we examined EMT-associated reactions in cholangiocytes in response to TGF-β1 *in vitro*, using a non-tumorigenic mouse 603B cholangiocyte cell line. Consistent with the results from cell fate mapping experiments *in vivo*, we found that TGF-β1 did not change the expression of FSP1 or vimentin in 603B cells. However, TGF-β1 induced EMT-like phenotypic

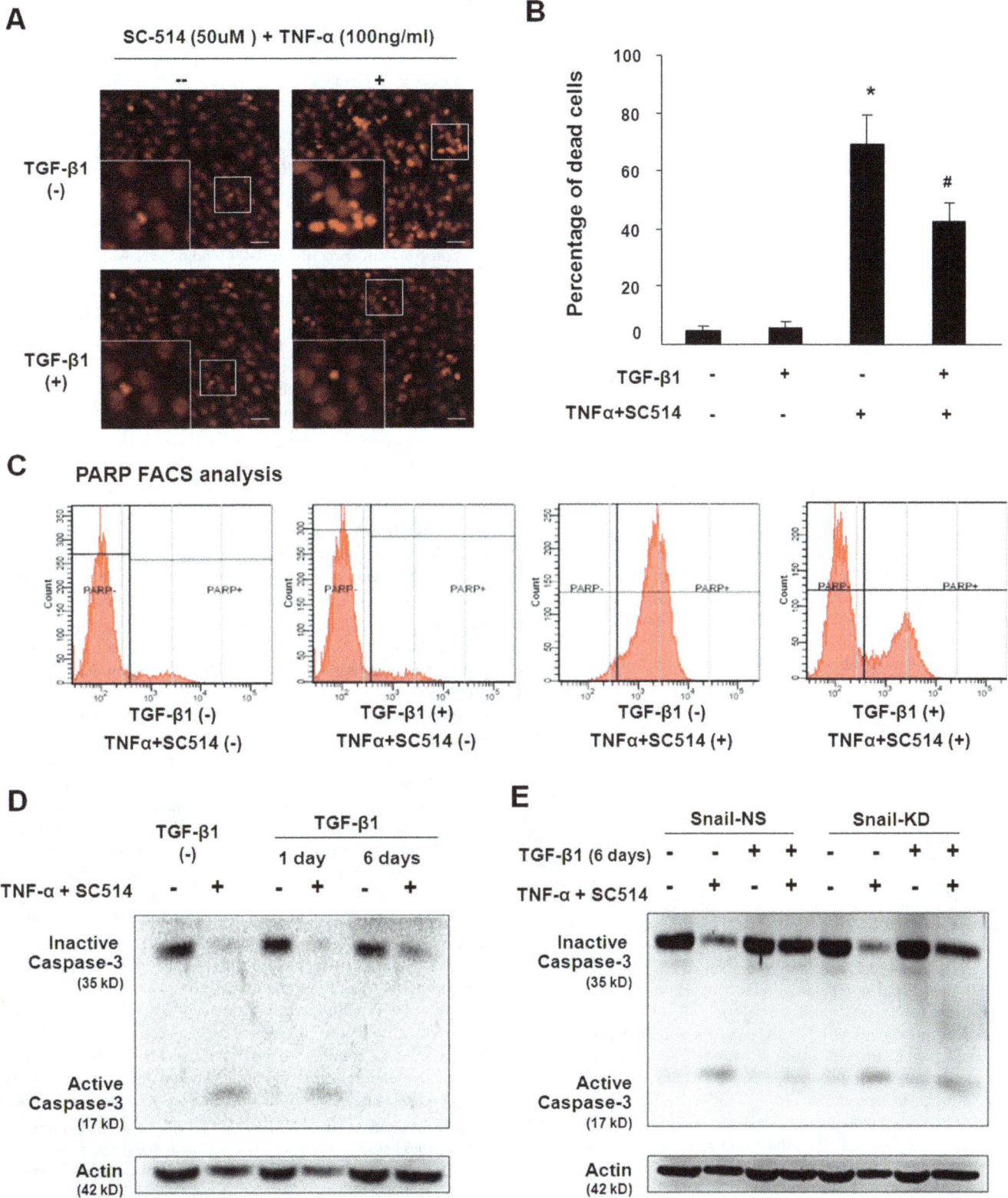

Figure 5. Snail1 is required for TGF-β1-induced apoptosis resistance in 603B cells. (A) TGF-β1 pretreatment inhibits TNF-α- and SC-514-induced cell death. Cells were culture in the absence or presence of TGF-β1 for 5 days and then treated with TNF-α plus SC-514 for additional 24 h. Apoptosis-associated nuclear decomposition in TGF-β1-pretrated or non-pretreated 603B cells as assessed by PI staining. Insets are higher magnifications of the boxed region. Bar = 10 μM. (B) Quantification of frequency of TNF-α/SC-514-induced cell death by trypan blue. Data are presented as percentage of total cell numbers. (C) The PARP cleavage assay for assessing apoptosis by flow cytometry. 603B cells were treated as described above. Both free-floating and attached cells were collected and stained with FITC-conjugated antibody against cleaved PARP followed by FACS analysis. (D) TGF-β1 pretreatment inhibits TNF-α- and SC-514-induced cleavage of caspase-3 in 603B cells. 603B cells were exposed to TGF-β1 for 1 and 5 days, followed by TNF-α plus SC-514 treatment for additional 24 h. The activation of caspase-3 was assessed by Western blot using

antibody recognizing both the full-length caspase-3 and cleaved caspase-3 forms. (E) Snai1 is required for the inhibitory effects of TGF-β1 pretreatment on TNF-α- and SC-514-induced cleavage of caspase-3 in 603B cells. 603B stably cells expressing control shRNA or Snail1 shRNA were stimulated with TGF-β1 for 5 days, followed by TNF-α plus SC-514 treatment for 24 h. The activation of caspase-3 was assessed by Western blot. Representative blots in D and E are from three independent experiments and actin was blotted to ensure equal loading. Values are means ± SE. *$p<0.05$ compared to non- TNF-α/SC514 treated cells; #$p<0.05$ compared to non-TGF-β1 pretreated cells. shRNA-NS = non specific shRNA control; Snail1-KD = snail shRNA knockdown.

alterations, promoted Col1A1 production and increased apoptotic resistance in 603B cells. Interestingly, TGF-β1-induced Col1A1 production appears to be independent of EMT-like alternations. These data suggest that TGF-β1 induces EMT-like differentiation in 603B cells. However, EMT-like differentiation of cholangiocytes may not be required for collagen production; rather, it promotes cell survival capacity.

Previous studies indicate that TGF-β1 is significantly elevated during liver fibrosis and plays a pivotal role in the development of liver fibrosis [16]. Our results showed that 603B clearly lost the epithelial morphological features after TGF-β1 treatment. Specifically, these cholangiocytes underwent morphological changes to become spindle-shaped cells in response to continuous TGF-β1 stimulation, which might reflect cholangiocyte shape changes observed during liver fibrosis [18]. More importantly, treated cells also gradually lost the expression of E-cadherin, an important protein to mediate the formation of tight junctions between epithelial cells [20]. TGF-β1 treatment also significantly increased N-cadherin expression in 603B cells, suggesting EMT-like differentiation. Of note, TGF-β1 stimulated 603B cells to enhance expression of Snail1, which is mechanically a critical downstream mediator for TGF-β1-induced EMT [15]. Consistently, we found that downregulation of E-cadherin, upregulation of N-cadherin and morphological alterations were largely dependent on the Snail1 signaling.

Liver fibrosis is characterized by the accumulation of excessive amounts of ECM proteins, which leads to the destruction of hepatic architecture. There is increasing interest in investigating whether epithelial cells undergoing EMT directly contribute to the ECM deposition, because uncovering the unique EMT signaling molecules associated with collagen production might help to identify novel therapeutic targets. Data from this study indicate that development of EMT is not a prerequisite for collagen production in cholangiocytes in response to TGF-β1 stimulation in vitro. Consistent with results from previous studies [17,19,35,36], we found that 603B cells increased Col1A1 production in response to TGF-β1 stimulation. However, Col1A1 expression was only transiently induced by TGF-β1 stimulation, and not paralleled with the persistent upregulation of N-cadherin or downregulation of E-cadherin in 603B cells undergoing EMT-like alterations. Moreover, upregulation of Col1A1 appears to be independence of Snail1 signaling. In fact, although most TGF-β1-induced EMT-like alterations were abolished in Snial-1 knockdown cells, these cells were still responsive to TGF-β1 to increase Col1A1 expression. It's possible that TGF-β1 might activate distinct pathways to induce Col1A1 production and EMT-like changes in cholangiocytes. Similar to our results, TGF-β1-induced Col1A1 production in mouse hepatocytes did not parallel the occurrence of EMT [36].

Recent studies demonstrated that miRNAs, such as miR-29 family members, might play a role in the control of cardiac and liver fibrosis [23,24]. It has experimentally been confirmed that miR-29s can target the 3′UTRs of several collagen mRNAs and suppress the expression of multiple collagens including Col1A1 [24]. Down-regulation of miR-29s has been reported in fibrotic areas of cardiac and liver fibrosis. The precise molecular

mechanisms underlying miR-29 dysregulation during fibrosis are unknown. TGF-β1 has been demonstrated to suppress miR-29 expression in the cardiac fibroblast and HSC cells in vitro [23,24]. We found that the luciferase activity in 603B cells transfected with the construct covering the miR-29 binding sites within the 3′UTR of Col1A1 was significant suppressed, indicating that endogenous miR-29 might help to prevent excessive expression of Col1A1. Nevertheless, expression of miR-29a/b/c in 603B cells was unaffected in response to TGF-β1 stimulation. Therefore, TGF-β1 may regulate miR-29 expression in a cell type-specific manner. Moreover, TGF-β1-induced Col1A1 expression in 603B cells in vitro is independent of miR-29 expression.

Cholangiocyte accumulation is a poor predictor for hepatic fibrosis. Our study demonstrated that TGF-β1-treated 603B cells were more resistant to TNF-α/SC-514-induced apoptosis. Snail1 knockdown significantly attenuated the protective effects of TGF-β1 on 603B cells, suggesting that TGF-β1-induced EMT-like alterations might contribute to cholangiocyte accumulation during liver fibrosis via suppressing apoptotic cell death. Increasing evidence supports that induction of EMT is generally associated with reduced apoptosis and the molecular mechanisms are not fully understood. We found a modest downregulation of multiple pro-apoptotic genes, including Bax, Bid, Bim, Pten, and Puma, in 603B cells after continuous TGF-β1 stimulation. Snail1 knockdown abolished down-regulation of Bid, Bim and Puma induced by TGF-β1 exposure, further supporting the involvement EMT-associated signaling in the development of apoptotic resistance in TGF-β1-treated cells. Genome-wide ChIP analysis suggested that Snail1 can bind the promoters of many apoptosis-associated genes when it was overexpressed in ovarian cancer cells [34]. Whether TGF-β1-induced Snail1 can directly silence these pro-apoptotic genes merits further investigation. In addition, the regulatory effects of Snail1 on apoptosis might not limit to silencing pro-apoptotic genes. A recent study suggested that snail1 knockdown prevented the upregulation of anti-apoptotic molecules, Bcl-xL and Mcl-1, in mouse hepatocytes induced by TGF-β1 [27]. Obviously, many anti-apoptotic and pro-apoptotic molecules and activation of multiple EMT-associated signal pathways are involved. Targeting accumulated proliferative cholangiocytes has been shown to attenuate liver fibrosis in mice [38]. A comprehensive evaluation of the role for EMT signaling in cholangiocyte apoptotic resistance during liver fibrosis may help to identify new targets for therapeutic intervention. It will be also of interest to extend these studies to other cholangiocyte cell lines, as well as to determine the role of TGF-β1-induced cholangiocyte EMT in ECM production during liver fibrosis in vivo.

Acknowledgments

We thank Drs. Guoku Hu, Rui Zhou, Ai-Yu Gong for technical assistance and Ms. Barbara L. Bittner for her assistance in editing the manuscript. We are very grateful to Drs. Patrick C. Swanson, Jason C. Bartz, Kristen M. Drescher, and Garrett A. Soukup for helpful and stimulating discussions.

A

B

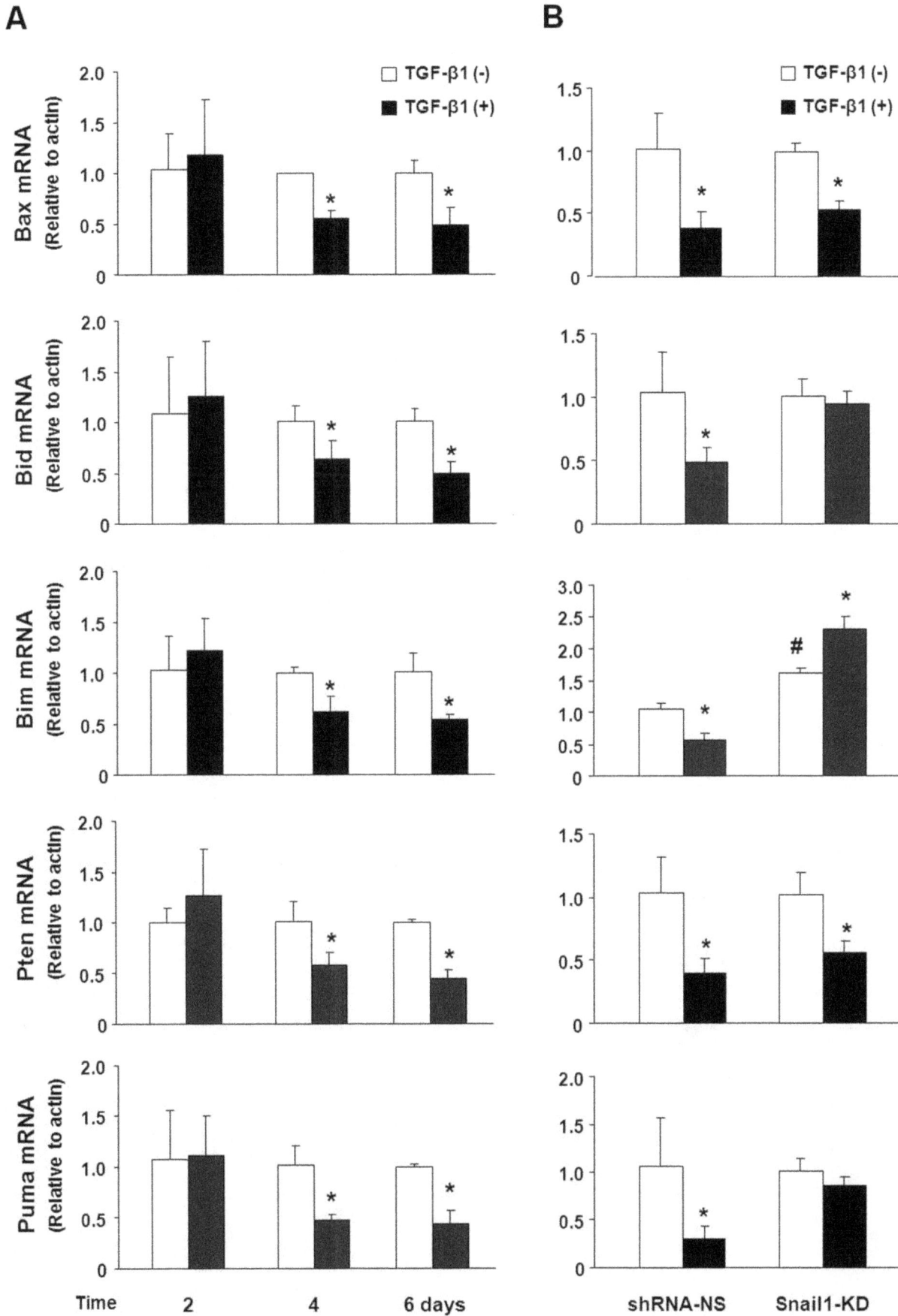

Figure 6. Snail1 contributes to the down-regulation of pro-apoptotic genes induced by TGF-β1. (A) 603B cells were treated with TGF-β1 for indicated periods of time. Alterations of mRNA expression for pro-apoptotic genes Pten, Bim, Bax, Bid and Puma were assessed by qRT-PCR. (B) 603B cells stably expressing control shRNA or Snail1 shRNA were treated with TGF-β1 for 6 days. Changes of pro-apoptotic gene mRNA levels were determined by qRT-PCR. Data represent an average of three independent experiments. Values are means ± SE. *$p<0.05$ compared to non-TGF-β1 treated cells; #$p<0.05$ compared to shRNA-NS control. shRNA-NS = non specific shRNA control; Snail1-KD = snail shRNA knockdown.

Author Contributions

Conceived and designed the experiments: JL XMC. Performed the experiments: JL AE. Analyzed the data: JL XMC. Wrote the paper: JL XMC.

References

1. Bataller R, Brenner DA (2005) Liver fibrosis. J Clin Invest: 115: 209–218.
2. Friedman SL (2008) Mechanisms of hepatic fibrogenesis. Gastroenterology. 134: 1655–1669.
3. Beaussier M, Wendum D, Schiffer E, Dumont S, Rey C, et al. (2007) Prominent contribution of portal mesenchymal cells to liver fibrosis in ischemic and obstructive cholestatic injuries. Lab Invest 87: 292–303.
4. Wells RG (2008) Cellular sources of extracellular matrix in hepatic fibrosis. Clin Liver Dis 12: 759–768.
5. Priester S, Wise C, Glaser SS (2010) Involvement of cholangiocyte proliferation in biliary fibrosis. World J Gastrointest Pathophysiol 1: 30–37.
6. Glaser SS, Gaudio E, Miller T, Alvaro D, Alpini G (2009) Cholangiocyte proliferation and liver fibrosis. Expert Rev Mol Med 11: e7. Available: http://journals.cambridge.org/action/displayAbstract?fromPage=online&aid=4187152. Accessed 2009 Apr 30.
7. Omenetti A, Porrello A, Jung Y, Yang L, Popov Y, et al. (2008) Hedgehog signaling regulates epithelial-mesenchymal transition during biliary fibrosis in rodents and humans. J Clin Invest 118: 3331–3342.
8. Rygiel KA, Robertson H, Marshall HL, Pekalski M, Zhao L, et al. (2008) Epithelial-mesenchymal transition contributes to portal tract fibrogenesis during human chronic liver disease. Lab Invest 88: 112–123.
9. Sato Y, Harada K, Ozaki S, Furubo S, Kizawa K, et al. (2007) Cholangiocytes with mesenchymal features contribute to progressive hepatic fibrosis of the polycystic kidney rat. Am J Pathol 171: 1859–1871.
10. Thiery JP, Acloque H, Huang RY, Nieto MA (2009) Epithelial-mesenchymal transitions in development and disease. Cell 39: 871–890.
11. Acloque H, Adams MS, Fishwick K, Bronner-Fraser M, Nieto MA (2009) Epithelial-mesenchymal transitions: the importance of changing cell state in development and disease. J Clin Invest 119: 1438–1449.
12. Kalluri R, Weinberg RA (2009) The basics of epithelial-mesenchymal transition. J Clin Invest 119: 1420–1428.
13. Jung Y, Brown KD, Witek RP, Omenetti A, Yang L, et al. (2008) Accumulation of hedgehog-responsive progenitors parallels alcoholic liver disease severity in mice and humans. Gastroenterology 134: 1532–1543.
14. Omenetti A, Yang L, Li YX, McCall SJ, Jung Y, et al. (2007) Hedgehog-mediated mesenchymal-epithelial interactions modulate hepatic response to bile duct ligation. Lab Invest 87: 499–514.
15. Xu J, Lamouille S, Derynck R (2009) TGF-beta-induced epithelial to mesenchymal transition. Cell Res 19: 156–172.
16. Inagaki Y, Okazaki I (2007) Emerging insights into Transforming growth factor beta Smad signal in hepatic fibrogenesis. Gut 56: 284–292.
17. Kaimori A, Potter J, Kaimori JY, Wang C, Mezey E, et al. (2007) Transforming growth factor-beta1 induces an epithelial-to-mesenchymal transition state in mouse hepatocytes in vitro. J Biol Chem 282: 22089–22101.
18. Xia JL, Dai C, Michalopoulos GK, Liu Y (2006) Hepatocyte growth factor attenuates liver fibrosis induced by bile duct ligation. Am J Pathol 168: 1500–1512.
19. Zeisberg M, Yang C, Martino M, Duncan MB, Rieder F, et al. (2007) Fibroblasts derive from hepatocytes in liver fibrosis via epithelial to mesenchymal transition. J Biol Chem 282: 23337–23347.
20. Zeisberg M, Neilson EG (2009) Biomarkers for epithelial-mesenchymal transitions. J Clin Invest 119: 1429–1437.
21. Gregory PA, Bracken CP, Bert AG, Goodall GJ (2008) MicroRNAs as regulators of epithelial-mesenchymal transition. Cell Cycle 7: 3112–3118.
22. Maurer B, Stanczyk J, Jüngel A, Akhmetshina A, Trenkmann M, et al. (2010) MicroRNA-29, a key regulator of collagen expression in systemic sclerosis. Arthritis Rheum 62: 1733–1743.
23. Roderburg C, Urban GW, Bettermann K, Vucur M, Zimmermann H,et al. (2011) Micro-RNA profiling reveals a role for miR-29 in human and murine liver fibrosis. Hepatology 53: 209–218.
24. Van Rooij E, Sutherland LB, Thatcher JE, DiMaio JM, Naseem RH, et al. (2008) Dysregulation of microRNAs after myocardial infarction reveals a role of miR-29 in cardiac fibrosis. Proc Natl Acad Sci U S A 105: 13027–13032.
25. Song J (2007) EMT or apoptosis: a decision for TGF-beta. Cell Res 17: 289–290.
26. Valdés F, Murillo MM, Valverde AM, Herrera B, Sánchez A, et al. (2004) Transforming growth factor-beta activates both pro-apoptotic and survival signals in fetal rat hepatocytes. Exp Cell Res 292: 209–18.
27. Franco DL, Mainez J, Vega S, Sancho P, Murillo MM, et al. (2010) Snail1 suppresses TGF-beta-induced apoptosis and is sufficient to trigger EMT in hepatocytes. J Cell Sci 123: 3467–3477.
28. Hanada S, Harada M, Koga H, Kawaguchi T, Taniguchi E, et al. (2003) Tumor necrosis factor-alpha and interferon- gamma directly impair epithelial barrier function in cultured mouse cholangiocytes. Liver Int 23: 3–11.
29. Decker P, Isenberg D, Muller S (2000) Inhibition of caspase-3-mediated poly(ADP-ribose) polymerase (PARP) apoptotic cleavage by human PARP autoantibodies and effect on cells undergoing apoptosis. J Biol Chem 275: 9043–9046.
30. Clotman F, Jacquemin P, Plumb-Rudewiez N, Pierreux CE, Van der Smissen P, et al. (2005) Control of liver cell fate decision by a gradient of TGF beta signaling modulated by Onecut transcription factors. Genes Dev 19: 1849–1854.
31. Escrivà M, Peiró S, Herranz N, Villagrasa P, Dave N, et al. (2008) Repression of PTEN phosphatase by Snail1 transcriptional factor during gamma radiation-induced apoptosis. Mol Cell Biol 28: 1528–1540.
32. Kajita M, McClinic KN, Wade PA (2004) Aberrant expression of the transcription factors snail and slug alters the response to genotoxic stress. Mol Cell Biol 24: 7559–7566.
33. Kurrey NK, Jalgaonkar SP, Joglekar AV, Ghanate AD, Chaskar PD, et al. (2009) Snail and slug mediate radioresistance and chemoresistance by antagonizing p53-mediated apoptosis and acquiring a stem-like phenotype in ovarian cancer cells. Stem Cells 27: 2059–2068.
34. Popov Y, Schuppan D (2010) Epithelial-to-mesenchymal transition in liver fibrosis: dead or alive? Gastroenterology 139: 722–725.
35. Scholten D, Osterreicher CH, Scholten A, Iwaisako K, Gu G, et al. (2010) Genetic labeling does not detect epithelial-to-mesenchymal transition of cholangiocytes in liver fibrosis in mice. Gastroenterology 139: 987–998.
36. Taura K, Miura K, Iwaisako K, Osterreicher CH, Kodama Y, et al. (2010) Hepatocytes do not undergo epithelial-mesenchymal transition in liver fibrosis in mice. Hepatology 51: 1027–1036.
37. Chu AS, Diaz R, Hui JJ, Yanger K, Zong Y, et al. (2011) Lineage tracing demonstrates no evidence of cholangiocyte epithelial-to-mesenchymal transition in murine models of hepatic fibrosis. Hepatology 53: 1685–1695.
38. Patsenker E, Popov Y, Stickel F, Jonczyk A, Goodman SL, et al. (2008) Inhibition of integrin alphavbeta6 on cholangiocytes blocks transforming growth factor-beta activation and retards biliary fibrosis progression. Gastroenterology 135: 660–670.

3

NDRG2 Ameliorates Hepatic Fibrosis by Inhibiting the TGF-β1/Smad Pathway and Altering the MMP2/TIMP2 Ratio in Rats

Jiandong Yang[1,2◊], Jin Zheng[3◊], Lin Wu[2◊], Ming Shi[4◊], Hongtao Zhang[1], Xing Wang[1], Ning Xia[1], Desheng Wang[1], Xinping Liu[2], Libo Yao[2], Yan Li[2]*, Kefeng Dou[1]*

1 Department of Hepatobiliary Surgery, Xijing Hospital, The Fourth Military Medical University, Xi'an, China, 2 Department of Biochemistry and Molecular Biology, State Key Laboratory of Cancer Biology, The Fourth Military Medical University, Xi'an, China, 3 Department of Traditional Chinese and Western Medicine of Oncology, Tangdu Hospital, The Fourth Military Medical University, Xi'an, China, 4 Department of Neurology, Xijing Hospital, The Fourth Military Medical University, Xi'an, China

Abstract

Liver fibrosis is a worldwide clinical issue. It has been well established that activated hepatic stellate cells (HSCs) are responsible for excessive extracellular matrix (ECM) deposition in chronically damaged livers. The identification of key elements that control HSCs activation will help to further our understanding of liver fibrosis and improve the outcome of clinical treatment. This study demonstrates that N-Myc downstream-regulated gene 2 (NDRG2) is a potential regulator of liver fibrosis as NDRG2 mRNA and protein levels were reduced during HSCs activation. In addition, enhanced NDRG2 expression reduced *Smad3* transcription and phosphorylation, which inhibited HSCs activation by blocking the TGF-β1 signal. Moreover, NDRG2 contributed to an increase in the ratio of matrix metalloproteinase 2 (MMP2) to tissue inhibitor of matrix metalloproteinase 2 (TIMP2), which may facilitate the degradation of the ECM. In dimethylnitrosamine (DMN)-induced fibrotic rat livers, adenovirus-mediated NDRG2 overexpression resulted in decreased ECM deposition and improved liver function compared with controls. In conclusion, the present findings indicate that the modulation of NDRG2 is a promising strategy for the treatment of liver fibrosis.

Editor: Ching-Ping Tseng, Chang Gung University, Taiwan

Funding: This work was supported by the National Natural Science Foundation of China Grants 81072973; 81100764; 30830054; 31070681; 81170400. The funders had no role in study design, data collection and analysis, decision to publish, or preparation of the manuscript.

Competing Interests: The authors have declared that no competing interests exist.

* E-mail: lsqfmmu@fmmu.edu.cn (YL); doukef@163.com (KD)

◊ These authors contributed equally to this work.

Introduction

Liver fibrosis is a major medical problem of liver diseases, especially in Asian countries. Chronic hepatitis, metabolic disorders, genetic mutations and cholestatic diseases are common causes of liver fibrosis and even cirrhosis and hepatocellular carcinoma (HCC) [1,2]. Substantial improvements in the treatment of liver fibrosis have been achieved due to continued studies [3,4,5], thereby prompting us to explore the mechanisms involved in the development of liver fibrosis and potential therapies that could inhibit the progression of fibrosis.

HSCs play a central role in liver fibrosis. In normal liver, HSCs are in a quiescent state and their main function is to store retinoids. However, during the development of hepatic fibrosis, chronic liver damage leads to HSCs activation, characterized by a transformation from the quiescent state to a proliferative, contractile and fibrogenic myofibroblast-like phenotype that terminates in excessive hepatic matrix deposition, liver function impairment, cirrhosis and organ failure [6,7].

The activation of HSCs is finely regulated by multiple pathways and factors, and of these, TGF-β1/Smad signaling is one of the major pathways in charge of HSCs activation, type I collagen expression and deposition. TGF-β1 binds to its receptor, leading to the phosphorylation of the intracellular mediators Smad2 and Smad3, which then form hetero-oligomers with a common mediator, Smad4. The complex then translocates from the cytoplasm to the nucleus to regulate gene transcription. The expression of inhibitory Smad7, which interacts with a group of ubiquitin ligases termed Smurf and degrades the TGF-β receptors through proteasomal and lysosomal pathways, is also induced by TGF-β signaling as part of a negative feedback loop [8,9]. In addition, TGF-β1 regulates the expression of matrix metalloproteinases (MMPs) and tissue inhibitor of matrix metalloproteinases (TIMPs). MMPs are endogenous peptidases capable of degrading various components of the basement membrane while TIMPs inhibit collagen degradation. In the fibrotic liver, the expression of MMPs and TIMPs are both increased [10] and it is the balance of MMPs and their tissue inhibitors that determines the progression and regression of ECM accumulation and liver fibrosis [11,12].

Recently, several studies have revealed that NDRG2 is a potent factor in regulating liver embryonic development, tissue remodeling and carcinogenesis. *NDRG2* (GenBank Accession No. AF159092) belongs to the *NDRG* family, which comprises four members, *NDRG1-4*. Our laboratory initially identified human NDRG2, a cytoplasmic protein that is down-regulated by MYC and is involved in cell growth and differentiation, stress and hormonal responses [13,14,15]. Accumulated data suggest that NDRG2 is closely involved in liver histogenesis and organogenesis as NDRG2 mRNA and protein levels are generally lower in the early stages and markedly higher during the later stages of histogenesis in mouse and human fetal livers of different gestational ages [16,17]. Our previous study demonstrated that NDRG2 could regulate liver regeneration by serving as a cell cycle and apoptosis regulator. As a new tumor suppressor gene [18,19,20], NDRG2 also plays a critical role in HCC, in which it is significantly down-regulated compared to adjacent normal tissues. Furthermore, high NDRG2 expression levels correlate positively with tumor differentiation and negatively with clinical parameters relevant to tumor metastasis. In vitro, it has been shown that NDRG2 affects the proliferative abilities of HCC cell lines [21] and antagonizes TGF-β1–mediated HCC cell invasion by down-regulating MMP2 [22]. Additionally, when determine the gene expression profile for the whole liver during development of DMN-induced hepatic fibrosis, Takahara et al [23] found that NDRG2 was down-regulated in hepatocytes following fibrogenesis. Taken together, these data implicate the multiple functions of NDRG2 in liver under both normal and pathological conditions. However, to date, the significance of NDRG2 in the development of liver fibrosis has been little studied.

In the current study, we demonstrated that NDRG2 expression exhibited an inverse relationship with HSCs activation. In addition, we have shown that NDRG2 inhibited basal and TGF-β1–mediated HSCs activation via a reduction in Smad3 phosphorylation. Furthermore, adenovirus-mediated NDRG2 overexpression attenuated rat liver fibrosis and improved liver function by enhancing ECM degradation via the alteration of MMP2 and TIMP2 expression. In conclusion, our study is the first to explore the anti-fibrotic effects of NDRG2 in liver.

Results

NDRG2 shows an inverse relationship with HSCs activation

The spontaneously immortalized human HSCs cell line, LX-2, exhibits features typical of stellate cells, while the immortalized rat HSCs cell line, HSC-T6, exhibits features typical of myofibroblasts [24]. In this study, NDRG2 was expressed in LX-2 cells and was mainly localized to the cytoplasm, together with alpha smooth muscle actin (α-SMA), a marker of HSCs activation (Figure 1A). Previous studies have demonstrated that HSCs undergo further activation during growth and expansion on a plastic surface [25], and using this model we were able to assess the relationship between NDRG2 expression and LX-2 cell activation. After LX-2 cells grew to confluence, they were trypsinized and replated in 100 mm dishes for further activation. Over the next 12 days, increased expression of α-SMA was detected, indicating LX-2 activation while, in contrast, NDRG2 mRNA and protein expression decreased (Figure 1B and C). Similar results were observed in HSC-T6 cells (Figure S1).

TGF-β1 is a classic stimulator for HSCs activation and collagen production [26,27]. To confirm the relationship between NDRG2 and HSCs activation further, LX-2 cells were treated with TGF-β1 for 24 h after serum starvation. As expected, TGF-β1 increased LX-2 activation, as indicated by enhanced α-SMA levels compared to controls, while NDRG2 expression was inhibited (Figure 1D and E).

NDRG2 inhibits HSCs activation

Since NDRG2 was down-regulated during HSCs activation, adenovirus vectors were used to elevate NDRG2 expression

transiently in LX-2 cells to determine the effect of NDRG2 on HSCs activation. The results showed that adenoviral vectors expressing NDRG2 (AdNDRG2) enhanced the level of NDRG2 compared to the negative control β-galactosidase (AdLacZ) group (Figure 2A and B). Next, the activation level of LX-2 cells was examined by treating the cells with adenovirus and/or TGF-β1. After treatment, both the basal and TGF-β1–induced α-SMA protein levels were decreased by NDRG2 overexpression (Figure 2C and D). These results indicated that NDRG2 could inhibit HSCs activation, even when mediated by TGF-β1.

NDRG2 inhibits the TGF-β1/Smad signaling pathway and alters the relative levels of MMP2 to TIMP2

TGF-β1 signaling is essential for HSCs activation and liver fibrosis. To gain a better understanding of the molecular mechanisms involved in the NDRG2-mediated inhibition of HSCs activation, the mRNA levels of the intracellular mediators of TGF-β1 signal transduction Smad2, Smad3 and Smad7 were analyzed. The results demonstrated that the transcription of all three Smads increased in TGF-β1–treated LX-2 cells; however, AdNDRG2 only attenuated the increase in Smad3 induced by TGF-β1, while Smad2 and Smad7 showed no differences among compared groups (Figure 3A). Furthermore, the protein levels of Smad2/3/7 as well as the phosphorylation of Smad 2/3 were upregulated in the presence of TGF-β1 stimulation, while AdNDRG2 treatment only inhibited the protein level and the phosphorylation status of Smad3 (Figure 3B).

MMPs and TIMPs contribute to both the progression and regression of liver fibrosis. In this study, the expression of both MMP2 and TIMP2 increased during LX-2 activation induced by TGF-β1; however, after AdNDRG2 infection, MMP2 was enhanced while TIMP2 levels decreased (Figure 3C) compared with AdLacZ controls (MMP9 and TIMP1 were undetectable). Consequently, the ratio of MMP2 to TIMP2 was increased (Table 1), which is helpful for the regression of ECM accumulation.

NDRG2 attenuates DMN-induced liver fibrosis

To explore the anti-fibrosis role of NDRG2 in vivo, a rat liver fibrosis model was established by DMN injection. Rats receiving DMN treatment developed severe fibrosis as shown in a representative hematoxylin and eosin (H&E) and Sirius Red stained image (Figure 4A). In addition, the expression of NDRG2 in liver cells decreased while α-SMA positive cells increased dramatically (Figure 5A), indicating that HSCs had been activated following DMN treatment.

To determine the infection efficiency of the adenovirus, rats were injected first with phosphate buffered saline (PBS) or a single dose of adenoviral vector (4×10^9 plaque forming units [PFU]) expressing enhanced green fluorescent protein (AdEGFP) via the tail vein. Forty-eight hours after injection, over 80% of liver cells were EGFP-positive compared with the PBS group (Figure S2A), showing that the adenovirus had a high infection efficiency. In addition, we found that after administration of the same dose of AdNDRG2, NDRG2 levels were significantly enhanced in rat liver from day three to day 14 (Figure S2B) while AdLacZ treatment had no effect on NDRG2 expression (Figure S2C). Thus, a single dose of adenovirus was enough to enhance NDRG2 expression, which lasted long enough to produce a therapeutic effect on liver fibrosis.

After treatment, we observed that, compared with PBS or AdLacZ injection, AdNDRG2 administration not only elevated NDRG2 expression in liver cells but also inhibited the expression of α-SMA (Figure 5), which demonstrated further that NDRG2

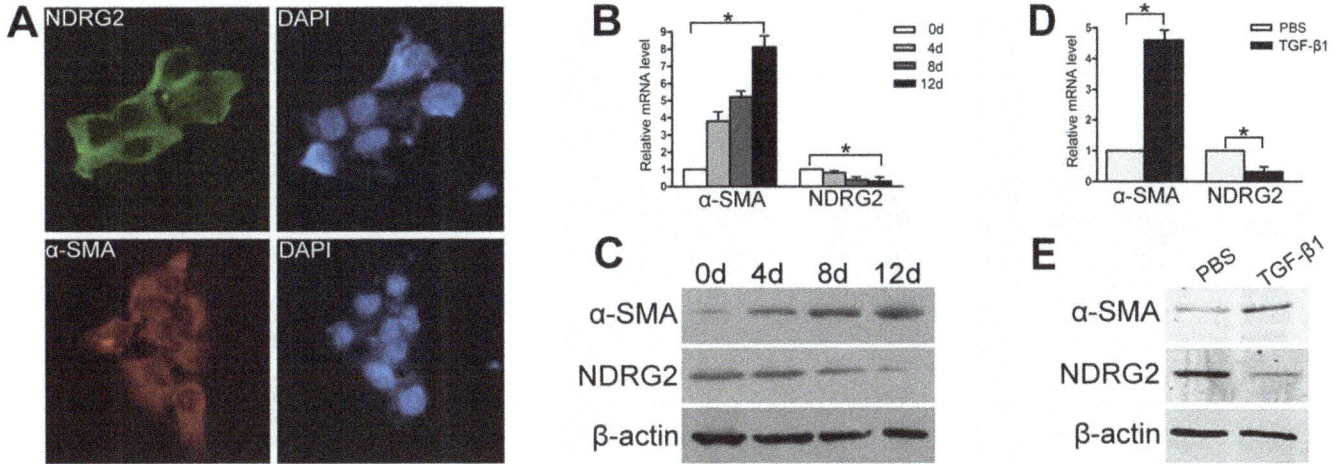

Figure 1. NDRG2 is decreased during LX-2 activation. (A) Green (FITC conjugated) represented NDRG2 expression while red (CY3 conjugated) represented α-SMA expression in LX-2 cells, DAPI (blue)-stained nuclei (400×). Real-time PCR (B) and Western blotting (C) were used to detect the expression of α-SMA and NDRG2 in LX-2 cells grown to confluence and then replated on 100 mm dishes for 12 days. Real-time PCR (D) and Western blotting (E) were used to detect the expression of α-SMA and NDRG2 in LX-2 cells following serum starvation and supplementing with 0.2% BSA for 48 hours prior to PBS or TGF-β1 treatment (2.5 ng/ml for 24 hours). β-actin was used as a loading control. All experiments were performed independently in triplicate. *P<0.05 between compared groups.

could suppress HSCs activation. In addition, the degree of fibrosis was significantly attenuated as revealed by H&E and Sirius Red staining (Figure 4A and B). Meanwhile, after AdNDRG2 injection, the hydroxyproline content, which is an indicator for ECM deposition, was decreased in the AdNDRG2-treated fibrotic livers (199.69±8.23 μg/mg) compared with the AdLacZ group

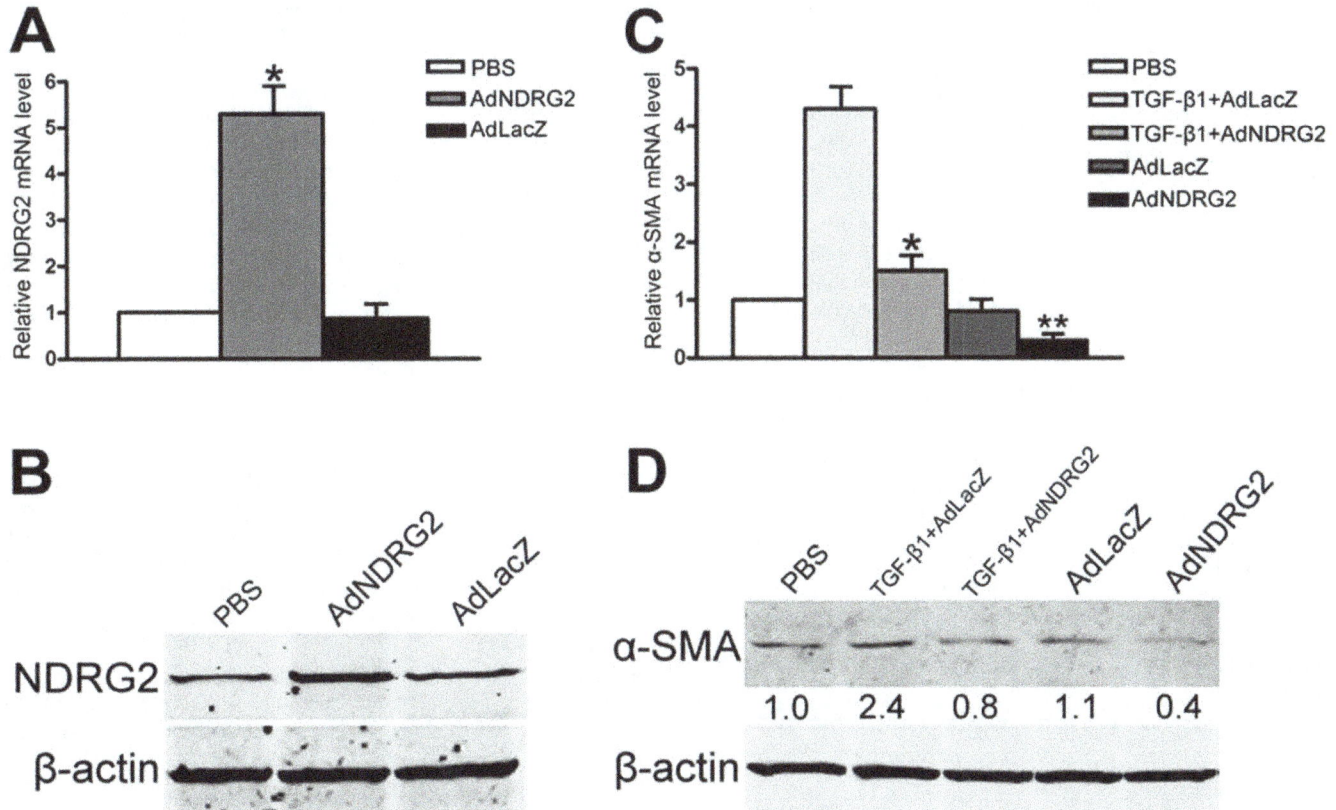

Figure 2. NDRG2 inhibits HSCs activation. NDRG2 mRNA (A) and protein (B) level in LX-2 cells assessed 48 hours after PBS or adenovirus infection. α-SMA mRNA (C) and protein (D) level in LX-2 cells assessed after PBS, TGF-β1 and/or adenovirus infection. β-actin was used as a loading control. Relative quantifications of α-SMA band intensities, normalized to β-actin levels, were shown below blots. All experiments were performed independently in triplicate. In (A), *P<0.05 compared with the PBS or AdLacZ group. In (C), *P<0.05 compared with the TGF-β1+AdLacZ group; **P<0.05 compared with the AdLacZ or PBS group.

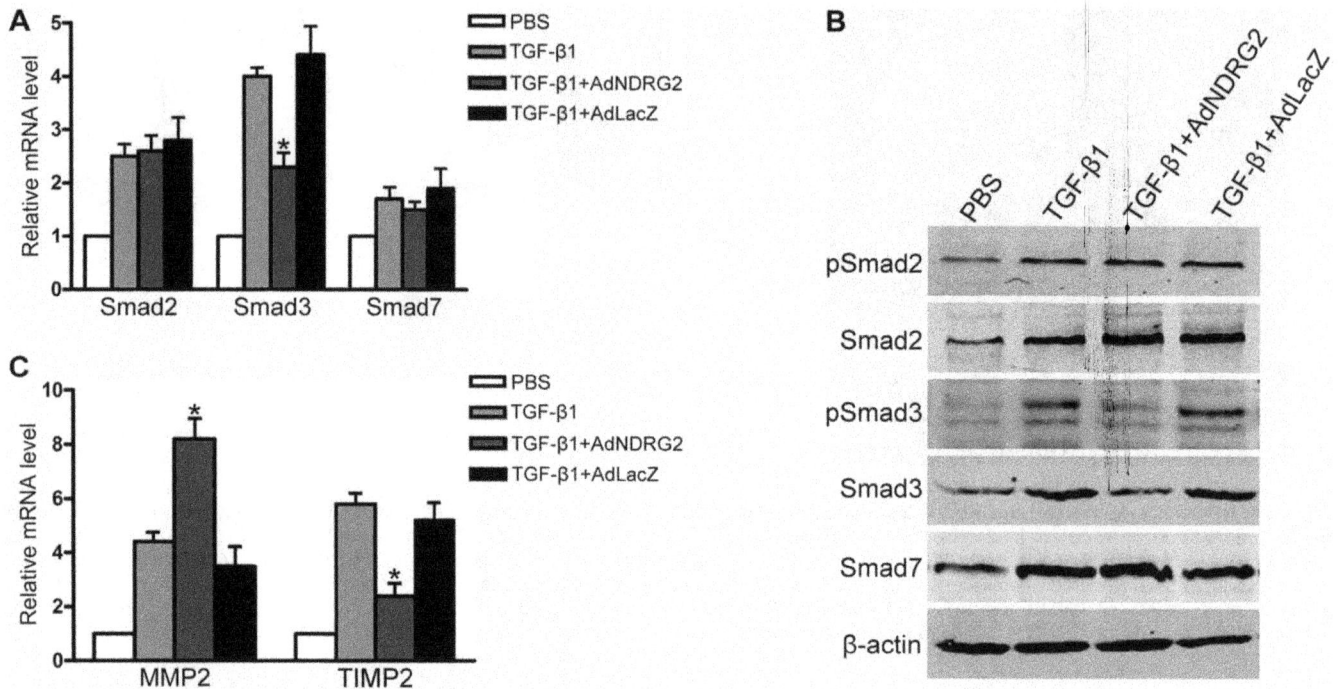

Figure 3. NDRG2 affects TGF-β1/Smad signaling pathway and the ratio of MMP2 to TIMP2 in LX-2 cells. (A) Real-time PCR was used to detect the expression of Smad2, Smad3 and Smad7 in LX-2 cells with TGF-β1 and/or adenovirus treatment. (B) Western blotting was used to detect the expression of Smad2, phospho-Smad2, Smad3, phospho-Smad3 and Smad7 in LX-2 cells with TGF-β1 and/or adenovirus treatment. (C) Real-time PCR was used to detect the expression of MMP2 and TIMP2 in LX-2 cells following TGF-β1 and/or adenovirus treatment. β-actin was used as a loading control. All experiments were performed independently in triplicate. *P<0.05 compared with the TGF-β1 or TGF-β1+AdLacZ group.

(295.06±17.14 μg/mg) or the PBS group (287.46±20.09 μg/mg) (Figure 4C).

In line with the *in vitro* results, the data obtained from fibrotic rats indicated that, following AdNDRG2 treatment, the expression and phosphorylation of Smad3 decreased while the ratio of MMP2 to TIMP2 increased (Figure 6) (Table 2), confirming that the regulatory role of NDRG2 in TGF-β1/Smad signaling and in the regulation of MMP2 and TIMP2 expression contributes towards its therapeutic effects in the fibrotic liver.

NDRG2 increases hepatocyte proliferation and improves liver function

Our previous data demonstrated that AdNDRG2 treatment induced hepatocyte cell cycle arrest and apoptosis *in vitro* [28]. However, in the present study, it is important to note that hepatocytes responded differently to AdNDRG2 in DMN-induced liver fibrosis. Proliferating cell nuclear antigen (PCNA) staining and BrdU staining increased in AdNDRG2 group compared with

Table 1. NDRG2 affects the ratio of MMP2 to TIMP2 in LX-2 cells.

Group	MMP2/TIMP2
PBS	1
TGF-β1	0.764±0.0003
TGF-β1+AdNDRG2	3.418±0.3124*
TGF-β1+AdLacZ	0.669±0.0639

*P<0.05 compared with the TGF-β1 or TGF-β1+AdLacZ group.

PBS or AdLacZ group while TUNEL analysis revealed that AdNDRG2 had no effect on inducing hepatocyte apoptosis (Figure 7) (Figure S3), which indicating that AdNDRG2 not only inhibited HSCs activation and ECM accumulation, but also facilitated the regression of liver fibrosis by enhancing the proliferation of hepatocytes without inducing apoptosis. Moreover, AdNDRG2 injection significantly improved hepatic serum biochemical parameters in the DMN-induced rat fibrotic model (Table 3).

Discussion

HSCs can undergo further activation either by cultured on uncoated plastic or treated with TGF-β1. These two models are well-established techniques for studying hepatic fibrogenesis at the cellular level. The present data demonstrated a decrease in NDRG2 expression using both of these methods for HSCs activation. Previous studies have revealed that the level of NDRG2 expression is linked positively to cell differentiation and negatively to cell proliferation [16,17,29,30,31], and it is well known that during chronic liver injury, HSCs activation involves the process of transdifferentiating from quiescent into proliferative and ECM-producing myofibroblasts [32]. Thus, the decrease in NDRG2 levels during the HSCs activation process is another evidence for the regulatory role of NDRG2 on cell differentiation and proliferation. Taking this into account, whether or not NDRG2 regulates the proliferative ability and transdifferentiation process of HSCs merits further investigation.

TGF-β1 is a profibrogenic cytokine in the liver. The current study has shown that NDRG2 inhibited HSCs activation in the absence and presence of TGF-β1, and in addition, increased the expression of MMP2 in HSCs. These results differ partly from

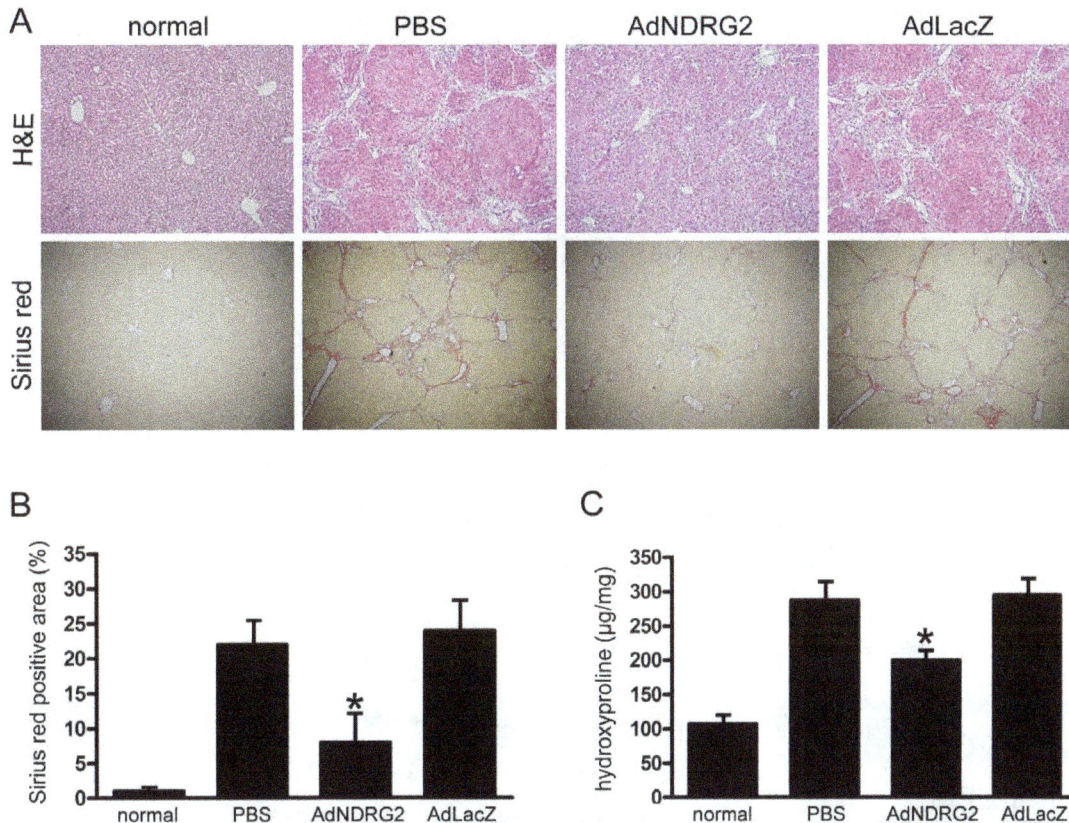

Figure 4. NDRG2 attenuates DMN-induced liver fibrosis. PBS or adenovirus was injected four weeks after DMN treatment and rats were sacrificed two weeks after injection. (A) Liver fibrosis was assessed by H&E staining (100×) and Sirius Red staining (40×). (B) Semiquantitative analysis of the Sirius Red staining result. (C) Assay of hydroxyproline content. The data are expressed as hydroxyproline (μg)/wet liver weight (mg). Three samples were determined from each group. "normal" means rats without treatment. *P<0.05 compared with PBS or AdLacZ group.

research into HCC, which revealed that overexpression of NDRG2 antagonized TGF-β1–mediated HCC invasion by down-regulating MMP2 expression [22]. However, the previous study was based on the HCC cell line PLC/PRF/5. Most cases of HCC develop on a liver fibrosis background [33] and a fibrous capsule surrounds a typical HCC at an early stage [34]. HCC cells have to degrade the ECM and basement membrane during the process of metastasis [35]. Therefore, overexpression of NDRG2 leads to reduced MMP2 and ECM degradation, which subsequently, confined HCC to its fibrous septa. Yet, in our study, AdNDRG2 treatment produced an increase in MMP2 as well as a decrease of TIMP2. MMP2 activity is regulated at the cell surface and involves the formation of a tri-molecular complex consisting of pro-MMP2, MT1-MMP and TIMP-2. All three components of this complex are expressed by activated HSCs [36]. An increase in MMPs and TIMPs is common in fibrotic diseases, while an alteration in the MMP/TIMP expression ratio is known to be critical in determining matrix remodeling [10]. In this study, the data from LX-2 cells demonstrated that over-expressing NDRG2 inhibited the expression of TIMP2 and increased MMP2. Consequently, NDRG2 administration reduced ECM deposition within the liver parenchyma and alleviated liver fibrosis.

Considering the significance of the TGF-β1/Smad signaling pathway in regulating fibrogenesis, researchers are trying to block the TGF-β1/Smad signal in order to suppress liver fibrosis. Importantly, Smad2 and Smad3 exert their functions depending on the status of HSCs. TGF-β1 induces the phosphorylation and nuclear translocation of Smad2 in quiescent HSCs and of Smad3

in transdifferentiated HSCs [37]. In addition, data obtained from infecting cultured rat HSCs with adenoviruses expressing Smad2 or Smad3 revealed that Smad3 plays a more important role than Smad2 in the morphological and functional maturation of myofibroblasts [38]. In the present study, LX-2 cells could be regarded as partially activated based on the fact that they expressed α-SMA under all culture conditions [25]. By infecting LX-2 cells with adenovirus expressing NDRG2, we found that an increase in NDRG2 in LX-2 cells caused a decrease in Smad3 and its phosphorylation in the presence of TGF-β1. In contrast, the status of Smad2 and Smad7 were not affected. Data obtained from fibrotic rat livers were also consistent with the in vitro study. Therefore, the decreased activation and inhibited transdifferentiation of HSCs depend on the suppression of Smad3 after AdNDRG2 treatment.

A recent study from our laboratory revealed that the overexpression of NDRG2 in a hepatocyte cell line resulted in G_1/S arrest and apoptosis induction. During the early phase of liver regeneration in a rat partial hepatectomy (PH) model, NDRG2 was down-regulated, which may have facilitated hepatocyte proliferation [28]. Based on these data, we wondered whether AdNDRG2 treatment could inhibit hepatocyte proliferation and cause apoptosis in fibrotic rat liver, which were harmful for liver fibrosis treatment. However, in our current study, enhanced PCNA and BrdU staining in the fibrotic liver implied that AdNDRG2 injection increased the proliferation of hepatocytes. In addition, TUNEL analysis revealed that there were no significant differences between the numbers of apoptotic cells in

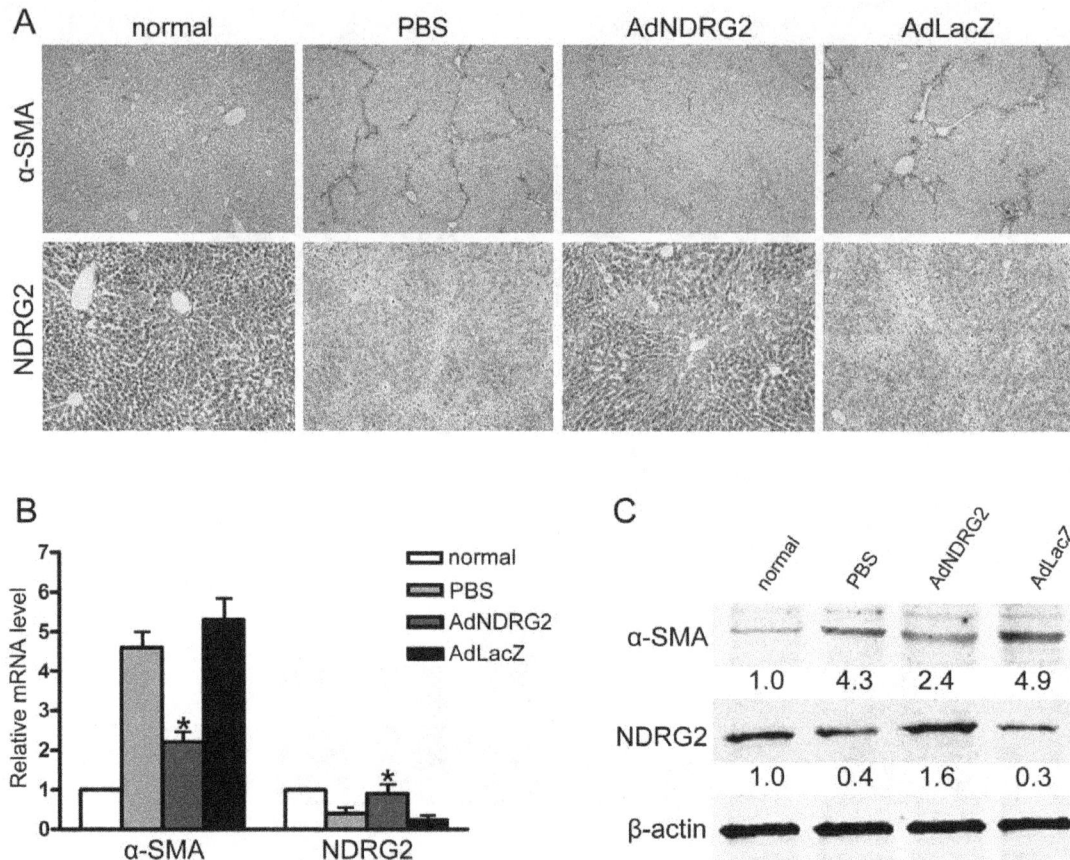

Figure 5. NDRG2 inhibits HSCs activation in DMN-induced liver fibrosis. (A) Immunohistochemistry was used to determine the expression of NDRG2 (200×) and α-SMA (100×). Real-time PCR (B) and Western blotting (C) were used to detect the expression of α-SMA and NDRG2 in liver tissues. β-actin was used as a loading control. Relative quantifications of band intensities, normalized to β-actin levels, were shown below blots. "normal" means rats without treatment. *P<0.05 compared with the PBS or AdLacZ group.

the AdNDRG2 group and the PBS and AdLacZ-treated groups. The discrepancies between these two studies may be attributed to the complexity of the NDRG2 regulation network in different liver tissue remodeling microenvironments (PH-induced liver regeneration compared to DMN-induced liver fibrosis). In addition, both TGF-β1 and ECM deposition have an anti-proliferative and pro-apoptotic effect on hepatocytes [39]. Thus, in the current study, it is possible that AdNDRG2 treatment exerted its therapeutic function by antagonizing TGF-β1 and subsequently increasing hepatocyte proliferation without inducing cell apoptosis, processes essential for treating liver fibrosis and improving liver function.

Collectively, the data reported in this study have demonstrated, for the first time, that NDRG2 is involved in the regulation of liver fibrosis. NDRG2 expression correlated inversely with HSCs activation and, in addition, inhibited TGF-β1–induced HSCs activation by suppressing Smad3 expression and phosphorylation. Furthermore, the *in vivo* study indicated that adenovirus-mediated NDRG2 treatment could effectively attenuate liver fibrosis and improve liver function. Thus, it is conceivable that modulating NDRG2 expression may provide a novel therapy for intervention in liver fibrosis.

Materials and Methods

Cell lines and cell culture

LX-2 and HSC-T6 cells [24] were kindly provided by Dr Scott Friedman. Cells were maintained in Dulbecco's modified Eagle's

medium (DMEM, Invitrogen Life Technologies, Carlsbad, CA, USA) supplemented with 10% fetal bovine serum (FBS, Invitrogen) in a humidified atmosphere of 5% CO_2 at 37°C.

Immunofluorescence analysis

Cells were seeded in 24-well plates and treated with 4% paraformaldehyde for 15 min at 4°C. After blocking with 1% bovine serum albumin (BSA) in PBS containing 0.1% Triton X-100 for 1 hour at room temperature, the cells were incubated with primary NDRG2 (Abnova, Taiwan, China) or α-SMA (Abcam, Cambridge, MA, USA) antibodies overnight at 4°C, followed by three washes with PBS and incubation for 2 hours with FITC- or CY3-conjugated secondary antibodies (Boster, Wuhan, China). Cell nuclei were stained with 4,6-diamidino-2-phenylindole (DAPI; Molecular Probes, OR).

TGF-β1 treatment

Cells were plated in 100 mm dishes. Once they reached 70% confluence, the cells were serum starved and supplemented with 0.2% BSA for 48 hours. Next, TGF-β1 (2.5 ng/ml, PeproTech, Rocky Hill, NJ, USA) was added for 24 hours.

Adenovirus infection

Adenoviral vectors expressing human or rat *NDRG2* (AdNDRG2), the negative control, β-galactosidase (AdLacZ), and enhanced green fluorescent protein (AdEGFP) were pur-

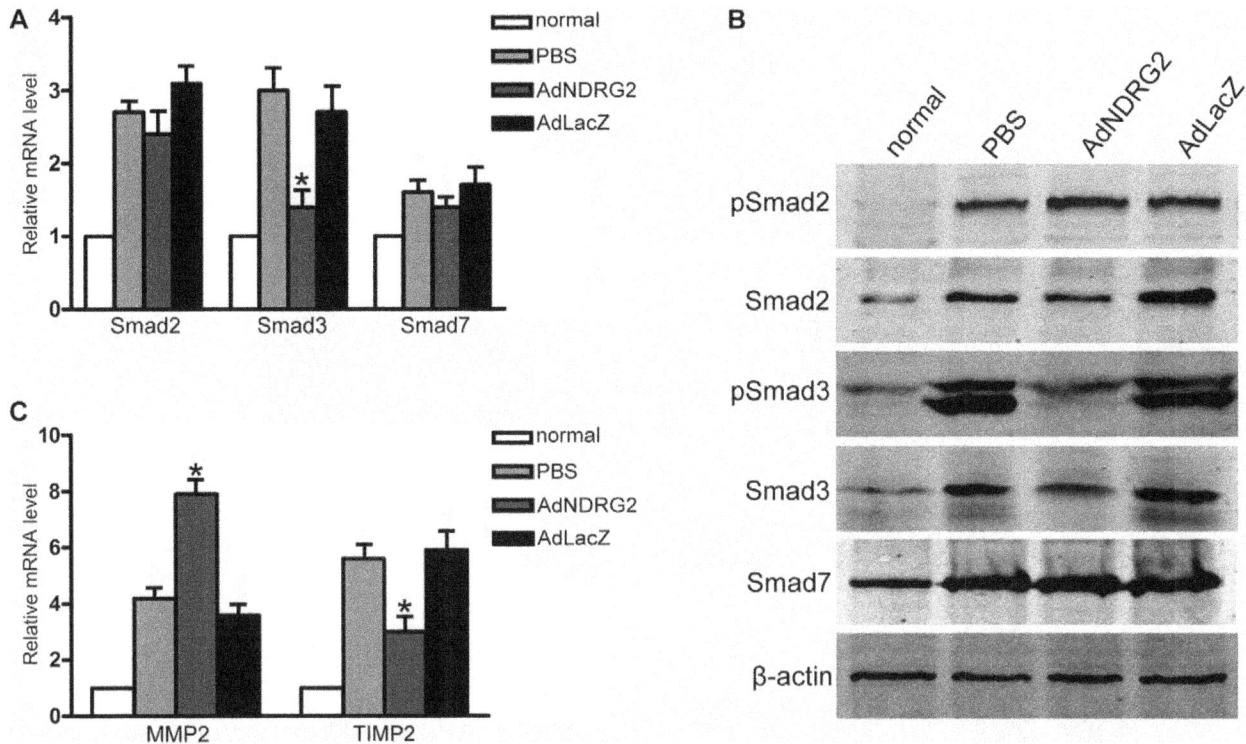

Figure 6. NDRG2 affects the TGF-β1/Smad signaling pathway and the ratio of MMP2 to TIMP2 in rats. (A) Real-time PCR was used to detect the expression of Smad2, Smad3 and Smad7 in rats with PBS or adenovirus treatment. (B) Western blotting was used to detect the expression of Smad2, phospho-Smad2, Smad3, phospho-Smad3 and Smad7 in rats with PBS or adenovirus treatment. (C) Real-time PCR was used to detect the expression of MMP2 and TIMP2 in rats following PBS or adenovirus treatment. β-actin was used as a loading control. "normal" means rats without treatment. *$P < 0.05$ compared with the PBS or AdLacZ group.

chased from Benyuan Zhengyang Company (Beijing, China). Cells were seeded in 100 mm dishes and treated with AdNDRG2, AdLacZ or PBS in serum-free DMEM for 2 hours. The medium was replaced with fresh DMEM supplemented with 10% FBS and incubated for 48 hours. The multiplicity of infection (MOI) was 40, which was determined according to preliminary experimental results.

Animals

Seven-week-old male Sprague-Dawley rats weighing between 200 and 225 g were housed individually in cages with a 12 hour light-dark cycle and given free access to water and standard rat chow throughout the study. All experimental procedures were conducted in accordance with the 'Detailed Rules for the Administration of Animal Experiments for Medical Research Purposes' issued by the Ministry of Health of China and had

Table 2. NDRG2 affects the ratio of MMP2 to TIMP2 in rats.

Group	MMP2/TIMP2
normal	1
PBS	0.749 ± 0.0076
AdNDRG2	$2.640 \pm 0.2891^{*}$
AdLacZ	0.615 ± 0.0125

*$P < 0.05$ compared with the PBS or AdLacZ group. "normal" means rats without treatment.

received ethical approval (Permit number: SCXK 2007-007) by the Animal Experiment Administration Committee of the Fourth Military Medical University (Xi'an, P.R., China). All efforts were made to minimize animals' suffering and to reduce the number of animals used.

Fibrosis model and tissue preparation

Rats were injected intraperitoneally with 1% DMN (10 µg/kg) for three consecutive days per week for up to five weeks. After 12 DMN injections, rats were infused with PBS or a single dose of 4×10^{9} PFU of AdLacZ or AdNDRG2 via the tail vein (ten rats in each group). Two weeks after gene delivery, animals were sacrificed and liver samples were collected. For 5'-Bromo-2'-deoxyuridine (BrdU) staining, one hour before sacrifice, 100 mg BrdU (Sigma, St. Louis, MO) per kg body weight was injected intraperitoneally. RNA and protein were extracted directly with standard techniques described below as soon as the liver samples were excised. For immunohistochemistry analysis, samples were fixed in 4% phosphate-buffered formalin for two days and then embedded in paraffin before 3 µm sections were cut and collected on glass slides. For apoptosis analysis, samples were fixed with neutral buffered 4% paraformaldehyde overnight at 4°C, and liver sections of 10 µm thickness were prepared using a cryostat microtome (Leica, Solms, Germany) and fixed to poly-L-lysine–coated glass slides. Sections were stored at -20°C until required.

Immunohistochemistry analysis

Sections were deparaffinized in xylene and dehydrated through a graduated alcohol series. After incubating with 0.3% H_2O_2 in

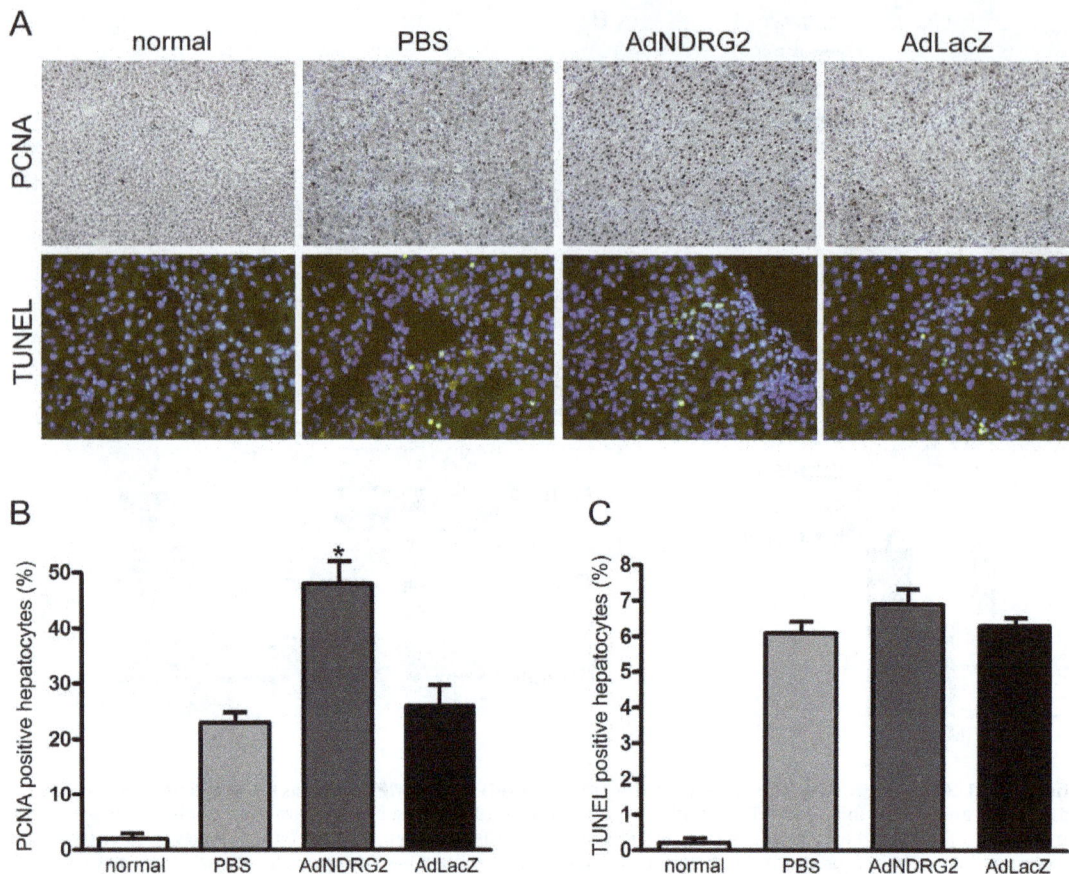

Figure 7. NDRG2 promotes hepatocyte proliferation without inducing apoptosis. (A) Immunohistochemistry and TUNEL staining were used to determine the expression of PCNA (200×) and cell apoptosis (400×) in normal and DMN-induced fibrotic rat livers following PBS or adenovirus treatment. Semiquantitative analysis of PCNA staining (B) and TUNEL staining (C). "normal" means rats without treatment. *P<0.05 compared with the PBS or AdLacZ group.

methyl alcohol for 15 min, sections were treated with citrate buffer (pH 6.0) for antigen retrieval and incubated with 10% normal goat serum in PBS for 1 hour at room temperature to block nonspecific binding. Then, the sections were incubated with the following primary antibodies in PBS at 4°C overnight: mouse anti-NDRG2 (1:100; Abnova), mouse anti-PCNA (1:2000; Cell Signaling Technology, Danvers, MA, USA), rabbit anti-α-SMA (1:100; Abcam), and mouse anti-BrdU (1:100; Santa Cruz Biotechnology, CA, USA). After equilibrating to room temperature, sections were first incubated with biotinylated goat anti-mouse/rabbit IgG (1:400, Sizhengbo, Beijing, China) for 2 hours and then treated with a streptavidin-horseradish peroxidase complex (Sizhengbo)

for 1 h at room temperature. Staining was examined by incubation with 3,3′-diaminobenzidine (DAB) and the sections were counterstained with hematoxylin and viewed under a light microscope.

Sirius Red staining

Sections were deparaffinized and the slides were incubated for 10 min in celestine blue solution and washed with distilled water three times. Next, the slides were placed in a solution of saturated picric acid containing 0.05% Sirius Red for 30 min. After washing with 100% ethanol, slides were mounted in mounting media and covered with a coverslip. The results of Sirius Red staining were quantified with Image-Pro Plus software 6.0 (Media Cybernetics, L.P., Silver Spring, MD).

Apoptotic cell staining

For apoptosis detection in frozen liver tissue sections, terminal deoxynucleotidyl transferase-mediated deoxyuridine triphosphate nick-end labeling (TUNEL) staining was performed as described in the manufacturer's instructions (Roche, Indianapolis, IN, USA). Staining was visualized by fluorescence microscopy (Olympus, Center Valley, PA).

Hepatic function and hydroxyproline content

An automated analyzer at the Department of Pharmacology in the Fourth Military Medical University was used to analyze serum

Table 3. NDRG2 improves hepatic serum biochemical parameters.

Group	ALB(g/l)	ALT(U/l)	AST(U/l)
normal	36.5±3.2	43.1±7.2	92.4±14.9
PBS	15.4±1.6	208.2±9.8	251.4±32.7
AdNDRG2	26.6±4.8*	156.6±25.7*	173.8±10.0 *
AdLacZ	13.1±0.7	218.7±12.4	279.2±35.5

*P<0.05 compared with the PBS or AdLacZ group. "normal" means rats without treatment.

Table 4. Primers for Real-time PCR.

Genes	Forward primer (5'- 3')	Reverse primer (5'- 3')
Human NDRG2	GAGATATGCTCTTAACCACCCG	GCTGCCCAATCCATCCAA
α-SMA	GACAATGGCTCTGGGCTCTGTAA	CTGTGCTTCGTCACCCACGTA
Smad2	TTAACCGAAATGCCACGGTAGAA	GCTCTGCACAAAGATTGCACTATCA
Smad3	AGGCGTGCGGCTCTACTACATC	CAGCGAACTCCTGGTTGTTGAA
Smad7	TGCTGTGCAAAGTGTTCAGGTG	CCATCGGGTATCTGGAGTAAGGA
MMP2	ATGACATCAAGGGCATTCAGGAG	TCTGAGCGATGCCATCAAATACA
TIMP2	GACGGCAAGATGCACATCAC	GAGATGTAGCACGGGATCATGG
β-actin	AGCGAGCATCCCCCAAAGTT	GGGCACGAAGGCTCATCATT
Rat NDRG2	ATGGCAGAGCTTCAGGAGG	CGGGTGGTTCAGAGCGTAT
α-SMA	CCGAGATCTCACCGACTACC	TCCAGAGCGACATAGCACAG
Smad2	TTACAGATCCATCGAACTCGGAGA	CACTTAGGCACTCGGCAAACAC
Smad3	CCAGATGAACCACAGCATGGA	CTACTGTCATGGACGGCTGTGAA
Smad7	CCTTACTCCAGATACCCGATGG	CTTGTTGTCCGAATTGAGCTGT
MMP2	TCCCGAGATCTGCAAGCAAG	AGAATGTGGCCACCAGCAAG
TIMP2	GACACGCTTAGCATCACCCAGA	CTGTGACCCAGTCCATCCAGAG
β-actin	ACCGTGAAAAGATGACCCAGAT	AACCCTCATAGATGGGCACAGT

biochemical parameters, and 100 mg of wet liver samples were subjected to acid hydrolysis to measure the hydroxyproline content according to the Hydroxyproline Testing Kit (Jiancheng, Nanjing, China) protocol.

Real-time PCR

Total RNA was isolated from each sample using TRIzol reagent (Invitrogen) and then quantified. The cDNA was synthesized from 5 μg of each RNA sample with a Taqman reverse transcriptase reagent kit (Applied Biosystems, UK) primed with oligo(dT) and was then used as a template for real-time quantitative PCR analysis. The sequences of the primers are listed in Table 4. The mRNAs were detected with SYBR Green PCR Master Mix and an ABI PRISM 7500 Sequence Detection System (Applied Biosystems) using the comparative threshold cycle method for relative quantification. The PCR reaction consisted of 12.5 μl SYBR Green PCR Master Mix, 10 pmol of the forward and reverse primers, and 5 μl of template cDNA in a total volume of 25 μl. The thermal cycling conditions comprised an initial denaturation step at 95°C for 10 s, followed by 45 cycles at 95°C for 5 s and 60°C for 34 s.

Western blot analysis

Cells were harvested from 100 mm culture dishes. Both cells and liver tissues were lysed in 200 μl RIPA buffer (0.05 M Tris-HCl [pH 7.4], 0.15 M NaCl, 0.25% deoxycholic acid, 1% Nonidet P-40, 1 mM EDTA, 1 mM phenylmethylsulfonyl fluoride, 10 μg/ml aprotinin and 10 μg/ml leupeptin). Protein concentrations were measured using the bicinchoninic acid (BCA) protein assay (Pierce, Rockford, IL, USA). Proteins were resolved by SDS-PAGE and transferred to Hybond-ECL nitrocellulose membranes (Amersham Biosciences, Piscataway, NJ, USA). The blots were probed with the following primary antibodies: NDRG2 (Abnova), β-actin, Smad7 (Santa Cruz Biotechnology), α-SMA (Abcam), Smad2/phospho-Smad2 (pSmad2), Smad3/phospho-Smad3 (pSmad3) (Cell Signaling Technology), followed by incubation with species-matched

secondary antibodies. The bands were detected using enhanced chemiluminescence (Pierce) or the Odyssey Imaging System (Li-Cor Biosciences). Band intensities were quantified with Kodak Digital Science 1D 3.0 (Eastman Kodak, New Haven, CT).

Statistical analysis

Statistical analyses were performed with SPSS software (version 16.0; SPSS, Chicago, IL, USA) using the t-test and analysis of variance of independent groups. Statistical significance was based on a value of $P<0.05$.

Supporting Information

Figure S1   NDRG2 is decreased during HSC-T6 activation. (A) NDRG2 was expressed in LX-2 and HSC-T6 cells. Western blotting (B) and real-time PCR (C) were used to detect the expression of α-SMA and NDRG2 in HSC-T6 cells grown to confluence and then replated on 100 mm dishes for 12 days. β-actin was used as a loading control. All experiments were performed independently in triplicate. *P<0.05 between compared groups.

Figure S2   Adenovirus has a high infection efficiency and significantly enhanced NDRG2 expression in rat liver. (A) Rats were injected with PBS or a single dose (4×10^9 PFU) of AdEGFP via the tail vein. Then, 48 hours after injection, rats were sacrificed and liver samples were fixed with neutral buffered 4% paraformaldehyde overnight at 4°C in the dark. Liver sections (10 μm thick) were prepared on a cryostat microtome and fixed to glass slides. Sections were examined directly under a fluorescent microscope (100×). (B) Rats were treated with a single dose (4×10^9 PFU) of AdNDRG2 or AdLacZ via the tail vein. Over the next 14 days, rats were sacrificed at the time points indicated. Liver samples were collected and proteins were extracted directly. NDRG2 expression was examined by Western blotting. β-actin was used as a loading control.

Figure S3 NDRG2 promotes hepatocyte proliferation.
(A) Immunohistochemistry staining was used to determine the expression of BrdU (200×) in DMN-induced fibrotic rat livers following PBS or adenovirus treatment. (B) Semiquantitative analysis of BrdU staining. *P<0.05 compared with the PBS or AdLacZ group.

Acknowledgments

We especially thank Dr Scott Friedman for providing HSC-T6 and LX-2

cell lines. We thank Prof. Huijie Bian for insightful suggestions and technical help with the cell culture and treatment.

Author Contributions

Conceived and designed the experiments: JY LY KD. Performed the experiments: JY JZ YL MS LW NX. Analyzed the data: JY HZ XW. Contributed reagents/materials/analysis tools: DW XL LY KD. Wrote the paper: JY JZ YL MS.

References

1. Farazi PA, DePinho RA (2006) Hepatocellular carcinoma pathogenesis: from genes to environment. Nat Rev Cancer 6: 674–687.
2. Bruix J, Boix L, Sala M, Llovet JM (2004) Focus on hepatocellular carcinoma. Cancer Cell 5: 215–219.
3. Hadziyannis SJ, Tassopoulos NC, Heathcote EJ, Chang TT, Kitis G, et al. (2006) Long-term therapy with adefovir dipivoxil for HBeAg-negative chronic hepatitis B for up to 5 years. Gastroenterology 131: 1743–1751.
4. Bruno S, Stroffolini T, Colombo M, Bollani S, Benvegnu L, et al. (2007) Sustained virological response to interferon-alpha is associated with improved outcome in HCV-related cirrhosis: a retrospective study. Hepatology 45: 579–587.
5. Veldt BJ, Heathcote EJ, Wedemeyer H, Reichen J, Hofmann WP, et al. (2007) Sustained virologic response and clinical outcomes in patients with chronic hepatitis C and advanced fibrosis. Ann Intern Med 147: 677–684.
6. Bataller R, Brenner DA (2005) Liver fibrosis. J Clin Invest 115: 209–218.
7. Friedman SL (2004) Mechanisms of disease: Mechanisms of hepatic fibrosis and therapeutic implications. Nat Clin Pract Gastroenterol Hepatol 1: 98–105.
8. Dooley S, Streckert M, Delvoux B, Gressner AM (2001) Expression of Smads during in vitro transdifferentiation of hepatic stellate cells to myofibroblasts. Biochem Biophys Res Commun 283: 554–562.
9. Inagaki Y, Okazaki I (2007) Emerging insights into Transforming growth factor beta Smad signal in hepatic fibrogenesis. Gut 56: 284–292.
10. Iredale JP (2001) Hepatic stellate cell behavior during resolution of liver injury. Semin Liver Dis 21: 427–436.
11. Okamoto K, Mimura K, Murawaki Y, Yuasa I (2005) Association of functional gene polymorphisms of matrix metalloproteinase (MMP)-1, MMP-3 and MMP-9 with the progression of chronic liver disease. J Gastroenterol Hepatol 20: 1102–1108.
12. Senties-Gomez MD, Galvez-Gastelum FJ, Meza-Garcia E, Armendariz-Borunda J (2005) [Hepatic fibrosis: role of matrix metalloproteases and TGFbeta]. Gac Med Mex 141: 315–322.
13. Wang L, Liu N, Yao L, Li F, Zhang J, et al. (2008) NDRG2 is a new HIF-1 target gene necessary for hypoxia-induced apoptosis in A549 cells. Cell Physiol Biochem 21: 239–250.
14. Boulkroun S, Fay M, Zennaro MC, Escoubet B, Jaisser F, et al. (2002) Characterization of rat NDRG2 (N-Myc downregulated gene 2), a novel early mineralocorticoid-specific induced gene. J Biol Chem 277: 31506–31515.
15. Shen L, Zhao ZY, Wang YZ, Ji SP, Liu XP, et al. (2008) Immunohistochemical detection of Ndrg2 in the mouse nervous system. Neuroreport 19: 927–931.
16. Hu XL, Liu XP, Deng YC, Lin SX, Wu L, et al. (2006) Expression analysis of the NDRG2 gene in mouse embryonic and adult tissues. Cell Tissue Res 325: 67–76.
17. Hu XL, Yao LB, Zhang YQ, Deng YC, Liu XP (2006) [Distribution characteristic of NDRG2 expression in human fetal tissues.]. Sheng Li Xue Bao 58: 331–336.
18. Hu XL, Liu XP, Lin SX, Deng YC, Liu N, et al. (2004) NDRG2 expression and mutation in human liver and pancreatic cancers. World J Gastroenterol 10: 3518–3521.
19. Liu N, Wang L, Liu X, Yang Q, Zhang J, et al. (2007) Promoter methylation, mutation, and genomic deletion are involved in the decreased NDRG2 expression levels in several cancer cell lines. Biochem Biophys Res Commun 358: 164–169.
20. Shon SK, Kim A, Kim JY, Kim KI, Yang Y, et al. (2009) Bone morphogenetic protein-4 induced by NDRG2 expression inhibits MMP-9 activity in breast cancer cells. Biochem Biophys Res Commun 385: 198–203.
21. Wu GQ, Liu XP, Wang LF, Zhang WH, Zhang J, et al. (2003) Induction of apoptosis of HepG2 cells by NDRG2. Xi Bao Yu Fen Zi Mian Yi Xue Za Zhi 19: 357–360.
22. Lee DC, Kang YK, Kim WH, Jang YJ, Kim DJ, et al. (2008) Functional and clinical evidence for NDRG2 as a candidate suppressor of liver cancer metastasis. Cancer Res 68: 4210–4220.
23. Takahara Y, Takahashi M, Wagatsuma H, Yokoya F, Zhang QW, et al. (2006) Gene expression profiles of hepatic cell-type specific marker genes in progression of liver fibrosis. World J Gastroenterol 12: 6473–6499.
24. Xu L, Hui AY, Albanis E, Arthur MJ, O'Byrne SM, et al. (2005) Human hepatic stellate cell lines, LX-1 and LX-2: new tools for analysis of hepatic fibrosis. Gut 54: 142–151.
25. Taimr P, Higuchi H, Kocova E, Rippe RA, Friedman S, et al. (2003) Activated stellate cells express the TRAIL receptor-2/death receptor-5 and undergo TRAIL-mediated apoptosis. Hepatology 37: 87–95.
26. Chen A, Davis BH (2000) The DNA binding protein BTEB mediates acetaldehyde-induced, jun N-terminal kinase-dependent alphaI(I) collagen gene expression in rat hepatic stellate cells. Mol Cell Biol 20: 2818–2826.
27. Seki E, De Minicis S, Osterreicher CH, Kluwe J, Osawa Y, et al. (2007) TLR4 enhances TGF-beta signaling and hepatic fibrosis. Nat Med 13: 1324–1332.
28. Yang J, Li Y, Wu L, Zhang Z, Han T, et al. (2010) NDRG2 in rat liver regeneration: role in proliferation and apoptosis. Wound Repair Regen 18: 524–531.
29. Zhang J, Liu J, Li X, Li F, Wang L, et al. (2007) The physical and functional interaction of NDRG2 with MSP58 in cells. Biochem Biophys Res Commun 352: 6–11.
30. Choi SC, Kim KD, Kim JT, Kim JW, Yoon DY, et al. (2003) Expression and regulation of NDRG2 (N-myc downstream regulated gene 2) during the differentiation of dendritic cells. FEBS Lett 553: 413–418.
31. Nichols NR, Agolley D, Zieba M, Bye N (2005) Glucocorticoid regulation of glial responses during hippocampal neurodegeneration and regeneration. Brain Res Brain Res Rev 48: 287–301.
32. Friedman SL (2008) Mechanisms of hepatic fibrogenesis. Gastroenterology 134: 1655–1669.
33. Theret N, Musso O, Turlin B, Lotrian D, Bioulac-Sage P, et al. (2001) Increased extracellular matrix remodeling is associated with tumor progression in human hepatocellular carcinomas. Hepatology 34: 82–88.
34. Ozaki I, Mizuta T, Zhao G, Yotsumoto H, Hara T, et al. (2000) Involvement of the Ets-1 gene in overexpression of matrilysin in human hepatocellular carcinoma. Cancer Res 60: 6519–6525.
35. Bodey B, Bodey B, Jr., Siegel SE, Kaiser HE (2001) Immunocytochemical detection of the expression of members of the matrix metalloproteinase family in adenocarcinomas of the pancreas. In Vivo 15: 71–76.
36. Arthur MJ, Friedman SL, Roll FJ, Bissell DM (1989) Lipocytes from normal rat liver release a neutral metalloproteinase that degrades basement membrane (type IV) collagen. J Clin Invest 84: 1076–1085.
37. Liu C, Gaca MD, Swenson ES, Vellucci VF, Reiss M, et al. (2003) Smads 2 and 3 are differentially activated by transforming growth factor-beta (TGF-beta) in quiescent and activated hepatic stellate cells. Constitutive nuclear localization of Smads in activated cells is TGF-beta-independent. J Biol Chem 278: 11721–11728.
38. Uemura M, Swenson ES, Gaca MD, Giordano FJ, Reiss M, et al. (2005) Smad2 and Smad3 play different roles in rat hepatic stellate cell function and alpha-smooth muscle actin organization. Mol Biol Cell 16: 4214–4224.
39. Arendt E, Ueberham U, Bittner R, Gebhardt R, Ueberham E (2005) Enhanced matrix degradation after withdrawal of TGF-beta1 triggers hepatocytes from apoptosis to proliferation and regeneration. Cell Prolif 38: 287–299.

4

Traditional Herbal Medicine use Associated with Liver Fibrosis in Rural Rakai, Uganda

Brandon J. Auerbach[1,2]*, Steven J. Reynolds[3,4], Mohammed Lamorde[1,5], Concepta Merry[1,5,6], Collins Kukunda-Byobona[8], Ponsiano Ocama[2,7], Aggrey S. Semeere[1,7], Anthony Ndyanabo[9], Iga Boaz[9], Valerian Kiggundu[9], Fred Nalugoda[9], Ron H. Gray[9,10], Maria J. Wawer[9,10], David L. Thomas[4], Gregory D. Kirk[11], Thomas C. Quinn[3,4], Lara Stabinski[3,11], on behalf of the Rakai Health Sciences Program

1 Infectious Diseases Institute, College of Health Sciences, Makerere University, Kampala, Uganda, 2 Harvard Medical School, Boston, Massachusetts, United States of America, 3 Division of Intramural Research, National Institute of Allergy and Infectious Diseases, National Institutes of Health, Bethesda, Maryland, United States of America, 4 Division of Infectious Diseases, Department of Medicine, School of Medicine, Johns Hopkins University, Baltimore, Maryland, United States of America, 5 Department of Pharmacology and Therapeutics, School of Medicine, University of Dublin, Trinity College, Dublin, Ireland, 6 St James's Hospital, Dublin, Ireland, 7 Department of Medicine, College of Health Sciences, Makerere University, Kampala, Uganda, 8 Department of Botany, Makerere University, Kampala, Uganda, 9 Rakai Health Sciences Program, Entebbe, Uganda, 10 Department of Population, Family, and Reproductive Health, Bloomberg School of Public Health, Johns Hopkins University, Baltimore, Maryland, United States of America, 11 Department of Epidemiology, Bloomberg School of Public Health, Johns Hopkins University, Baltimore, Maryland, United States of America

Abstract

Background: Traditional herbal medicines are commonly used in sub-Saharan Africa and some herbs are known to be hepatotoxic. However little is known about the effect of herbal medicines on liver disease in sub-Saharan Africa.

Methods: 500 HIV-infected participants in a rural HIV care program in Rakai, Uganda, were frequency matched to 500 HIV-uninfected participants. Participants were asked about traditional herbal medicine use and assessed for other potential risk factors for liver disease. All participants underwent transient elastography (FibroScan®) to quantify liver fibrosis. The association between herb use and significant liver fibrosis was measured with adjusted prevalence risk ratios (adjPRR) and 95% confidence intervals (CI) using modified Poisson multivariable logistic regression.

Results: 19 unique herbs from 13 plant families were used by 42/1000 of all participants, including 9/500 HIV-infected participants. The three most-used plant families were Asteraceae, Fabaceae, and Lamiaceae. Among all participants, use of any herb (adjPRR = 2.2, 95% CI 1.3–3.5, p = 0.002), herbs from the Asteraceae family (adjPRR = 5.0, 95% CI 2.9–8.7, p<0.001), and herbs from the Lamiaceae family (adjPRR = 3.4, 95% CI 1.2–9.2, p = 0.017) were associated with significant liver fibrosis. Among HIV infected participants, use of any herb (adjPRR = 2.3, 95% CI 1.0–5.0, p = 0.044) and use of herbs from the Asteraceae family (adjPRR = 5.0, 95% CI 1.7–14.7, p = 0.004) were associated with increased liver fibrosis.

Conclusions: Traditional herbal medicine use was independently associated with a substantial increase in significant liver fibrosis in both HIV-infected and HIV-uninfected study participants. Pharmacokinetic and prospective clinical studies are needed to inform herb safety recommendations in sub-Saharan Africa. Counseling about herb use should be part of routine health counseling and counseling of HIV-infected persons in Uganda.

Editor: John E. Tavis, Saint Louis University, United States of America

Funding: The study was primarily funded by the United States National Institutes of Health (NIH) Bench to Bedside Program. Additional support was provided by the Division of Intramural Research, National Institutes of Allergy and Infectious Diseases, National Institutes of Health. Support was also provided by the National Institute on Drug Abuse (PI: DLT, R01-AI-16078) and the American Cancer Society (PI: GDK, MRSG-07-284-01-CCE). The study was jointly conducted and benefited from close collaboration of researchers from the intramural NIH Laboratory of Immunoregulation, Johns Hopkins University, the Infectious Diseases Institute of Makerere University, and the Rakai Health Sciences Program. Support for the RHSP HIV Care Program was provided by the President's Emergency Fund for AIDS Relief (PEPFAR) and support for the Rakai Community Cohort Study was provided by the Department of the Army, United States Army Medical Research and Material Command Cooperative Agreement DAMD17-98-2-8007; grants R01 A134826 and R01 A134265 from the National Institute of Allergy and Infectious Diseases; grant R01 016078 (DLT) from the National Institute on Drug Abuse; and grant 5P30HD06826 from the National Institute of Child and Health Development. BJA and ASS were funded by the Fogarty International Clinical Research Scholars (FICRS) program of the NIH, administered by the Vanderbilt University Institute for Global Health (R24 TW007988). The funders had no role in study design, data collection and analysis, decision to publish, or preparation of the manuscript.

Competing Interests: The authors have declared that no competing interests exist.

* E-mail: brandon_auerbach@hms.harvard.edu

Introduction

Traditional herbal medicines are commonly used for HIV/ AIDS and other health conditions in Uganda and sub-Saharan Africa, often in parallel with programs that provide antiretroviral therapy (ART). In the 1990's an estimated 80% of Ugandans living in rural villages used traditional healers for primary health care [1]. A study of 137 HIV-infected Ugandans receiving ART found that 60% used herbs concurrently with ART [2].

In Uganda traditional herbal medicines are usually boiled extracts of herbs taken orally [3]. Some potentially hepatotoxic traditional herbal medicines used in Uganda and sub-Saharan Africa include *Hoodia gordoni* [4], kava [5], *Phytolacca dioica* [6], and herbs from the Asteraceae family [7]. Little is known about the hepatotoxicity of other commonly used herbs or the contribution of herbs to the burden of liver fibrosis and hepatocellular carcinoma in sub- Saharan Africa, including when used concomitantly with ART. Data on the specific types of herbs taken by HIV-infected persons in Uganda is limited, as is information about their components, side effects, toxicities, and ART interactions [8].

In Rakai, Uganda, liver toxicity associated with herbal medicine may be of particular concern given the high prevalence of significant liver disease (17%) among HIV-infected persons in Rakai recently identified by transient elastography (FibroScan®, Echosense, Paris, France) [9]. In the aforementioned study, reported herbal medicine use was associated with a two-fold increased risk of significant liver disease, defined as a transient elastography score equivalent to METAVIR liver fibrosis stage 2 (portal fibrosis with few septa) or greater [9]. The study presented here follows up on this prior investigation with an in-depth analysis of the herbs used by study participants and their relation to liver fibrosis.

Methods

This cross-sectional study enrolled 500 HIV-infected participants receiving care at five HIV care clinics within the Rakai Health Sciences Program (RHSP) HIV Care Program. 500 HIV-uninfected participants from the Rakai Community Cohort Study (RCCS) were frequency- matched to these participants by age, gender, and community. Begun in 1994 in one of Uganda's hardest-hit regions by the HIV epidemic, the RCCS conducts annual surveys in a population of 10,000–15,000 people aged 15–49 years, and is described in detail elsewhere [10]. Participants underwent a detailed liver-disease focused risk factor questionnaire which included an assessment of herbal drug use, venous blood collection, and transient elastography (FibroScan®, Echosense, Paris, France) to quantify liver fibrosis.

Ethics Statement

Written informed consent was obtained from all participants. Institutional Review Boards of theNational Institute of Allergy and Infectious Diseases, the Johns Hopkins Medical Institutions, the Scientific and Ethics Committee of the Uganda Virus Research Institute, and the Uganda National Council for Science and Technology approved this study. The study protocol conforms to the ethical guidelines of the 1975 Declaration of Helsinki, and is registered on clinicaltrials.gov (#NCT00782158).

Herb Use Assessment

Participants were asked about any current herb use and then to name the two herbs they used most often. Scientific names were assigned to local herb names in consultation with local traditional medicine practitioners and a member of Makerere University

Botany Department (CKB). The Makerere University Herbarium database was also used to validate herb identities. Some participants reported non-plant substances such as clay and spiritual charms as herb use. Participants reporting use of non-plant based entities were reclassified as non-herb users in this analysis.

Laboratory Assays

HIV-1 serology was determined by two HIV-1 enzyme immuno-assays: Vironostika HIV-1 (OrganonTeknika, Charlotte, North Carolina, USA) and Cambridge Biotech (Worcester, Massachusetts, USA). Participants with discrepant HIV-1 enzyme immune assay results were tested with western blot (HIV-1 Western Blot; Bio-Merieux-Vitek, St. Louis, Missouri, USA). For HIV-infected participants, current CD4 count (within 12 months) and CD4 count nadir were abstracted from the RHSP HIV Care Program database. CD4 counts were measured by FACSCalibur flow cytometer (software version 1.4, Becton Dickinson, San Jose, California, USA). Hepatitis B virus surface antigen (HBsAg) was determined using ELISA (ETI-MAK-2 Plus, Diasorin, Vercelli, Italy). Alanine aminotransferase (ALT) was tested using standard methods (COBAS CII; Roche, Basel, Switzerland), and hepato-toxicity was defined by ALT elevations and classified according to AIDS Clinical Trial Group criteria [11]. The upper limit of normal for ALT was defined as 19 IU/L in women and 39 IU/L in men [12,13].

Transient Elastography

Transient elastography or FibroScan® is a novel, validated, noninvasive technology for the evaluation of fibrosis in chronic liver disease [14]. A FibroScan® is approximately the size of an ultrasound unit. A probe placed over a patient's abdomen produces vibration and the speed of the responding elastic wave is detected by ultrasound. The propagation of these waves through the liver is directly correlated to the degree of liver stiffness. The results are instantaneously received as a single, quantitative parameter of liver stiffness measurement (LSM, reported in kPa). Each transient elastography scan takes ten liver stiffness measurements in rapid succession over several seconds. The median of the ten measurements is reported as the final liver stiffness measurement. The procedure is non-invasive, painless, has no side effects, and requires only a few minutes to perform. The device requires minimal training and does not need to be performed by advanced medical personnel.

In this study a conservative liver stiffness measurement cutoff of ≥9.3 kPa, from a validation study in persons of predominantly African descent, was used to define significant fibrosis equivalent to METAVIR fibrosis stage 2 (portal fibrosis with few septa) or greater [15]. Two study nurses at the Rakai Health Science Program study site conducted all transient elastography scans after receiving certification from the manufacturer. According to manufacturer recommendations, scans with high variability—defined as an interquartile range greater than 30% of the median LSM value from an individual examination—were not considered valid and were excluded from the analysis. Participants with invalid scans on an initial attempt were repositioned and rescanned up to 4 times to achieve a valid scan.

Statistics

Baseline demographic, behavioral and clinical characteristics were compared by HIV status. Differences in continuous variables were assessed using t-tests and Wilcoxon-Mann-Whitney tests. Categorical variables were compared using Pearson's chi squared test.

Table 1. Baseline characteristics of study participants.

Characteristic	HIV-infected pts (n = 500) n (% or IQR)	HIV-uninfected pts (n = 500) n (% or IQR)	p value
Median Age, years	38 (IQR 31–44)	37 (IQR 32–44)	0.025
Female	312 (67%)	333 (67%)	0.89
Heavy Liquor use (>1.25 L/week)	11 (2%)	9 (2%)	0.65
Lifetime occupational fishing	5 (1%)	1 (0.2%)	0.65
HBsAg positive	23 (5%)	14 (3%)	0.10
Valid TE scan	468 (94%)	494 (99%)	<0.001
Herb Use			
Current herb use	8 (2%)	33 (7%)	0.0001
Known herbs	5 (0.9%)	16 (3%)	0.015
Unknown herbs	4 (0.9%)	17 (3%)	0.004
Asteraceae family	2 (0.4%)	6 (1%)	0.16
Fabaceae family	0 (0%)	6 (1%)	0.014
Lamiaceae family	1 (0.2%)	4 (0.8%)	0.18
ACTG Heptatotoxicty Criteria			
Median ALT (U/L)	22 (IQR 16–31)	19 (IQR 15–25)	<0.001
Grade 0 (<1.25×ULN) by ALT	354 (71%)	414 (83%)	
Grade 1 (1.25–2.5×ULN) by ALT	122 (24%)	77 (15%)	
Grade 2 (2.6–5×ULN) by ALT	19 (4%)	9 (2%)	
Grade 3 (5.1–10×ULN) by ALT	5 (1%)	0 (0%)	
Grade 4 (>10×ULN) by ALT	0 (0%)	0 (0%)	
CD4 and ART Characteristics			
Current CD4 count (cells/uL)	449 (IQR 320–642)		
Nadir CD4 count (cells/uL)	214 (IQR 130–350)		
Nadir CD4 count <100 cells/uL	95 (19%)		
On ART	302 (60%)		
ART duration (months)	19 (IQR 9–38)		

HIV (Human Immunodeficiency Virus), IQR (Interquartile Range), HBsAg (Hepatitis B Surface Antigen), ACTG (AIDS Clinical Trials Group), CD4 (Cluster of Differentiation 4 positive Helper T cells), ART (Antiretroviral Therapy).

The primary outcome measure was liver fibrosis. Because odds ratios may overestimate the magnitude of association between variables if the outcome of interest is common, adjusted prevalence risk ratios (adjPRR) with 95% confidence intervals (95% CI) were estimated using modified Poisson regression [16]. The multivariable models adjusted for HIV, gender, occupation in the fishing industry, chronic hepatitis B infection (positive hepatitis B surface antigen), and drinking ≥1.25 liters per week of liquor, as these risk factors were associated with liver disease in previous analysis of this study population [9]. Age was included in all models and nadir CD4 cell count and ART status were included in models restricted to HIV- infected participants for reasons of biologic plausibility. STATA version 11.0 (STATA Corp, College Station, TX) was used for statistical analysis.

Results

Baseline Characteristics

The HIV-infected and uninfected groups each had 67% females (see table 1). The median age of 38 years in the HIV-infected

group was close to the median age of 37 years in the HIV-uninfected group (p = 0.025). Only 2% of both HIV-infected and uninfected participants were heavy liquor drinkers (p = 0.65). The prevalence of chronic HBV infection was similar in both groups, 5% in HIV-infected participants and 3% in HIV-uninfected participants (p = 0.010). 29% of HIV-infected participants and 17% of HIV-uninfected participants had any grade 1 or higher hepatotoxicity by AIDS Clinical Trial Group (ACTG) criteria (p<0.001). No participants demonstrated grade 4 hepatotoxicity.

At the time of enrolment HIV-infected participants had a median CD4 count of 449 cells/μL (IQR 320–642) and 60% were receiving ART with a median duration of 19 months (IQR 9–38). Demographics of the HIV-infected group were also similar to participants in the Rakai Health Sciences HIV Care Program, in which 65% of participants are female, 64% are on ART, and the median CD4 count is 480 cells/μL.

468/500 (94%) of HIV-infected participants and 494/500 (99%) of HIV-uninfected participants had valid elastography scans. Those with valid scans were included in the assessment of liver fibrosis and were included in the regression models.

Table 2. Characteristics of participants reporting current herb use.

Characteristic	Using Herbs (n = 42) n (% or IQR)	Not Using Herbs (n = 958) n (% or IQR)	p value
Median Age, years	39 (32–44 IQR)	38 (31–44 IQR)	0.61
Female	27 (64%)	643 (67%)	0.15
Heavy Liquor use (>1.25 L/week)	3 (7%)	17 (2%)	0.015
Lifetime occupational fishing	1 (2%)	5 (0.5%)	0.13
HBsAg positive	2 (5%)	35 (4%)	0.73
HIV infected	9 (20%)	491 (50%)	0.0001

L (Liters), HBsAg (Hepatitis B Surface Antigen), HIV (Human Immunodeficiency Virus).

Characteristics of Herb Users

42/1000 (4%) of all participants reported current use of traditional herbal medicines, including 9/500 (2%) of HIV-infected participants and 33/500 (7%) HIV-uninfected participants (table 1). 21/42 (50%) of participants could name at least one herb they were taking. 4/46 (9%) of participants reporting

Table 3. Characteristics of known herbs in the Asteraceae, Fabaceae, and Lamiaceae families.

Family (n taking)	Scientific Name	Local Names (n taking)	English Name	Taken in Rakai for:	Known Pharmacology	Known Liver Toxicity and/or ART Interaction
Asteraceae (8)	Vernonia amygdalina	Mululuza (4)	Bitter leaf	Fever, fever with jaundice	Contains alkaloids, saponins, tannins, flavonoids, steroid glycosides, sesquiterpine lactone [32]	Hepatotoxic at high doses (750 mg/kg) [24]. One herb from the Veronia genus (V. lasiopus) was hepatotoxic in an in-vitro rat precision cut liver slice model [33]. Many herbs in the Asteraceae family contain pyrrolizidine alkaloids, which are associated with veno-occlusive liver disease [17]
	Vernonia genus	Kiluluuza (2)				
	Microglossa densiflora	Kafugankande, Akafugankande (1)		Fever, indigestion, loose stools, parasites	Microglossa family contains clerodane diterpenoids [34]	A similar herb from the Microglossa family (M. pyrifolia) was hepatotoxic in an in-vitro rat precision cut liver slice model [33]. Many herbs in the Asteraceae family contain pyrrolizidine alkaloids, which are associated with veno-occlusive liver disease [17]
	Aspilia africana	Makaayi (1)	Wild sunflower	Fever with jaundice	Contains saponins, tannins, terpenoids, Sesquiterpenes, monoterpenes [35,36]	No hepatoxicity in rat in vivo model [38]. Many herbs in the Asteraceae family contain pyrrolizidine alkaloids, which are associated with veno-occlusive liver disease [17]
Fabaceae (6)	Pseudarthria hookeri	Bikakala, Kikakala, Omukakala, Mukakala (4)		Fever, fever with jaundice, allergy, cough, wounds	May have estrogenic activity [37]	Many herbs in the Fabaceae family contain pyrrolizidine alkaloids, which are associated with veno-occlusive liver disease [17]
	Indigofera congesta	Namasumi (2)	Indigo	Fever with jaundice, antenatal health	Indigofera family members contain flavonoids, saponins, quinones, sterols/triterpenes, tannins, gallic acid, caffeic acid, rutin and myricetin [38]	Many herbs in the Fabaceae family contain pyrrolizidine alkaloids, which are associated with veno-occlusive liver disease [17]
Lamiaceae (5*)	Ocimum gratissimum	Mujaaja, Omujaaja (3)	African basil	Epigastric pain	Contains tannin phlobaphenes, flavones, flavonols, xanthones, chalcones, aurones, terpenes, flavononols, leucoanthocyanidins, catechins [39]	Herb from Ocimum genus (O. lamiifolium) was hepatotoxic in an in-vitro rat precision cut liver slice model [33], Ocimum gratissimum caused hepatoxicity in-vivo rabbit liver model [25]
	Hoslundia opposita	Kamunye (3)		To replace blood, postnatal health, vomiting during fever and jaundice	Contains sesquiterpenes and sesquiterpene alcohols [40]	

*one patient took both Ocimum gratissimum and Hoslundia oopposita. mg (milligrams), kg (kilograms).

Table 4. Characteristics of known herbs in remainder of plant families.

Family (n taking)	Scientific Name	Local Names (n taking)	English Name	Taken in Rakai for:	Known Pharmacology	Known Liver Toxicity and/or ART Interaction
Anacardiaceae (2)	Rhus vulgaris or Rhus natalenis	Olukansokanso, akakwansokwanso (1)		Antenatal health, aphrodisiac, gastrointestinal ulcers, back pain	No published information about contents	
	Mangifera indica	Mango Tree Bark (1)	Mango tree bark		Leaves contains flavonoids [41], Peel contains phenolic compounds and carotenoids [42]	
Primulaceae (2)	Maesa lanceolata	Oluwongwa, Oluwongo (2)		Neonatal jaundice	Contains Saponins [43], benzoquinone [44]	
Euphorbiaceae (2)	Sapium ellipticum	Musasa, Omusiisa, Musanvuma (2)	Jumping tree seed	Hypertension, antenatal health, sexually transmitted infections, epigastric pain	Contains phenols [45]	
Amaryllidaceae (1)	Allium sativum	Garlic (1)	Garlic	—	Contians diallyl disulfide [46]	Induces CYP3A4 and Pgp and should not be taken with the following antiretrovirals: APV, ATV, AZT, EFV, IDV, LPV, NFV, NVP, SQV [27]
Bignoniaceae (1)	Spathodea campanulata	Ekifabakazi (1)	African tulip tree	Dysmennorrhea, antenatal health	Contains 3β-acetoxyoleanolic acid, siaresinolic acid, oleanolic acid, others [47]	
Solanaceae (1)	Solanum incanum	Akatengotengo (1)	Sodom apple	Cough, chest pain	Contains alkaloids, saponins, solanine; High concentrations cause hemolysis of erythrocytes [48]	Herbs containing pyrrolizidine alkaloids are associated with veno-occlusive liver disease [17].
Vitaceae (1)	Cyphostemma adenocaule	Kamombo (1)		Peptic ulcers	Contain carotenoids (carotenes), xanthophylls, Vitamin C, Tocopherols, and Tocotrienols [49]	
Myrtaceae (1)	Callistemon citrinus	Bottlebrush (1)	Bottlebrush tree	Rhino-sinusitis	Contains 1,8-cineole, apha-pinene [50]	
		Kagulukandayi, Katangulucumu (1)		Epilepsy		
		Kakubamusolo (1)				

APV (amprenavir), ATV (atazanavir), AZT (zidovudine), EFV (efavirenz), IDV indinavir), LPV (lopinavir), NFV (nelfinavir), NVP (nevirapine), SQV (saquinavir).

herb use were reclassified as not taking herbs because they only reported use of inert, non-plant substances including clay. Herb users did not differ by age (p = 0.61) or gender (p = 0.15) from those who did not report herb use (see table 2). Herb users were not more likely to work in the fishing industry (p = 0.13) or have chronic hepatitis B infection (p = 0.73). 7% of participants reporting herb use drank liquor heavily (≥1.25 L/week), compared to 2% of participants who did not report herb use (p = 0.015). 19 unique herbs from 13 families were used, and are characterized in tables 3 and 4. The most common families were Asteraceae, Fabaceae, and Lamiaceae, which were used by eight, six and five participants, respectively.

Herb Use and Liver Fibrosis

Among the 137/962 (14%) subjects with significant liver fibrosis, 12/137 (9%) reported herb use. Of the 825/962 (86%) subjects without significant liver fibrosis, 29/825 (4%) reported current herb use (p = 0.005). 56/494 (11%) of HIV-uninfected participants had significant fibrosis, compared to 81/468 (17%) of HIV-infected participants (p = 0.008).

In multivariable analysis that adjusted for age, fishing occupation, HIV infection, positive HBsAg, gender, and heavy liquor use, herb use was associated with two to five fold increases in significant liver fibrosis (see table 5). Among all participants, use of any herb (adjPRR = 2.2, 95% CI 1.3–3.5, p = 0.002), herbs from the Asteraceae family (adjPRR = 5.0, 95% CI 2.9–8.7, p<0.001), and herbs from the Lamiaceae family (adjPRR = 3.4, 95% CI 1.2–

Table 5. Association of herbs with significant liver fibrosis in all participants.

Herb (n taking)	Univariate			Multivariate		
	PRR	95% CI	P value	adjPRR	95% CI	P value
Any current herb use (41)	2.2	1.3–3.6	0.003	2.2	1.3–3.5	0.002
Asteraceae (8)	5.5	3.6–8.4	<0.001	5.0	2.9–8.7	<0.001
Fabaceae (6)	1.2	0.19–7.1	0.86	1.6	0.26–10.3	0.60
Lamiaceae (5)	2.8	0.96.0–8.4	0.060	3.4	1.2–9.2	0.017
Unknown herb (21)	1.0	0.35–2.9	0.995	1.2	0.40–3.3	0.79

Multivariate model for all participants adjusts for: age, occupational fishing, HIV infection, positive Hepatitis B surface antigen, gender, heavy liquor use (≥1.25 L/week). Only participants with a valid TE scan (962/1000) were included in the model. CI (Confidence Interval).

9.2, p = 0.017) were associated with increased significant fibrosis. Use of herbs from the Fabaceae family was not associated with significant liver fibrosis (adjPRR = 1.6, 95% CI 0.26–10.3, p = 0.60).

Of 81 HIV-infected subjects with significant liver fibrosis, 4 (5%) reported herb use (see table 6). Among 387 HIV-infected subjects without significant liver fibrosis, 4 (1%) reported herb use (p = 0.014). In the multivariable analysis of HIV-infected participants adjusted for age, occupational fishing, positive HBsAg, gender, heavy liquor use, ART, and CD4 nadir, the associations between herb use and significant liver fibrosis were similar to findings among all participants. Among HIV-infected participants the use of any herb (adjPRR = 2.3, 95% CI 1.0–5.0, p = 0.044) and the use of herbs from the Asteraceae family (adjPRR = 5.0, 95% CI 1.7–14.7, p = 0.004) were associated with increased liver fibrosis.

Among all participants as well as HIV-infected participants, herb use was not associated with increased hepatotoxicity. 8/41 (20%) of participants reporting herb use had ACTG grade 1–4 ALT elevations, compared to 216/961 (23%) who did not report herb use (p = 0.56). Among HIV-infected participants reporting herb use, 6/33 (18%) had grade 1–4 ALT elevations, compared to 79/461 (17%) who did not report herb use (p = 0.88).

Table 7 shows the proportion of participants who took individual herbs in the Asteraceae, Lamiaceae, and Fabaceae families who had significant liver fibrosis. 6/8 participants taking herbs in the Asteraceae family had significant liver fibrosis. 4/6

Table 6. Association of herbs with significant liver fibrosis in HIV-infected participants.

Herb (n taking)	Univariate			Multivariate		
	PRR	95% CI	P value	adjPRR	95% CI	P value
Any current herb use (8)	3.0	1.4–6.2	0.003	2.3	1.0–5.0	0.044
Asteraceae (2)	6.0	4.9–7.3	<0.001	5.0	1.7–14.7	0.004
Unknown herb (5)	1.2	0.20–6.8	0.87	1.0	0.15–6.7	0.998

Multivariate model for HIV-infected participants adjusts for: age, occupational fishing, positive Hepatitis B surface antigen, gender, heavy liquor use (≥1.25 L/week), ART, and CD4 nadir. Only participants with a valid TE scan (468/500) were included in the model. CI (Confidence Interval).

Table 7. Use of specific herbs and significant liver fibrosis.

Herb used	Proportion of participants taking with significant liver fibrosis
Asteraceae Family	**6/8**
Vernonia amygdalina	2/4
Vernonia, species unknown	2/2
Microglossa densiflora	1/1
Aspilia Africana	1/1
Fabaceae Family	**2/6**
Pseudarthria hookeri	1/4
Indigofera congesta	1/2
Lamaceae Family	**2/5 ***
Ocimum gratissimum	1/3
Hoslundia opposita	1/3

*One participant took both Ocmum gratissimum and Hoslundia opposite. Only participants with a valid TE scans are shown.

subjects who used herbs in the *Vernonia* genus of the Asteraceae family had significant liver fibrosis.

Discussion

This study indicates that traditional herbal medicine use may contribute to liver disease in Uganda. Use of traditional herbal medicines was independently associated with two to five fold increases in significant liver fibrosis. Herbs from the Asteraceae family were the most often used and showed the strongest association with significant liver fibrosis: a five-fold increase in all participants (p<0.001) and HIV-infected participants (p = 0.004).

Six of eight participants who took herbs in the Asteraceae family had significant liver fibrosis (see table 5). Many plants in the Asteraceae and Fabaceae families contain pyrrolizidine alkaloids, a known risk factor for veno-occlusive liver disease [7,17]. Although none of the alkaloid-containing herbs used by participants in this study have been confirmed to contain pyrrolizidine alkaloids, ingestion of plants containing pyrrolizidine alkaloids caused outbreaks of veno-occlusive liver disease in Jamaica, India, Egypt, and South Africa [17,18]. No outbreaks of veno-occlusive liver disease associated with pyrrolizidine alkaloids have been reported to our knowledge in East Africa. Pyrrolizidine alkaloids are inert until dehydrogenation by cytochrome P450 3A4 (CYP3A4) in the liver [19], where reactive toxic pyrrolic and N-oxide metabolites directly damage liver sinusoidal endothelial cells and hepatocytes (zone III of the liver acinus) [20]. Pyrroles cause chromosomal damage in a dose-dependent manner, resulting in an inflammatory response that culminates in fibrin deposition [17,20,21].

Although plants in both the Asteraceae and Fabaceae families ingested by study participants may contain pyrrolizidine alkaloids, our data shows a strong association between significant liver fibrosis and use of herbs in the Asteraceae family but not the Fabaceae family. The literature about African traditional herbal medicines is limited and does not explain why this difference might exist. Traditional herbal medicine remedies used in Rakai and throughout Uganda are often mixtures containing multiple herbs [8,22]. It is possible that herbs in the Asteraceae family are taken at high doses, or potentiate the toxicity of other herbs or hepatotoxins.

Two participants with fibrosis reported use of *Vernonia amygdalina* in the Asteraceae family. This particular herb is commonly used in Africa is thought to have hepatoprotective properties [23]. However, animal studies show that at higher doses, this member of the Asteracaae family may be hepatotoxic. In an *in-vivo* rat CCl_4 liver injury model, low doses (250–500 mg/kg) of *Vernonia amygdalina* were hepatoprotective, but a high dose (750 mg/kg) caused increased hepatotoxicity [24].

Herbs from the Lamiaceae family were associated with a 3.4 fold increase in significant liver fibrosis among all participants in our study (p = 0.017). Herbs in the Lamiaceae family have been associated with hepatoxicity in an *in-vivo* rabbit model [25]. In addition, Aloe, taken by two participants in our study, has been linked in case reports to severe hepatitis [26]. However, data about the potential hepatotoxicity of many herbs used by participants in this study do not exist, or come from animal model studies only that should be interpreted cautiously.

The risk of significant fibrosis associated with herb use was similar in the overall and HIV- infected study populations. Data on herb use was limited in the HIV-infected population, and plant family specific analysis was only possible for the Asteraceae family. Only two HIV- infected participants reported using herbs in the Asteraceae family.

Despite the small number of HIV-infected participants in this study who reported herb use, it is important to note that ART may alter the toxicity profile of co-administered herbs. CYP3A4 is a major pathway for metabolism of a wide range of chemically distinct foreign compounds including phytochemicals and antiretroviral drugs [27]. Antiretroviral drugs of the non- nucleoside reverse transcriptase inhibitor (NNRTI) and protease inhibitor (PI) classes are also inducers or inhibitors of CYP3A4 activity [28,29]. Therefore, these drugs have potential to influence phytochemical toxification or detoxification pathways in the liver. For example, commonly used NNRTI in initial ART regimens in Uganda (efavirenz and nevirapine) are inducers of CYP3A4 and therefore have potential to increase generation of toxic metabolites of pyrrolizidine alkaloids [27,28]. Inhibitors of CYP3A4 may lead to accumulation of phytochemicals or their metabolites in the liver which may also result in toxicity.

Conversely, herbs may potentiate ART toxicities by influencing antiretroviral drug disposition in the liver, kidney, and gut. Herbs may affect NNRTI and PI metabolism by CPY3A4 and alter activity of cellular drug transporters and glucuronidation pathways [27]. Existing evidence from Africa about herb-ART interactions is limited to two herb families commonly used in South Africa: *Hypoxis* (African potato) and *Sutherlandia*, neither of which were taken by participants in this study. Hypoxis causes a dose-dependent inhibition of CYP3A4 up to 86% of the normal activity of CYP3A4 and 50% reduction of the expression of P-glycoprotein. Sutherlandia *frutescens* also causes a dose dependent inhibition of CYP3A4 up to 96% of CYP3A4 activity [30]. One participant in this study reported garlic use, which is known to significantly reduce concentrations of a PI (saquinavir), most likely by induction of CYP3A4 [31]. Since nevirapine and efavirenz are also eliminated by CYP3A4, garlic may reduce plasma levels of these drugs, but there are no clinical data on these interactions.

Limitations

This study had limitations. The study was cross-sectional and only information about current herb use was available for analysis. Only 4% of participants in this study reported using herbs, compared to other studies in Uganda in which 60% of HIV-infected persons reported concurrent use of ART and herbs [2]. Some misclassification of herb exposure could have occurred due to a social desirability or reporting bias, especially among HIV-infected persons on ART who are counseled to avoid herbs in the communities around Rakai. Only 2% of HIV- infected participants reported herb use. While this lower number of HIV-infected participants reporting herb use could represent effective counseling, the difference in herb use among those on ART and those not on ART was not significant (1% vs. 2%, p = 0.42). The small number of participants reporting herb use limited many comparisons (e.g., herb-ART interactions) and suggests that our findings should be interpreted cautiously.

An important limitation of this study is the potential for reverse causality. Although the most frequently used families of herbs in this study contain known hepatotoxins (see table 3), it is possible that the association of fibrosis with herb use could represent reverse causality, or persons with symptomatic liver disease being more likely to use herbal medicines. According to consultations with local traditional practitioners, some of the herbs in Asteraceae and other families are sometimes prescribed for "fever with jaundice". However, none of the study participants had been previously diagnosed with liver disease within the formal medical system or by traditional healers. Most herbs used in this study to treat fever are usually taken for general fever ("fever" or "malaria"), not fever with jaundice ("yellow fever").

Conclusions

More studies are needed to assess the impact of traditional herbal medicines in sub-Saharan Africa. Phytochemical, pharmacokinetic and prospective clinical studies are needed to investigate herb contents, benefits, side effects, direct toxicity, and herb-ART interactions. Plants in the Asteraceae family reported in this study should be prioritized for these investigations.

The risk of liver disease associated with herb use was similar in the overall study population and among HIV-infected participants. Given the potential of at least additive risk of hepatotoxicity with long term use of some antiretroviral drugs, as well as the potential for herbs to alter the pharmacology of antiretroviral drugs, it may be prudent to counsel HIV-infected persons against herb use in sub-Africa until there is data about the safety of specific herbs. Counseling about herb use should be part of routine health counseling and counseling of HIV- infected persons in sub-Africa.

Author Contributions

Conceived and designed the experiments: LS SJR TCQ PO GDK. Performed the experiments: LS SJR IB PO. Analyzed the data: BJA LS GDK AN. Contributed reagents/materials/analysis tools: CKB. Wrote the paper: BJA LS. Provided additional technical assistance and contributed to interpretation of the data: BJA CKB ML CM AS PO VK IB FN AN MJW RHG DLT.

References

1. Hamill FA, Apio S, Mubiru NK, Mosango M, Bukenya-Ziraba R, et al. (2000) Traditional herbal drugs of southern Uganda, I. J Ethnopharmacol 70: 281–300.
2. Langlois-Klassen D, Kipp W, Rubaale T (2008) Who's talking? Communication between health providers and HIV-infected adults related to herbal medicine for AIDS treatment in western Uganda. Soc Sci Med 67: 165–176.
3. Tabuti J, Lye K, Dhillion S (2003) Traditional herbal drugs of Bulamogi, Uganda: plants, use, and administration. J Ethnopharmacol 88: 19–44.
4. Dara L, Hewett J, Lim JK (2008) Hydroxycut hepatotoxicity: a case series and review of liver toxicity from herbal weight loss supplements. World J Gastroenterol 14: 6999–7004.
5. Teschke R, Fuchs J, Bahre R, Genthner A, Wolff A (2010). Kava hepatotoxicity: comparative study of two structured quantitative methods for causality assessment. J Clin Pharm Ther 35: 545–563.

6. Ashafa AO, Sunmonu TO, Afolayan AJ (2010) Toxicological evaluation of aqueous leaf and berry extracts of Phytolacca dioica L. in male Wistar rats. Food Chem Toxicol 48: 1886–1889.

7. Asres K, Sporer F, Wink M (2007) Identification and quantification of hepatotoxic pyrrolizidine alkaloids in the Ethiopian medicinal plant Solanecio gigas (Asteraceae). Pharmazie 62: 709–713.

8. Lamorde M, Tabuti JR, Obua C, Kukunda-Byobona C, Lanyero H, et al. (2010) Medicinal plants used by traditional medicine practitioners for the treatment of HIV/AIDS and related conditions in Uganda. J Ethnopharmacol 130: 43–53.

9. Stabinski L, Reynolds S, Ocama P, Laeyendecker O, Ndyanabo A, et al. (2011) High Prevalence of Liver Fibrosis Associated with HIV Infection: A Study in Rural Rakai, Uganda. Antiviral Therapy 16: 405–411.

10. Wawer MJ, Gray RH, Sewankambo NK, Serwadda D, Paxton L, et al. (1998) A randomized, community trial of intensive sexually transmitted disease control for AIDS prevention, Rakai, Uganda. AIDS 12: 1211–1225.

11. AIDS Clinical Trials Group (1994) Table for grading the severity of adult and pediatric adverse advents. Rockville (Maryland): National Institutes of Health, Division of AIDS.

12. Prati D, Taioli E, Zanella A, Della Torre E, Butelli S, et al. (2002) Updated definitions of healthy ranges for serum alanine aminotransferase levels. Ann Intern Med 137: 1–10.

13. Ruhl CE, Everhart JE. (2012) Upper limits of normal for alanine aminotransferase activity in the United States population. Hepatology 55: 447–454.

14. Andersen ES, Christensen PB, Weis N (2009) Transient elastography for liver fibrosis diagnosis. Eur J Intern Med 20: 339–342.

15. Kirk GD, Astemborski J, Mehta SH, Spoler C, Fisher C, et al. (2009) Assessment of liver fibrosis by transient elastography in persons with hepatitis C virus infection or HIV- hepatitis C virus coinfection. Clin Infect Dis 48: 963–972.

16. Barros AJ, Hirakata VN (2003) Alternatives for logistic regression in cross-sectional studies: an empirical comparison of models that directly estimate the prevalence ratio. BMC Med Res Methodol 3: 21.

17. Chen Z, Huo JR (2010) Hepatic veno-occlusive disease associated with toxicity of pyrrolizidine alkaloids in herbal preparations. Neth J Med 68: 252–260.

18. Ridker PM, McDermott WV (1989) Comfrey herb tea and hepatic veno-occlusive disease. Lancet 1: 657–658.

19. Prakash AS, Pereira TN, Reilly PE, Seawright AA (1999) Pyrrolizidine alkaloids in human diet. Mutat Res 443: 53–67.

20. Chen T, Mei N, Fu PP (2010) Genotoxicity of pyrrolizidine alkaloids. J Appl Toxicol 30: 183–196.

21. Yeong ML, Wakefield SJ, Ford HC (1993) Hepatocyte membrane injury and bleb formation following low dose comfrey toxicity in rats. Int J Exp Pathol 74: 211–217.

22. Tabuti J, Collins B, Kukunda C, Waako P (2010) Medicinal plants used by traditional medicine practitioners in the treatment of tuberculosis and related ailments in Uganda. J Ethnopharmacol 127: 130–136.

23. Iwalokun BA, Efedede BU, Alabi-Sofunde JA, Oduala T, Magbagbeola OA, et al. (2006) Hepatoprotective and antioxidant activities of Vernonia amygdalina on acetaminophen- induced hepatic damage in mice. J Med Food 9: 524–530.

24. Adesanoye O, Farombi E (2009) Hepatoprotective effects of Vernonia amygdalina (Asteraceae) in rats treated with carbon tertachloride. Exp Toxicol Pathol 62: 197–206.

25. Effraim K, Jacks T, Sodipo O (2002) Histopathological studies on the toxicity of Ocimum gratissimum leave extract on some organs of rabbit. African Journal of Biomedical Research 6: 21–25.

26. Yang HN, Kim DJ, Kim YM, Kim BH, Sohn KM, et al. (2010) Aloe-induced toxic hepatitis. J Korean Med Sci 25: 492–495.

27. van den Bout-van den Beukel CJ, Koopmans PP, van der Ven AJ, De Smet PA, Burger DM (2006) Possible drug-metabolism interactions of medicinal herbs with antiretroviral agents. Drug Metab Rev 38: 477–514.

28. Barry M, Mulcahy F, Merry C, Gibbons S, Back D (1999) Pharmacokinetics and potential interactions amongst antiretroviral agents used to treat patients with HIV infection. Clin Pharmacokinet 36: 289–304.

29. Dickinson L, Khoo S, Back D (2010) Pharmacokinetics and drug-drug interactions of antiretrovirals: an update. Antiviral Res 85: 176–189.

30. Mills E, Foster BC, van Heeswijk R, Phillips E, Wilson K, et al. (2005) Impact of African herbal medicines on antiretroviral metabolism. AIDS 19: 95–97.

31. Piscitelli SC, Burstein AH, Welden N, Gallicano KD, Falloon J (2002) The effect of garlic supplements on the pharmacokinetics of saquinavir. Clin Infect Dis 34: 234–238.

32. Akah P, Okafor C (1992) Blood sugar lowering effect of Vernonia amygdalina (del) in an experimental rabbit model. Phytotherapy Research 6: 171–173.

33. Mukazayire MJ, Allaeys V, Buc Calderon P, Stevigny C, Bigendako MJ, et al. (2010) Evaluation of the hepatotoxic and hepatoprotective effect of Rwandese herbal drugs on in vivo (guinea pigs barbiturate-induced sleeping time) and in vitro (rat precision-cut liver slices, PCLS) models. Exp Toxicol Pathol 62: 289–299.

34. Tamokou JD, Kuiate JR, Tene M, Tane P (2009) Antimicrobial clerodane diterpenoids from Microglossa angolensis Oliv. et Hiern. Indian J Pharmacol 41: 60–63.

35. Kuiate J, Zollo PA, Lamaty G, Mentu C, Besseiere J (1999) Composition of essential oils from the leaves of two varieties of Aspilia africana (Pers) C.D Adams from Cameroon. Flavor and Fragrance 14: 167–169.

36. Taziebou LC, Etoa FX, Nkegoum B, Pieme CA, Dzeufiet DP (2006) Acute and subacute toxicity of Aspilia africana leaves. Afr J Tradit Complement Altern Med 4: 127–134.

37. Njamen D, Magne Nde CB, Tanee Fomum Z, Vollmer G (2008) Effects of the extracts of some tropical medicinal plants on estrogen inducible yeast and Ishikawa screens, and on ovariectomized Wistar rats. Pharmazie 63: 164–168.

38. Bakasso S, Lamien-Meda A, Lamien CE, Kiendrebeogo M, Millogo J, et al. (2008) Polyphenol contents and antioxidant activities of five Indigofera species (Fabaceae) from Burkina Faso. Pak J Biol Sci 11: 1429–1435.

39. Matias EF, Santos KK, Almeida TS, Costa JG, Coutinho HD (2010) Phytochemical screening and modulation of antibiotic activity by Ocimum gratissimum L. Biomed Pharmacother 23: 23.

40. Gundidza GM, Deans SG, Svoboda KP, Mavi S (1992) Antimicrobial activity of essential oil from Hoslundia opposita. Cent Afr J Med 38: 290–293.

41. Kanwal Q, Hussain I, Latif Siddiqui H, Javaid A (2010) Antifungal activity of flavonoids

42. Ajila CM, Rao LJ, Rao UJ (2010) Characterization of bioactive compounds from raw and ripe Mangifera indica L. peel extracts. Food Chem Toxicol 48: 3406–3411.

43. Foubert K, Cuyckens F, Vleeschouwer K, Theunis M, Vlietinck A, et al. (2010) Rapid quantification of 14 saponins of Maesa lanceolata by UPLC-MS/MS. Talanta 81: 1258–1263.

44. Arot Manguro LO, Midiwo JO, Kraus W, Ugi I (2003) Benzoquinone derivatives of Myrsine africana and Maesa lanceolata. Phytochemistry 64: 855–862.

45. Adesegun SA, Elechi NA, Coker HA (2008) Antioxidant activities of methanolic extract of Sapium ellipticum. Pak J Biol Sci 11: 453–457.

46. Nahdi A, Hammami I, Brasse-Lagnel C, Pilard N, Hamdaoui MH, et al. (2010) Influence of garlic or its main active component diallyl disulfide on iron bioavailability and toxicity. Nutr Res 30: 85–95.

47. Ngouela S, Tsamo E, Sondengam BL (1988) Extractives from bignoniaceae: constituents of the stem bark of Spathodea campanulata. Planta Med 54: 476.

48. Beaman-Mbaya V, Muhammed SI (1976) Antibiotic action of Solanum incanum Linnaeus.

49. Al-Duais M, Hohbein J, Werner S, Bohm V, Jetschke G (2009) Contents of vitamin C, carotenoids, tocopherols, and tocotrienols in the subtropical plant species Cyphostemma digitatum as affected by processing. J Agric Food Chem 57: 5420–5427.

50. Oyedeji OO, Lawal OA, Shode FO, Oyedeji AO (2009) Chemical composition and antibacterial activity of the essential oils of Callistemon citrinus and Callistemon viminalis from South Africa. Molecules 14: 1990–1998.

5

HIV-1 Tropism and Liver Fibrosis in HIV–HCV Co-Infected Patients

Florence Abravanel[1,2]*, Stéphanie Raymond[1,2], Elodie Pambrun[3], Maria Winnock[3], Philippe Bonnard[4], Philippe Sogni[5,6], Pascale Trimoulet[7,8], François Dabis[3], Dominique Salmon-Ceron[6,9], Jacques Izopet[1,2], ANRS CO13 HEPAVIH Study Group[¶]

1 INSERM, U1043, Centre de Physiopathologie de Toulouse Purpan, Toulouse, France, 2 CHU Toulouse Purpan, Laboratoire de Virologie, Institut Fédératif de Biologie de Purpan, France, 3 INSERM, U897 and ISPED, Université Victor Segalen, Bordeaux, France, 4 Service des Maladies Infectieuses et Tropicales, Hôpital Tenon, AP-HP, Paris, France, 5 Unité d'Hépatologie, Hôpital Cochin, AP-HP, Paris, France, 6 Université Paris Descartes, Paris, France, 7 CHU Pellegrin, Laboratoire de virologie, Bordeaux, France, 8 CNRS, UMR 5234, Microbiologie fondamentale et pathogénicité, Université Bordeaux Segalen, Bordeaux, France, 9 Service des Maladies Infectieuses et Tropicales, Hôpital Cochin, AP-HP, Paris, France

Abstract

Background and Aims: Hepatic stellate cells, the major producers of extracellular matrix in the liver, and hepatocytes bear CXCR4 and CCR5, the two main co-receptors for entry of the human immunodeficiency virus (HIV). *In vitro* studies suggest that HIV-envelope proteins can modulate the replication of hepatitis C virus (HCV) and fibrogenesis. We investigated the influence of HIV tropism on liver fibrosis and the concentration of HCV RNA in HIV–HCV co-infected patients.

Methods: We used a phenotypic assay to assess HIV tropism in 172 HCV–HIV co-infected patients: one group (75 patients) had mild fibrosis (score ≤F2) and the other (97 patients) had severe fibrosis (score >F2). We also assessed the relationship between HIV tropism and HCV RNA concentration in all these patients. We also followed 34 of these patients for 3 years to determine the evolution of HIV tropism and liver fibrosis, estimated by liver stiffness.

Results: Initially, most patients (91.8%) received a potent antiretroviral therapy. CXCR4-using viruses were found in 29% of patients. The only factor associated with a CXCR4-using virus infection in multivariate analysis was the nadir of CD4 cells: $<200/mm^3$ (OR: 3.94, 95%CI: 1.39–11.14). The median HCV RNA concentrations in patients infected with R5 viruses, those with dual-mixed viruses and those with X4 viruses, were all similar. The prevalence of CXCR4-using viruses in patients with mild fibrosis (≤F2) (31%) and those with severe fibrosis (F3–F4) (28%, $p = 0.6$) was similar. Longitudinal analyses showed that the presence of CXCR4-using viruses did not increase the likelihood of fibrosis progression, evaluated by measuring liver stiffness.

Conclusions: The presence of CXCR4-using viruses in patients receiving a potent antiretroviral therapy does not influence HCV RNA concentration or liver fibrosis.

Editor: Michael Alan Polis, National Institute of Allergy and Infectious Diseases, United States of America

Funding: This work was supported by the Agence Nationale de Recherche contre le SIDA et les Hepatites Virales (ANRS). The funders had no role in study design, data collection and analysis, decision to publish, or preparation of the manuscript.

Competing Interests: The ANRS CO13 HEPAVIH cohort is sponsored by Abbott France, Glaxo-Smith-Kline, Roche and Schering-Plough, and INSERM's "Programme cohortes TGIR."

* E-mail: abravanel.f@chu-toulouse.fr

¶ Membership of the ANRS CO13 HEPAVIH Study Group is provided in Appendix S1.

Introduction

Liver disease has emerged as a leading cause of death among people in Europe and the United States infected with the human immunodeficiency virus (HIV), and most of these deaths are caused by chronic viral hepatitis [1]. Co-infection with hepatitis C virus (HCV) and HIV is common because these viruses share the same transmission route. HIV infection modifies the natural course of HCV infection in several ways [2,3,4,5]. HCV RNA concentrations are increased in HIV-infected patients [6]. Infection with HIV enhances HCV transmission, particularly mother-to-child transmission [7], and decreases the rates of spontaneous HCV clearance, which leads to higher rates of chronic HCV infection [6]. Lastly, liver disease progresses more rapidly in HIV–HCV co-infected patients than in patients infected with HCV alone [3,8,9]. However, the mechanisms by which HIV infection increase the risk of liver disease are poorly understood and are probably multi-factorial [2].

HIV enters CD4-expressing cells using one or both of the chemokine receptors: C–C chemokine receptor type 5 (CCR5) and C–X–C chemokine receptor type 4 (CXCR4). CCR5-using viruses are classified as R5 variants, CXCR4-using viruses are classified as X4 variants, and viruses that can use both co-receptors are classified as dual-mixed variants (D/M) [10]. Hepatic stellate

Table 1. Demographic and clinical data for the patients according to their HIV tropism.

	n	CCR5-using viruses (n=122)	CXCR4-using viruses (n=50)	P-value
Age	172	45 (33–65)	44 (35–64)	0.397
Gender (male)	172			0.349
Male		92 (75)	41 (82)	
Female		30 (25)	9 (18)	
Geographic origin	160			0.50
Europe		81 (71)	34 (74)	
North Africa		23 (20)	8 (17)	
Sub-Saharan Africa		7 (6)	1 (2)	
Other				
Body-mass index	167	22.4 (13.9–37.0)	22.0 (17.4–29.4)	0.521
Insulin resistance	138			0.767
HOMA <3.8		71 (71)	26 (68)	
HOMA ≥3.8		29 (29)	12 (32)	
Alcohol consumption	171			0.988
Never		23 (19)	9 (18)	
Ongoing		43 (36)	18 (36)	
Past		55 (45)	23 (46)	
Age at infection				
HCV infection	172	21 (14–43)	21 (13–42)	0.614
HIV infection	171	29 (10–59)	29 (20–46)	0.517
Duration of infection				
HCV infection (years)	172	23 (1–42)	23 (1–35)	0.714
HIV infection (years)	171	18 (1–24)	18 (1–23)	0.793
Source of HCV infection	162			0.185
IVDU		97 (84)	34 (74)	
Other		19 (16)	12 (26)	
Source of HIV infection	171			0.20
IVDU		93 (77)	37 (74)	
Other		27 (23)	13 (26)	
CDC clinical stage	172			0.218
A		61 (50)	21 (42)	
B		35 (29)	12 (24)	
C		26 (21)	17 (34)	
Plasma HIV RNA concentration	149			0.319
Undetectable (<50 copies/mL)		70 (66)	32 (74)	
Detectable (≥50 copies/mL)		36 (34)	11 (26)	
HIV RNA concentration (when detectable) ($\log_{10}$)	47	3.1 (1.7–5.8)	2.8 (1.7–4.3)	0.735
CD4-cell count at inclusion	171	403 (48–1878)	342 (55–1327)	0.011
Nadir CD4-cell count	153	169 (1–520)	61 (1–405)	<10-4
ART at inclusion	172			0.246
Naive		7 (6)	0 (-)	
Pre-treated patients		7 (6)	2 (4)	
Ongoing treatment		108 (88)	48 (96)	
Class of ART at inclusion	172			
PI	172	69 (57)	42 (84)	0.001
NNRTI	172	29 (24)	6 (12)	0.082
NRTI	172	103 (84)	46 (92)	0.185
Cumulative duration under ART before inclusion (months)	165	116.9 (1.2–233.8)	119.3 (0.9–243.7)	0.908
Cumulative duration under PI before inclusion (months)	144	60.1 (1.1–137.9)	59.4 (0.9–199.3)	0.278
Cumulative duration of NNRTI before inclusion (months)	109	21.8 (0.3–118.9)	24.3 (0.3–106.3)	0.810

Table 1. Cont.

	n	CCR5-using viruses ($n=122$)	CXCR4-using viruses ($n=50$)	P-value
Cumulative duration of NRTI before inclusion (months)	165	110.4 (1.2–214.0)	116.5 (0.9–243.7)	0.890
HCV genotype	171			0.606
1		74 (61)	34 (70)	
2		2 (2)	0 (-)	
3		25 (20)	10 (20)	
4		21 (17)	5 (10)	
Plasma HCV RNA concentration ($\log_{10}$; UI/mL)	145	6.2 (3.3–7.8)	6.2 (1.6–7.6)	0.320
Fibrosis	172			0.685
F0–F2		52 (43)	23 (46)	
F3–F4		70 (57)	27 (54)	

Abbreviations: ART: antiretroviral therapy; CDC: Centers for Disease Control; HOMA: homeostasis model assessment of insulin resistance score; PI: protease inhibitors; NNRTI: non-nucleoside reverse-transcriptase inhibitors; NRTI: nucleoside reverse-transcriptase inhibitors; IQR: inter-quartile range; IVDU: intravenous drug user.

cells (HSCs), the major producers of the extracellular matrix in the liver [11], bear functional CXCR4 and CCR5 receptors [12,13]. Primary hepatocytes also bear both co-receptors and can be infected by HIV [14].

In vitro studies suggest that the HIV gp120 protein modulates fibrogenesis and the concentration of HCV RNA in HIV–HCV co-infected patients [15,16,17,18,19]. HIV increases the replication of HCV in the JFH1 model and in HCV subgenomic replicons *in vitro* [16]. This increase is mediated by the interaction of the HIV-envelope glycoprotein, gp120, with CCR5 and CXCR4, and depends on transforming growth factor beta 1 [16]. The HSCs respond to exposure to CCR5-tropic recombinant gp120 by increasing chemotaxis and expression of genes that encode for the proinflammatory chemokine, the monocyte chemoattractant protein-1, interleukin 6 and the tissue inhibitor of metalloprotease-1 [15]: however, collagen production increases only slightly [15]. In contrast, HSCs infected with the X4 virus increase collagen synthesis and secrete more monocyte chemoattractant protein-1 [17].

CXCR4-tropic recombinant gp120 promotes the synthesis of fibrogenic markers in HSCs [20]. Other studies using various recombinant gp120 proteins or entire HIV virions with different types of tropism indicate that HIV enhances apoptosis of hepatocytes, which is mediated by the CXCR4 receptor [18,19]. The HCV-envelope proteins, E2, act in cooperation with CXCR4-tropic gp120 HIV-envelope proteins to trigger apoptosis in hepatocytes via an innocent bystander mechanism [21]. There is also evidence that the phagocytotic clearance of apoptotic debris may directly stimulate fibrogenesis [22,23,24]. Thus, there seems to be a direct pathway linking HIV infection with liver fibrogenesis via the envelope proteins.

We analysed these *in vitro* data and developed a working hypothesis that CXCR4-using viruses are more pathogenic in terms of liver damage than the R5 virus. We then investigated the influence of HIV tropism on liver fibrosis by assessing the prevalence of CXCR4-using viruses in two groups of HCV–HIV co-infected patients: one with mild fibrosis (score $\leq$F2) and the other with severe fibrosis (score >F2). We also followed 34 patients for 3 years and assessed the influences of HIV tropism on fibrosis progression by studying liver stiffness. Lastly, we assessed the influence of HIV-1 tropism on the plasma concentration of HCV RNA.

Patients and Methods

Participants

Patients were enrolled from the ANRS CO13 HEPAVIH nationwide cohort of HIV–HCV co-infected individuals [25]. They all had HIV-1 antibodies and a chronic HCV infection that had been confirmed by Western blotting and plasma HCV-RNA assays. Patients who agreed to participate gave their written informed consent.

Based on the *in vitro* studies, we postulated that CXCR4-using viruses have a more deleterious impact on liver disease than CCR5-using viruses. We calculated the sample size required in a cross-sectional study, which detected a 20% difference in the prevalence of CXCR4-using viruses between patients with mild fibrosis (score: F0–F2) and those with severe fibrosis (score: F3–F4) using a one-sided test, with 80% power and a 0.05 alpha risk. According to several studies, the prevalence of CXCR4-using viruses in HIV patients at similar stages of infection is estimated to be approximately 30% [26,27]. Thus, if the prevalence of CXCR4-using viruses is 30% in patients with mild fibrosis, each group should contain 73 patients in order to detect a 20% difference in prevalence (one-sided test, 80% power, 0.05 alpha risk). Thus, we recruited a total of 195 patients: 90 with mild fibrosis and 105 with severe fibrosis.

These patients met the following inclusion criteria: patients had either had a liver biopsy the year before inclusion or a clinician has confirmed liver cirrhosis at inclusion, they had a blood sample available at inclusion, and their dates of HCV and HIV acquisition were known. We estimated the date of HCV infection to be 1 year after the onset of being an intravenous drug user (IVDU), whereas the date of HIV infection was based on the first positive serological test. The day of inclusion into the cohort, and the clinical and biological data, were entered into a clinical research form completed by the medical staff at the respective clinical centres.

HIV tropism was determined using a phenotypic assay in 172 patients (75 with mild fibrosis, 97 with a fibrosis score of F3–F4). We failed to determine HIV tropism in 23 patients for technical reasons. In 34 of these patients, we also determined the evolution of HIV tropism and liver fibrosis, estimated by measuring liver stiffness, after a median period of 36 months (IQR: 35–36 months).

Table 2. Factors associated with the presence of CXCR4-using viruses.

	Univariate analyses		Multivariate analyses	
	OR (95%CI)	P-value	OR (95%CI)	P-value
Age (per additional year)	0.89 (0.66–1.21)	0.46	–	
Gender (male)	1.48 (0.64–3.41)	0.35	–	
Age at infection (per additional year)				
HCV infection	1.04 (0.81–1.32)	0.75	–	
HIV infection	0.91 (0.71–1.15)	0.42	–	
Duration of infection (per additional year)				
HCV infection	0.91 (0.72–1.13)	0.38	–	
HIV infection	1.07 (0.79–1.45)	0.66	–	
Source of HCV infection				
IVDU vs. other	0.55 (0.24–1.26)	0.16	–	
Source of HIV infection				
IVDU vs. other	0.85 (0.40–1.83)	0.69	–	
CDC clinical stage				
B vs. A	0.99 (0.43–2.26)	0.99	–	
C vs. A	1.9 (0.86–4.1)	0.11	–	
Plasma HIV RNA concentration ($\geq$50 copies/mL)	0.66 (0.30–1.47)	0.32	–	
CD4-cell count at inclusion ($<$200/mm^3)	2.72 (1.23–6.03)	0.01	–	
Nadir CD4-cell count ($<$200/mm^3)	5.08 (1.85–13.91)	0.002	3.94 (1.39–11.14)	0.01
ART at inclusion (treated vs. untreated-naive)	3.11 (0.68–14.22)	0.14	–	
Class of ART at inclusion				
PI	4.03 (1.74–9.31)	0.001	–	
NNRTI	0.43 (0.17–1.13)	0.09	–	
NRTI	2.12 (0.68–6.58)	0.19	–	
Cumulative duration under ART before inclusion (months)	1.0 (0.97–1.02)	0.98	–	
Cumulative duration under PI before inclusion (months)	1.02 (0.99–1.04)	0.17	–	
Cumulative duration of NNRTI before inclusion (months)	1.0 (0.96–1.04)	0.99	–	
Cumulative duration of NRTI before inclusion (months)	1.0 (0.98–1.02)	0.94	–	
HCV genotype				
2–3 vs. 1–4	0.90 (0.39–2.04)	0.80	–	
Plasma HCV RNA concentration (log$_{10}$; IU/mL)	1.11 (0.73–1.70)	0.60	–	

Abbreviations: ART: antiretroviral therapy; CDC: Centers for Disease Control; PI: protease inhibitors; NNRTI: non-nucleoside reverse-transcriptase inhibitors; NRTI: nucleoside reverse-transcriptase inhibitors; IQR: inter-quartile range; IVDU: intravenous drug user.

Liver fibrosis

Most (103) patients underwent a liver biopsy the year before their inclusion. The grade and stage of chronic hepatitis were assessed in the liver biopsies according to the Metavir classification [28]. The remaining 69 patients were classified as having a fibrosis score of F4 because their clinical signs of cirrhosis were verified by the examining clinician (oesophageal varices, ascites, liver encephalopathy or intestinal bleeds). We also used transient elastography with a Fibroscan machine (EchoSens) to determine liver stiffness at inclusion and after a median period of 36 months (inter-quartile range [IQR]: 35–36 months) in the 34 patients followed-up long term [29].

HIV tropism

Blood samples were collected on the day of inclusion. A recombinant virus phenotypic entry assay was used to determine HIV-1 co-receptor usage [30,31,32]. This test is suitable for use with blood plasma and cell samples. A fragment encompassing the gp120 and ectodomain of gp41 was amplified from HIV RNA in the plasma by RT-PCR, or from HIV DNA within a whole-blood sample using PCR. HIV-1 tropism was determined by amplifying HIV DNA in the cells of 145 patients whose HIV RNA was $\leq$400 copies/mL and by amplifying the HIV RNA from 27 patients whose plasma HIV RNA was $>$400 copies/mL. HIV tropism was also determined from HIV DNA in blood samples from the 34 long-term follow-up patients collected 36 months after their inclusion.

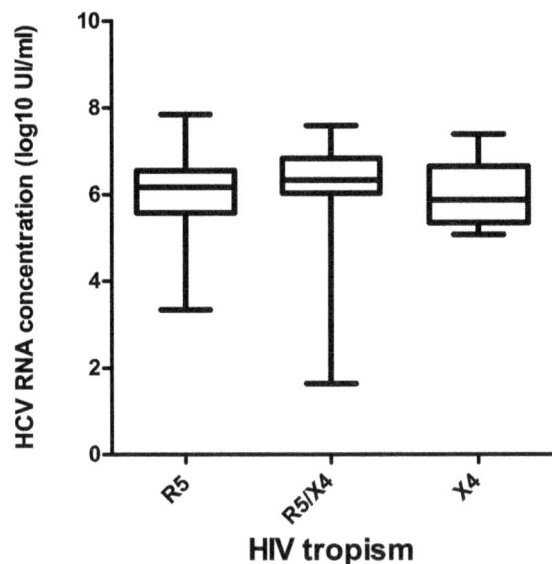

Figure 1. HCV RNA concentrations according to HIV-1 tropism.

Plasma HCV RNA

We determined the concentration of HCV RNA in the plasma of blood samples collected at cohort inception using the Cobas Ampliprep-Cobas Taqman test (Roche Diagnostics, Meylan, France).

Statistical analyses

Descriptive values are expressed as medians with their IQRs. Non-parametric tests were used to compare the differences between the groups (Wilcoxon test for continuous variable, χ^2 test for qualitative variables). A p-value of <0.05 was considered significant. Baseline predictors of CXCR4 tropism were evaluated by univariate and multivariate analyses.

The following covariates were analysed at inclusion: age, gender, age at HCV and HIV infections, duration of HCV and HIV infections, source of HCV and HIV infections, liver steatosis, CD4-cell count at inclusion, nadir of CD4-cell count, type of antiretroviral therapy, but also the type and duration of any previous antiretroviral therapy before inclusion into the cohort, HCV genotype, HCV RNA plasma concentration, and plasma HIV RNA concentration. Variables with a p-value of ≤ 0.25 after univariate analyses were entered into multivariate, backward, stepwise logistic regression analyses to identify significant variables independently associated with the presence of CXCR4-using viruses. Odds ratios (OR) were estimated from the model and are given with their 95% confidence intervals (CI).

The same methods and covariates, including HIV tropism (classified as CCR5 or CXCR4-using viruses), geographic origin of the patients, body-mass index, alcohol consumption in the past or at cohort inception, insulin resistance (stratified with the homeostasis model assessment of insulin resistance score (HOMA) of ≥ 3.8 or <3.8) [33], and infection with hepatitis B virus, were used to determine factors associated with severe fibrosis (F3–F4).

Results

Main characteristics of the study population and HIV tropism

We studied 172 HIV–HCV co-infected patients from the ANRS HEPAVIH CO13 cohort: 75 with mild liver fibrosis (F0–

F2) and 97 with severe fibrosis (F3–F4). Their median age was 45 years (IQR: 42–48 years) and 133 (77.3%) were males. Most of the patients were former IVDUs ($n = 128$, 76.2%) infected with HCV genotype 1 ($n = 108$, 63.2%). The median duration of HCV infection was 23 years (IQR: 19–27 years) and the median duration of HIV infection was 18 years (IQR: 13–20 years). The majority (91.8%) had received successful antiretroviral therapy (HIV RNA concentration <50 copies/mL in 70.8% of patients). No patient was taking a CCR5 antagonist at inclusion or had already taken a CCR5 antagonist before inclusion into the cohort.

A total of 122 patients (71%) were infected with the R5 virus, 40 with the D/M virus (23%) and 10 with the pure X4 virus (6%). The proportions of CXCR4-using viruses, found by testing the tropism of HIV DNA (24.8%) and HIV RNA (22%), were similar ($p = 0.60$). Because there were so few cases of purely X4 virus infection, the tropism was dichotomized as either a CCR5- or CXCR4-using virus (Table 1).

Univariate analyses revealed three factors associated with infection by CXCR4-using viruses: the current CD4-cell count, the nadir CD4-cell count and current treatment with protease inhibitors (Table 2). The only factor associated with the presence of CXCR4-using viruses in multivariate analyses was a nadir of CD4-positive cells $<200/\text{mm}^3$ (OR: 3.94, 95% CI: 1.39–11.14, $p = 0.01$) (Table 2).

Plasma HCV RNA

We investigated the influence of HIV tropism on the plasma concentration of HCV RNA. The median HCV RNA concentration in patients infected with R5 viruses was 6.2 $\log_{10}$ IU/mL (IQR: 3.3–7.8 $\log_{10}$ IU/mL); it was 6.3 $\log_{10}$ IU/mL (1.6–7.6 $\log_{10}$ IU/mL) in patients infected with D/M viruses, and was 5.9 $\log_{10}$ IU/mL (5.1–7.4 $\log_{10}$ IU/mL) in patients infected with X4 viruses ($p = 0.28$) (Figure 1).

Predictors of advanced fibrosis

A liver biopsy or clinical signs of cirrhosis indicated that 75 HIV–HCV co-infected patients had mild liver fibrosis (F0–F2) and 97 had severe fibrosis (F3–F4). The proportion of mild fibrosis patients infected with CXCR4-using viruses ($n = 23$, 31%) was similar to that of the severe fibrosis patients ($n = 27$, 28%, $p = 0.6$) (Table 3). Univariate analyses showed several factors associated with severe fibrosis: age, gender, insulin resistance, alcohol consumption, duration of HCV and HIV infections, HCV infection caused by IVDU, current CD4-cell count, nadir CD4-cell count, the duration of exposure to antiretroviral therapy (ART), especially nucleoside reverse-transcriptase inhibitors and steatosis (Table 4).

Multivariate analyses identified five factors associated with severe fibrosis (F3–F4): increasing age, insulin resistance (HOMA ≥ 3.8), past alcohol consumption, duration of HIV infection of ≥ 10 years and a nadir CD4-cell count of $<200/\text{mm}^3$ (Table 4).

Changes in liver stiffness and HIV tropism

We assessed the influence of HIV tropism on the progress of fibrosis in a subgroup of 34 patients. HIV tropism and liver fibrosis, estimated by measuring liver stiffness, were determined at inclusion and at 3 years later. At inclusion, 12/34 were infected with CXCR4-using viruses and 22/34 were infected with CCR5-using viruses. They were all given ART.

The HIV RNA of 24 (73%) patients was <50 copies/mL throughout the 3-year period. The median HIV RNA concentration in all 34 patients was 2.7 $\log_{10}$ copies/mL (IQR: 1.9–3.7 $\log_{10}$ copies/mL), it was 3.2 $\log_{10}$ copies/mL (IQR: 2.0–4.0 $\log_{10}$ copies/mL) in patients with CXCR4-using viruses and 2.5 $\log_{10}$

Table 3. Demographic and clinical data for the patients according to liver fibrosis.

	n	F0–F2 (n=75)	F3–F4 (n=97)	P-value
Age	172	43 (33–63)	46 (39–65)	0.005
Gender (male)	172			0.003
Male		50 (67)	83 (86)	
Female		25 (33)	14 (14)	
Geographic origin	160			0.76
Europe		49 (69)	66 (75)	–
North Africa		14 (20)	17 (19)	–
Sub-Saharan Africa		5 (7)	3 (3)	
Other		3 (4)	3 (3)	
Body-mass index	167	22.2 (17.4–32.2)	22.4 (13.9–37.0)	0.967
Insulin resistance	138			0.01
HOMA <3.8		49 (82)	48 (62)	
HOMA ≥3.8		11 (18)	30 (38)	
Alcohol consumption	171			0.019
Never		17 (23)	15 (16)	
Ongoing		18 (24)	43 (45)	
Past		40 (53)	38 (39)	
Age at infection				
HCV infection	172	21 (14–43)	21 (13–43)	0.693
HIV infection	171	28 (10–49)	29 (19–59)	0.506
Duration of infection				
HCV infection (years)		22 (1–37)	24 (1–42)	0.004
HIV infection (years)		18 (1–23)	18 (1–24)	0.11
Source of HCV infection				0.02
IVDU		55 (73)	76 (87)	
Other		20 (27)	11 (13)	
Source of HIV infection	171			0.010
IVDU		49 (66)	81 (84)	
Other		25 (34)	16 (16)	
CDC clinical stage	172			0.423
A		40 (53)	42 (43)	
B		18 (24)	29 (30)	
C		17 (23)	26 (27)	
Plasma HIV RNA concentration				0.874
Undetectable (<50 copies/mL)		42 (68)	60 (69)	
Detectable (≥50 copies/mL)		20 (32)	27 (31)	
HIV RNA concentration (when detectable) ($\log_{10}$)		3.1 (1.8–4.9)	3.1 (1.7–5.8)	0.855
CD4-cell count at inclusion	171	396 (55–1878)	356 (48–1185)	0.032
Nadir CD4-cell count	153	185 (4–520)	110 (1–480)	0.002
HIV tropism	172			0.685
(CCR5-using virus)		52 (69)	70 (72)	
(CXCR4-using virus)		23 (31)	27 (28)	
ART at inclusion	172			0.516
Naïve		4 (5)	3 (3)	
Pre-treated patients		5 (7)	4 (4)	
Ongoing treatment		66 (88)	90 (93)	
Class of ART at inclusion	172			
PI		47 (63)	64 (66)	0.653
NNRTI		17 (23)	18 (19)	0.507
NRTI		64 (85)	85 (88)	0.661

Table 3. Cont.

	n	F0–F2 (n=75)	F3–F4 (n=97)	P-value
Cumulative duration under ART before inclusion (months)	165	108.1 (0.9–192.1)	120.4 (4.0–243.7)	0.024
Cumulative duration under PI before inclusion (months)	144	50.3 (0.9–141.7)	67.6 (1.1–199.3)	0.121
Cumulative duration of NNRTI before inclusion (months)	109	28.2 (0.3–118.9)	20.3 (0.3–117.6)	0.724
Cumulative duration of NRTI before inclusion (months)	165	105.0 (0.9–192.1)	120.4 (4.0–243.7)	0.027
HCV genotype	171			0.064
1		47 (63)	61 (63)	
2		0 (-)	2 (2)	
3		11 (15)	24 (25)	
4		16 (22)	10 (10)	
Plasma HCV RNA concentration (log$_{10}$; UI/mL)	145	6.3 (1.6–7.8)	6.1 (3.3–7.8)	0.173
Steatosis	112			0.725
≤10%		53 (72)	26 (68)	
>10%		21 (28)	12 (32)	

Abbreviations: ART: antiretroviral therapy; CDC: Centers for Disease Control; HOMA: homeostasis model assessment of insulin resistance score; PI: protease inhibitors; NNRTI: non-nucleoside reverse-transcriptase inhibitors; NRTI: nucleoside reverse-transcriptase inhibitors; IQR: inter-quartile range; IVDU: intravenous drug user.

copies/mL (1.9–3.4 log$_{10}$ copies/mL) in patients with CCR5-using viruses ($p = 0.27$). HIV tropism did not evolve in 32 patients, but two patients infected with the R5 virus at inclusion had the R5X4 virus by 36 months later. The median changes in the patients' liver stiffness values relative to baseline values after 36 months were 0.45 kPa (IQR: -2.25, 2.9 kPa) for the 20 patients with a CCR5-using virus and -0.4 kPa (IQR: -0, 0.8 kPa) for the 14 patients with a CXCR4-using virus ($p = 0.3$) (Figure 2).

Discussion

We assessed the prevalence of CXCR4-using viruses in a population of HIV–HCV co-infected patients and investigated the influence of HIV-1 tropism on plasma concentration of HCV RNA and HCV-related liver fibrosis. The plasma HCV RNA concentrations of patients infected with CCR5-using and CXCR4-using viruses were similar. We also found no relationship between HIV tropism and severe fibrosis in either the cross-sectional study or the longitudinal substudy.

We determined HIV-1 tropism in 172 HIV–HCV co-infected patients at their inclusion into the ANRS CO13 cohort using a phenotypic assay that had been validated for cell-associated HIV-1 DNA or plasma HIV-1 RNA to determine HIV-1 co-receptor usage [32].

Data on HIV tropism from HCV–HIV co-infected subjects are scarce, and there are none on the prevalence of CXCR4-using viruses in this population. A recent study reported that CXCR4-using viruses are more frequently transmitted in HCV-infected IVDUs [31]. CXCR4-using viruses appeared to be less prevalent in our patients compared to highly experienced treatment patients (39–50% of CXCR4-using viruses) [34,35,36]. Multivariate analysis indicated that the nadir CD4-cell count was the only factor associated with the presence of CXCR4-using viruses, as previously reported for HIV monoinfected patients [37,38]. The nadir CD4-cell count was a better marker of HIV disease progression and the presence of CXCR4-using viruses in this population than the current CD4-cell count.

The HCV RNA concentration is higher in HIV–HCV co-infected patients compared to patients with HCV alone [2]. Lin et al. reported that inactivated HIV or recombinant gp120 increased

HCV replication *in vitro* [16]. This effect on HCV replication was neutralized by antibodies to CCR5 or CXCR4. This is why we investigated the influence of HIV tropism on HCV RNA concentration *in vivo*. However, our data show that HCV RNA concentrations in patients infected with R5, D/M and X4 viruses were all similar.

We also studied the relationship between HIV tropism and liver fibrosis. Multivariate analyses of the 172 patients in the cross-sectional study identified five factors associated with severe fibrosis: age, alcohol consumption, insulin resistance, the nadir of CD4-cell count and the duration of HIV infection. This supports the current recommendation that these patients limit their alcohol consumption as much as possible. We also found that insulin resistance, estimated using the HOMA score, was associated with liver fibrosis. Insulin resistance has been identified as a factor that promotes steatosis and progression of fibrosis in HCV mono-infected patients [39,40] and HIV–HCV co-infected patients [41,42].

It is unclear whether the CD4-cell count or the CD4 nadir is associated with the progression of liver disease. Some have found that lower CD4-cell counts or the CD4 nadir is associated with more severe liver fibrosis and liver outcomes [41,43,44,45,46], whereas others have found no such association [9,47]. Nevertheless, HIV-induced immune suppression should be considered a major factor in the progression of liver fibrosis. This supports the recommendation that antiretroviral therapy should be started earlier for HIV–HCV co-infected patients in order to slow down the progression of fibrosis [48].

Having an HIV infection for >10 years is associated with severe fibrosis. However, the estimated durations of infections in the ANRS CO13 cohort differed. The duration of HCV infection was estimated from the year IVDU began, whereas the duration of HIV infection was based on the first positive serological test. This difference may have introduced a bias in the durations of HCV infection. This variable is probably linked to the duration of HCV infection, a major factor associated with the progression of fibrosis [49].

In vitro studies have indicated a direct link between HIV tropism and markers for liver fibrogenesis. We postulated that CXCR4-using viruses have a more deleterious impact on liver disease than

Table 4. Factors associated with severe fibrosis (F3–F4).

	Univariate analyses		Multivariate analyses	
	OR (95%CI)	P-value	OR (95%CI)	P-value
Age (per additional year)	1.6 (1.17–2.20)	0.003	1.12 (1.02–1.24)	0.02
Gender (male)	2.96 (1.41–6.22)	0.004	_	
Geographic origin				
Europe vs. North Africa	1.011 (0.49–2.46)	0.79	_	
Sub-Saharan Africa vs. North Africa	0.49 (0.10–2.44)	0.38	_	
Body-mass index	1.001 (0.92–1.10)	0.91	_	
Insulin resistance (HOMA ≥3.8)	2.78 (1.25–6.17)	0.012	5.56 (1.29–23.9)	0.02
Alcohol consumption		0.02		
Ongoing vs. never	1.07 (0.47–2.45)	0.86	_	
Past vs. never	2.707 (1.11–6.56)	0.02	6.4 (1.26–32.7)	0.02
Age at infection				
HCV infection	0.91 (0.72–1.14)	0.42	_	
HIV infection	1.13 (0.91–1.39)	0.26	_	
Duration of infection				
HCV infection (≥10 years)	6.47 (1.35–30.9)	0.02	_	
HIV infection (≥10 years)	2.62 (1.08–6.3)	0.03	33.3 (2.21–503.1)	0.01
Source of HCV infection				
IVDU vs. other	2.5 (1.11–5.66)	0.02	_	
Source of HIV infection				
IVDU vs. other	2.58 (1.25–5.31)	0.01	_	
CDC clinical stage				
B vs. A	1.53 (0.73–3.18)	0.25	_	
C vs. A	1.45 (0.68–3.08)	0.32	_	
Plasma HIV RNA concentration (≥50 copies/mL)	0.94 (0.46–1.90)	0.87	_	
CD4 cell-count at inclusion (<200/mm^3)	3.68 (1.87–7.25)	<0.01	_	
Nadir CD4-cell count (<200/mm^3)	4.08 (1.94–8.58)	<0.01	17.5 (4.08–74.9)	<0.01
HIV tropism (CXCR4-using virus)	0.87 (0.45–1.69)	0.68	_	
ART at inclusion (treated vs. untreated)	1.75 (0.62–4.94)	0.29	_	
Class of ART at inclusion				
PI	1.15 (0.61–2.16)	0.65	_	
NNRTI	0.77 (0.37–1.63)	0.50	_	
NRTI	1.21 (0.50–2.93)	0.66	_	
Cumulative duration under ART before inclusion	1.02 (1.003–1.043)	0.026	_	
Cumulative duration under PI before inclusion	1.02 (0.99–1.04)	0.12	_	
Cumulative duration of NNRTI before inclusion	0.99 (0.96–1.03)	0.81	_	
Cumulative duration of NRTI before inclusion	1.02 (1.00–1.04)	0.028		
HCV genotype				
1–2–4 vs. 3	0.53 (0.24–1.17)	0.11	_	
Plasma HCV RNA concentration (log$_{10}$; UI/mL)	0.83 (0.56–1.23)	0.37	_	
Steatosis (>10%)	1.16 (0.49–2.72)	0.72	_	

Abbreviations: ART: antiretroviral therapy; CDC: Centers for Disease Control; HOMA: homeostasis model assessment of insulin resistance score; PI: protease inhibitors; NNRTI: non-nucleoside reverse-transcriptase inhibitors; NRTI: nucleoside reverse-transcriptase inhibitors; IQR: inter-quartile range; IVDU: intravenous drug user.

R5-tropic viruses because of their pro-apoptotic effect on hepatocytes [18,19] and their stimulation of collagen production by HSCs [17,20]. However, our cross-sectional study shows that the prevalence of CXCR4-using viruses, in patients with severe fibrosis and in those with mild fibrosis, were similar. The longitudinal follow-up of 34 patients also showed no relationship between HIV tropism and the progression of liver fibrosis. However, the majority of patients in the cross-sectional and longitudinal studies were receiving an antiretroviral therapy. HIV tropism may not affect the progression of fibrosis in patients receiving a potent antiretroviral therapy.

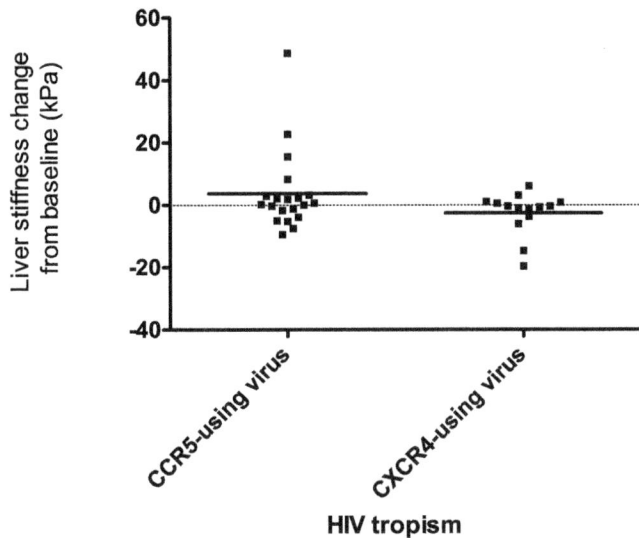

Figure 2. Changes in liver stiffness according to HIV-1 tropism of the 34 patients in the longitudinal study (medians are indicated by bars).

These results agree with those from a recent study by Lin et al. [50], who demonstrated that X4-tropic HIV and R5-tropic HIV trigger the formation of reactive oxygen species in HSC and Huh7.5.1 cells, and that this effect is enhanced by HCV. The production of reactive oxygen species in HSCs, when triggered by HIV, activates profibrogenic genes that encode collagen and the tissue inhibitor metalloprotease-1, as well as down-regulating matrix metallo-protease 3 synthesis. Both X4-tropic HIV and R5-tropic HIV stimulated the production of reactive oxygen species and profibrogenic gene expression to about the same extent [50]. In addition, both X4 and R5 viral infections increased HCV-induced apoptosis of hepatocytes [51]. Therefore, the CXCR4 pathway contributes to liver fibrosis, but the CCR5 pathway has also been demonstrated to play a role in mouse models of liver fibrosis [52]. Moreover, a recent *in vitro* study has demonstrated

that a CCR5 antagonist inhibits the migration, proliferation and synthesis of chemokines and collagen secretion by stellate cells in culture [53]. It is perhaps important that a CCR5 antagonist has been shown to greatly ameliorate liver fibrosis in a mouse model [53].

Our study has some limitations. HIV-1 tropism was determined by amplifying HIV DNA from the cells of 145 patients and by amplifying HIV RNA from 27 patients for the cross-sectional study. Nevertheless, a positive correlation has been demonstrated between the abundance of CXCR4-using variants, determined by ultra-deep sequencing in circulating HIV, and the amount of proviral HIV in these cells [54]. As sequential liver biopsies are now rarely taken in clinical practice, we used liver stiffness to estimate changes in liver fibrosis and to assess the influence of HIV tropism on liver fibrosis. This procedure is valid for assessing liver fibrosis in patients with chronic HCV infection, regardless of if it is HIV-negative or HIV-positive [55,56,57].

Only a small number of patients were included in our longitudinal study. Yet, the results of this study agree well with those of the cross-sectional study, which supports our conclusion. However, further longitudinal studies on more patients are needed.

In conclusion, we found no relationship between the presence of CXCR4-using viruses and the severity of liver fibrosis or the concentration of HCV RNA in HIV–HCV patients receiving a potent antiretroviral therapy. Recent work suggests that the CCR5 pathway could be antagonized to block fibrosis progression, and further evaluation of the action of CCR5 antagonists in HIV–HCV patients should be assessed.

Author Contributions

Conceived and designed the experiments: FA JI FD DSC PB PS. Performed the experiments: FA SR PT. Analyzed the data: EP MW. Contributed reagents/materials/analysis tools: FA SR JI. Wrote the paper: FA JI.

References

1. Weber R, Sabin CA, Friis-Moller N, Reiss P, El-Sadr WM, et al. (2006) Liver-related deaths in persons infected with the human immunodeficiency virus: the D:A:D study. Arch Intern Med 166: 1632–1641.
2. Rotman Y, Liang TJ (2009) Coinfection with hepatitis C virus and human immunodeficiency virus: virological, immunological, and clinical outcomes. J Virol 83: 7366–7374.
3. Thein HH, Yi Q, Dore GJ, Krahn MD (2008) Natural history of hepatitis C virus infection in HIV-infected individuals and the impact of HIV in the era of highly active antiretroviral therapy: a meta-analysis. Aids 22: 1979–1991.
4. Graham CS, Baden LR, Yu E, Mrus JM, Carnie J, et al. (2001) Influence of human immunodeficiency virus infection on the course of hepatitis C virus infection: a meta-analysis. Clin Infect Dis 33: 562–569.
5. Mohsen AH, Easterbrook PJ, Taylor C, Portmann B, Kulasegaram R, et al. (2003) Impact of human immunodeficiency virus (HIV) infection on the progression of liver fibrosis in hepatitis C virus infected patients. Gut 52: 1035–1040.
6. Soriano V, Mocroft A, Rockstroh J, Ledergerber B, Knysz B, et al. (2008) Spontaneous viral clearance, viral load, and genotype distribution of hepatitis C virus (HCV) in HIV-infected patients with anti-HCV antibodies in Europe. J Infect Dis 198: 1337–1344.
7. Marine-Barjoan E, Berrebi A, Giordanengo V, Favre SF, Haas H, et al. (2007) HCV/HIV co-infection, HCV viral load and mode of delivery: risk factors for mother-to-child transmission of hepatitis C virus? Aids 21: 1811–1815.
8. Balagopal A, Philp FH, Astemborski J, Block TM, Mehta A, et al. (2008) Human immunodeficiency virus-related microbial translocation and progression of hepatitis C. Gastroenterology 135: 226–233.
9. Bonnard P, Lescure FX, Amiel C, Guiard-Schmid JB, Callard P, et al. (2007) Documented rapid course of hepatic fibrosis between two biopsies in patients

coinfected by HIV and HCV despite high CD4 cell count. J Viral Hepat 14: 806–811.
10. Berger EA, Doms RW, Fenyo EM, Korber BT, Littman DR, et al. (1998) A new classification for HIV-1. Nature 391: 240.
11. Jiao J, Friedman SL, Aloman C (2009) Hepatic fibrosis. Curr Opin Gastroenterol 25: 223–229.
12. Hong F, Tuyama A, Lee TF, Loke J, Agarwal R, et al. (2009) Hepatic stellate cells express functional CXCR4: role in stromal cell-derived factor-1alpha-mediated stellate cell activation. Hepatology 49: 2055–2067.
13. Schwabe RF, Bataller R, Brenner DA (2003) Human hepatic stellate cells express CCR5 and RANTES to induce proliferation and migration. Am J Physiol Gastrointest Liver Physiol 285: G949–958.
14. Xiao P, Usami O, Suzuki Y, Ling H, Shimizu N, et al. (2008) Characterization of a CD4-independent clinical HIV-1 that can efficiently infect human hepatocytes through chemokine (C-X-C motif) receptor 4. Aids 22: 1749–1757.
15. Bruno R, Galastri S, Sacchi P, Cima S, Caligiuri A, et al. (2010) gp120 modulates the biology of human hepatic stellate cells: a link between HIV infection and liver fibrogenesis. Gut 59: 513–520.
16. Lin W, Weinberg EM, Tai AW, Peng LF, Brockman MA, et al. (2008) HIV increases HCV replication in a TGF-beta1-dependent manner. Gastroenterology 134: 803–811.
17. Tuyama AC, Hong F, Saiman Y, Wang C, Ozkok D, et al. (2010) Human immunodeficiency virus (HIV)-1 infects human hepatic stellate cells and promotes collagen I and monocyte chemoattractant protein-1 expression: Implications for the pathogenesis of HIV/hepatitis C virus-induced liver fibrosis. Hepatology 52: 612–622.
18. Babu CK, Suwansrinon K, Bren GD, Badley AD, Rizza SA (2009) HIV induces TRAIL sensitivity in hepatocytes. PLoS One 4: e4623.

19. Vlahakis SR, Villasis-Keever A, Gomez TS, Bren GD, Paya CV (2003) Human immunodeficiency virus-induced apoptosis of human hepatocytes via CXCR4. J Infect Dis 188: 1455–1460.

20. Hong F, Saiman Y, Si C, Mosoian A, Bansal MB (2012) X4 Human Immunodeficiency Virus Type 1 gp120 Promotes Human Hepatic Stellate Cell Activation and Collagen I Expression through Interactions with CXCR4. PLoS One 7: e33659.

21. Munshi N, Balasubramanian A, Koziel M, Ganju RK, Groopman JE (2003) Hepatitis C and human immunodeficiency virus envelope proteins cooperatively induce hepatocytic apoptosis via an innocent bystander mechanism. J Infect Dis 188: 1192–1204.

22. Canbay A, Feldstein AE, Higuchi H, Werneburg N, Grambihler A, et al. (2003) Kupffer cell engulfment of apoptotic bodies stimulates death ligand and cytokine expression. Hepatology 38: 1188–1198.

23. Canbay A, Friedman S, Gores GJ (2004) Apoptosis: the nexus of liver injury and fibrosis. Hepatology 39: 273–278.

24. Canbay A, Taimr P, Torok N, Higuchi H, Friedman S, et al. (2003) Apoptotic body engulfment by a human stellate cell line is profibrogenic. Lab Invest 83: 655–663.

25. Loko MA, Salmon D, Carrieri P, Winnock M, Mora M, et al. (2010) The French national prospective cohort of patients co-infected with HIV and HCV (ANRS CO13 HEPAVIH): Early findings, 2006–2010. BMC Infect Dis 10: 303.

26. Recordon-Pinson P, Soulie C, Flandre P, Descamps D, Lazrek M, et al. (2010) Evaluation of the genotypic prediction of HIV-1 coreceptor use versus a phenotypic assay and correlation with the virological response to maraviroc: the ANRS GenoTropism study. Antimicrob Agents Chemother 54: 3335–3340.

27. Raymond S, Delobel P, Mavigner M, Cazabat M, Souyris C, et al. (2008) Correlation between genotypic predictions based on V3 sequences and phenotypic determination of HIV-1 tropism. Aids 22: F11–16.

28. Bedossa P, Poynard T (1996) An algorithm for the grading of activity in chronic hepatitis C. The METAVIR Cooperative Study Group. Hepatology 24: 289–293.

29. Sandrin L, Fourquet B, Hasquenoph JM, Yon S, Fournier C, et al. (2003) Transient elastography: a new noninvasive method for assessment of hepatic fibrosis. Ultrasound Med Biol 29: 1705–1713.

30. Raymond S, Delobel P, Izopet J (2012) Phenotyping methods for determining HIV tropism and applications in clinical settings. Curr Opin HIV AIDS.

31. Raymond S, Delobel P, Mavigner M, Cazabat M, Encinas S, et al. (2010) CXCR4-using viruses in plasma and peripheral blood mononuclear cells during primary HIV-1 infection and impact on disease progression. Aids 24: 2305–2312.

32. Raymond S, Delobel P, Mavigner M, Cazabat M, Souyris C, et al. (2010) Development and performance of a new recombinant virus phenotypic entry assay to determine HIV-1 coreceptor usage. J Clin Virol 47: 126–130.

33. Ascaso JF, Romero P, Real JT, Lorente RI, Marti, et al. (2003) Abdominal obesity, insulin resistance, and metabolic syndrome in a southern European population. Eur J Intern Med 14: 101–106.

34. Wilkin TJ, Su Z, Kuritzkes DR, Hughes M, Flexner C, et al. (2007) HIV type 1 chemokine coreceptor use among antiretroviral-experienced patients screened for a clinical trial of a CCR5 inhibitor: AIDS Clinical Trial Group A5211. Clin Infect Dis 44: 591–595.

35. Melby T, Despirito M, Demasi R, Heilek-Snyder G, Greenberg ML, et al. (2006) HIV-1 coreceptor use in triple-class treatment-experienced patients: baseline prevalence, correlates, and relationship to enfuvirtide response. J Infect Dis 194: 238–246.

36. Gulick RM, Lalezari J, Goodrich J, Clumeck N, DeJesus E, et al. (2008) Maraviroc for previously treated patients with R5 HIV-1 infection. N Engl J Med 359: 1429–1441.

37. Soulie C, Fourati S, Lambert-Niclot S, Malet I, Wirden M, et al. (2010) Factors associated with proviral DNA HIV-1 tropism in antiretroviral therapy-treated

patients with fully suppressed plasma HIV viral load: implications for the clinical use of CCR5 antagonists. J Antimicrob Chemother 65: 749–751.

38. Hunt PW, Harrigan PR, Huang W, Bates M, Williamson DW, et al. (2006) Prevalence of CXCR4 tropism among antiretroviral-treated HIV-1-infected patients with detectable viremia. J Infect Dis 194: 926–930.

39. Fartoux L, Poujol-Robert A, Guechot J, Wendum D, Poupon R, et al. (2005) Insulin resistance is a cause of steatosis and fibrosis progression in chronic hepatitis C. Gut 54: 1003–1008.

40. Halfon P, Penaranda G, Carrat F, Bedossa P, Bourliere M, et al. (2009) Influence of insulin resistance on hepatic fibrosis and steatosis in hepatitis C virus (HCV) mono-infected compared with HIV-HCV co-infected patients. Aliment Pharmacol Ther 30: 61–70.

41. Blanco F, Barreiro P, Ryan P, Vispo E, Martin-Carbonero L, et al. (2011) Risk factors for advanced liver fibrosis in HIV-infected individuals: role of antiretroviral drugs and insulin resistance. J Viral Hepat 18: 11–16.

42. Ryan P, Berenguer J, Michelaud D, Miralles P, Bellon JM, et al. (2009) Insulin resistance is associated with advanced liver fibrosis and high body mass index in HIV/HCV-coinfected patients. J Acquir Immune Defic Syndr 50: 109–110.

43. Benhamou Y, Bochet M, Di Martino V, Charlotte F, Azria F, et al. (1999) Liver fibrosis progression in human immunodeficiency virus and hepatitis C virus coinfected patients. The Multivirc Group. Hepatology 30: 1054–1058.

44. Brau N, Salvatore M, Rios-Bedoya CF, Fernandez-Carbia A, Paronetto F, et al. (2006) Slower fibrosis progression in HIV/HCV-coinfected patients with successful HIV suppression using antiretroviral therapy. J Hepatol 44: 47–55.

45. Martin-Carbonero L, Benhamou Y, Puoti M, Berenguer J, Mallolas J, et al. (2004) Incidence and predictors of severe liver fibrosis in human immunodeficiency virus-infected patients with chronic hepatitis C: a European collaborative study. Clin Infect Dis 38: 128–133.

46. Pineda JA, Gonzalez J, Ortega E, Tural C, Macias J, et al. (2011) Prevalence and factors associated with significant liver fibrosis assessed by transient elastometry in HIV/hepatitis C virus-coinfected patients. J Viral Hepat 17: 714–719.

47. Collazos J, Carton JA, Asensi V (2011) Immunological Status Does Not Influence Hepatitis C Virus or Liver Fibrosis in HIV-Hepatitis C Virus-Coinfected Patients. AIDS Res Hum Retroviruses 24: 383–389.

48. Hammer SM, Eron JJ Jr, Reiss P, Schooley RT, Thompson MA, et al. (2008) Antiretroviral treatment of adult HIV infection: 2008 recommendations of the International AIDS Society-USA panel. JAMA 300: 555–570.

49. Thein HH, Yi Q, Dore GJ, Krahn MD (2008) Estimation of stage-specific fibrosis progression rates in chronic hepatitis C virus infection: a meta-analysis and meta-regression. Hepatology 48: 418–431.

50. Lin W, Wu G, Li S, Weinberg EM, Kumthip K, et al. (2011) HIV and HCV cooperatively promote hepatic fibrogenesis via induction of reactive oxygen species and NFkappaB. J Biol Chem 286: 2665–2674.

51. Jang JY, Shao RX, Lin W, Weinberg E, Chung WJ, et al. (2011) HIV infection increases HCV-induced hepatocyte apoptosis. J Hepatol 54: 612–620.

52. Seki E, De Minicis S, Gwak GY, Kluwe J, Inokuchi S, et al. (2009) CCR1 and CCR5 promote hepatic fibrosis in mice. J Clin Invest 119: 1858–1870.

53. Berres ML, Koenen RR, Rueland A, Zaldivar MM, Heinrichs D, et al. (2010) Antagonism of the chemokine Ccl5 ameliorates experimental liver fibrosis in mice. J Clin Invest 120: 4129–4140.

54. Abbate I, Rozera G, Tommasi C, Bruselles A, Bartolini B, et al. (2011) Analysis of co-receptor usage of circulating viral and proviral HIV genome quasispecies by ultra-deep pyrosequencing in patients who are candidates for CCR5 antagonist treatment. Clin Microbiol Infect 17: 725–731.

55. Kirk GD, Astemborski J, Mehta SH, Spoler C, Fisher C, et al. (2009) Assessment of liver fibrosis by transient elastography in persons with hepatitis C virus infection or HIV-hepatitis C virus coinfection. Clin Infect Dis 48: 963–972.

56. Martinez SM, Crespo G, Navasa M, Forns X (2010) Noninvasive assessment of liver fibrosis. Hepatology 53: 325–335.

57. de Ledinghen V, Vergniol J (2010) Transient elastography for the diagnosis of liver fibrosis. Expert Rev Med Devices 7: 811–823.

6

The Progression of Liver Fibrosis is Related with Overexpression of the miR-199 and 200 Families

Yoshiki Murakami[1]*, Hidenori Toyoda[2], Masami Tanaka[3], Masahiko Kuroda[3], Yoshinori Harada[4], Fumihiko Matsuda[1], Atsushi Tajima[5¤], Nobuyoshi Kosaka[6], Takahiro Ochiya[6], Kunitada Shimotohno[7]

1 Center for Genomic Medicine, Kyoto University Graduate School of Medicine, Kyoto, Japan, 2 Department of Gastroenterology, Ogaki Municipal Hospital, Ogaki, Japan, 3 Department of Molecular Pathology, Tokyo Medical University, Tokyo, Japan, 4 Department of Pathology and Cell Regulation, Kyoto Prefectural University of Medicine, Kyoto, Japan, 5 Department of Molecular Life Science, Tokai University School of Medicine, Isehara, Japan, 6 Division of Molecular and Cellular Medicine, National Cancer Center Research Institute, Tokyo, Japan, 7 Research Institute, Chiba Institute of Technology, Narashino, Japan

Abstract

Background: Chronic hepatitis C (CH) can develop into liver cirrhosis (LC) and hepatocellular carcinoma (HCC). Liver fibrosis and HCC development are strongly correlated, but there is no effective treatment against fibrosis because the critical mechanism of progression of liver fibrosis is not fully understood. microRNAs (miRNAs) are now essential to the molecular mechanisms of several biological processes. In order to clarify how the aberrant expression of miRNAs participates in development of the liver fibrosis, we analyzed the liver fibrosis in mouse liver fibrosis model and human clinical samples.

Methodology: In a CCL_4-induced mouse liver fibrosis model, we compared the miRNA expression profile from CCL_4 and olive oil administrated liver specimens on 4, 6, and 8 weeks. We also measured expression profiles of human miRNAs in the liver biopsy specimens from 105 CH type C patients without a history of anti-viral therapy.

Principle Findings: Eleven mouse miRNAs were significantly elevated in progressed liver fibrosis relative to control. By using a large amount of human material in CH analysis, we determined the miRNA expression pattern according to the grade of liver fibrosis. We detected several human miRNAs whose expression levels were correlated with the degree of progression of liver fibrosis. In both the mouse and human studies, the expression levels of miR-199a, 199a*, 200a, and 200b were positively and significantly correlated to the progressed liver fibrosis. The expression level of fibrosis related genes in hepatic stellate cells (HSC), were significantly increased by overexpression of these miRNAs.

Conclusion: Four miRNAs are tightly related to the grade of liver fibrosis in both human and mouse was shown. This information may uncover the critical mechanism of progression of liver fibrosis. miRNA expression profiling has potential for diagnostic and therapeutic applications.

Editor: Chad Creighton, Baylor College of Medicine, United States of America

Funding: This work was supported by the Japanese Ministry of Health, Labour and Welfare (Y.M, and K.S). This work was also supported by the 'Strategic Research-Based Support' Project for private universities; with matching funds from the Ministry of Education, Culture, Sports, Science and Technology (M.K). The funders had no role in study design, data collection and analysis, decision to publish, or preparation of the manuscript.

Competing Interests: The authors have declared that no competing interests exist.

* E-mail: ymurakami@genome.med.kyoto-u.ac.jp

¤ Current address: Department of Human Genetics and Public Health, Institute of Health Biosciences, The University of Tokushima Graduate School, Tokushima, Japan

Introduction

Chronic viral hepatitis is a major risk factor for hepatocellular carcinoma (HCC) [1]. Worldwide 120–170 million persons are currently chronically Hepatitis C Virus (HCV) infected [2]. Due to repetitive and continuous inflammation, these patients are at increased risk of developing cirrhosis, subsequent liver decompensation and/or hepatocellular carcinoma. However, the current standard of care; pegylated interferon and rivabirin combination therapy is unsatisfied in the patients with high titre of HCVRNA and genotype 1b. Activated human liver stellate cells (HSC) with chronic viral infection, can play a pivotal role in the progression of liver fibrosis [3]. Activated HSC produce a number of profibrotic cytokines and growth factors that perpetuate the fibrotic process through paracrine and autocrine effects.

MicroRNAs (miRNAs) are endogenous small non-coding RNAs that control gene expression by degrading target mRNA or suppressing their translation [4]. There are currently 940 identifiable human miRNAs (The miRBase Sequence Database - Release ver. 15.0). miRNAs can recognize hundreds of target genes with incomplete complementary; over one third of human genes appear to be conserved miRNA targets [5][6]. miRNA is associated several pathophysiologic events as well as fundamental cellular processes such as cell proliferation and differentiation. Aberrant expression of miRNA can be associated with the liver diseases [7][8][9][10]. Recently reported miRNAs can regulate the activation of HSCs and thereby regulate liver fibrosis. miR-29b, a negative regulator for the type I collagen and SP1, is a key regulator of liver fibrosis [11]. miR-27a and 27b allowed culture-activated rat HSCs to switch to a more quiescent HSC phenotype, with restored cytoplasmic lipid droplets and decreased cell proliferation [12].

In this study, we aimed to reveal the association between miRNA expression patterns and the progression of liver fibrosis by using a chronic liver inflammation model in mouse. We also sought to identify the miRNA expression profile in chronic hepatitis (CH) C patients according to the degree of liver fibrosis, and to clarify how miRNAs contribute to the progression of liver fibrosis. We observed a characteristic miRNA expression profile common to both human liver biopsy specimens and mouse CCL_4 specimens, comprising the key miRNAs which are associated with the liver fibrosis. This information is expected to uncover the mechanism of liver fibrosis and to provide a clearer biomarker for diagnosis of liver fibrosis as well as to aid in the development of more effective and safer therapeutic strategies for liver fibrosis.

Results

The expression level of several mouse miRNAs was increased by introducing mouse liver fibrosis

In order to identify changes in the miRNA expression profile between advanced liver fibrosis and non-fibrotic liver, we intra-peritoneally administered CCL_4 in olive oil or olive oil alone twice a week for 4 weeks and then once a week for the next 4 weeks. Mice were sacrificed at 4, 6, or 8 weeks and then the degree of mouse liver fibrosis was determined by microscopy (Figure S1). miRNA expression analysis was performed from the liver tissue collected at the same time. Histological examination revealed that the degree of liver fibrosis progressed in mice that received CCL_4 relative to mice receiving olive oil alone (Figure 1A). Microarray analysis revealed that in CCL_4 mice, the expression level of 11 miRNAs was consistently higher than that in control mice (Figure 1B).

miRNA expression profile in each human liver fibrosis grade

We then established human miRNAs expression profile by using 105 fresh-frozen human chronic hepatitis (CH) C liver tissues without a history of anti-viral therapy, classified according to the grade of the liver fibrosis (F0, F1, F2, and F3 referred to METAVIR fibrosis stages)(Figure 2, Table S2). Fibrosis grade F0 was considered to be the negative control because these samples were derived from patients with no finding of liver fibrosis. In zebrafish, most highly tissue-specific miRNAs are expressed during embryonic development; approximately 30% of all miRNAs are expressed at a given time point in a given tissue [13]. In mammals, the 20–30% miRNA call rate has recently been validated [14]. Such analysis revealed that the diversity of miRNA expression level among specimens was small. Therefore, we focused on miRNAs with a fold change in mean expression level greater than 1.5 (p<0.05) in the two arbitrary groups of liver fibrosis.

Expression of several miRNAs was dramatically different among grades of fibrosis. In the mice study 11 miRNAs were related to the progression of liver fibrosis (mmu-let-7e, miR-125-5p, 199a-5p, 199b, 199b*, 200a, 200b, 31, 34a, 497, and 802). In the human study 10 miRNAs were extracted, and the change in their expression level varied significantly between F0 and F3 (F0<F3: hsa-miR-146b, 199a, 199a*, 200a, 200b, 34a, and 34b, F0>F3: hsa-miR-212, 23b, and 422b). The expression level of 6 miRNAs was significantly different between F0 and F2 (F0<F2: hsa-miR-146b, 200a, 34a, and 34b, F0>F2: hsa-miR-122 and 23b). 5 extracted miRNAs had an expression level that was significantly different between F1 and F2 (F1<F2: hsa-miR-146b, F1>F2: hsa-miR-122, 197, 574, and 768-5p). The expression level of 9 miRNAs changed significantly between F1 and F3 (F1<F3:

hsa-miR-146b, 150, 199a, 199a*, 200a, and 200b, F1>F3: hsa-miR-378, 422b, and 768-5p). The miRNAs related to liver fibrosis were extracted using two criteria: similar expression pattern in both the human and the mice specimens and shared sequence between human and mouse. We compared the sequences of mouse miRNAs as described on the Agilent Mouse MiRNA array Version 1.0 (miRbase Version 10.1) and human miRNAs as described on the Agilent Human MiRNA array Version 1.5 (miRbase Version 9.1). The sequences of mmu-miR-199a-5p, mmu-miR-199b, mmu-miR-199b, mmu-miR-200a, and mmu-miR-200b in mouse miRNA corresponded to the sequences of hsa-miR-199a, hsa-miR-199a*, hsa-miR-199a, hsa-miR-200a, and hsa-miR-200b in human miRNA, respectively (Table S3).

Validation of the microarray result by real-time qPCR

The 4 human miRNAs (miR-199a, miR-199a*, miR-200a, and miR-200b) with the largest difference in fold change between the F1 and F3 groups were chosen to validate the microarray results using stem-loop based real-time qPCR. The result of real-time qPCR supported the result of that microarray analysis. The expression level of these 4 miRNAs was significantly different between F0 and F3 and spearman correlation analysis also showed that the expressions of these miRNAs were strongly and positively correlated with fibrosis grade (n = 105, r = 0.498(miR-199a), 0.607(miR-199a*), 0.639(miR-200a), 0.618(miR-200b), p-values<0.0001) (Figure 3).

Over expression of miR-199a, 199a*, 200a, and 200b was associated with the progression of liver fibrosis

In order to reveal the function of miR-199a, miR-199a*, miR-200a, and miR-200b, we investigated the involvement of these miRNAs in the modulation of fibrosis-related gene in LX-2 cells. The endogenous expression level of these 4 miRNAs in LX2 and normal liver was low according to the microarray study (Figure S2). Transforming growth factor (TGF)β is one of the critical factors for the activation of HSC during chronic inflammation [15] and TGFβ strongly induced expression of three fibrosis-related genes include a matrix degrading complex comprised of α1 procollagen, matrix remodeling complex, comprised of metallo-proteinases-13 (MMP-13), tissue inhibitors of metalloproteinases-1 (TIMP-1) in LX-2 cells (Figure 4A). Furthermore, overexpression of miR-199a, miR-199a*, miR-200a and miR-200b in LX-2 cells resulted significant induction of above fibrosis-related genes compared with control miRNA (Figure 4B). Finally we validated the involvement of TGFβ in the modulation of these miRNAs. In LX-2 cells treated with TGFβ, the expression levels of miR-199a and miR-199a* were significantly higher than in untreated cells; the expression levels of miR-200a and miR-200b were significantly lower than in untreated cells. Thus, our in vitro analysis suggested a possible involvement of miR-199a, 199a*, 200a, and 200b in the progression of liver fibrosis.

Discussion

Our comprehensive analysis showed that the aberrant expression of miRNAs was associated with the progression of liver fibrosis. We identified that 4 highly expressed miRNAs (miR-199a, miR-199a*, miR-200a, and miR-200b) that were significantly associated with the progression of liver fibrosis both human and mouse. Coordination of aberrant expression of these miRNAs may contribute to the progression of liver fibrosis.

Prior studies have discussed the expression pattern of miRNA found in liver fibrosis samples between previous and present study. In this report and prior mouse studies and the expression pattern of

A

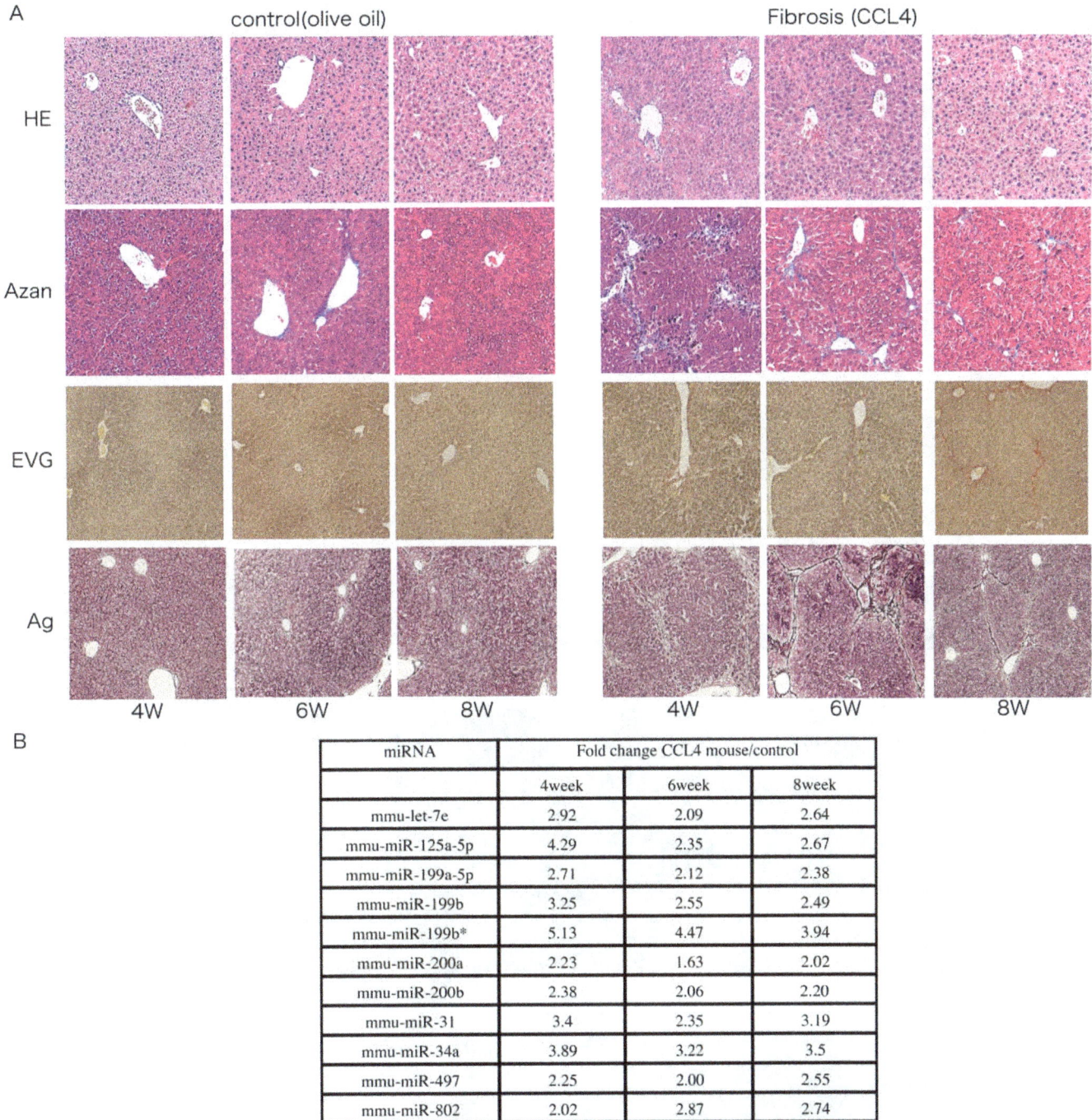

B

miRNA	Fold change CCL4 mouse/control		
	4week	6week	8week
mmu-let-7e	2.92	2.09	2.64
mmu-miR-125a-5p	4.29	2.35	2.67
mmu-miR-199a-5p	2.71	2.12	2.38
mmu-miR-199b	3.25	2.55	2.49
mmu-miR-199b*	5.13	4.47	3.94
mmu-miR-200a	2.23	1.63	2.02
mmu-miR-200b	2.38	2.06	2.20
mmu-miR-31	3.4	2.35	3.19
mmu-miR-34a	3.89	3.22	3.5
mmu-miR-497	2.25	2.00	2.55
mmu-miR-802	2.02	2.87	2.74

Figure 1. The change of liver fibrosis in mouse model. A. Representative H&E-stained, Azan-stained, Ag-stained, and EVG-stained histological sections of liver from mice receiving olive oil alone or CCL$_4$ in olive oil. Magnification is ×10. B. The expression level of mmu-miRNA in mouse liver with olive oil or CCL$_4$ at 4W, 6W, and 8W respectively, by microarray analysis.

3 miRNAs (miR-199a-5p, 199b*, 125-5p) was found to be similar while the expression pattern of 11 miRNAs (miR-223, 221, 24, 877, 29b, 29a, 29c, 30c, 365, 148a, and 193) was partially consistent with fibrosis grade [16]. In low graded liver fibrosis, the low expression pattern of 3 miRNAs (miR-140, 27a, and 27b) and the high expression pattern of 6 miRNAs in rat miRNAs (miR-29c*, 143, 872, 193, 122, and 146) in rat miRNA was also similar to our mouse study (GEO Series accession number GSE19865) [11] [12] [17].

The results in this study and previously completed human studies reveal that the expression level of miR-195, 222, 200c, 21,

and let-7d was higher in high graded fibrotic liver tissue than in low graded fibrotic liver tissue. Additionally, the expression level of miR-301, 194, and 122 was lower in the high graded fibrotic liver tissue than in low graded fibrotic liver tissue [18] [19] [20](GEO Series accession number GSE16922). This difference in miRNA expression pattern may be contributed to (1) the difference of microarray platform, (2) difference of analytic procedure, and (3) the difference of the species (rat, mouse, and human).

The miR-199 and miR-200 families have are circumstantially related to liver fibrosis. TGFβ-induced factor (TGIF) and SMAD

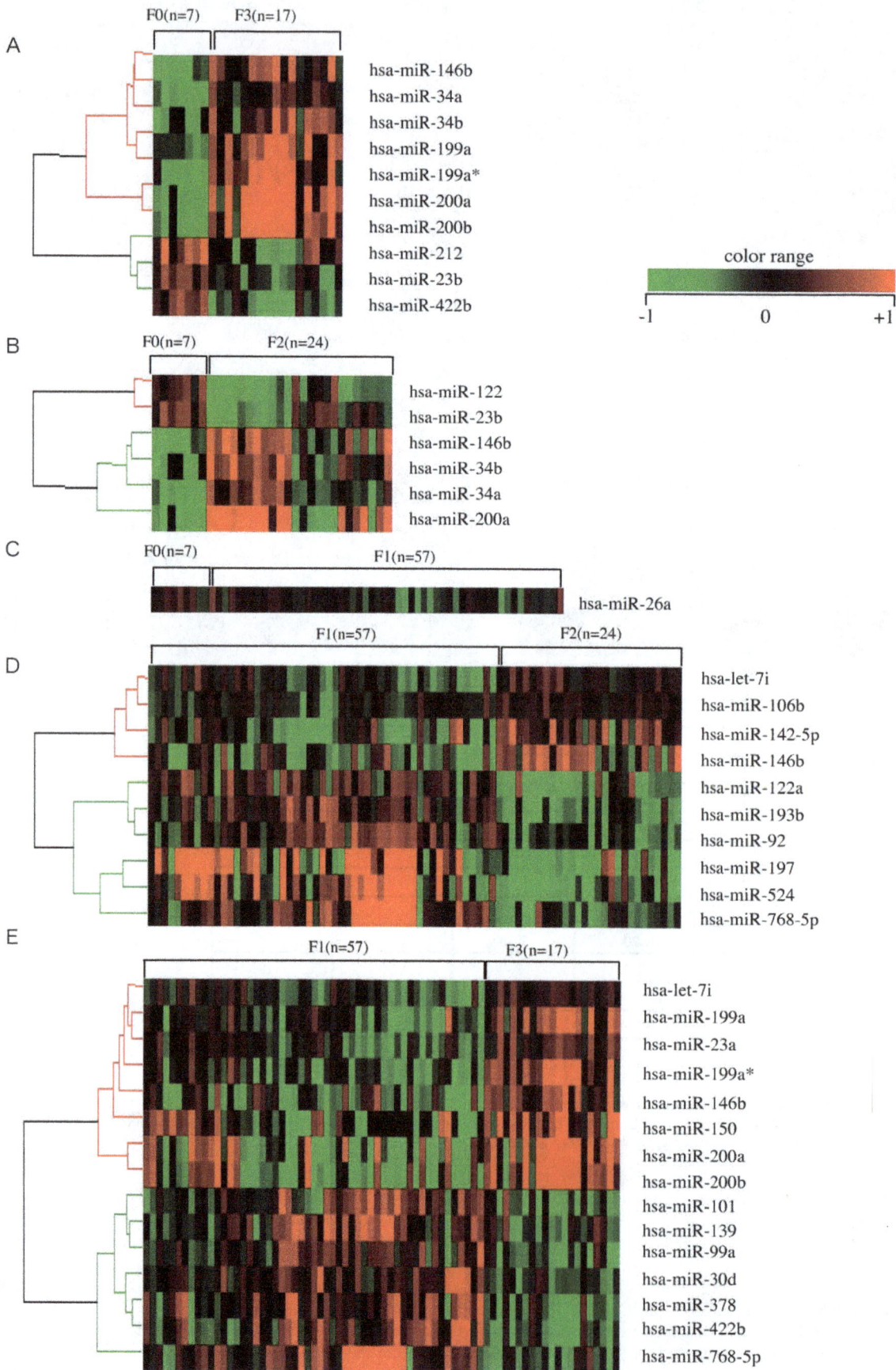

Figure 2. Liver fibrosis in human liver biopsy specimen. A. B. C. D. and E. miRNAs whose expression differs significantly between F0 and F3, F0 and F1, F0 and F2, F1 and F2, and F1 and F3, respectively. Relative expression level of each miRNA in human liver biopsy specimen by microarray. Data from microarray were also statistically analyzed using Welch's test and the Bonferroni correction for multiple hypotheses testing. Fold change, p-value are listed in Table S2.

specific E3 ubiquitin protein ligase 2 (SMURF2), both of which play roles in the TGFβ signaling pathway, are candidate targets of miR-199a* and miR-200b, respectively, as determined by the Targetscan algorithm. The expression of miR-199a* was silenced in several proliferating cell lines excluding fibroblasts [21]. Down regulation of miR-199a, miR-199a* and 200a in chronic liver injury tissue was associated with the hepatocarcinogenesis [9]. miR-199a* is also one of the negative regulators of the HCV replication [22]. According to three target search algorithms (Pictar, miRanda, and Targetscan), the miRNAs that may be associated with the liver fibrosis can regulate several fibrosis-related genes (Table S4). Aberrant expression of these miRNAs may be closely related to the progress of the chronic liver disease.

Epithelial-mesenchymal transition (EMT) describes a reversible series of events during which an epithelial cell loses cell-cell contacts and acquires mesenchymal characteristics [23]. Although EMT is not a common event in adults, this process has been implicated in such instances as wound healing and fibrosis. Recent reports showed that the miR-200 family regulated EMT by targeting EMT accelerator ZEB1 and SIP1 [24]. From our

observations, overexpression of miR-200a and miR-200b can be connected to the progression of liver fibrosis.

The diagnosis and quantification of fibrosis have traditionally relied on liver biopsy, and this is still true at present. However, there are a number of drawbacks to biopsy, including the invasive nature of the procedure and inter-observer variability. A number of staging systems have been developed to reduce both the inter-observer variability and intra-observer variability, including the METAVIR, the Knodell fibrosis score, and the Scheuer score. However, the reproducibility of hepatic fibrosis and inflammatory activity is not as consistent [25]. In fact, in our study, the degree of fibrosis of the two arbitrary fibrosis groups was classified using the miRNA expression profile with 80% or greater accuracy (data not shown). Thus, miRNA expression can be used for diagnosis of liver fibrosis.

In this study we investigated whether common miRNAs in human and mouse could influence the progression of the liver fibrosis. The signature of miRNAs expression can also serves as a tool for understanding and investigating the mechanism of the onset and progression of liver fibrosis. The miRNA expression profile has the potential to be a novel biomarker of liver fibrosis.

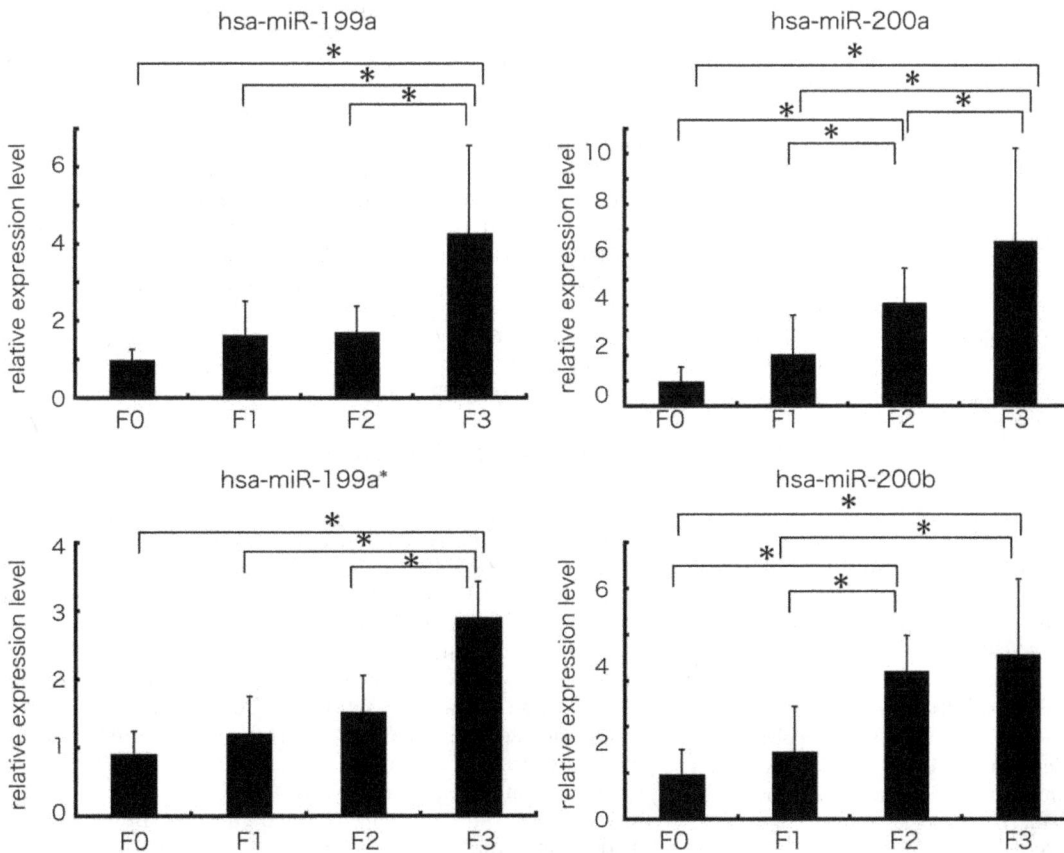

Figure 3. The expression level of miR-199 and 200 families in human liver biopsy specimen by real-time qPCR. Real-time qPCR validation of the 4 miRNAs (miR-199a, miR-199a*, miR-200a, and miR-200b). Each column represents the relative amount of miRNAs normalized to the expression level of U18. The data shown are the means+SD of three independent experiments. Asterisks indicates to a significant difference of p<0.05 (two-tailed Student-t test), respectively.

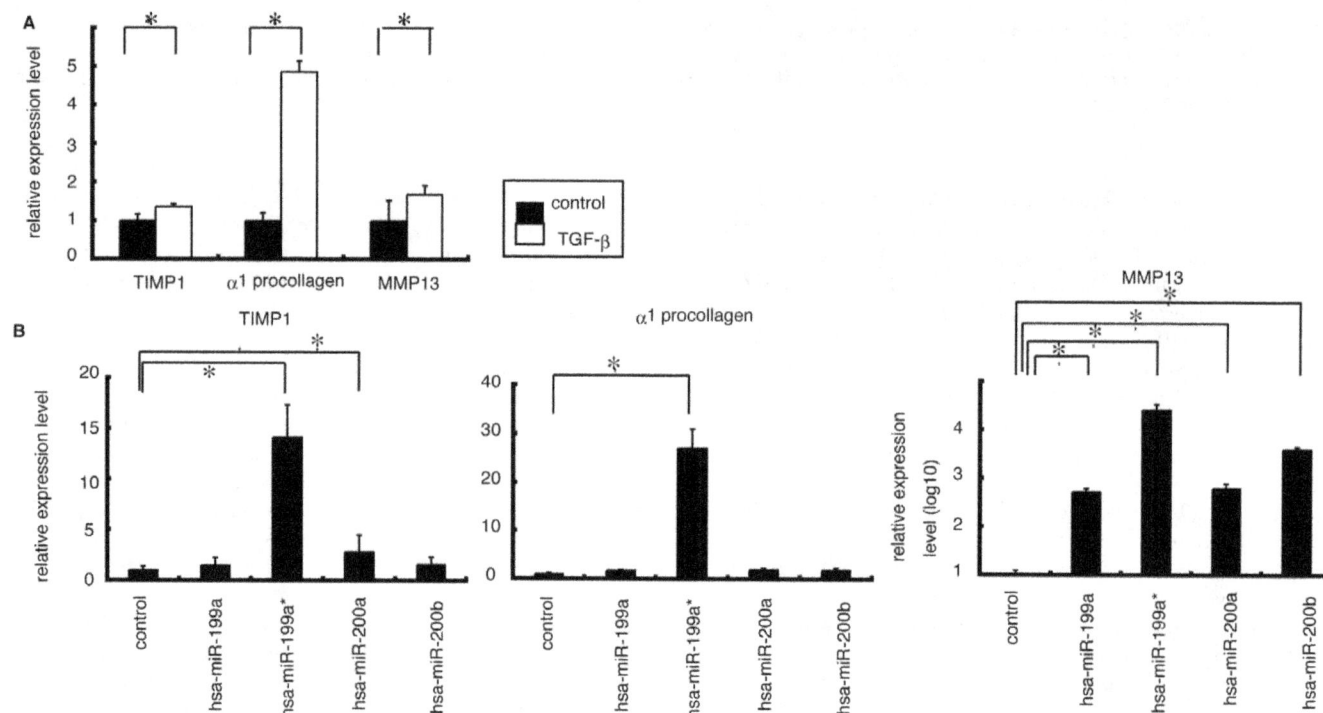

Figure 4. The relationship between expression level of miR-199 and 200 families and expression level of three fibrosis related genes. A. Administration of TGFβ in LX2 cells showed that the expression level of three fibrosis related genes were higher than that in non-treated cells. The data shown are the means+SD of three independent experiments. Asterisk was indicated to the significant difference of p<0.05 (two-tailed Student-t test). B. The expression levels of 3 fibrosis related genes in LX2 cells with overexpressing miR-199a, 199a*, 200a, or 200b, respectively were significantly higher than that in cells transfected with control miRNA (p<0.05; two-tailed Student t-test).

Moreover miRNA expression profiling has further applications in novel anti-fibrosis therapy in CH.

Materials and Methods

Sample preparation

105 liver tissues samples from chronic hepatitis C patients (genotype 1b) were obtained by fine needle biopsy (Table S1). METAVIR fibrosis stages were F0 in 7 patients, F1 in 57, F2 in 24 and F3 in 17. Patients with autoimmune hepatitis or alcoholic liver injury were excluded. None of the patients were positive for hepatitis B virus associated antigen/ antibody or anti human immunodeficiency virus antibody. No patient received interferon therapy or immunomodulatory therapy prior to the enrollment in this study. We also obtained normal liver tissue from the Liver Transplantation Unit of Kyoto University. All of the patients or their guardians provided written informed consent, and Kyoto University Graduate School and Faculty of Medicine's Ethics Committee approved all aspects of this study in accordance with the Helsinki Declaration.

RNA preparation and miRNA microarray

Total RNA from cell lines or tissue samples was prepared using a *mir*Vana miRNA extraction Kit (Ambion, Austin, TX, USA) according to the manufacturer's instruction. miRNA microarrays were manufactured by Agilent Technologies (Santa Clara, CA, USA) and 100 ng of total RNA was labeled and hybridized using the Human microRNA Microarray Kit protocol for use with Agilent microRNA microarrays Version 1.5 and Mouse microRNA Microarray Kit protocol for use with Agilent microRNA microarrays Version 1.0. Hybridization signals were detected with a DNA microarray scanner G2505B (Agilent Technologies) and

the scanned images were analyzed using Agilent feature extraction software (v9.5.3.1). Data were analyzed using GeneSpring GX 7.3.1 software (Agilent Technologies) and normalized as follows: (i) Values below 0.01 were set to 0.01. (ii) In order to compare between one-color expression profile, each measurement was divided by the 75th percentile of all measurements from the same species. The data presented in this manuscript have been deposited in NCBI's Gene Expression Omnibus and are accessible through GEO Series accession number GSE16922 (human) and accession number GSE19865 (mouse).

Real-time qPCR for human miRNA

For detection of the miRNA level by real-time qPCR, TaqMan® microRNA assay (Applied Biosystems) was used to quantify the relative expression level of miR-199a (assay ID. 002304), miR-199a* (assay ID. 000499), miR-200a (assay ID. 000502), miR-200b (assay ID. 002251), and U18 (assay ID. 001204) was used as an internal control. cDNA was synthesized using the Taqman miRNA RT Kit (Applied Biosystems). Total RNA (10 ng/ml) in 5ml of nuclease free water was added to 3 ml of 5× RT primer, 10× 1.5μl of reverse transcriptase buffer, 0.15 μl of 100 mM dNTP, 0.19 μl of RNase inhibitor, 4.16 μl of nuclease free water, and 50U of reverse transcriptase in a total volume of 15 μl. The reaction was performed for 30 min at 16°C, 30 min at 42°C, and 5 min at 85°C. All reactions were run in triplicate. Chromo 4 detector (BIO-RAD) was used to detect miRNA expression.

Animal and Chronic Mouse Liver Injury Model

Each 5 adult (8-week-old) male C57BL/6J mice were given a biweekly intra-peritoneal dose of a 10% solution of CCL$_4$ in olive oil (0.02 ml/g/ mouse) for the first 4 weeks and then once a week for the next 4 weeks. At week 4, 6 or 8, the mice were sacrificed. Partial livers were fixed, embedded in paraffin, and processed for histology. Serial liver sections were stained with hematoxylin-eosin, Azan staining, Silver (Ag) staining, and Elastica van Gieson (EVG) staining, respectively. Total RNA from mice liver tissue was prepared as described previously. All animal procedures concerning the analysis of liver injury were performed in following the guidelines of the Kyoto University Animal Research Committee and were approved by the Ethical Committee of the Faculty of Medicine, Kyoto University.

Cell lines and Cell preparation

The human stellate cell lines LX-2, was provided by Scott L. Friedman. LX-2 cells, which viable in serum free media and have high transfectability, were established from human HSC lines [26]. LX-2 cells were maintained in D-MEM (Invitrogen, Carlsbad, CA, USA) with 10% fetal bovine serum, plated in 60 mm diameter dishes and cultured to 70% confluence. Huh-7 and Hela cells were also maintained in D-MEM with 10% fetal bovine serum. HuS-E/2 immortalized hepatocytes were cultured as described previously [27]. LX-2 cells were then cultured in D-MEM without serum with 0.2% BSA for 48 hours prior to TGFβ1 (Sigma-Aldrich, Suffolk, UK) treatment (2.5 ng/ml for 20 hours). Control cells were cultured in D-MEM without fetal bovine serum.

miRNA transfection

LX-2 cells were plated in 6-well plates the day before transfection and grown to 70% confluence. Cells were transfected with 50 pmol of Silencer® negative control siRNA (Ambion) or double-stranded mature miRNA (Hokkaido System Science, Sapporo, Japan) using lipofectamine RNAiMAX (Invitrogen). Cells were harvested 2 days after transfection.

Real-time qPCR

cDNA was synthesized using the Transcriptor High Fidelity cDNA synthesis Kit (Roche, Basel, Switzerland). Total RNA (2 μg) in 10.4 μl of nuclease free water was added to 1 μl of 50mM random hexamer. The denaturing reaction was performed for 10min at 65°C. The denatured RNA mixture was added to 4 μl of 5× reverse transcriptase buffer, 2 μl of 10 mM dNTP, 0.5 μl of 40U/μl RNase inhibitor, and 1.1 μl of reverse transcriptase (FastStart Universal SYBR Green Master (Roche) in a total volume of 20 μl. The reaction ran for 30 min at 50°C (cDNA synthesis), and five min at 85°C (enzyme denaturation). All reactions were run in triplicate. Chromo 4 detector (BIO-RAD, Hercules, CA, USA) was used to detect mRNA expression. The primer sequences are follows; MMP13 s; 5'-gaggctccgagaaatgcagt-3', as; 5'-atgccatcgtgaagtctggt-3', TIMP1 s; 5'-cttggcttctgcactgatgg-3', as; 5'-acgctggtataaggtggtct-3', α1-procollagen s; 5'-aacatgaccaaaaaccaaaagtg-3', as; 5'-catt-

gtttcctgtgtcttctgg-3', and β-actin s; 5'-ccactggcatcgtgatggac-3', as; 5'-tcattgccaatggtgatgacct-3'. Assays were performed in triplicate, and the expression levels of target genes were normalized to expression of the β-actin gene, as quantified using real-time qPCR as internal controls.

Statistical analyses

Statistical analyses were performed using Student's t-test; p values less than 0.05 were considered statistically significant. Microarray data were also statistically analyzed using Welch's test and Bonferroni correction for multiple hypotheses testing.

Supporting Information

Figure S1 Time line of the induction of chronic liver fibrosis. Upward arrow indicated administration of olive oil or CCL_4. Downward arrow indicates when mice were sacrificed.

Figure S2 Comparison of the expression level of miR-199 and 200 familes in several cell lines and human liver tissue. Endogenous expression level of miR-199a, 199a*, 200a, and 200b in normal liver and LX2 cell as determined by microarray analysis (Agilent Technologies). Endogenous expression level of same miRNAs in Hela, Huh-7 and, immortalized hepatocyte: HuS-E/2 by previously analyzed data [9].

Table S1 Clinical characteristics of patients by the grade of fibrosis.

Table S2 Extracted human miRNAs related to liver fibrosis.

Table S3 Corresponding human and mouse miRNAs.

Table S4 Hypothetical miRNA target genes according to in silico analysis.

Author Contributions

Conceived and designed the experiments: YM KS. Performed the experiments: YM HT YH NK. Analyzed the data: MT MK. Contributed reagents/materials/analysis tools: YM HT YH NK. Wrote the paper: YM MT AT FM NK TO.

References

1. Wasley A, Alter MJ (2000) Epidemiology of hepatitis C: geographic differences and temporal trends. Semin Liver Dis 20: 1–16.
2. Shepard CW, Finelli L, Alter MJ (2005) Global epidemiology of hepatitis C virus infection. Lancet Infect Dis 5: 558–567.
3. Gressner AM, Weiskirchen R (2006) Modern pathogenetic concepts of liver fibrosis suggest stellate cells and TGF-beta as major players and therapeutic targets. J Cell Mol Med 10: 76–99.
4. Nilsen TW (2007) Mechanisms of microRNA-mediated gene regulation in animal cells. Trends Genet 23: 243–249.
5. Zamore PD, Haley B (2005) Ribo-gnome: the big world of small RNAs. Science 309: 1519–1524.
6. Pillai RS (2005) MicroRNA function: multiple mechanisms for a tiny RNA? Rna 11: 1753–1761.
7. Ura S, Honda M, Yamashita T, Ueda T, Takatori H, et al. (2009) Differential microRNA expression between hepatitis B and hepatitis C leading disease progression to hepatocellular carcinoma. Hepatology 49: 1098–1112.

8. Yamamoto Y, Kosaka N, Tanaka M, Koizumi F, Kanai Y, et al. (2009) MicroRNA-500 as a potential diagnostic marker for hepatocellular carcinoma. Biomarkers 14: 529–538.
9. Murakami Y, Yasuda T, Saigo K, Urashima T, Toyoda H, et al. (2006) Comprehensive analysis of microRNA expression patterns in hepatocellular carcinoma and non-tumorous tissues. Oncogene 25: 2537–2545.
10. Jin X, Ye YF, Chen SH, Yu CH, Liu J, et al. (2008) MicroRNA expression pattern in different stages of nonalcoholic fatty liver disease. Dig Liver Dis.
11. Ogawa T, Iizuka M, Sekiya Y, Yoshizato K, Ikeda K, et al. (2009) Suppression of type I collagen production by microRNA-29b in cultured human stellate cells. Biochem Biophys Res Commun.
12. Ji J, Zhang J, Huang G, Qian J, Wang X, et al. (2009) Over-expressed microRNA-27a and 27b influence fat accumulation and cell proliferation during rat hepatic stellate cell activation. FEBS Lett 583: 759–766.
13. Wienholds E, Kloosterman WP, Miska E, Alvarez-Saavedra E, Berezikov E, et al. (2005) MicroRNA expression in zebrafish embryonic development. Science 309: 310–311.

14. Landgraf P, Rusu M, Sheridan R, Sewer A, Iovino N, et al. (2007) A mammalian microRNA expression atlas based on small RNA library sequencing. Cell 129: 1401–1414.

15. Friedman SL (2008) Hepatic fibrosis-Overview. Toxicology.

16. Roderburg C, Urban GW, Bettermann K, Vucur M, Zimmermann H, et al. (2010) Micro-RNA profiling reveals a role for miR-29 in human and murine liver fibrosis. Hepatology.

17. Venugopal SK, Jiang J, Kim TH, Li Y, Wang SS, et al. (2010) Liver fibrosis causes downregulation of miRNA-150 and miRNA-194 in hepatic stellate cells, and their overexpression causes decreased stellate cell activation. Am J Physiol Gastrointest Liver Physiol 298: G101–106.

18. Jiang J, Gusev Y, Aderca I, Mettler TA, Nagorney DM, et al. (2008) Association of MicroRNA expression in hepatocellular carcinomas with hepatitis infection, cirrhosis, and patient survival. Clin Cancer Res 14: 419–427.

19. Jiang X, Tsitsiou E, Herrick SE, Lindsay MA (2010) MicroRNAs and the regulation of fibrosis. Febs J 277: 2015–2021.

20. Marquez RT, Bandyopadhyay S, Wendlandt EB, Keck K, Hoffer BA, et al. (2010) Correlation between microRNA expression levels and clinical parameters associated with chronic hepatitis C viral infection in humans. Lab Invest.

21. Kim S, Lee UJ, Kim MN, Lee EJ, Kim JY, et al. (2008) MicroRNA miR-199a* regulates the MET proto-oncogene and the downstream extracellular signal-regulated kinase 2 (ERK2). J Biol Chem 283: 18158–18166.

22. Murakami Y, Aly HH, Tajima A, Inoue I, Shimotohno K (2009) Regulation of the hepatitis C virus genome replication by miR-199a. J Hepatol 50: 453–460.

23. Gibbons DL, Lin W, Creighton CJ, Rizvi ZH, Gregory PA, et al. (2009) Contextual extracellular cues promote tumor cell EMT and metastasis by regulating miR-200 family expression. Genes Dev 23: 2140–2151.

24. Gregory PA, Bert AG, Paterson EL, Barry SC, Tsykin A, et al. (2008) The miR-200 family and miR-205 regulate epithelial to mesenchymal transition by targeting ZEB1 and SIP1. Nat Cell Biol 10: 593–601.

25. Oberti F, Valsesia E, Pilette C, Rousselet MC, Bedossa P, et al. (1997) Noninvasive diagnosis of hepatic fibrosis or cirrhosis. Gastroenterology 113: 1609–1616.

26. Xu L, Hui AY, Albanis E, Arthur MJ, O'Byrne SM, et al. (2005) Human hepatic stellate cell lines, LX-1 and LX-2: new tools for analysis of hepatic fibrosis. Gut 54: 142–151.

27. Aly HH, Watashi K, Hijikata M, Kaneko H, Takada Y, et al. (2007) Serum-derived hepatitis C virus infectivity in interferon regulatory factor-7-suppressed human primary hepatocytes. J Hepatol 46: 26–36.

7

Truncated Active Human Matrix Metalloproteinase-8 Delivered by a Chimeric Adenovirus-Hepatitis B Virus Vector Ameliorates Rat Liver Cirrhosis

Jinxia Liu[1,9], Xin Cheng[1,9], Zhengrong Guo[1,9], Zihua Wang[1], Dong Li[1], Fubiao Kang[1], Haijun Li[1], Baosheng Li[1], Zhichen Cao[2], Michael Nassal[3]*, Dianxing Sun[1]*

1 The Liver Diseases Diagnosis and Treatment Center of PLA, Bethune International Peace Hospital, Shijiazhuang, People's Republic of China, 2 Department of Traditional Chinese Medicine and Liver Disease, The Third Affiliated Hospital of Hebei Medical University, Shijiazhuang, People's Republic of China, 3 University Hospital Freiburg, Internal Medicine II/Molecular Biology, Freiburg, Germany

Abstract

Background: Liver cirrhosis is a potentially life-threatening disease caused by progressive displacement of functional hepatocytes by fibrous tissue. The underlying fibrosis is often driven by chronic infection with hepatitis B virus (HBV). Matrix metalloproteinases including MMP-8 are crucial for excess collagen degradation. In a rat model of liver cirrhosis, MMP-8 delivery by an adenovirus (Ad) vector achieved significant amelioration of fibrosis but application of Ad vectors in humans is subject to various issues, including a lack of intrinsic liver specificity.

Methods: HBV is highly liver-specific and its principal suitability as liver-specific gene transfer vector is established. HBV vectors have a limited insertion capacity and are replication-defective. Conversely, in an HBV infected cell vector replication may be rescued *in trans* by the resident virus, allowing conditional vector amplification and spreading. Capitalizing on a resident pathogen to help in its elimination and/or in treating its pathogenic consequences would provide a novel strategy. However, resident HBV may also reduce susceptibility to HBV vector superinfection. Thus a size-compatible truncated MMP-8 (tMMP8) gene was cloned into an HBV vector which was then used to generate a chimeric Ad-HBV shuttle vector that is not subject to superinfection exclusion. Rats with thioacetamide-induced liver cirrhosis were injected with the chimera to evaluate therapeutic efficacy.

Results: Our data demonstrate that infectious HBV vector particles can be obtained via *trans*-complementation by wild-type virus, and that the tMMP8 HBV vector can efficiently be shuttled by an Ad vector into cirrhotic rat livers. There it exerted a comparable beneficial effect on fibrosis and hepatocyte proliferation markers as a conventional full-length MMP-8Ad vector.

Conclusions: Though the rat cirrhosis model does not allow assessing *in vivo* HBV vector amplification these results advocate the further development of Ad-HBV vectors for liver-specific gene therapy, including and perhaps particularly for HBV-related disease.

Editor: Haitao Guo, Drexel University College of Medicine, United States of America

Funding: This work was supported by National Natural Science Foundation of China (grant numbers: 30872255; 30571667, URL of the funder's website, http://isisn.nsfc.gov.cn/egrantweb/) and Chinese Foundation for Hepatitis Prevention and Control, Wang Baoen Liver Fibrosis Foundation (grant number: 20070001, URL of funder's website, http://www.wbelff.org/keti.php). The funders had no role in study design, data collection and analysis, decision to publish, or preparation of the manuscript.

Competing Interests: The authors have declared that no competing interests exist.

* E-mail: sundianxing@hotmail.com (DS); nassal2@ukl.uni-freiburg.de (MN)

9 These authors contributed equally to this work.

Introduction

Liver cirrhosis is a chronic, progressive condition characterized by fibrosis and the conversion of normal liver architecture into structurally abnormal nodules [1,2]. Frequently, liver cirrhosis precedes hepatocellular carcinoma [3]. Prevention, detection and therapy pose serious challenges to clinical management and engender major health costs worldwide [4,5]. The etiologies of liver injury resulting in cirrhosis are diverse, but globally 30%, and in China up to 66% of cirrhosis are attributed to hepatitis B virus

(HBV) infection [6]. Cirrhosis emerges successively from liver fibrosis [7], a progressive imbalance between fibrogenesis and fibrolysis leading to deposition of extracellular matrix (ECM) proteins, mostly from activated hepatic stellate cells [8]. Type I collagen accounts for 60%–70% of the total collagen in fibrotic livers [9,10,11].

Progression of experimental liver cirrhosis is accompanied by a gradual loss of collagenolytic activity in liver tissue [12,13]. The major collagenases are the matrix metalloproteinases (MMPs) MMP-1, MMP-8, MMP-13 [14,15]. They are synthe-

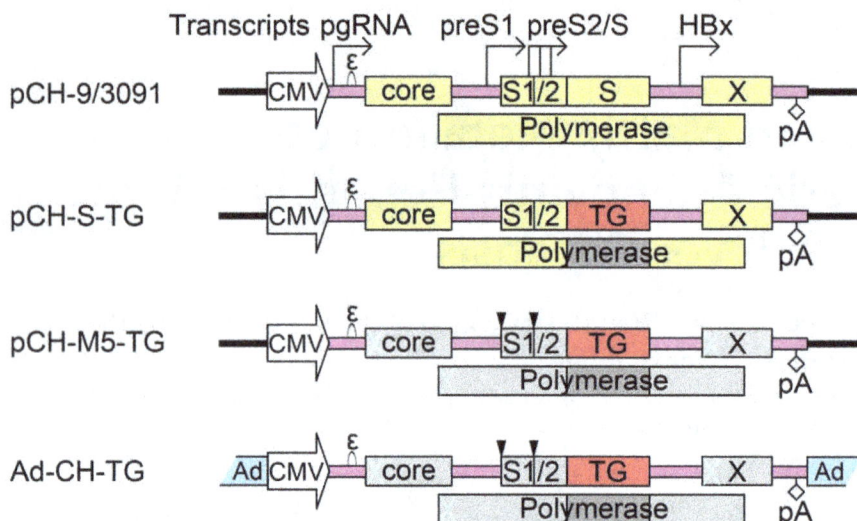

Figure 1. HBV vector constructs used. All constructs were based on the wild-type HBV expression plasmid pCH-9/3091 which contains a complete HBV genome. Open reading frames are depicted as yellow boxes. Transcription of the pregenomic (pg) RNA is under control of the CMV-IE promoter. The start sites for transcripts controlled by the endogenous preS1, preS2/S and HBx promoters are indicated by the rightward pointing arrows. "ε" denotes the RNA packaging signal whose interaction with the polymerase initiates pgRNA encapsidation and reverse transcription. The diamond labeled pA symbolizes the HBV polyadenylation signal. In first generation HBV vectors, represented by pCH-S-TG, the transgene (TG) replaced the viral S gene. Here, eGFP, RFP2 and Luc were used as transgenes. These vectors still produce core and X protein, plus truncated forms of polymerase (region covered with dark slash lines) and PreS1/PreS2 (pS1, pS2) gene products. For vector production, functional polymerase and surface proteins are provided in trans by a helper plasmid, e.g. pCH3142 which is identical to pCH-9/3091 except it lacks the "ε" signal. In the pCH-M5-TG vectors, expression of the endogenous HBV gene products was ablated by premature stop codons (blue crosses), or mutation of the preS1 and preS2 initiation codons (downward pointing triangles) so as to engage all preS/S transcripts as TG mRNAs; here TG included truncated MMP-8 (tMMP8). For the chimeric Ad-HBV vectors, Ad-CH-TG, the entire HBV vector expression cassettes from the pCH-M5-TG plasmids were incorporated into ΔE1/ΔE3 Ad-vector backbones. Ad-C-MMP8 contained full-length MMP-8 under CMV promoter control, but no HBV sequences.

sized as about 470 amino acid latent preproproteins which are activated by removal of the prepro sequences comprising the first 100 residues. Activation of MMPs is controlled by the tissue inhibitors of metalloproteinases (TIMPs) [16,17]. Failure to degrade excessive ECM can thus result from insufficient expression and/or activation of MMPs, or from up-regulation of TIMPs. Plausible therapeutic approaches beyond removal of the fibrotic stimuli underlying liver injury [7] might hence include inhibition of TIMPs or increased expression of collagenases [7,18,19].

Experimental proof of concept for the latter strategy has been obtained in two studies that employed adenovirus (Ad) vector-mediated delivery of MMP-1 and MMP-8 genes into experimental rat models of fibrosis [20]. The results showed indeed regression of fibrosis and, as an additional benefit, induction of hepatocyte proliferation [21,22].

Hence MMP delivery as such appears promising for treatment of liver fibrosis and cirrhosis yet application of Ad vectors in human liver gene therapy is currently restricted by issues of safety, and efficacy and sustainability of heterologous gene transduction [23]. At high doses favoring efficient trans-duction, the Ad vector particles may trigger excessive innate and adaptive immune responses. Less vigorous responses upon lower dose administration may still prevent repeated application of the vector although this may often be desirable due to the transient expression of Ad vector-transduced genes. Intrave-neously administered Ad vectors accumulate preferentially in the liver [24], but they have an intrinsically broad tropism for epithelial-derived cells in other tissues [25], especially the upper respiratory tract, which may increase the risk of systemic delivery [23]. In contrast, HBV has a strict hepatocyte tropism making it a principally useful vehicle for liver-specific gene

transfer. Moreover, transgenes controlled by the endogenous HBV promoter/enhancer elements may preferentially be expressed in hepatocytes, thus contributing to liver specificity. HBV and its related animal viruses, e.g. duck HBV (DHBV), are small (genome size about 3 kb) enveloped DNA viruses that replicate through reverse transcription [26,27]. This requires that the greater-than-genome length pregenomic (pg) RNA be co-packaged with the viral polymerase into newly forming nucleocapsids, inside of which reverse transcription occurs. This and the extremely compact genome organization (see Fig. 1) with numerous overlapping open reading frames (ORFs) and regulatory cis-elements has hampered early attempts to harness HBV into a gene-transfer vector by simple insertion of foreign sequences. However, replacement of the S gene by similarly sized heterologous sequences turned out as a viable strategy [28]. Once the vector has entered the target cell and the incoming relaxed-circular (RC) DNA is converted into nuclear covalently closed circular DNA (cccDNA), transcription of the foreign gene is then controlled by the endogenous HBV preS1 and preS2/S promoters which in the authentic virus direct synthesis of the mRNAs for the L protein (PreS1/PreS2/S), and the M (PreS2/S) and S proteins (Fig. 1); especially the preS1 promoter shows a high specificity for differentiated hepatocyte-derived cells [29]. The simultaneous loss of functional surface proteins and polymerase is rescued by cotransfection of the vector with a helper plasmid such as pCH3142, which harbors a slightly truncated HBV genome that provides all necessary viral proteins in trans but itself is not packaged because the 5' proximal RNA encapsidation signal ε is deleted [30]. HBV vectors obtained in this way selectively accumulated in the liver after inoculation into peripheral vessels, efficiently infected quiescent hepatocytes, and successfully transduced genes for green fluorescent protein (GFP) and type I interferon (IFN-α). The IFN-α vector substantially suppressed replication of resident HBV. These data suggested that HBV-based vectors may also become useful against other liver diseases [31]. However, appropriate effector genes have to be smaller than about 1 kb.

HBV vectors produced in this way are infectious but replication-defective, i.e. they cannot reproduce and transgene expression is transient. However, analogous to *trans*-complementation by a helper plasmid during vector production, a vector entering a wild-type HBV-infected hepatocyte may be rescued *in trans*, leading to a second generation of recombinant virions that can infect surrounding hepatocytes. Hence the therapeutic vector might be amplified *in situ* and maintain transgene expression as long as wild-type HBV is present. The most obvious application would be vectors that directly target the resident wild-type HBV because vector spread would be self-limited by the progressive loss of HBV infected cells capable of trans-complementation. The potential helper functions of wild-type HBV might also be capitalized upon when targeting the sequelae of chronic HBV infection such as liver cirrhosis, especially in the light of the large number of patients suffering from this condition.

At present, however, this concept is theoretical because several basic issues have not yet been experimentally addressed. Particularly important are the unknown ability of the HBV vector to be complemented by wild-type HBV rather than a designed helper construct, and overcoming superinfection exclusion by which a resident virus impairs infection of its host cell by another virus using the same infection route. For DHBV, this phenomenon is well established [32]. Not the least, therapeutic benefit of an HBV vector-based therapy has not yet been demonstrated in an *in vivo* disease model.

The aim of this study was therefore to address several of these outstanding questions, using the *in vivo* fibrosis model data available for full-length MMP-8 transduction by a conventional Ad vector [33] as a reference.

Several prior studies facilitated in realization of the current approach. First, previous data on HBV vector design [28,34] provided a basis for further vector improvements. Second, a truncated MMP-8 encompassing aa 100–262, a-tMMP-8 (for simplicity termed tMMP8 below) can be recombinantly expressed and secreted and is still capable of degrading exogenously accumulated extracellular type I collagen [35]. Lacking the prosequence it does not require proteolytic activation, and with about 600 bp the coding region easily accomodates into HBV vectors. Third, we and others have previously demonstrated that complete wild-type HBV genomes can be incorporated into conventional Ad vectors and efficiently be transduced into human cell lines and primary hepatocytes, with production of HBV cccDNA, and into animals [36,37]. This might also hold for recombinant HBV vector genomes. The different infection route of adenovirus vs. HBV should circumvent any superinfection exclusion problems, enabling efficient initial deposition of the Ad vector-shuttled HBV vector also in HBV infected cells. The results shown below strongly suggest that the concept of Ad-vector shuttled HBV vector delivery into the liver is feasible. Importantly, the truncated tMMP8 embedded into the HBV part of the chimeric Ad-HBV vector maintained key therapeutic features previously seen with conventional Ad vector delivery of full-length MMP-8 [33,38], namely a similarly efficient reduction of fibrosis and cirrhosis, and in addition the activation of signals promoting hepatocyte proliferation.

Materials and Methods

Ethics Statement

This study was performed in strict accordance with the recommendations in the guidelines (Animal Research: Reporting *In vivo* Experiments) developed by the National Center for the Replacement, Refinement and Reduction of Animal's in Research, London, UK. The protocols for animal experiments were approved by the Medical Ethics Committee of Bethune International Peace Hospital (Permit Number: 2009–19). Only the minimal number of required animals was used. All rats were kept under species-appropriate conditions, with sufficient supply and convenient access of food and water. All surgery was performed under sodium pentobarbital anesthesia, and every effort was made to minimize suffering.

Cell Culture, Transfection, and HepaRG Cell Infection

HepG2 cells (American Type Culture Collection) were cultured in high glucose Dulbecco's minimal essential medium (Thermo Scientific) supplemented with 10% heat-inactivated fetal bovine serum (Thermo Scientific), 2 mM L-glutamine, 100 μg streptomycin/ml, and 100 U of penicillin G ml^{-1} and buffered with sodium bicarbonate (complete medium), 1% (v/v) non-essential amino acid (Invitrogen), in a fully humidified atmosphere containing 5% CO_2, 95% air at 37°C. Fugene HD (Roche) was used for plasmid transfection. HepaRG cells (Biopredic International, France) were cultured and differentiated as described [39]. For infection, viral particles in the culture supernatants from HepG2 cells cotransfected with a 1:1 mixture of plasmids pCH-M5-GFP and pCH-9/3091 were concentrated by PEG 8000 precipitation. Prior to precipitation, DNase I (Takara) and micrococcal nuclease (Fermentas) were used to minimize residual plasmid DNA so as to exclude uptake and potential gene expression from internalized plasmids. Nominal viral titers, reflecting the sum of wild-type and recombinant virus, were determined by quantitative PCR (qPCR) with a commercial HBV DNA quantification kit (Shanghai Kehua Bio-engineering Co., Ltd, Shanghai, China) and expressed as viral genome equivalents (vge) per ml. Inoculation of the HepaRG cells was performed in the presence of 4% PEG 8000 as described [39], using about 5×10^8 vge per 10^5 cells in one well of a six-well plate. The virus inoculum was left on the cells for 48 hours and then replaced by fresh medium.

Fluorescence Imaging and Luciferase Activity Assay

GFP expression was detected using a fluorescence microscope (Leica, Germany), 48 hours after transfection of HepG2 cells, or six days after infection of HepaRG cells. Expression of red fluorescent protein 2 (RFP2) in frozen sections of recombinant adenovirus infected rat liver was also detected by fluorescence microscopy. Firefly luciferase (pGL3-control, Promega) and Renilla luciferase activity were measured 48 hours after co-transfection by the Dual-Luciferase Reporter Assay System (Promega, USA) as recommended by the manufacture.

Plasmid Construction

Plasmid pCH-S-GFP had been derived from the wild-type HBV (Genbank accession no: V01460, formerly J02203) expression vector pCH-9/3091 [40] by replacing the S gene with a gene of eGFP [28]. To prevent expression of endogenous HBV proteins, the following mutations were introduced into pCH-S-GFP, yielding plasmid pCH-M5-GFP (nucleotide numbers refer to the position of the A in core gene initiation codon): G28T (GGA to TGA), T444A (TTG to TAG), C2677T (CAA to TAA). These mutations introduce premature stop codons in the core, polymerase, and X gene respectively. Knock-out of the PreS1 and PreS2 start codons involved mutations T949C (ATG to ACG) and T1273C (ATG to ACG) [41]. Plasmids pCH-S-RFP2 and pCH-M5-RFP2, and the corresponding firefly luciferase constructs pCH-S-Luc and pCH-M5-Luc were obtained by appropriate gene substitution in pCH-S-GFP and pCH-M5-GFP, respectively. Vector pCH-M5-tMMP8 was analogously constructed by introduction of the PCR product obtained using the primers tMMP8Nco(+): 5'GGC GCC ATG GTA ACC CCA GGA AAC C and tMMP8Spe(−): 5'GCC GAC TAG TCA TCC ATA GAT GGC CTG AAT G on plasmid pGW1GH-MMP8 encoding full-length MMP-8 (Genbank accession no. NP_002415.1; kindly provided by Professor Christopher M. Overall, Canada) as template [42].

For Ad vector construction, the NheI fragments from pCH-M5-tMMP8 and pCH-M5-RFP2 comprising the CMV promoter plus the complete HBV vector part were transferred into plasmid pDC312-hrGFP, a derivative of the shuttle plasmid pDC312 (AdMax system; Microbix, Canada), yielding plasmids pDC-CH-tMMP8 and pDC-CH-RFP2. The corresponding shuttle plasmid for full-length MMP-8, pDC-C-MMP8, was obtained by subcloning the Spe I to BamH I fragment from pGW1GH-MMP8, comprising CMV promoter, full-length MMP8 coding sequence and SV40 polyA signal, into pDC312-hrGFP.

Recombinant Ad-vectors and Ad-HBV Chimeric Vectors

Shuttle plasmids pDC-CH-tMMP8, pDC-C-MMP8 and pDC-CH-RFP2 were recombined with adenovirus rescue plasmid pBHGloxΔ-E1,3Cre in HEK293 cells according to the protocols provided with the AdMax system. Briefly, HEK293 cells were seeded in 6-well plates (1.2×10^6 cells per well) 24 h ahead of transfection and cultured with 10% (v/v) fetal bovine serum supplemented DMEM (Invitrogen,USA) at 37°C, 5% CO_2. Cells were then co-transfected with 5 μg shuttle plasmid and 25 μg rescue plasmid using FuGene 6 reagent (Roche). When visible plaques formed 15 to 20 days post transfection, cells and medium were harvested for virus preparation as previously described [36]. These viruses were then used to infect HEK293 cells in thirty 150 mm dishes. When more than 90% of the cells showed complete cytopathic effect (48–72 h later), viral particles were released from the pelleted cells by three freeze/thaw cycles and purified using cesium chloride density gradients. After removing CsCl from the viral stocks using NAP-25 columns (Sephadex G-25 Medium, Pharmacia), physical titers were determined via optical absorbance at 260 nm. The concentration was calculated using the formula1 OD_{260} unit = 1.1×10^{12} virus particles/ml.

Southern Blotting of HBV Constructs in Cells Transfected by Recombinant HBV

Southern blotting was performed as previously described [43,44,45]. Briefly, cytoplasmic extracts were obtained by suspending the cells in lysis buffer containing 10 mM Tris-HCl (pH8.0), 1 mM EDTA (pH8.0), 150 mM NaCl, 0.2% NP-40 and removing nuclei and cellular debris by centrifugation for 2 min at 13000 rpm, 4°C. The supernatants were adjusted to 6 mM magnesium acetate, 200 μg/ml DNase I, 20 U/ml micrococcal nuclease and 1 mg/ml RNase A, and the reactions were incubated at 37°C for 45 min to digest nonencapsidated DNA. After adding EDTA to 10 mM final concentration, capsid-protected DNA was released by incubation for 3–5 h at 45°C with 800 μg/ml proteinase K and 5% SDS. Following phenol/chloroform extraction, HBV DNA was precipitated using 0.1 volumes of 10 M ammonium acetate, 60 μg/ml GlycogenBlue (Ambion) and 1 volume isopropanol, and washed using 70% ethanol. After gel

electrophoresis, HBV specific DNAs were detected using a ^{32}P-labeled probe obtained by random priming (NEBlot^{TM} Kit) on a 3.2 kb EcoR I fragment containing a complete linear HBV genome.

MMP8 and tMMP8 Detection by Immunoblotting

HepG2 cells were inoculated with Ad-CH-tMMP8, Ad-C-MMP8 and, for control, Ad-CH-RFP2. Four days later, immunoblotting after SDS-PAGE was performed as described [36] using a rabbit polyclonal MMP-8 antibody (Novus Biologicals, USA) which recognizes the segment (aa 107~178) shared between MMP-8 and tMMP-8. Bands were visualized using a peroxidase-conjugated goat anti-rabbit IgG secondary antibody (ZSGB-Bio, China) and the enhanced chemiluminescence kit (Santa Cruz, USA). Tubulin on the same blot was detected as loading control.

Rat Model of Liver Cirrhosis and Infection with Recombinant Adenoviruses

All animal experiments were approved by the Medical Ethics Committee of Bethune International Peace Hospital. Male Wistar rats were acquired from the Laboratory Animal Center of Hebei Medical University. To achieve cirrhosis, drinking water of the treatment group was adjusted to 0.03% (w/v) thioacetamide (TAA; Sigma-Aldrich) for 16 weeks [46]. Rats of the control group were reared in the same way but received normal tap water feeding. After validation of the cirrhosis model, the rats treated with TAA for 16 weeks were randomly divided into four experimental groups of 8 animals each. Ad virus particles were injected at 1.5×10^{11} VP/kg bodyweight through the tail vein.

Detection of mRNAs for Full-length and Truncated MMP-8, Hepatocyte Growth Factor and c-Met

Total RNA from was extracted from HepG2 cells, or 100–150 mg rat liver tissue which was snap frozen and stored at −70°C prior to extraction, using TRIzol Reagent (Invitrogen) following the manufacturer's instructions. Remaining DNA was removed by incubation with RNase-free Dnase I. First-strand cDNA was synthesized from 2 μg total RNA by SuperScript III reverse transcriptase (Invitrogen) with oligo(dT)$_{15}$ primers as recommended by the manufacturer. Quantitative PCR (qPCR) was performed in an SLAN^{TM} Real-Time PCR System (Hongshi, Shanghai, China) using the primers specific for MMP-8, tMMP8, hepatocyte growth factor (HGF; also known as scatter factor), c-Met, and glyceraldehyde-3-phosphate dehydrogenase (GAPDH) as listed in Table 1. Thermal cycling conditions comprised a predenaturation step at 94°C for 5 min and 45 cycles for amplification (denaturation at 94°C for 30 s, annealing at 52~54°C for 30 s, extension and data collection at 72°C for 30 s). PCR was performed using the standard curve method for relative quantification of gene expression. Results for each sample were calculated as a ratio of the GAPDH concentration.

Hepatic Hydroxyproline Determination

Liver samples of rats were obtained at the moment of sacrifice, and 150 mg of tissue were frozen, weighed and minced to homogeneity. Hepatic tissue (1 mg) was hydrolyzed with 2 ml 6N HCl for 12 h at 100°C. Hydroxyproline (HYP) content was determined by colorimetric assay at a wavelength of 560 nm as described [47]. The quantity of HYP was calculated against a calibration curve obtained using HYP standards

Table 1. PCR primers for MMP8, tMMP8, HGF, c-Met, and GAPDH mRNA.

Primers		Sequences
tMMP-8	Forward	5-GGCGCCATGGTAACCCCAGGAAACC-3
	Reverse	5-GCCGACTAGTCATCCATAGATGGCCTGAATG-3
MMP-8	Forward	5-CCATCTATGGACTTTCAAGCAAC-3
	Reverse	5-TTGGAAGGGATGGCCAGAATAG-3
HGF	Forward	5-TCAAATGCCAGCCTTGGAATTCC-3
	Reverse	5-TCAAGAGTGTAGCACCATGGC-3
c-Met	Forward	5-AGCTGTACCTTGACCTTAAGC-3
	Reverse	5-TTCAGGGTCTTCCCAATACC-3
GAPDH	Forward	5-TCAAATGCCAGCCTTGGAATTCC-3
	Reverse	5-TCAAGAGTGTAGCACCATGGC-3

(Sigma-Aldrich). Finally, the HYP content in each sample was normalized to the weight of liver tissue in which HYP was quantified.

Sirius Red and Hematoxylin-eosin Staining

Liver tissues were fixed overnight in buffered formaldehyde (10%). After paraffin embedding, the liver tissues were sectioned at 5 μm in thickness. Sections were stained with 0.1% Sirius red in saturated picric acid to visualize collagen deposition [48] with a polarizing microscope. Area-density percent of collagen in fibrotic livers of rats was calculated using the Histogram module of Photoshop 8.0 software (Adobe). Hematoxylin–eosin (HE) staining was simultaneously performed to evaluate the degree of inflammation and pathological progression in liver with standard procedures. Modified Knodell scores for liver fibrosis [49] were determined to stage the inflammation and fibrosis of livers from rats of the different groups.

Immunohistochemistry for Type I Collagen, MMP-8 and tMMP-8

Paraffin-embedded rat liver tissue sections were deparaffinized in xylene, rehydrated in alcohol, and incubated in 3% H_2O_2 to block endogenous peroxidase activity. Each section was incubated with normal goat serum for 30 min at room temperature to block nonspecific antibody-binding sites, then the slides were incubated at 4°C overnight with 1:200 diluted mouse anti rat type I collagen antibody (Abcam), or 1:200 diluted rabbit polyclonal antibody against human MMP-8 aa 107–178, respectively. After subsequent incubation with biotinylated goat anti-mouse IgG (Abcam) for 30 min at 37°C, each slide was twice rinsed in PBS. Peroxidase labeled streptavidin was applied and incubated for 20 min at room temperature according to manufacturer's protocol. Sections were counterstained with hematoxylin (Sigma-Aldrich) for 1 min, then dehydrated and mounted.

Statistical Analysis

All data are presented as mean ± standard deviation unless otherwise stated. Statistical analysis for parametric data was performed using Student's t-test or, where appropriate, ANOVA, and for non-parametric data using Mann–Whitney's U test. Differences were considered statistically significant at P values<0.05. All analyses were processed by SPSS for Windows ver 13.0 (SPSS, Chicago, IL, USA).

Results

Construction of HBV Vectors

The plasmid for the first transgene encoding HBV vector, pCH-S-GFP [28], was derived from the CMV promoter driven wild-type HBV expression vector pCH-9/3091 (Fig. 1A; [40]) by replacing the S gene with a gene for GFP such that GFP encoding mRNAs could be produced from the endogenous HBV sp1 and sp2 promoters normally controlling transcription of the 2.4 kb L protein (PreS1/PreS2/S) mRNA and the 2.1 kb M (PreS2/S) and S protein mRNAs [50]. Here we first generated additional analogous vectors encoding RFP2 and Renilla luciferase, termed pCH-S-RFP and pCH-S-Luc, respectively. A potential drawback of these vectors is that they can still express core protein and HBx protein, as well as C terminally truncated forms of the polymerase and L and M protein which may evoke undesired immune responses or act as transcriptional transactivators [51]. Similar to but not identical with (see below) a previous study [34] we therefore generated a second set of vectors that do not express endogenous HBV gene products. This was achieved by introducing artificial stop codons shortly after the initiation codons of the core, polymerase and X ORFs. For the preS1 and preS2 ORFs, rather than introducing premature stops codons [34], we mutated the initiation codons (Fig. 1). In this way, the transgene initiation codon becomes the first ATG also on the longer PreS2/S and PreS1 promoter driven RNAs which could then contribute to transgene expression (see below). The corresponding plasmids were termed pCH-M5, followed by the name of the encoded transgene. The pCH-S and pCH-M5 plasmids were later on used to generate the respective chimeric Ad-HBV vectors (Fig. 1).

To assess the ability of the new vectors to be trans-complemented, the GFP and RFP2 encoding pCH-S and pCH-M5 vectors were co-transfected into HepG2 cells with the helper plasmid pCH3142 at a 1:1 molar ratio. Previous data had already shown that on their own the pCH-S vectors (due to the massive alterations of the polymerase gene) and the helper plasmid (due to the deletion of the encapsidation signal) are unable to replicate [28,30]. Cells transfected with the wild-type HBV vector pCH-9/3091 served as reference. Subsequently, DNA from intracellular nucleocapsids was analyzed by Southern blotting. As shown in Fig. 2A, trans-complemented pCH-S-GFP generated the typical DNA replication intermediates, i.e. relaxed circular (RC), double-strand linear (DS) and single-stranded (ss) DNA. The lower signal intensities compared to pCH-9/3091 transfected cells likely results from the preferential cis-packaging of the pgRNA from which polymerase is translated [52]. Essentially the same DNA patterns and similar signal intensities were produced by co-transfection of pCH3142 with the new pCH-M5 vectors. Hence neither replacement of the eGFP gene by the gene for RFP2 nor the mutations causing the knock-out of the endogenous HBV genes had a major impact on encapsidation or reverse transcription of the recombinant pgRNAs. Altogether, the modified vectors were as efficiently trans-complemented as the original pCH-S-GFP vector.

Enhanced Transgene Expression by Abolishing the preS1 and preS2 Initiation Codons

Knocking out production of a functional gene product by premature termination will, in most cases, not allow translation initiation at downstream ATGs on the RNA and may even promoted nonsense-mediated mRNA decay [53]. Mutation of the preS1 and preS2 start codons should, in contrast, allow

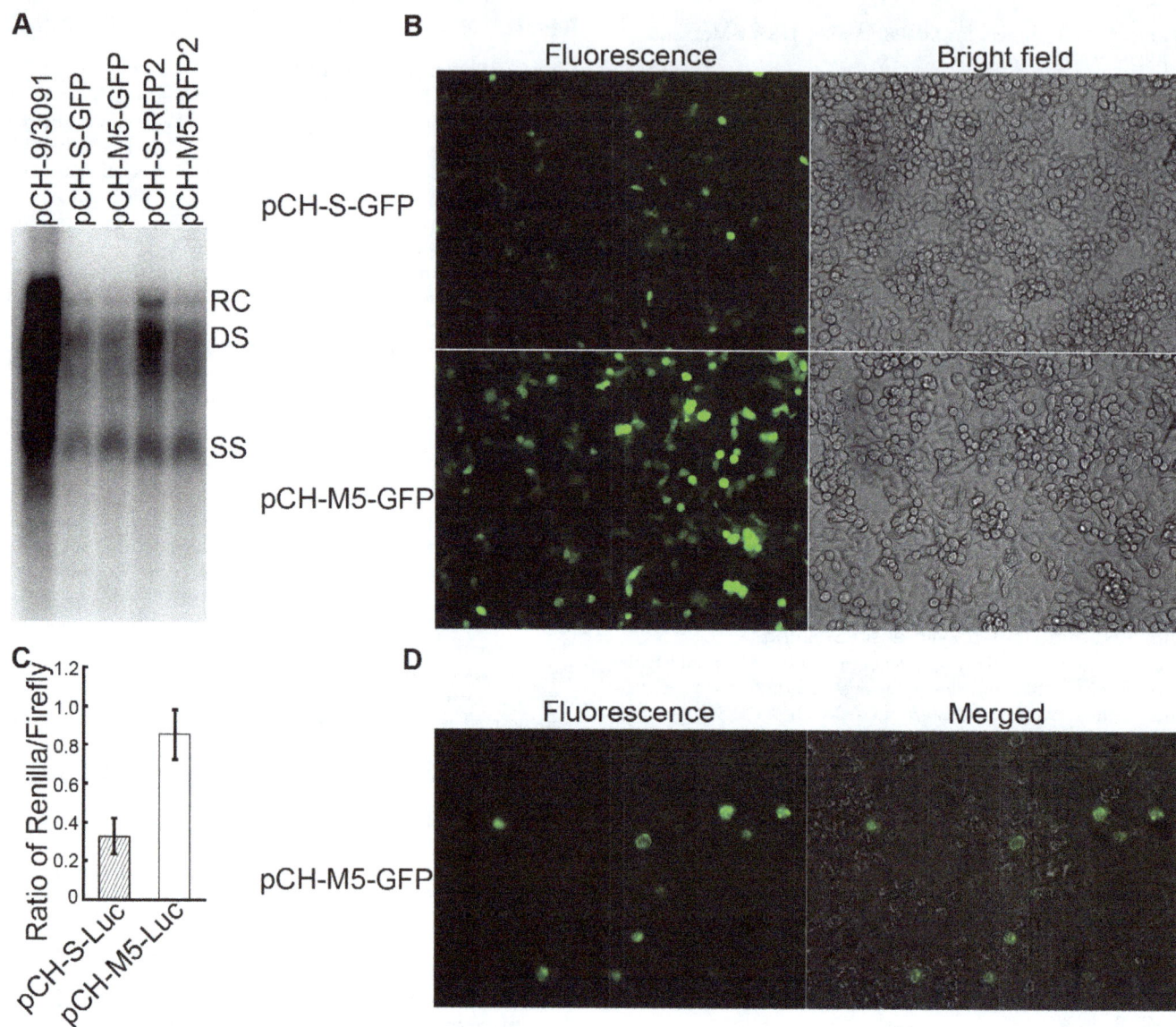

Figure 2. Trans-complementation rescues HBV vectors lacking endogenous gene products into infectious virions with enhanced transgene expression. (A) Rescue of replication in intracellular nucleocapsids by helper plasmid pCH3142. HepG2 cells were cotransfected with equal amounts of pCH3142 and the indicated pCH-S or pCH-M5 plasmids. Transfection with the wild-type HBV expression plasmid pCH-9/3091 served as reference. DNA from cytoplasmic nucleocapsids was analyzed by Southern blotting using a ^{32}P-labeled HBV-specific probe. The positions of the major replicative intermediates, i.e. relaxed circular (RC) DNA, double-stranded linear DNA (DS) and single-stranded DNA (SS) are indicated. **(B) and (C) Enhanced transgene expression by HBV vectors devoid of endogenous gene products.** HepG2 cells were transfected with either the first generation pCH-S-GFP plasmid, or the new pCH-M5-GFP vector and GFP expression at 48 h post transfection was monitored by fluorescence microscopy (B). Alternatively, HepG2 cells were cotransfected with the Renilla luciferase encoding plasmids pCH-S-Luc or pCH-M5-Luc plus a plasmid encoding firefly luciferase (pGL3-control). At 48 h post transfection, Renilla luciferase activity from the HBV vector was then normalized to firefly luciferase activity in the same cells (C). **(D) Rescue of infectious HBV vector particle formation by wild-type HBV.** HepG2 cells were cotransfected with the vector pCH-M5-GFP and, instead of the helper plasmid pCH3142 as in (A), with the wild-type HBV expression plasmid pCH-9/3091. Viral particles from the supernatant were then tested for infectivity on differentiated HepaRG cells, using a nominal moi of 5,000 vge/cell. GFP expression indicating the presence of infectious vector particles was assessed by fluorescence microscopy 6 days post infection (panel "Fluorescence"). An overlay with the brightfield image of the same field is shown in panel "Merged".

transgene expression from all preS1 and preS2/S promoter transcripts and may thus enhance transgene expression. To test this assumption, we transfected the fluorescent protein encoding pCH-S versus pCH-M5 vectors in the absence of helper plasmid into HepG2 cells and monitored the cells by fluorescence microscopy. As shown in Fig. 2B for the eGFP expressing vectors, the pCH-M5 vector caused a visibly stronger fluorescence. For quantitative assessment, we cotransfected

HepG2 cells with a firefly luciferase expression plasmid (pGL3) plus either the pCH-S or pCH-M5 vector encoding Renilla luciferase. When normalized to the firefly luciferase control, Renilla luciferase activity was about 2.6-fold higher in pCH-M5-Luc than in pCH-S-Luc transfected cells (Fig. 2C); the difference was statistically significant ($p<0.05$). While other explanations are not excluded, these data were consistent with the intended increase in transgene expression level.

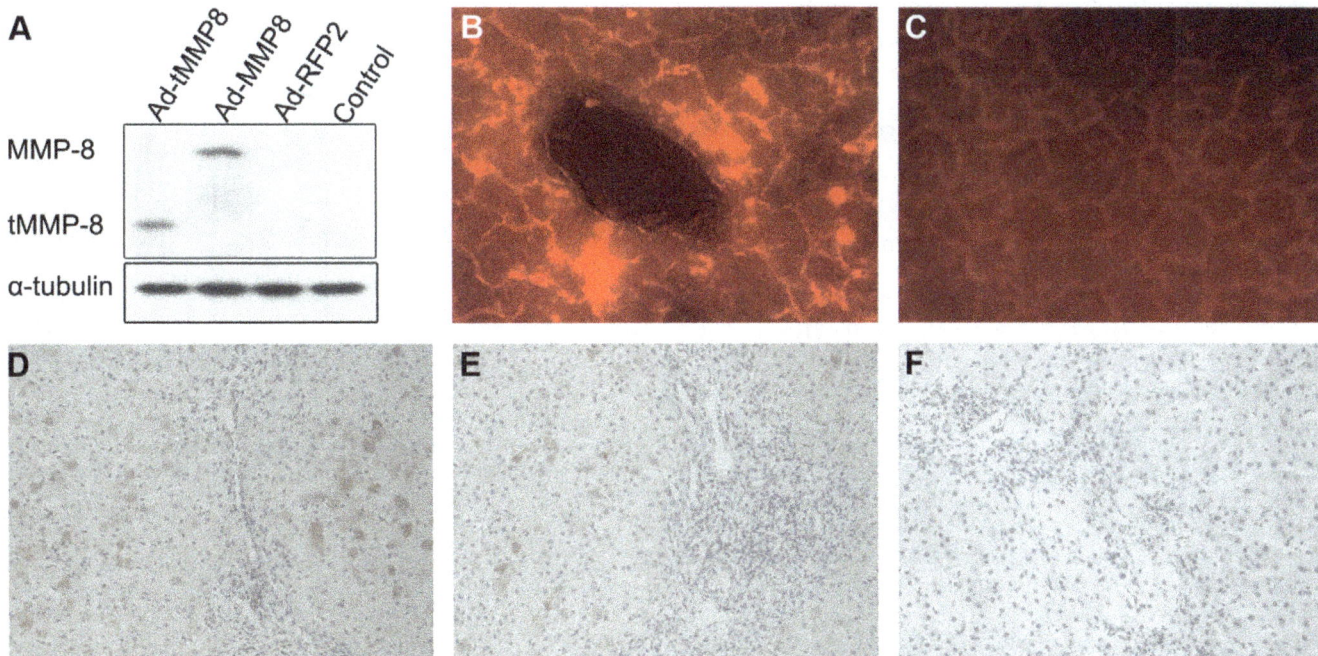

Figure 3. *In vitro* and *in vivo* transgene expression by chimeric Ad-HBV vectors. (A) tMMP8 expression in HepG2 cells. HepG2 cells were inoculated with the chimeric virus particles Ad-CH-tMMP8 (Ad-tMMP8) and Ad-CH-RFP2 (Ad-RFP2), or the conventional Ad-C-MMP8 particles; untreated HepG2 cells served as control. Four days later, cell lysates were analyzed by immunoblotting using a polyclonal MMP-8 antibody that recognizes an amino acid segment present in both MMP-8 and tMMP-8. Detection of tubulin on the same blot served as loading control. **(B)** and **(C)** Ad-HBV vector encoded transgene delivery into the liver. Ad-CH-RFP2 particles were injected into the tail vein of normal rats, with rats injected with saline as control. Two weeks later, liver tissues were immediately freeze-sectioned and analyzed for RFP2 expression by fluorescence microscopy. Strong red fluorescence was detected in rats treated with the Ad-HBV vector (B) whereas only limited autofluorescence was seen in rats treated with saline (C). **(D)**, **(E)** and **(F)** Rats with liver fibrosis were treated with Ad-CH-tMMP8 (D), Ad-C-MMP8 (E), or Ad-CH-RFP2 (F), respectively. Two weeks later, rat livers were sectioned and immunohistochemically stained with MMP-8 antibody. MMP-8 and tMMP-8 were visualized as brown precipitates.

Wild-type HBV can Support Formation of Infectious Recombinant Hepatitis B Virions *in trans*

Next we addressed whether the endogenous gene knockout HBV vectors could be rescued into infectious virions by wild-type HBV. To this end, we cotransfected HepG2 cells with equal amounts of the vector pCH-M5-GFPand the wild-type HBV plasmid pCH-9/3091; the GFP vector was chosen to allow direct detection of even a low percentage of infected cells. Successful *trans*-complementation should yield a mixture of wild-type and recombinant virions. Next we enriched viral particles from the culture supernatants and tested their infectivity in an *in vitro* infection system that is strictly dependent on an intact envelope, namely differentiated HepaRG cells [39]. About 10^5 prediffer-entiated HepaRG cells per well of a six-well plate were incubated with about 5×10^8 vge per well; this corresponds, combined for wild-type and potential recombinant virions, to a nominal multiplicity of infection (moi) of 5,000. As shown in Fig. 2D, in the range of 1% to 3% of the cells developed easily detectable green fluorescence which peaked around day 6 to day 8 post inoculation. Though seemingly low, this infection efficiency is not much below that reported for HepaRG cell infection with wild-type HBV which likely accounted for the majority of virions in the inoculum. For instance, at moi 1.25×10^4 around 1% and even at moi 40×10^4 not more than 7% of the cells became infected [54]. Similarly, others reported that at most 20% of the cells could be infected regardless of the amount of virions used [55]. While we have not directly tested the percentage of exclusively wild-type virus infected cells in our experiments, an additional factor may be the lack of intact HBx expression from the pCH-M5-GFP vector.

Though not required for cccDNA formation, HBx appears to strongly promote transcriptional activity of the cccDNA [56]. This also implies that HBx was provided by co-infecting wild-type virus and/or that HBx dependence of cccDNA transcription is not absolute, as also suggested by previous data [34]. Also, other host factors might be crucial for cccDNA formation [57]. Clearly, however, GFP expression demonstrated that *cis*-preferential encapsidation of the wild-type pgRNA [52] did not abolish packaging and reverse transcription of the recombinant pgRNA, that the recombinant nucleocapsids received an intact envelope, and that the vector particles generated transcriptionally active cccDNA, all at levels allowing to easily detect recombinant virus infected cells. Infection-independent GFP expression from internalized vector plasmid is extremely unlikely (see Discussion).

Based on these data, we next generated an analogous vector for tMMP8, termed pCH-M5-tMMP8. With about 500 bp in length, the tMMP8 transgene is even smaller than the genes for eGFP (about 750 bp) and IFN-α (about 600 bp) that previously have) successfully been transduced using HBV vectors [28]. Subsequently, we used the pCH-M5 vectors for eGFP, RFP2, and tMMP8 to construct chimeric E1/E3-deleted (ΔE1/ΔE3) Ad-HBV vectors (Fig. 1), all of which were termed Ad-CH followed by the name of the HBV-embedded trans-gene. For reference, we generated a conventional Ad vector, Ad-C-MMP8, which encodes full-length MMP-8 under CMV promoter control (Fig. 1), as previously described [33]. To validate transgene expression by the Ad-HBV vectors, HepG2 cells were inoculated with Ad-CH-tMMP8, Ad-C-MMP8 or Ad-CH-RFP2; untreatedHepG2 cells served as negative control. Immunoblotting demonstrated that tMMP8 from the chimeric Ad-HBV vector was expressed at comparable levels as MMP8 from the conventional Ad vector (Fig. 3A). Successful liver transduction of the chimeric Ad-HBV vector encoded transgene, upon tail vein injection, was demonstrated by the development of strong fluorescence in liver sections from the RFP2 vector injected compared to non-injected rats (Fig. 3B and C).

Rat Model of Liver Cirrhosis and Treatment Set-up

Long-term oral administration of 0.03% TAA in drinking water generates a well-established rat model of liver fibrosis and cirrhosis [20]. To confirm cirrhosis development in our setting, two animals each from the TAA treatment group were sacrificed at 4, 8, 12 and 16 weeks after initiation of treatment and their livers were tested by hematoxylin-eosin (HE) staining. Severe cirrhosis was confirmed in both animals sacrificed at the 16 week time point. Thirty-two of the remaining rats were then randomly divided into 4 groups (A, B, C and D) of 8 animals each. Rats of group A, B, and C were injected with 1.5×10^{11} virus particles (VP)/kg bodyweight of Ad-CH-tMMP8, Ad-C-MMP8, or Ad-CH-RFP2, respectively, through the tail vein. Animals from group D received physiological saline by the same route. The normal control group E consisted of eight weight-matched rats that had received normal drinking water without TAA.

To confirm expression of MMP8 and tMMP8, respectively, in fibrotic liver, liver tissue sections from TAA-treated rats of group A, B and C were immunohistologically evaluated with a polyclonal MMP-8 antibody recognizing an amino acid segment of MMP-8 that is also present in tMMP-8. Two weeks post virus injection, comparable cytoplasmic MMP-8 staining was seen in the livers of rats injected with Ad-C-MMP8 or Ad-CH-tMMP8 but not those having received Ad-CH-RPF2. (Fig. 3D, E and F). These data suggested the practical applicability of the chimeric Ad-HBV vectors in fibrotic livers.

Because the cirrhotic phenotype is reportedly maintained for at least 2 months after termination of TAA feeding [21,58], rats were sacrificed 2, 4, 8 weeks after Ad vector or saline injection to evaluate potential therapeutic effects. Fibrosis was assessed by determining standard parameters, including hepatic hydroxyproline content, morphological and histological changes, Sirius red staining, and Knodell histologic activity index as modified by Wang et al. [49,59].

Similar Reduction in Elevated Hydroxyproline Content of Cirrhotic Livers by Ad-C-tMMP8 and Ad-CH-tMMP8 Treatment

Hydroxylation of prolines stabilizes collagen, and increased HYP content is a marker for fibrosis. As shown in Fig. 4, the HYP contents in the control group E remained constant over time at around 5–7 µg/g liver whereas they were significantly higher in all TAA treated rats, with a gradual decline from week 2 to week 8 after Ad vector or saline administration (Fig. 4). The highest values (around 40 µg/g) were found in the animals that had received the Ad-CH-RFP2 vector or saline (p<0.05 compared to the normal group at all time points). The lack of significant difference between these two groups showed that the Ad vector as such had no measurable effect. Much in contrast, HYP contents in the rats injected with either Ad-CH-tMMP8 or Ad-C-MMP8 were two-fold lower already at two weeks after vector administration, and around three-fold lower at the 8 week timepoint (p<0.05 at all three time points). Notably, with about 10 µg/g the levels at week 8 were only slightly higher than in the normal control compared to still around 30 µg/g in the Ad-CH-RFP2 and saline injected rats

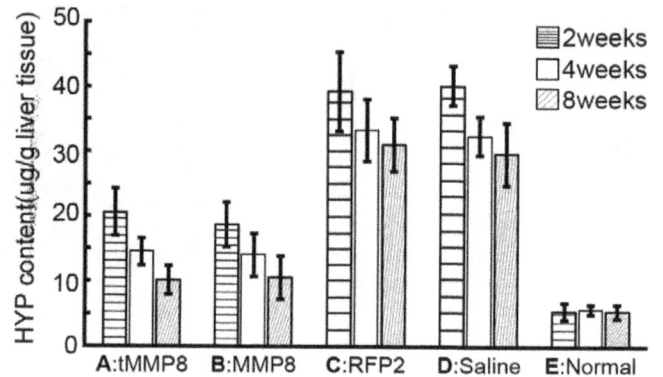

Figure 4. Chimeric Ad-HBV vector delivering truncated MMP-8 achieves similar reduction of hydroxyproline content in cirrhotic liver as a conventional full-length MMP-8 Ad vector. Hydroxyproline (HYP) contents in livers from normal rats (group E), or rats with TAA-induced cirrhosis (groups A–D) and treated with the chimeric Ad-HBV vectors Ad-CH-tMMP8 (group A) or Ad-CH-RFP2 (group C), or the conventional Ad vector Ad-C-MMP8 (group B) or saline (group D) were determined 2 weeks, 4 weeks, 8 weeks after treatment, using a standard colorimetric assay. Both MMP-8 vectors achieved a significant reduction in HYP content compared to the Ad-CH-RFP2 vector and saline. Error bars represent standard deviation (n = 3).

(p<0.05 compared to the normal controls). Hence the conventional full-length MMP-8 Ad vector and the chimeric Ad-HBV vector for truncated tMMP-8 were similarly effective in reducing the fibrosis marker HYP.

Similar Amelioration of Cirrhotic Phenotype by Ad-C-MMP8 and Ad-CH-tMMP8 Vector Administration

Visual inspection of the gross liver morphologies eight weeks after Ad vector or saline administration (Fig. 5A, panel Gross view) revealed massive changes compared to the normal control, particularly for the TAA treated rats that had received the Ad-CH-RFP2 vector or saline. While the normal livers exhibited ordinary reddish-rufous color, perfectly smooth surface, and regular shape, livers from the latter two groups showed more or less shrinkage, abnormal color, irregular outlines, and a strikingly uneven surface with protruding mixed-sized fibrotic nodules. Histology confirmed numerous regenerative parenchyma nodules surrounded by septa of fibrous tissue, and a significant increase in fat storing cells, Kupffer cells and bile ductules. In contrast, livers of rats injected with Ad-CH-tMMP8 or Ad-C-MMP8 presented with much milder patho-morphological progression, with fewer and smaller fibrotic nodules on the liver surface and softer hepatic parenchyma. HE-staining eight weeks after Ad-CH-tMMP8 or Ad-C-MMP8 administration (Fig. 5A, panel HE staining) showed a relatively normal aspect and subcellular structure of hepatocytes, with well-preserved cytoplasm and prominent nuclei and nucleoli. Appreciable histological regeneration was indicated by a reduced extent of fibrous septa and an increase in the extension of normal hepatic parenchyma. Knodell scores of livers from rats injected with Ad-CH-tMMP8 or Ad-C-MMP8 were evidently lower than in rats treated by Ad-CH-RFP2 or saline (Fig. 5B), and the differences were statistically significant at all time points (p<0.05). No significant histological differences were observed between Ad-CH-tMMP8 and Ad-C-MMP8 injected animals. Sirius red staining eight weeks after Ad vector or saline administration followed by polarized light microscopy can be used to visualize the collagen in fibrotic or cirrhotic livers (Fig. 5A, panel Sirius red), and to semi-quantitatively calculate the collagen content by area-density percentage of collagen in liver sections [48]. As shown in Fig. 5C, compared to the normal control these values were strongly increased (around 30%) in livers of TAA treated animals that had received Ad-CH-RFP2 or saline, indicating severe destruction of hepatic lobules and frequent pseudolobuli formation accompanied by impaired hepatic function. In contrast, significantly ($p<0.05$) lower values (around 17% at week 2, declining to around 10% at week 8) were observed in the groups that had received Ad-C-MMP8 and Ad-CH-tMMP8. These data further supported that tMMP8 embedded in the Ad-HBV vector was

similarly efficient in reducing pathological collagen deposition as the conventional full-length MMP8 Ad vector.

This was further confirmed by immunocytochemistry using a type I collagen-specific antibody eight weeks after Ad vector or saline administration (Fig. 5A, panel Collagen I). Livers from the control group E showed only weak brownish staining that was sporadically distributed around vessel walls. In all TAA treated animals, abundant positively staining structures accumulated in portal areas, portal veins, fibrous septa and hepatic stellate cells. In contrast, type I collagen congestion in rats injected with Ad-CH-tMMP8 and Ad-C-MMP8 was markedly reduced when compared to the RFP2 vector and saline injected controls, and further

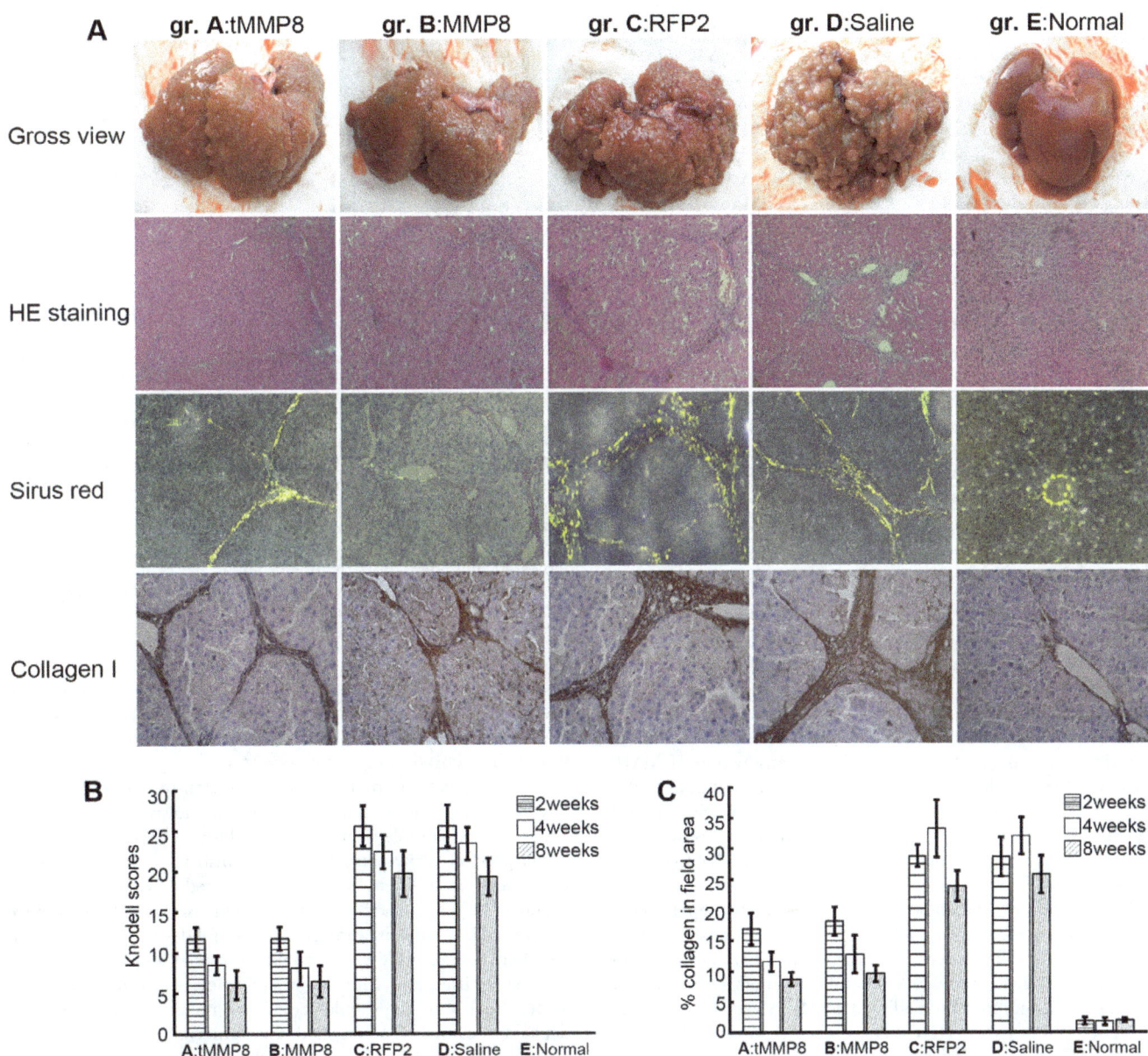

Figure 5. Chimeric Ad-HBV vector delivering truncated MMP-8 achieves similar amelioration of fibrosis and cirrhosis as a conventional full-length MMP-8 Ad vector. (**A**) Gross morphology and histology. Livers and liver sections from rats of the same treatment groups as in Fig. 4 were analyzed for gross morphology (Gross view), and by hematoxylin - eosin (HE) staining, Sirius red collagen staining, or immunohistochemical staining specific for type I collagen. (**B**) Overall collagen contents. Sirius red staining followed by polarizing microscopy was used to determine the collagen positive areas per liver sections. (**C**) Knodell fibrosis scores. The highly elevated collagen levels and Knodell scores in the cirrhotic animals treated with the RFP2 Ad vector or saline were strongly reduced by treatment with either the full-length MMP-8 Ad vector or the chimeric Ad-HBV vector delivering truncated tMMP8. Error bars represent standard deviations (n = 3).

decreased gradually from week 2 to week 8 after treatment. Furthermore, the therapeutic effect was extended up to 8 weeks after adenovirus infection (Fig. 5A, panel Collagen I).

Similar Elevated Hepatocyte Growth Factor and c-Met mRNA Levels in Ad-C-MMP8 and Ad-CH-tMMP8 Transduced Livers

Removal of excess ECM not only frees physical space for hepatocytes but also acts negatively on activated HSC, the main ECM producers, and positively on hepatocyte proliferation [18], possibly by liberating ECM-bound HGF. Because Ad vector-mediated transduction of full-length MMP-1 and MMP-8 was reported to induce hepatocyte proliferation [21,33] and HGF upregulation, we investigated whether truncated tMMP8 delivered by the chimeric Ad-HBV vector would have a similar effect. In addition, we included the HGF receptor c-Met [60] into the analysis, considering that activation of the HGF/c-Met signaling pathway is one of the earliest events towards hepatocyte regeneration following partial hepatectomy [60,61,62,63].

To this end, we used qPCR to determine the levels of c-Met and HGF mRNA relative to the levels of the mRNA for the house-keeping gene product GAPDH. Compared to the normal control, relative mRNA levels for both HGF and c-Met were slightly elevated in the TAA cirrhotic animals injected with Ad-CH-RFP2 or saline, but were markedly higher in the rats that had received the Ad-C-MMP8 and the Ad-CH-tMMP8 vector, especially at the early timepoints after administration (Fig. 6A and B). The differences to the Ad-CH-RFP2 and saline controls were significant (p<0.05), while those between the two MMP-8 vectors were not (Fig. 6A and B, Group A,B vs Group C,D, p<0.05). Upregulation of HGF and c-Met mRNA could be detected as long as 8 weeks after injection of the MMP-8 vectors, implying a similarly sustained hepatocyte proliferation promoting effect by the chimeric Ad-HBV vector encoding truncated tMMP8 as by the conventional Ad-vector encoding full-length MMP-8.

Discussion

Liver fibrosis prepares the ground for cirrhosis and, especially in the context of chronic hepatitis B, may directly progress into hepatocellular carcinoma in some 40% of the patients [2]. Removing the injurious stimuli underlying liver fibrosis appears to promote fibrosis regression and possibly even reversion [2] but treatment of advanced fibrosis and cirrhosis probably require more direct means of ECM remodeling. Transduction of MMP genes by Ad vectors has shown promise [18,21,33] yet application of conventional Ad vectors in humans has met with several concerns [23], particularly when high doses of vector are required to reach a sufficient fraction of liver cells without affecting other tissues.

The previous demonstration that the naturally hepatotropic HBV can be engineered into a liver-specific gene transfer vehicle [28,34] suggests HBV-based vectors as a potential alternative in the treatment of liver diseases. A general restriction is their limited insertion capacity, requiring finding a suitably sized effector gene. A second, relevant for HBV-related diseases, is superinfection exclusion. Though not absolute, as shown experimentally [28] and by the frequent takeover in chronic HBV carriers by resistant virus variants during treatment with early generation nucleoside analogs [64], resident HBV might substantially reduce transduction by HBV-based vectors, as shown for DHBV [32]. Conversely, once in an HBV-infected cell, a replication-defective HBV vector might be amplified and spread until the supply of wild-type virus ceases, e.g. by antiviral treatment. Thus, an appropriately designed HBV

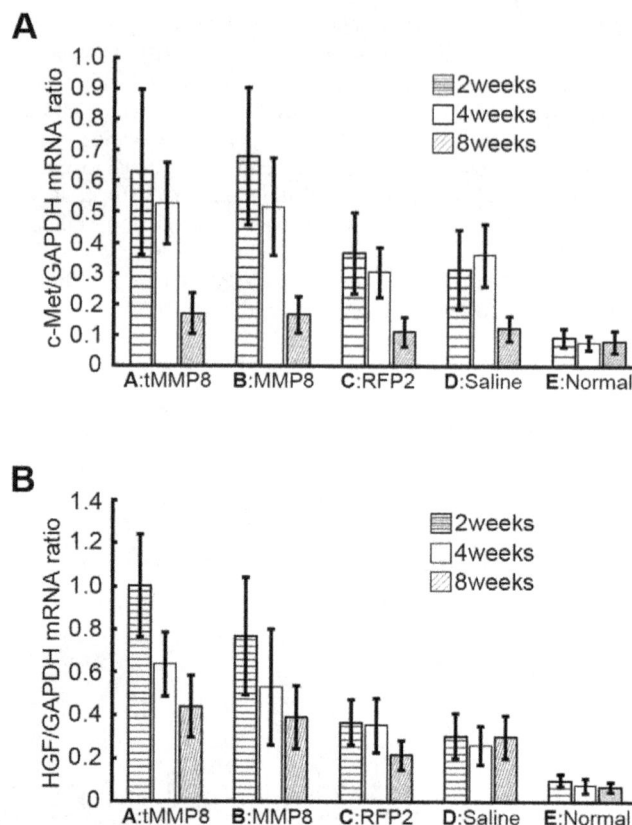

Figure 6. Similar enhancement of hepatocyte proliferation promoting factors by chimeric Ad-HBV vector for truncated MMP-8 and conventional full-length MMP-8 Ad vector. (A) c-Met mRNA. (B) Hepatocyte growth factor mRNA. mRNA levels for c-Met, hepatocyte growth factor (HGF) and glyceraldehyde 3-phosphate dehydrogenase (GAPDH) in liver tissue from the same treatment groups as in Fig. 3 were determined by quantitative RT-PCR at the indicated timepoints post treatment. Values for c-Met and HGF were then correlated with those for GAPDH in the same sample. Error bars represent standard deviations (n = 3).

vector treatment might achieve a longer term expression of therapeutic genes than high-dose administration of conventional Ad-vectors, yet avoid the risks associated with permanently integrating retroviral or lentiviral vectors.

However, various prerequisites for seriously considering such advanced application regimens were unknown. These include whether *trans*-complementation by wild-type HBV rather than a purposefully engineered helper construct would occur to practically useful levels, whether a truncated MMP-8, sufficiently small to fit into an HBV vector, would exert similarly positive effects against fibrosis and cirrhosis as full-length MMP-8, and whether such an HBV-vector could be shuttled into liver cells and express the transgene with similar efficiency as a conventional Ad-vector. Such shuttling should provide the means for efficient initial deposition of the HBV vector despite superinfection exclusion.

The current study addresses, for the first time in an *in vivo* liver disease model, several of these questions. Given the lack of animal models that combine susceptibility to HBV infection with human-like disease progression, some aspects had to be assessed using surrogate models. Hence it remains to be shown whether vector complementation by resident wild-type HBV occurs *in vivo*, and whether potential vector spreading can occur in fibrotic/cirrhotic liver, an issue that is currently unclear even for wild-type HBV.

Altogether, however, our other data strongly suggest that further investments into developing HBV-vectors for liver diseases including, but not limited to, fibrosis and cirrhosis are warranted.

Improved HBV Vector Design and Trans-complementation by Wild-type HBV

The first generation HBV vectors retained the potential to generate core and HBx protein, as well as truncated forms of polymerase and L and M protein [28]. For application in HBV-infected cells anti-HBV vector immune responses would be of less concern, but undesired side-effects could arise from the reported transactivation activity of truncated M and L protein [65,66]. Similar to a previous study [34], we therefore knocked out expression of all residual vector encoded viral gene products, including intact HBx (see below). However, different from that study we prevented expression of the preS1 and preS2 ORFs by mutating the respective start codons such that all transcripts from the preS1 and preS2/S promoters would be usable as mRNAs for the transgenes. Indeed, the pCH-M5-GFP vector produced visibly more GFP than the parental pCH-S-GFP vector, as was quantitatively confirmed using the corresponding luciferase constructs (Fig. 2B and 2C). In addition, the distinct hepatocyte specificity especially of the preS1 promoter [29] should contribute to liver-specific transgene expression. Alternatively, a previous study [34] as well as our own unpublished data indicate that transgene expression may be achieved by replacing the entire preS1, preS2 plus S regions with expression cassettes comprising a heterologous promoter, and that such cassettes are tolerated at a few other sites in the HBV genome. Such flexibility may turn out to be advantageous in further HBV vector improvement.

The knock out mutations in pCH-M5-GFP did not impair trans-complementation by the pCH3142 helper plasmid, as shown by the approximately equal amounts of replicative DNA intermediates obtained by cotransfection with the parental versus the new vectors (Fig. 2A). More relevant regarding potential vector amplification by wild-type HBV was the apparent formation of infectious, GFP-transducing vector particles by trans-complementation with the wild-type HBV vector pCH-9/3091, although only a low percentage of the inoculuated HepaRG cells became GFP-positive (Fig. 2D). Several factors are likely to contribute to this result. First, only a fraction of the HepaRG cells is susceptible even to wild-type HBV infection [54]. Second, given the choice, HBV polymerase packages the pgRNA from which it was translated at four- to ten-times higher efficiency than a simultaneously present pgRNA on which polymerase translation was ablated [52]; with the encapsdiation-deficient pCH3142 helper plasmid such competition for pgRNA packaging is deliberately excluded. Third, the pCH-M vector does not produce intact HBx which according to recent results with wild-type HBV infected HepaRG cells is not required for HBV cccDNA formation but strongly enhances its transcriptional activity [56]. One interpretation for visible GFP expression in our experiments is a low level HBx-independent cccDNA transcription, as previously seen with HBx-deficient vectors [28,34] and also with wild-type HBV [56]. Another is that the GFP-positive cells had been co-infected with wild-type HBV which was likely present in the inoculum in substantial excess and provided HBx. While additional experiments will be required for distinction, the data strongly suggest that vector trans-complementation by wild-type HBV is principally possible and comprises all processes required for infectious virion formation. A trivial explanation would be GFP expression from internalized pCH-M-GFP plasmid; however, we consider this extremely unlikely. First, the total amount of viral DNA inoculated was in the nanogram range (around 5×10^8 vge per well) whereas microgram

amounts plus an efficient transfection reagent are required to achieve expression of a plasmid-encoded gene in a substantial fraction cells (in the range of 20% for HepG2 cells which probably more easily transfected than HepaRG cells). Second, free DNAs not protected inside viral particles had been digested by DNase I and micrococcal nuclease prior to enrichment of the virions used for inoculation (see Materials and Methods).

Definite proof for vector trans-complementation by wild-type HBV in vivo would require an appropriate animal infection model such as uPA-SCID mice xenotransplanted with human or tupaia hepatocytes [67]. However, this model is highly complex and not readily available, and as yet no fibrosis or cirrhosis model based on this infection system has been reported.

Similar Therapeutic Benefit of an Ad-vector Shuttled HBV Vector Encoding TruncaTed tMMP8 as of a Conventional Ad-vector Encoding Full-length MMP-8

The previously observed benefits of full-length MMP-1 and MMP-8 delivery into rat models of liver cirrhosis by conventional Ad-vectors [21,33] provided a standard against which the performance of our Ad-vector-shuttled HBV tMMP8 vector could be compared. Initial experiments confirmed about equal expression of tMMP8 from the Ad-HBV vector versus MMP8 from the conventional Ad vector in infected HepG2 cells (Fig. 3A), and productive in vivo delivery of an Ad-HBV vector encoded reporter transgene into the liver of normal rats by tail-vein injection (Fig. 3B,C). Confirming earlier studies [20], 16 week administration of TAA induced severe fibrosis and cirrhosis in all rats tested, as shown by gross morphological and histological comparison with normal rat liver (Fig. 4 and Fig. 5). In particular, various qualitative and quantitative parameters reflecting the hallmark of fibrosis, i.e. excess interstitial collagen-containing ECM deposition, were strongly elevated in the TAA treated animals. Notably, in all assays, including HYP content (Fig. 4), area-density percentage of collagen (Fig. 5B) or Knodell score (Fig. 5C), the cirrhotic animals injected with the Ad-CH-RFP2 vector or saline showed significantly higher elevations than the Ad-C-MMP8 and Ad-CH-tMMP8 treated animals, correlating with detectable MMP8 expression in the latter but not the former groups (Fig. 6 D, E vs. F). In contrast, no significant differences were seen amongst the two control groups and amongst the two MMP-8 vector treated groups. The lack of difference between Ad-CH-RFP2 vs. saline injected rats implies that their assay parameters were representative for the degree of TAA-induced fibrosis in all animals of the cohort, and it further confirmed that the Ad-CH vector per se had no detectable influence. The equal reduction in fibrotic and cirrhotic parameters in the tMMP-8 versus MMP8 vector-treated groups indicated that both caused a significant and comparable therapeutic benefit compared to the RFP2 vector or saline controls. This may suggest that vector amplification by resident HBV, not testable in this rat model, would even further enhance therapeutic efficacy of the HBV vector yet proof will require a disease model that is susceptible to HBV infection.

Notably, however, in another, testable, aspect the tMMP8 chimeric Ad-HBV vector proved again as effective as the conventional full-length MMP8 Ad vector. In the previous studies on MMP-1 and MMP-8 transduction the induction of hepatocyte proliferation [38] was noted as an additional benefit accompanying fibrosis regression. Though various mechanisms may account for this effect, the ECM itself probably plays an important part. Excessive ECM further stimulates activated HSCs, whereas ECM reduction favors hepatocyte proliferation, possibly by liberating ECM-bound HGF [18]. HGF signaling through its receptor kinase c-Met [60] is indeed the major initial stimulus for liver regeneration after partial hepatectomy [61,62,63]. Our corresponding qPCR analysis of HGF and c-Met mRNA (Fig. 6) revealed significantly (compared to the normal control) and about equally elevated levels of both mRNAs in the animals receiving the two different MMP-8 vectors. Smaller increases, compared to the normal control, were also observed in the cirrhotic animals injected with the RFP2 vector or saline, which may reflect spontaneous liver regeneration after cessation of the TAA treatment. Importantly, the lack of difference between the RFP2 and saline controls further confirmed that the elevated HGF and c-Met mRNA levels can be attributed to the vector-encoded MMP-8 genes.

Implications for Future Application of HBV-based Vectors Against Liver Diseases

Although efficient and safe delivery of therapeutic genes remains challenging, with none of the currently used viral and non-viral systems being ideal, HBV-based vectors offer distinct conceptual advantages for liver-specific gene therapy [31]. A unique feature is their potential for limited amplification by exploiting resident wild-type virus as a natural helper; however, this potential may be counteracted by superinfection exclusion.

Our study demonstrates that HBV vectors can exert therapeutic benefit in an *in vivo* model of liver fibrosis and cirrhosis, which are relevant liver diseases often associated with HBV infection; that HBV vectors can be complemented by wild-type HBV; and that an unrelated vector that is not subject to HBV-specific superinfection exclusion can efficiently shuttle an HBV vectors into the liver. Hence further development of this or similar strategies for efficient initial deposition of an HBV vector by a low, and consequently low-risk, dose of appropriate shuttling vectors appears highly warranted.

Acknowledgments

We thank Professor Christopher M. Overall (Canada) for kindly providing the pGW1GH-MMP8 plasmid. We are grateful to Jiwen Kang for technical support.

Author Contributions

Conceived and designed the experiments: DS MN XC. Performed the experiments: JL XC. Analyzed the data: DS MN XC. Wrote the paper: DS MN XC. Assisted with performing the experiments: ZG ZW DL FK HL BL ZC.

References

1. Anthony PP, Ishak KG, Nayak NC, Poulsen HE, Scheuer PJ, et al. (1978) The morphology of cirrhosis. Recommendations on definition, nomenclature, and classification by a working group sponsored by the World Health Organization. J Clin Pathol 31: 395–414.
2. Ellis EL, Mann DA (2012) Clinical evidence for the regression of liver fibrosis. J Hepatol 56: 1171–1180.
3. Forner A, Llovet JM, Bruix J (2012) Hepatocellular carcinoma. Lancet 379: 1245–1255.
4. Goyal N, Jain N, Rachapalli V, Cochlin DL, Robinson M (2009) Non-invasive evaluation of liver cirrhosis using ultrasound. Clin Radiol 64: 1056–1066.
5. Garcia-Tsao G, Friedman S, Iredale J, Pinzani M (2010) Now there are many (stages) where before there was one: In search of a pathophysiological classification of cirrhosis. Hepatology 51: 1445–1449.
6. Perz JF, Armstrong GL, Farrington LA, Hutin YJ, Bell BP (2006) The contributions of hepatitis B virus and hepatitis C virus infections to cirrhosis and primary liver cancer worldwide. J Hepatol 45: 529–538.
7. Mormone E, George J, Nieto N (2011) Molecular pathogenesis of hepatic fibrosis and current therapeutic approaches. Chem Biol Interact 193: 225–231.
8. Friedman SL (2008) Hepatic stellate cells: protean, multifunctional, and enigmatic cells of the liver. Physiol Rev 88: 125–172.
9. Gressner AM (1991) Liver fibrosis: perspectives in pathobiochemical research and clinical outlook. Eur J Clin Chem Clin Biochem 29: 293–311.
10. Rojkind M, Giambrone MA, Biempica L (1979) Collagen types in normal and cirrhotic liver. Gastroenterology 76: 710–719.
11. Schuppan D (1990) Structure of the extracellular matrix in normal and fibrotic liver: collagens and glycoproteins. Semin Liver Dis 10: 1–10.
12. Montfort I, Perez-Tamayo R (1978) Collagenase in experimental carbon tetrachloride cirrhosis in the rat. Am J Pathol 92: 411–420.
13. Perez-Tamayo R, Montfort I, Gonzalez E (1987) Collagenolytic activity in experimental cirrhosis of the liver. Exp Mol Pathol 47: 300–308.
14. Nagase H, Visse R, Murphy G (2006) Structure and function of matrix metalloproteinases and TIMPs. Cardiovasc Res 69: 562–573.
15. Page-McCaw A, Ewald AJ, Werb Z (2007) Matrix metalloproteinases and the regulation of tissue remodelling. Nat Rev Mol Cell Biol 8: 221–233.
16. Hemmann S, Graf J, Roderfeld M, Roeb E (2007) Expression of MMPs and TIMPs in liver fibrosis - a systematic review with special emphasis on anti-fibrotic strategies. J Hepatol 46: 955–975.
17. Moore CS, Crocker SJ (2012) An alternate perspective on the roles of TIMPs and MMPs in pathology. Am J Pathol 180: 12–16.
18. Iimuro Y, Brenner DA (2008) Matrix metalloproteinase gene delivery for liver fibrosis. Pharm Res 25: 249–258.
19. Iredale JP (2004) A cut above the rest? MMP-8 and liver fibrosis gene therapy. Gastroenterology 126: 1199–1201.
20. Tsukamoto H, Matsuoka M, French SW (1990) Experimental models of hepatic fibrosis: a review. Semin Liver Dis 10: 56–65.
21. Iimuro Y, Nishio T, Morimoto T, Nitta T, Stefanovic B, et al. (2003) Delivery of matrix metalloproteinase-1 attenuates established liver fibrosis in the rat. Gastroenterology 124: 445–458.
22. Siller-Lopez F, Sandoval A, Salgado S, Salazar A, Bueno M, et al. (2004) Treatment with human metalloproteinase-8 gene delivery ameliorates experimental rat liver cirrhosis. Gastroenterology 126: 1122–1133; discussion 1949.

23. Descamps D, Benihoud K (2009) Two key challenges for effective adenovirus-mediated liver gene therapy: innate immune responses and hepatocyte-specific transduction. Curr Gene Ther 9: 115–127.
24. Waddington SN, McVey JH, Bhella D, Parker AL, Barker K, et al. (2008) Adenovirus serotype 5 hexon mediates liver gene transfer. Cell 132: 397–409.
25. Ni S, Bernt K, Gaggar A, Li ZY, Kiem HP, et al. (2005) Evaluation of biodistribution and safety of adenovirus vectors containing group B fibers after intravenous injection into baboons. Hum Gene Ther 16: 664–677.
26. Beck J, Nassal M (2007) Hepatitis B virus replication. World J Gastroenterol 13: 48–64.
27. Nassal M (2008) Hepatitis B viruses: reverse transcription a different way. Virus Res 134: 235–249.
28. Protzer U, Nassal M, Chiang PW, Kirschfink M, Schaller H (1999) Interferon gene transfer by a hepatitis B virus vector efficiently suppresses wild-type virus infection. Proc Natl Acad Sci U S A 96: 10818–10823.
29. Raney AK, Milich DR, Easton AJ, McLachlan A (1990) Differentiation-specific transcriptional regulation of the hepatitis B virus large surface antigen gene in human hepatoma cell lines. J Virol 64: 2360–2368.
30. Junker-Niepmann M, Bartenschlager R, Schaller H (1990) A short cis-acting sequence is required for hepatitis B virus pregenome encapsidation and sufficient for packaging of foreign RNA. EMBO J 9: 3389–3396.
31. Ganem D (1999) An advance in liver-specific gene delivery. Proc Natl Acad Sci U S A 96: 11696–11697.
32. Walters KA, Joyce MA, Addison WR, Fischer KP, Tyrrell DL (2004) Superinfection exclusion in duck hepatitis B virus infection is mediated by the large surface antigen. J Virol 78: 7925–7937.
33. Siller-López F, Sandoval A, Salgado S, Salazar A, Bueno M, et al. (2004) Treatment with human metalloproteinase-8 gene delivery ameliorates experimental rat liver cirrhosis. Gastroenterology 126: 1122–1133.
34. Untergasser A, Protzer U (2004) Hepatitis B virus-based vectors allow the elimination of viral gene expression and the insertion of foreign promoters. Hum Gene Ther 15: 203–210.
35. Siller-Lopez F, Garcia-Banuelos J, Hasty KA, Segura J, Ramos-Marquez M, et al. (2000) Truncated active matrix metalloproteinase-8 gene expression in HepG2 cells is active against native type I collagen. J Hepatol 33: 758–763.
36. Ren S, Nassal M (2001) Hepatitis B virus (HBV) virion and covalently closed circular DNA formation in primary tupaia hepatocytes and human hepatoma cell lines upon HBV genome transduction with replication-defective adenovirus vectors. J Virol 75: 1104–1116.
37. Sprinzl MF, Oberwinkler H, Schaller H, Protzer U (2001) Transfer of hepatitis B virus genome by adenovirus vectors into cultured cells and mice: crossing the species barrier. J Virol 75: 5108–5118.
38. Iredale JP (2004) A cut above the rest? MMP-8 and liver fibrosis gene therapy. Gastroenterology 126: 1199–1201.
39. Gripon P, Rumin S, Urban S, Le Seyec J, Glaise D, et al. (2002) Infection of a human hepatoma cell line by hepatitis B virus. Proc Natl Acad Sci U S A 99: 15655–15660.
40. Nassal M (1992) The arginine-rich domain of the hepatitis B virus core protein is required for pregenome encapsidation and productive viral positive-strand DNA synthesis but not for virus assembly. J Virol 66: 4107–4116.

41. Liu JX, Sun DX, Cao ZC (2009) [Stable cell line for secretion of replication-defective hepatitis B virus vector expressing blasticidin resistant gene]. Zhonghua Shi Yan He Lin Chuang Bing Du Xue Za Zhi 23: 316–318.

42. Pelman GR, Morrison CJ, Overall CM (2005) Pivotal Molecular Determinants of Peptidic and Collagen Triple Helicase Activities Reside in the S3' Subsite of Matrix Metalloproteinase 8 (MMP-8): The role of hydrogen bonding potential of ASN188 and TYR189 and the connecting cis bond. Journal of Biological Chemistry 280: 2370–2377.

43. Li D, Liu J, Kang F, Guan W, Gao X, et al. (2011) Core-APOBEC3C chimerical protein inhibits hepatitis B virus replication. J Biochem 150: 371–374.

44. Sun D, Nassal M (2006) Stable HepG2- and Huh7-based human hepatoma cell lines for efficient regulated expression of infectious hepatitis B virus. J Hepatol 45: 636–645.

45. Sun D, Rosler C, Kidd-Ljunggren K, Nassal M (2010) Quantitative assessment of the antiviral potencies of 21 shRNA vectors targeting conserved, including structured, hepatitis B virus sites. J Hepatol 52: 817–826.

46. Bruck R, Weiss S, Traister A, Zvibel I, Aeed H, et al. (2007) Induced hypothyroidism accelerates the regression of liver fibrosis in rats. Journal of gastroenterology and hepatology 22: 2189–2194.

47. Rojkind M, González E (1974) An improved method for determining specific radioactivities of proline-14C and hydroxyproline-14C in collagen and in noncollagenous proteins. Analytical Biochemistry 57: 1–7.

48. Junqueira LC, Bignolas G, Brentani RR (1979) Picrosirius staining plus polarization microscopy, a specific method for collagen detection in tissue sections. Histochem J 11: 447–455.

49. Wang TL, Liu X, Zhou YP (1998) A semiquantitative scoring system for assessment of hepatic inflammation and fibrosis in chronic viral hepatitis. Chinese Journal of Hepatology 6: 195–197.

50. Schaller H, Fischer M (1991) Transcriptional control of hepadnavirus gene expression. Curr Top Microbiol Immunol 168: 21–39.

51. Hildt E, Hofschneider PH (1998) The PreS2 activators of the hepatitis B virus: activators of tumour promoter pathways. Recent Results Cancer Res 154: 315–329.

52. Bartenschlager R, Junker-Niepmann M, Schaller H (1990) The P gene product of hepatitis B virus is required as a structural component for genomic RNA encapsidation. J Virol 64: 5324–5332.

53. Nicholson P, Yepiskoposyan H, Metze S, Zamudio Orozco R, Kleinschmidt N, et al. (2010) Nonsense-mediated mRNA decay in human cells: mechanistic insights, functions beyond quality control and the double-life of NMD factors. Cell Mol Life Sci 67: 677–700.

54. Schulze A, Mills K, Weiss TS, Urban S (2012) Hepatocyte polarization is essential for the productive entry of the hepatitis B virus. Hepatology 55: 373–383.

55. Hantz O, Parent R, Durantel D, Gripon P, Guguen-Guillouzo C, et al. (2009) Persistence of the hepatitis B virus covalently closed circular DNA in HepaRG human hepatocyte-like cells. J Gen Virol 90: 127–135.

56. Lucifora J, Arzberger S, Durantel D, Belloni L, Strubin M, et al. (2011) Hepatitis B virus X protein is essential to initiate and maintain virus replication after infection. J Hepatol 55: 996–1003.

57. Guo H, Xu C, Zhou T, Block TM, Guo JT (2012) Characterization of the host factors required for hepadnavirus covalently closed circular (ccc) DNA formation. PLoS One 7: e43270.

58. Oren R, Dotan I, Papa M, Marravi Y, Aeed H, et al. (1996) Inhibition of experimentally induced cirrhosis in rats by hypothyroidism. Hepatology 24: 419–423.

59. Knodell RG, Ishak KG, Black WC, Chen TS, Craig R, et al. (1981) Formulation and application of a numerical scoring system for assessing histological activity in asymptomatic chronic active hepatitis. Hepatology 1: 431–435.

60. Gherardi E, Birchmeier W, Birchmeier C, Vande Woude G (2012) Targeting MET in cancer: rationale and progress. Nat Rev Cancer 12: 89–103.

61. Borowiak M, Garratt AN, Wustefeld T, Strehle M, Trautwein C, et al. (2004) Met provides essential signals for liver regeneration. Proc Natl Acad Sci U S A 101: 10608–10613.

62. Huh CG, Factor VM, Sanchez A, Uchida K, Conner EA, et al. (2004) Hepatocyte growth factor/c-met signaling pathway is required for efficient liver regeneration and repair. Proc Natl Acad Sci U S A 101: 4477–4482.

63. Paranjpe S, Bowen WC, Bell AW, Nejak-Bowen K, Luo JH, et al. (2007) Cell cycle effects resulting from inhibition of hepatocyte growth factor and its receptor c-Met in regenerating rat livers by RNA interference. Hepatology 45: 1471–1477.

64. Zoulim F, Durantel D, Deny P (2009) Management and prevention of drug resistance in chronic hepatitis B. Liver Int 29 Suppl 1: 108–115.

65. Hildt E, Saher G, Bruss V, Hofschneider PH (1996) The hepatitis B virus large surface protein (LHBs) is a transcriptional activator. Virology 225: 235–239.

66. Hildt E, Urban S, Hofschneider PH (1995) Characterization of essential domains for the functionality of the MHBst transcriptional activator and identification of a minimal MHBst activator. Oncogene 11: 2055–2066.

67. Dandri M, Burda MR, Zuckerman DM, Wursthorn K, Matschl U, et al. (2005) Chronic infection with hepatitis B viruses and antiviral drug evaluation in uPA mice after liver repopulation with tupaia hepatocytes. J Hepatol 42: 54–60.

8

NADPH Oxidase NOX4 Mediates Stellate Cell Activation and Hepatocyte Cell Death during Liver Fibrosis Development

Patricia Sancho[1], Jèssica Mainez[1], Eva Crosas-Molist[1], César Roncero[2], Conrado M. Fernández-Rodriguez[3], Fernando Pinedo[4], Heidemarie Huber[5], Robert Eferl[5,6], Wolfgang Mikulits[5], Isabel Fabregat[1,7]*

1 Biological Clues of the Invasive and Metastatic Phenotype Group, Bellvitge Biomedical Research Institute (IDIBELL), L'Hospitalet, Barcelona, Spain, 2 Departamento de Bioquímica y Biología Molecular II, Facultad de Farmacia, Universidad Complutense and Instituto de Investigación Sanitaria del Hospital Clínico San Carlos (IdISSC), Madrid, Spain, 3 Service of Gastroenterology, Hospital Universitario Fundación Alcorcón and Universidad Rey Juan Carlos, Alcorcón, Madrid, Spain, 4 Unit of Pathology, Hospital Universitario Fundación Alcorcón, Alcorcón, Madrid, Spain, 5 Department of Medicine I, Division: Institute of Cancer Research, Medical University of Vienna, Vienna, Austria, 6 Ludwig Boltzmann Institute for Cancer Research (LBI-CR), Vienna, Austria, 7 Department of Physiological Sciences II, University of Barcelona, Barcelona, Spain

Abstract

A role for the NADPH oxidases NOX1 and NOX2 in liver fibrosis has been proposed, but the implication of NOX4 is poorly understood yet. The aim of this work was to study the functional role of NOX4 in different cell populations implicated in liver fibrosis: hepatic stellate cells (HSC), myofibroblasts (MFBs) and hepatocytes. Two different mice models that develop spontaneous fibrosis ($Mdr2^{-/-}/p19^{ARF-/-}$, $Stat3^{\Delta hc}/Mdr2^{-/-}$) and a model of experimental induced fibrosis (CCl_4) were used. In addition, gene expression in biopsies from chronic hepatitis C virus (HCV) patients or non-fibrotic liver samples was analyzed. Results have indicated that NOX4 expression was increased in the livers of all animal models, concomitantly with fibrosis development and TGF-β pathway activation. In vitro TGF-β-treated HSC increased NOX4 expression correlating with transdifferentiation to MFBs. Knockdown experiments revealed that NOX4 downstream TGF-β is necessary for HSC activation as well as for the maintenance of the MFB phenotype. NOX4 was not necessary for TGF-β-induced epithelial-mesenchymal transition (EMT), but was required for TGF-β-induced apoptosis in hepatocytes. Finally, NOX4 expression was elevated in patients with hepatitis C virus (HCV)-derived fibrosis, increasing along the fibrosis degree. In summary, fibrosis progression both in vitro and in vivo (animal models and patients) is accompanied by increased NOX4 expression, which mediates acquisition and maintenance of the MFB phenotype, as well as TGF-β-induced death of hepatocytes.

Editor: Marie Jose Goumans, Leiden University Medical Center, The Netherlands

Funding: This work was supported by grants to IF from the Ministerio de Ciencia e Innovación (MICINN), Spain (BFU2009-07219 and ISCIII-RTICC RD06/0020) and AGAUR-Generalitat de Catalunya (2009SGR-312). The work of WM was supported by the European Union, FP7 Health Research project number HEALTH-F4-2008-202047. JM and EC-M were recipients of pre-doctoral fellowships from the FPI and FPU programs, respectively, MICINN, Spain. The funders had no role in study design, data collection and analysis, decision to publish, or preparation of the manuscript.

Competing Interests: The authors have declared that no competing interests exist.

* E-mail: ifabregat@idibell.cat

Introduction

Liver fibrosis is the final consequence of many chronic liver injuries [1]. Hepatic stellate cells (HSCs) are activated to myofibroblasts (MFBs), which are mainly responsible for collagen deposition during hepatic fibrogenesis. Once injured, hepatocytes undergo apoptosis. The transforming growth factor-beta (TGF-β), whose levels increase during the development of liver fibrosis, could be involved in both processes [2]. Thus, TGF-β inhibits growth and induces apoptosis of hepatocytes and also contributes to the activation of HSCs [3,4].

The generation of reactive oxygen species (ROS) plays relevant roles in hepatic fibrosis and recent works point to NADPH oxidases (NOX) as a key source of ROS in the fibrotic liver [5]. Two NOX isoforms, NOX1 and NOX2, mediate pro-fibrogenic effects in endogenous liver cells [6,7,8]. However, less is known about the possible role in liver fibrosis of another isoform, NOX4, which is highly expressed in hepatocytes and HSCs [8]. We

previously reported that NOX4 mediates TGF-β-induced apoptosis in hepatocytes in primary culture [9] and causes ROS production upon the in vitro transdifferentiation of activated HSCs to MFBs [3]. In other fibrotic models, NOX4 accounts for ROS-induced fibroblast and mesangial cell activation, playing an essential role in TGF-β1-mediated fibroblast differentiation into a profibrotic myofibroblast phenotype and matrix production [10]. Indeed, TGF-β induces NOX4 expression in lung mesenchymal cells, which mediates MFB activation and fibrogenic responses to lung injury [11]. In this same line of evidence, ROS signaling by NOX4 is required for TGF-β-induced differentiation of fibroblasts into MFB in heart [12], kidney [13] and diseased prostatic stroma [14].

The aim of this work was to analyze whether NOX4 expression is modulated in experimental animal models of liver fibrosis and during the development of human liver fibrogenesis. We demonstrate that NOX4 expression increases in parallel to liver fibrotic processes and may be required for TGF-β-induced activation of HSC and for the maintenance of the MFB phenotype. In hepatocytes, NOX4 causes cell death but does not mediate epithelial-mesenchymal transition (EMT). These results open new perspectives for the involvement of NOXes in liver fibrosis and for the potential development of new therapeutic targeted tools.

Materials and Methods

Ethics statement

Mice were housed in accordance with European laws and with the general regulations specified by the Good Scientific Practices Guidelines of the Medical University of Vienna. From Spain, the approval for all the experiments related to the study of liver fibrosis in experimental animal models was applied to the General Direction of Environment and Biodiversity, Government of Catalonia, and approved with the number #4589, 2011 (document enclosed). Human tissues were collected with the required approvals from the Institutional Review Board (Comité Ético de Investigación Clínica del Hospital Universitario Fundación Alcorcón) and patient's written consent conformed to the ethical guidelines of the 1975 Declaration of Helsinki (both documents are enclosed).

Reagents and antibodies

TGF-β was from Merck (Darmstadt, Germany). Fetal bovine serum was from Sera Laboratories International (Cinder Hill, UK). Glutathione-ethyl-ester (GEE), Diphenyleneiodonium chloride (DPI) and Butylated hydroxyanisole (BHA) were from Sigma (St Louis, USA). The caspase-3 substrate Ac-DEVD-AMC was from Pharmingen (San Diego, CA, USA). Antibodies: mouse anti-β-actin (clone AC-15, Sigma), rabbit anti-cleaved caspase-3 (Asp-175) from Cell Signaling Technology (Danvers, MA, USA), anti-F4/80 (Abcam, Cambridge, UK), mouse anti-E-cadherin (BD Pharmingen, NJ, USA), rabbit anti-ki67 (Abcam), mouse anti-NOX2 (Santa Cruz Biotechnology, CA, USA), anti-NOX4 raised by Sigma-Genosys against a peptide corresponding to the C-terminal loop region (aminoacids 499–511), mouse anti-α-SMA (Sigma, St Louis, USA), rabbit anti-phospho-Smad2 (Ser465/467) and rabbit anti-phospho-Smad3 (Ser423/425) from Cell Signaling Technology, goat anti-Smad2/3, anti-Smad7 and anti-TGF-β from Santa Cruz Biotechnology and mouse anti-vimentin (Sigma, St Louis, USA).

Mice

Three animal experimental models of liver fibrosis were used for this study: two genetically modified mice and one drug-induced model. Mdr2$^{-/-}$/p19$^{ARF-/-}$ double null mice [15] displayed a fibrotic phenotype comparable to Mdr2$^{-/-}$ mice, widely used as a model for experimental liver fibrosis [16,17], characterized by severe hepatic injury and large periductal accumulation of MFBs, but showed the additional advantage of allowing the isolation of immortal cells for in vitro experiments [15]. Stat3$^{\Delta hc}$/Mdr2$^{-/-}$ mice show Stat3 conditional inactivation specifically in hepatocytes and cholangiocytes in a Mdr2$^{-/-}$ background [18], which strongly aggravates liver injury and fibrosis. Animals were sacrificed to evaluate liver histology at 2 and 7 weeks of age. C.B-17/IcrHsd-Prkcd^{scid} (SCID) mice have been used as control. For CCl$_4$ experiments, CCl$_4$ (Sigma, St Louis, USA) was diluted 1:4 in ultrapure Olive Oil (Sigma, St Louis, USA) and injected intraperitoneally at a concentration of 1.5 mg per gram of body weight into 3-month old C57BL/6J mice. The treatment was performed two times a week for 6 weeks to induce hepatic fibrosis.

Mice were sacrificed 3 days after the last injection and liver samples were collected and processed for immunohistochemical analysis.

Cell models and cell culture conditions

No commercial cell lines have been used in this study. Mice stellate cells, myofibroblasts and hepatocytes were obtained in our or colleagues' laboratories and used in previous published works [14,18,19]: 1) By employing p19^{ARF} deficiency, we established a non-transformed murine HSC model to investigate their plasticity and the dynamics of HSC activation [19]. The immortal cell line, referred to as M1-4HSC, showed stellate cell characteristics including the expression of desmin, glial fibrillary acidic protein, alpha-smooth muscle actin and pro-collagen I [19]. Treatment of these non-tumorigenic M1-4HSC with pro-fibrogenic TGF-β1 provoked a morphological transition to a myofibroblastoid cell type which was accompanied by enhanced cellular turnover and impaired migration [19]. These cells have been used in this study to analyze the role of NOX4 in the in vitro activation of HSC to MFB; 2) In vivo-activated MFBs derived from physiologically inflamed livers of Mdr2/p19^{ARF} double-null mice were obtained as previously described [15] and used in this study in in vitro experiments to analyze the role of NOX4 in maintaining the myofibroblast phenotype; 3) Finally, hepatocytes from wild-type mice were isolated and immortalized with a puromycin-resistance retroviral vector pBabe encoding Simian virus 40 large T antigen (LTAg), as described [20] and were generously provided by Dr. AM Valverde (Madrid, Spain). These cells were used in this study to analyze the potential role of NOX4 in the TGF-β-induced effects related to fibrosis development, i.e., epithelial-mesenchymal transitions and apoptosis. For cell culture, cells were grown in DMEM (Lonza, Basel, Switzerland) supplemented with 10% FBS and maintained in a humidified atmosphere of 37°C, 5% CO2.

Human samples

Biopsies from 28 chronic hepatitis C virus (HCV) patients showing different degrees of fibrosis or control liver samples extracted in surgeries from colorectal cancer patients with hepatic metastasis were collected in the Hospital Universitario de Alcorcón (Madrid, Spain). The control group was formed by 10 patients in whom liver biopsy was performed by altered function test. Liver biopsy examination revealed normal histology or minimal change.

Immunohistochemistry and immunocytochemistry studies

For immunohistochemistry, sections of 4 μm-thick paraffin-embedded livers were stained with hematoxylin and eosine (H&E) or Trichrome (Sigma) for collagen staining using standard procedures. The immunostaining was performed by incubating primary antibodies (diluted from 1:50 to 1:100) overnight at 4°C and by visualization with the Vectastain ABC kit (Vector Laboratories, Burlingame, CA). Immunocytochemistry studies were performed as described previously [21]. Representative images were taken with a Spot 4.3 digital camera and edited in Adobe Photoshop. Cells were visualized in an Olympus BX-60 with the appropriate filters.

Analysis of cell number

Cell number was analyzed after crystal violet staining [4].

Total ROS production

Intracellular ROS content was measured by staining with the fluorescent probe H$_2$DCF-DA as described previously [22].

Analysis of caspase-3 activity

Caspase-3 activity was analyzed fluorimetrically upon incubation of 20 μg of cell lysates with 6.6 μg/mL Ac-DEVD-AMC for 2 hours at 37°C [22]. Results are calculated as units of caspase-3 activity per microgram of protein per hour.

Analysis of gene expression

RNeasy Mini Kit (Qiagen, Valencia, CA, USA) was used for total RNA isolation. Reverse transcription (RT) was carried out using the High Capacity Reverse Transcriptase kit (Applied Biosystems, Foster City, CA, USA), and 500 ng of total RNA from each sample for complementary DNA synthesis. PCR products in semiquantitative reactions were obtained after 30–35 cycles of amplification at annealing temperatures of 57–62°C, and analyzed by 1.5% agarose gel electrophoresis. Expression of *18S* was analyzed as a loading control, as indicated. The –RT channel contained RNA that had not been treated with the RT mixture.

For Real-Time quantitative PCR, expression levels were determined in duplicate in an ABIPrism7700 System, using the Sybr® Green PCR Master Mix (Applied Biosystems).

All the primers used for both semiquantitative PCR or Real-Time quantitative PCR reactions are listed in Suppl. Table 1 and 2, respectively.

Western blot analysis

Total protein extracts and Western Blot procedure were carried out as previously described [22,23]. Antibodies were used at 1:1000, except β-actin (1:3000). Protein concentration was measured with the BCA^{TM} Protein Assay kit (Pierce, Rockford, USA).

Knock-down assays

Cells at 70% confluence were transiently transfected with 50 nM siRNA during 8 hours using TransIT-siQuest following manufacturer's instructions (Mirus, Madison, USA). Oligos were obtained from Sigma-Genosys (Suffolk, UK). The oligo sequences were as follows: unsilencing: GUAAGACACGACUUAUCGC; mouse NOX4: CAAGAAGAUUGUUGGAUAA. The unsilencing siRNA used was selected from previous works [22]. Specific oligos with maximal knock-down efficiency were selected among three different sequences for each gene.

Statistics

All data represented at least three experiments and expressed as the mean ± SEM. Differences between groups were compared using either Student's t test or one-way ANOVA associated with the Dunnett's test. Statistical significance was assumed when $p < 0.05$.

Results

Activation of the TGF-β/NOX4 pathway in fibrosis development

Mdr2$^{-/-}$ mice represent a widely used model for experimental liver fibrosis [16,17] and are characterized by chronic liver injury and large periductal accumulation of MFBs. Similarly, Mdr2$^{-/-}$/p19$^{ARF-/-}$ double null mice [15] displayed a fibrotic phenotype comparable to Mdr2$^{-/-}$ mice which allows, on one hand, investigation of *in vivo* fibrosis development and, on the other hand, isolation of MFBs for *in vitro* experiments that become immortalized upon loss of p19^{ARF}, a gene involved in the negative control of cell cycle [15]. As observed in Mdr2$^{-/-}$ mice, Mdr2$^{-/-}$/p19$^{ARF-/-}$ mice developed spontaneous fibrosis characterized by

periductal accumulation of collagen and MFBs, as well as an increased number of Kupffer cells (F4/80 positive) (Suppl. Fig. 1). Importantly, these periductal changes were accompanied by damage of the hepatic parenchyma and compensatory hepatocyte proliferation, since we could not only detect increased apoptosis by cleaved caspase-3, but also increased numbers of Ki67 positive cells, (Fig. 1A). Fibrotic cells, easily recognized by their elongated form, condensed nuclei and positive expression for alpha-Smooth Muscle Actin (α-SMA) (Suppl. Fig. 1), stained for Ki67, but not for apoptosis. Of note, dying hepatocytes were mostly detected in the surrounding tissue of these fibrotic areas. Stat3^{Δhc}/Mdr2$^{-/-}$ mice represent a mouse model with conditional inactivation of Stat3 in hepatocytes and cholangiocytes of Mdr2$^{-/-}$ mice [18]. Loss of the hepatoprotective transcription factor Stat3 strongly aggravated liver injury and fibrosis of the Mdr2$^{-/-}$ fibrotic phenotype (Suppl. Fig. 2) leading to premature lethality. The compensatory hepatocyte proliferation due to parenchymal liver damage was severely reduced in this model (Suppl. Fig. 2, Fig. 1B).

Previous reports have indicated that several profibrotic genes are up-regulated at early stages of fibrosis development in Mdr2$^{-/-}$ mice, highlighting the major pro-fibrotic cytokine, TGF-β [24]. In agreement with these previous results, we found that both TGF-β and its downstream signal molecule, phospho-Smad2, were increased during fibrosis development in both animal models as analyzed by immunohistochemistry (Fig. 2 and Suppl. Fig. 3). Phospho-Smad2 staining intensity was higher at 2 weeks and decreased over time, inversely correlating with Smad7 level, a TGF-β pathway inhibitor. Importantly, NOX4 level was also found elevated in these fibrosis models in both hepatocytes and fibroblastoid cells. In the case of hepatocytes, NOX4 expression was more intense in those cells surrounding the MFBs area (Fig. 3A), which was coincident with the regions showing positive cells for cleaved caspase-3 (Suppl. Fig. 4). Interestingly, these observations were corroborated in a model of chemically-induced fibrosis by CCl$_4$ injection (Suppl. Fig. 5). CCl4 model has been widely used as an experimental model of chronic damage to the liver that produces fibrogenesis and may mimic the situation of human chronic liver diseases. These data together suggest that changes in the expression of NOX4 occur in different experimental animal models of hepatic fibrosis.

Since lack of p19^{ARF} allows the culture of spontaneously immortalized cells, we isolated and cultured both HSC in an inactive state from p19$^{ARF-/-}$ non fibrotic livers and activated MFB from Mdr2$^{-/-}$/p19$^{ARF-/-}$ fibrotic livers, as described in the Materials and Methods section. These MFB, which have suffered the activation process *in vivo* during spontaneous fibrosis development in Mdr2$^{-/-}$/p19$^{ARF-/-}$ mice, showed increased expression of NOX1, NOX2 and NOX4 at the mRNA level when compared to p19$^{ARF-/-}$ inactive HSC (Fig. 3B–D, left graphs). Thus, these results suggest that these NOX isoforms may be induced during the HSC activation process. In addition, and corroborating the results at the tissue level, immortalized hepatocytes showed very high NOX4 expression when compared to HSC or MFB, which was further up-regulated when they were treated with TGF-β (Fig. 3B, right graph). NOX1 expression was also predominantly expressed in hepatocytes, but was down-regulated by TGF-β in *in vitro* experiments (Fig. 3C, right graph). NOX2 was predominantly expressed in MFBs and was not affected by TGF-β in hepatocytes (Fig. 3D).

Role of NOX4 in HSC activation and MFBs phenotype maintenance

Since NOX4 seemed to increase during the transdifferentiation process of HSC to MFBs and its role in this process is completely

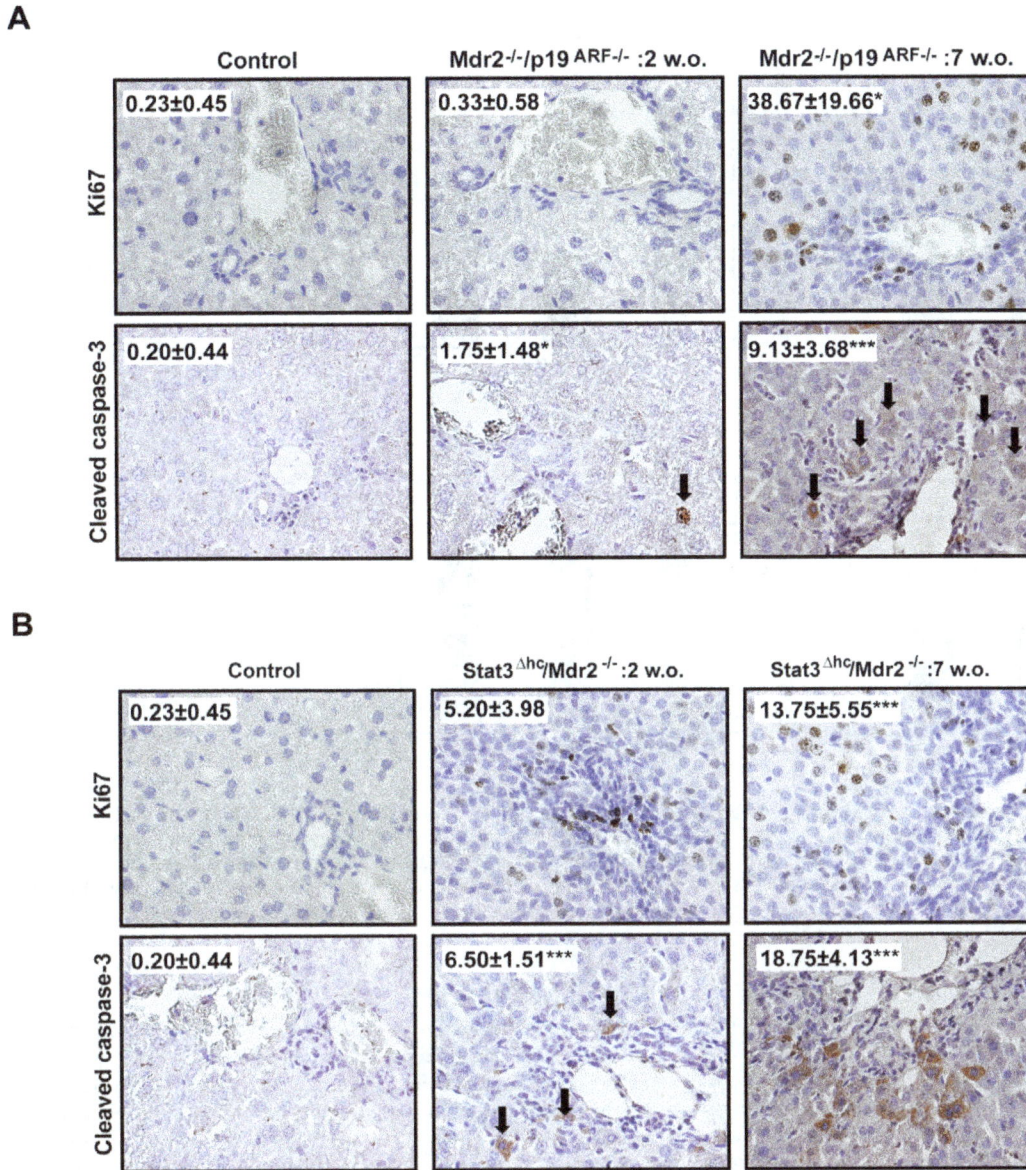

Figure 1. Fibrosis development in Mdr2$^{-/-}$/p19$^{ARF-/-}$ and Stat3$^{\Delta hc}$/Mdr2$^{-/-}$ mice is accompanied by hepatocellular proliferation and apoptosis. Representative 60x histological sections of livers from control or 2 or 7 weeks-old Mdr2$^{-/-}$/p19$^{ARF-/-}$ (A) and Stat3$^{\Delta hc}$/Mdr2$^{-/-}$ mice (B): Ki67 (upper row) and cleaved caspase-3 (lower row). Inset: quantification of positive cells for each marker. Data represent the mean ± SEM of the number of positive cells in at least ten different fields. Student's t test calculated versus control sections (*p<0.05; **p<0.01;***p<0.001).

unknown, we decided to focus our study on the potential role of NOX4 in the *in vitro* activation of HSC with TGF-β. As expected, TGF-β treatment induced HSC activation, featured by increase in α-SMA levels and E-cadherin down-regulation, which was accompanied by NOX1, NOX2 and NOX4 up-regulation (Fig. 4A). In the absence of TGF-β, this activation was not observed (Suppl. Fig. 6). Regulation of α-SMA at the protein level correlated with parallel changes at the mRNA level, along with up-regulation of vimentin and the extracellular matrix genes collagen I and fibronectin (Fig. 4B). The same panel shows that all these changes in gene expression induced by TGF-β were inhibited when NOX4 was knocked-down in cultured HSC cells. Importantly, phenotypical changes induced by TGF-β during the transdifferentiation process, such as morphological alterations and increased expression and reorganization of α-SMA and

vimentin, were impaired when NOX4 was targeted knock-down (Fig. 4C). No apparent changes in the viability of these cells were observed in NOX4 deficient cells (results not shown).

Since TGF-β and NOX4 appeared to play a crucial role in the activation of HSC, we next wondered if they could play a role in the maintenance of the activated MFB phenotype. For this purpose, firstly we treated isolated Mdr2$^{-/-}$/p19$^{ARF-/-}$ MFBs during 72 hours with LY364947, an inhibitor of the TGF-β receptor I (TβRI), in *in vitro* experiments. As shown in Figure 5A, inhibition of the TβRI reversed the MFB phenotype, measured as expression of pro-fibrotic genes, which correlated with a decrease in NOX4 mRNA levels. Importantly, this fact implicates plasticity of the MFB phenotype suggesting that it is possible to reverse the MFB activated state towards a more inactive HSC-like phenotype. It is worthy to note that blocking the TGF-β pathway down-

A

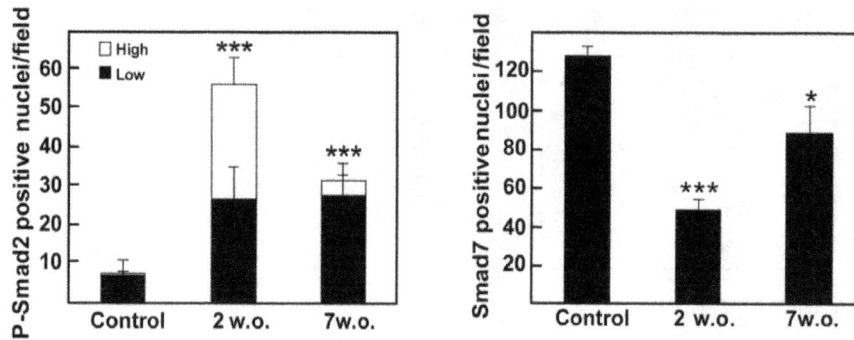

B

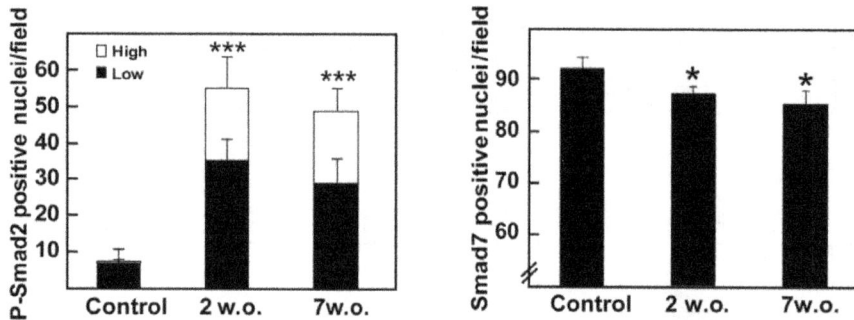

Figure 2. TGF-β pathway is activated at early stages of fibrosis in Mdr2$^{-/-}$/p19$^{ARF-/-}$ and Stat3$^{\Delta hc}$/Mdr2$^{-/-}$ mice. 60x histological sections of livers from control or 2 or 7 weeks-old Mdr2$^{-/-}$/p19$^{ARF-/-}$ (A) and Stat3$^{\Delta hc}$/Mdr2$^{-/-}$ mice (B) were stained with phospho-Smad2 or Smad7 and the number of positive cells was quantified. Left graph: positive nuclei for phospho-Smad2 with low or high signal intensity. Right graph: positive nuclei for Smad7. Data represent the mean ± SEM of cells in at least ten different fields. Student's t test calculated versus control sections (*p<0.05; **p<0.01;***p<0.001).

regulated TGF-β expression, indicating the existence of an autocrine positive feed-back loop implicated in the maintenance of the MFB properties. In addition, as shown in Fig. 5B, NOX4 knock-down produced a similar change as the one found with the TβRI inhibitor. Indeed, the expression of pro-fibrotic genes, as well as α-SMA and vimentin expression and organization, were significantly diminished when NOX4 was knocked-down, cells acquiring an HSC-like morphology (Fig. 5C). Furthermore, desmin expression, as a marker of activated stellate cells, decreased when NOX4 was knocked-down, correlating with the reversion of MFB phenotype. However, NOX4 silencing was unable to inhibit the expression of either TGF-β or its receptor (Fig. 5B, 5D), and it did not alter Smad2/3 phosphorylation status (Fig. 5D).

These results together suggest that NOX4 acts downstream TGF-β and controls the expression of different pro-fibrotic genes; however, autocrine expression of the cytokine in MFB, and activation of its downstream immediate signals, i.e., Smads, seems to be independent of NOX4.

It is interesting to point out that NOX4 expression at the mRNA level in both HSC and MFB was much higher than the expression of the other isoforms NOX1 and NOX2 (50-fold higher than NOX2 and 25-fold higher than NOX1 in hepatocytes; 80-fold higher than NOX2 and 60-fold higher than NOX1 in HSC: Suppl. Fig. 7), which may explain why neither NOX1 nor NOX2 replaces NOX4 function.

Role of NOX4 in hepatocytes

Finally, we decided to study the putative role of NOX4 in TGF-β-induced effects in hepatocytes. As shown in Fig. 6A, NOX4 expression was significantly up-regulated reaching the maximum mRNA levels at 12 h and the maximum protein level at 24–48 hours upon TGF-β treatment. As we and others have previously reported in several experimental models, induction of apoptosis by TGF-β was impaired when NOX4 was knocked-down (Fig. 6B). These in vitro data support the immunohistochemistry studies, where elevated NOX4 expression seemed to correlate with the areas of higher apoptosis of hepatocytes (Suppl. Fig 4). Interestingly, supplementation of cell culture medium with either antioxidants or a general inhibitor of NADPH oxidases (DPI) blocked TGF-β-induced ROS production and caspase-3 activation in hepatocytes (Suppl. Fig. 8A, B). In a similar way, a permeable form of GSH and DPI also attenuated changes in gene expression addressed by TGF-β in HSC (Suppl. Fig. 8C), highlighting the relevant role played by ROS in these processes.

We have previously reported that some liver cells are able to impair the pro-apoptotic effects of TGF-β and undergo EMT, characterized by cytoskeleton rearrangement and changes in gene expression leading to a mesenchymal phenotype with up-regulation of Snail, vimentin and α-SMA and loss of E-cadherin expression [21,25]. In view of the results regarding apoptosis, we next wondered whether NOX4 could be mediating TGF-β-induced EMT in vitro. NOX4 knock-down did not influence TGF-β-induced cytoskeletal changes, neither affected the expression of several EMT-related genes (Fig. 6C, D). In summary, NOX4 is

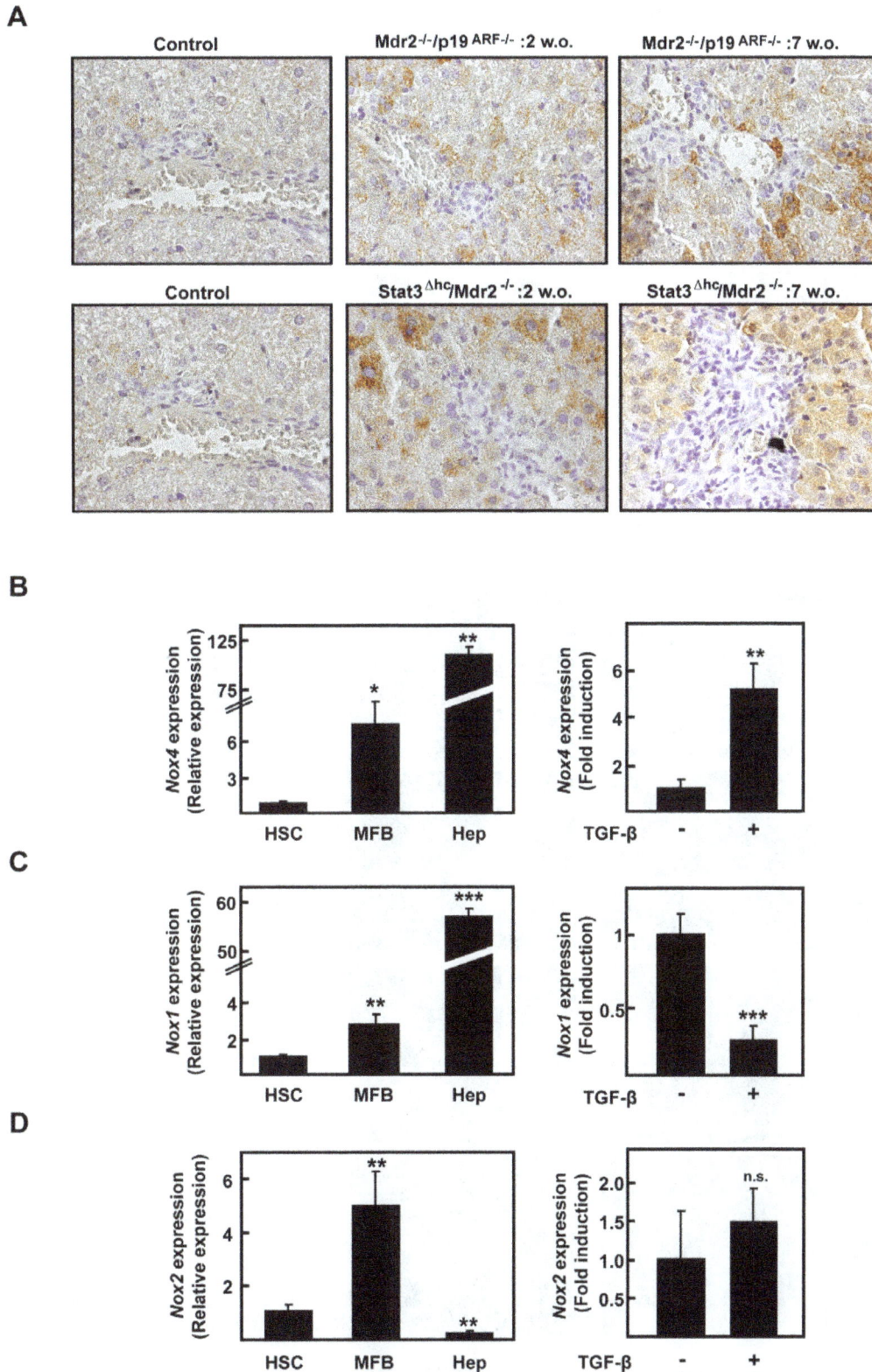

Figure 3. NOX4 expression is increased concomitant with fibrosis development in Mdr2$^{-/-}$/p19$^{ARF-/-}$ and Stat3$^{\Delta hc}$/Mdr2$^{-/-}$ mice.
(A) Representative 60x photographs from NOX4 immunohistochemistry performed in control or 2 or 7 weeks-old livers. (B, C, D) Real time PCR of NOX4, NOX1 or NOX2. Left: comparison of cultures of inactive stellate cells (HSC) isolated from p19$^{ARF-/-}$ mice, in vivo activated myofibroblats (MFB) isolated from fibrotic Mdr2$^{-/-}$/p19$^{ARF-/-}$ livers and wild type immortalized hepatocytes (Hep) (see Materials and Methods section). Right: immortalized hepatocytes treated or not with 2 ng/ml TGF-β. Data represent the mean ± SEM of three independent experiments, and were calculated relative to HSC (left) or untreated hepatocytes (right) respectively, which were given an arbitrary value of 1. Student's t test calculated versus HSC cells in the left column (*p<0.05; **p<0.01) or untreated hepatocytes in the right column (**p<0.01).

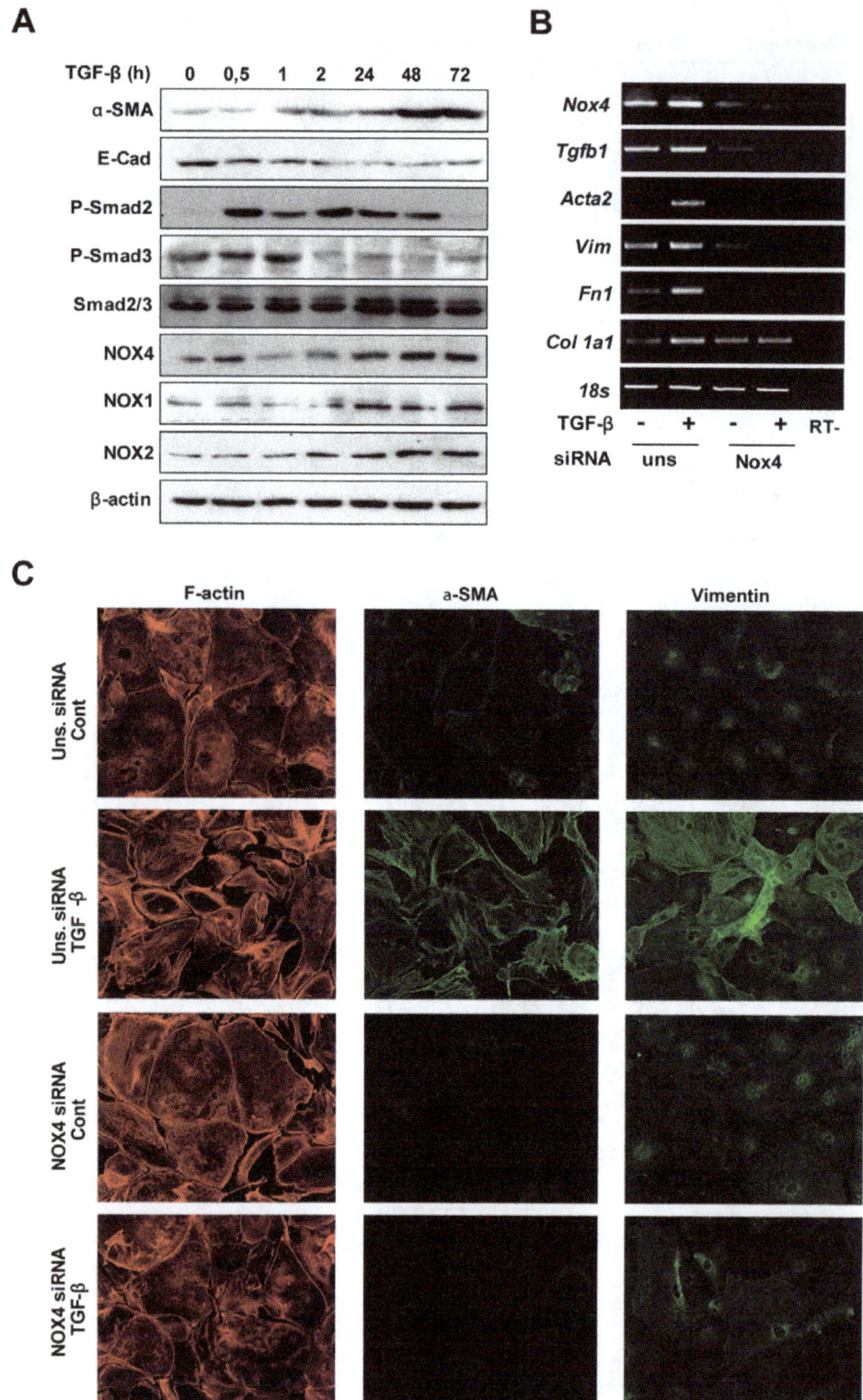

Figure 4. NOX4 knock-down inhibits TGF-β-dependent HSC activation. (A) p19[ARF−/−] HSC cells at early passages were treated for the indicated times with 2 ng/ml TGF-β and a Western blot of total extracts was performed. β-actin was used as loading control. Additional information to this experiment is presented in Suppl. Fig. 6, where the expression of the different proteins in HSC cultured for 24, 48 and 72 h in the absence of treatments is shown, as well as densitometric analysis of the Western blots. In (B) and (C), p19[ARF−/−] HSC cells were transfected with either an unsilencing siRNA (uns siRNA) or a specific siRNA for NOX4 (NOX4 siRNA) and then treated or not with 2 ng/ml TGF-β during 48 hours, when it was performed: (B) RT-PCR of NOX4, α-SMA (Acta2), vimentin (vim), fibronectin (Fn1) and collagen I (Col1a1); (C) immunofluorescence images of F-actin, α-SMA and vimentin. A representative image for each RT-PCR (B) or immunofluorescence staining (C) is shown. 18S was used as loading control in B. Since HSC are very sensitive to serum deprivation, all experiments were carried out in the presence of 10% FBS.

A

B

C

D

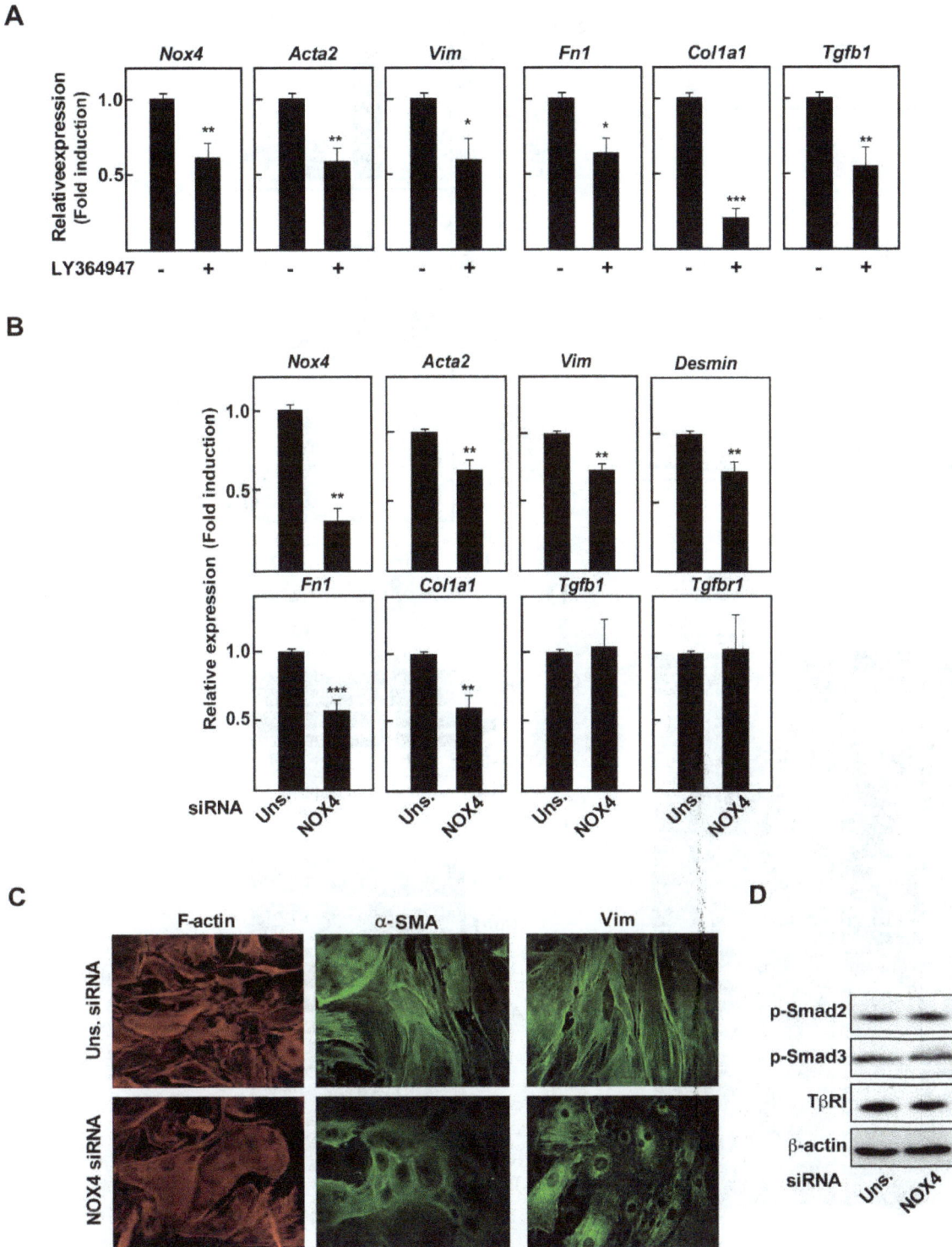

Figure 5. NOX4 downstream autocrine TGF-β is necessary to maintain the activated phenotype of cultured Mdr2$^{-/-}$/p19$^{ARF-/-}$ MFB. MFB isolated from fibrotic Mdr2$^{-/-}$/p19$^{ARF-/-}$ livers were used. *(A)* Real time PCR of Mdr2$^{-/-}$/p19$^{ARF-/-}$ MFB treated for 72 hours with 10 μM LY36494 (TRβI inhibitor): *NOX4*, α-SMA (*Acta2*), vimentin (*vim*), fibronectin (*Fn1*), collagen I (*Col1a1*) and TGF-β$_1$ (*Tgfb1*). In *B–D*, Mdr2$^{-/-}$/p19$^{ARF-/-}$ MFB were transfected with either an unsilencing siRNA (uns siRNA) or a specific siRNA for NOX4 (NOX4 siRNA) for 72 hours, when it was performed: *(B)* Real time PCR of the indicated genes. *(C)* Immunofluorescence staining of F-actin, α-SMA and vimentin. *(D)* Western blot of total lysates. β-actin was used as loading control. Data represent the mean ± SEM of three to six independent experiments, and were calculated relative to untreated MFB *(A)* or unsilencing-transfected cells *(B)* (*p<0.05; **p<0.01).

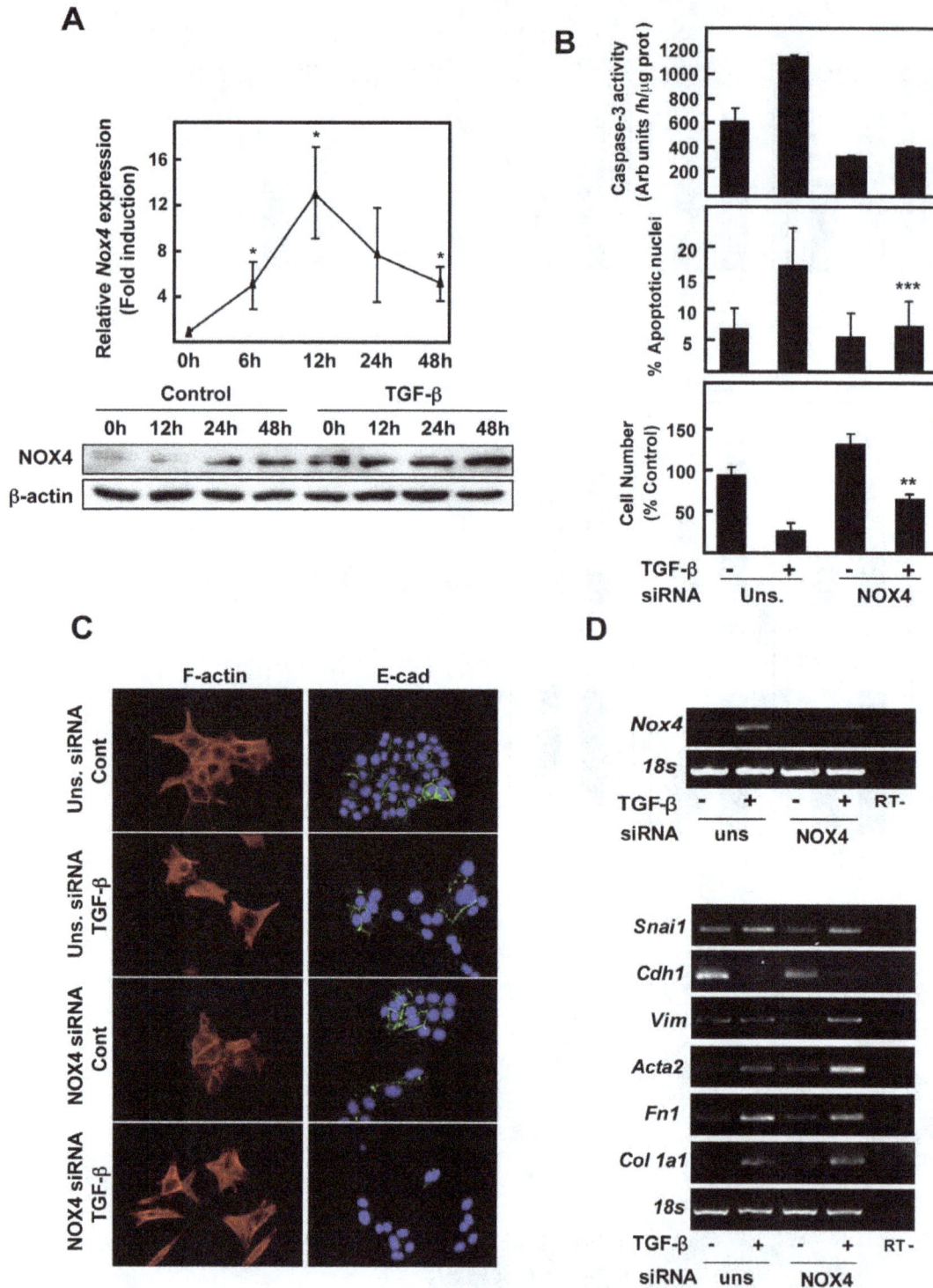

Figure 6. NOX4 is required for apoptosisbut not necessary for the EMT process, induced by TGF-β in hepatocytes. *(A)* TGF-β induces NOX4 expression in hepatocytes. NOX4 transript and protein levels were determined by Real time-PCR (upper panel) and western blot (lower panel), respectively, at the indicated times of treatment with 2 ng/ml TGF-β. In *B–D*, immortalized hepatocytes were transfected with either an unsilencing siRNA (uns siRNA) or a specific siRNA for NOX4 (NOX4 siRNA), serum-depleted for 4 hours and, finally, treated or not with 2 ng/ml TGF-β. *(B)* Cell death analysis: activation of caspase-3 activity at 16 hours, where the peak of maximal activation was found *(upper graph)*; percentage of cells with apoptotic nuclei at 48 h upon nuclear staining with DAPI *(middle graph)*; loss in cell viability at 48 h *(lower graph)*. Data represent the mean ± SEM of three independent experiments. Student's t test calculated comparing TGF-β-treated cells between the two conditions with the different siRNAs (**p<0.01; ***p<0.001). *(C)* Fluorescence microscopy staining for F-actin and E-cadherin at 48 hours. *(D)* Representative RT-PCR of the indicated genes after 3 h of treatment to observe the effects on *Nox4* expression (upper panel) and 48 h of treatment to analyze the effects on EMT-related genes (bottom panel). *18S* was used as loading control.

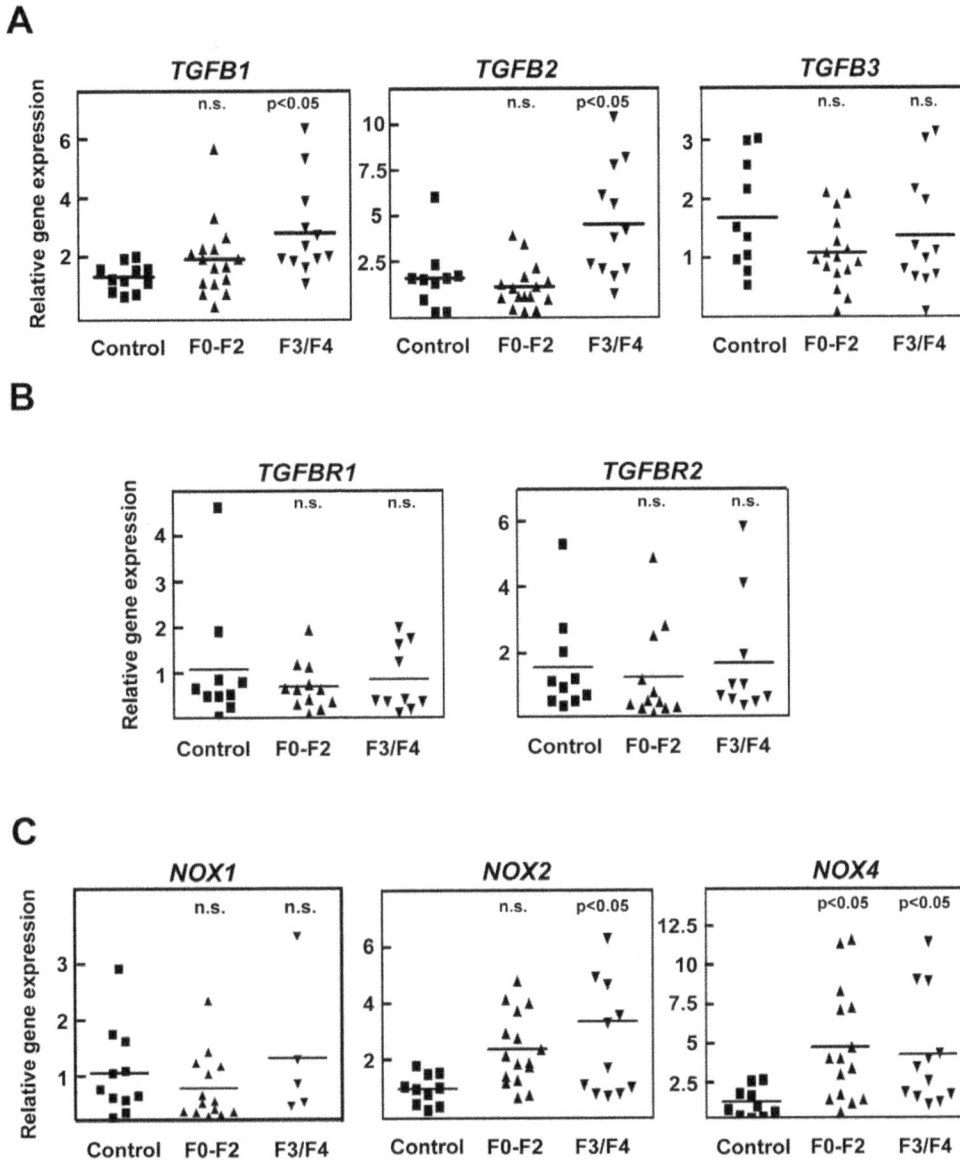

Figure 7. TGF-β1 and 2, NOX2 and NOX4 are up-regulated in human samples from patients with HCV-derived fibrosis. Samples from patients showing control livers (control; n = 10), low or mildly fibrotic livers (F0–F2; n = 16) or severely fibrotic and cirrhotic livers (F3/F4; n = 12). Real time determination of TGF-β$_1$(*TGFB1*), TGF-β$_2$ (*TGFB2*), TGF-β$_3$ (*TGFB3*) (*A*), TGFβRI and TGFβRII (*TGFBR1*, *TGFBR2*) (*B*), and *NOX1*, *NOX2* and *NOX4* (*C*). Statistic was calculated using one-way ANOVA associated with Dunnett's test.

implicated in apoptosis but not in the EMT process that TGF-β induces in hepatocytes.

Up-regulation of TGF-β and NOX4 in human samples from HCV infected patients

Since our *in vivo* and *in vitro* results in animal models pointed to a crucial role for NOX4 in fibrosis development, we next studied the situation in human samples. For this reason, we chose patients suffering from different degrees of liver fibrosis associated to HCV infection, who were classified as having mildly fibrotic livers (F0–F2) or severely fibrotic and cirrhotic livers (F3/F4) (Table 1). Comparing with samples from control livers, we performed real time PCR determinations of the three isoforms of TGF-β and the corresponding receptors, and also NOX1, NOX2 and NOX4. As shown in Fig. 7, TGF-β1 shows a clear tendency to increase from

F0/F2 stages, showing significant enhanced levels in F3/F4 patients. TGF-β2 was also significantly increased in the F3/F4 stage (Fig. 7A). No relevant changes in the expression of their receptors were observed. Interestingly, NOX1 expression did not show any significant change (Fig. 7C, left graph), but NOX2 and NOX4 were significantly up-regulated in fibrotic livers, being the relative increase in NOX4 higher than that observed for NOX2 (Fig. 7C).

Discussion

Chronic liver disease often progresses to fibrosis and finally to cirrhosis, which is a preneoplastic condition [1]. Thus far, there are no direct therapies aimed at liver fibrosis reversal, therefore innovative antifibrogenic approaches are needed [26]. Different models of hepatic fibrosis have been used to study the molecular

Table 1. Demographic, virological and histopathological characteristics of patients with chronic hepatitis C.

Age (yr) (Median and range)		46 (31–67)
Gender (M/F)		17/11
Baseline Viral load ($\times 10^3$ IU/ml) (Mean ± SD)		1.36±2.05
Genotype distribution (%)	Ia	7.14
	Ib	75.00
	II	3.57
	III	14.28
Activity distribution (n, %) (METAVIR)	0	0 (0)
	1	11 (39.28)
	2	14 (50.00)
	3	3 (10.71)
	4	0 (0)
Fibrosis distribution (n, %) (METAVIR)	0	1 (3.57)
	1	11 (39.28)
	2	4 (14.28)
	3	7 (25.00)
	4	5 (17.85)

Tissue of liver biopsies from 28 patients with chronic hepatitis C in different stages of liver fibrosis was examined for the gene expression analysis shown in Fig. 7.

pathogenesis of this disease. From these studies, several key generalizations have been done [1]: i) TGF-β is the most potent liver pro-fibrogenic cytokine; ii) oxidative stress induces liver fibrosis; iii) blocking normal liver regeneration by massive hepatocyte apoptosis turns out to be pro-fibrogenic. One of the most studied mechanisms of fibrogenesis actually influenced by ROS is myofibroblast activation. Previous reports and results presented in this manuscript have revealed that stellate cell transdifferentiation into myofibroblast is inhibited by antioxidants [27,28]. NOX4 downstream TGF-β has been described as the main mediator for myofibroblast activation in different organs such as heart [12], lung [11], kidney [13] and diseased prostatic stroma [14]. However, very few were known about the role of NOX4 in liver fibrosis. Results presented here indicate that induction of NOX4 occurs in three different animal models of liver fibrosis and in chronic HCV infection in humans, associated with activation of the TGF-β pathway, appearance of fibrotic areas and hepatocyte proliferation and apoptosis. NOX4 may play a key role in liver fibrosis development, downstream TGF-β, at two different levels: i) in vitro experiments reveal that NOX4 is required for both HSC activation and maintenance of the activated phenotype in MFBs and ii) hepatocytes respond to TGF-β by inducing NOX4 that is required for its pro-apoptotic response, which might be relevant to blunt regeneration and create a pro-fibrogenic microenvironment.

However, the role of NOX proteins in liver fibrogenesis is not only circumscribed to NOX4. Thus, studies performed in $Nox1^{-/-}$, $Nox2^{-/-}$ or $p47phox^{-/-}$ mice have pointed out the importance of NOX1 and NOX2 in fibrosis development [5,29,30]. Our results indicate that expression of NOX4 at the mRNA levels is much higher than those found for NOX1 and NOX2 in HSCs and hepatocytes, and functions are not redundant, since knock-down of NOX4 in these cells cause effects that cannot be prevented by the other NOXes. It is possible that

each isoform plays differential roles in liver fibrosis. Indeed, it has been suggested that NOX1 promotes myofibroblast proliferation by PTEN inactivation to positively regulate an Akt/FOXO4/p27 signaling pathway [29]. NOX2, highly expressed in macrophages and bone marrow-derived cells [8] may be acting in the process of phagocytosis of dead hepatocytes [30]. NOX1 activity might also contribute to the inflammatory process promoting COX-2 expression and prostaglandin synthesis in hepatocytes [31]. Interestingly, whereas the revised version of this manuscript was being prepared, evidences for the role of dual NOX4/NOX1 pharmacological inhibitors in decreasing both the apparition of fibrogenic markers and hepatocyte apoptosis in vivo, upon bile duct ligation, were reported [32], highlighting the relevant role of NOX1 and NOX4 in liver fibrosis and opening new perspectives for its treatment.

Hepatic fibrosis has been considered as an irreversible process but recent experimental and clinical data indicate that removal of the pro-fibrotic agent or condition may reverse liver fibrosis [33]. Results presented in this manuscript suggest that either TβRI inhibition or NOX4 silencing reverses the MFB phenotype, decreasing the expression of extracellular matrix genes, such as collagen I or fibronectin, down-regulating α-SMA and vimentin expression and changing cell morphology, which loses myofibroblastic appearance. Since it has been recently proposed that NOX4 modulates α-SMA and procollagen I (alpha1) expression in pulmonary fibrosis by controlling activation of Smad2/3 [34], we checked the effect of silencing NOX4 on TGF-β levels and Smad2/3 phosphorylation. Our results have indicated that NOX4 clearly acts downstream TGF-β-independently from Smads activation. It also has been described that NOX4 is critical for maintenance of smooth muscle gene expression in vascular smooth muscle cells [35], where ROS production impairs the TGF-β-induced phosphorylation of Ser103 on serum response factor (SRF) and reduces its transcriptional activity. Thus, NOX4 may play an important role associated with the α-SMA phenotype, being not only important in fibrotic processes, but also in cardiovascular physiology.

We have previously described that liver cells respond to TGF-β in vitro undergoing EMT [25,36]. The role of EMT is perhaps the most intriguing and controversial of recent hypothesis on the origin mechanisms of liver fibrosis [37]. Strong evidences indicate that hepatocytes from transgenic animals that overexpress Snail (a master gene involved in EMT through its capacity to repress E-cadherin gene, among others) fully undergo EMT [38] and may propagate liver fibrosis progression [39]. However, under normal genetic background, data from different experimental approaches in animals and humans show controversy [40]. Our results show that EMT occurs in hepatocytes in vitro, but NOX4 is not required for this process. However, NOX4 mediates TGF-β-induced cell death that is prevented in the presence of antioxidants. In agreement with these results, it has been recently proposed a role for NOX4 in epithelial cell death during development of bleomycin-induced lung fibrosis [41]. Using a model of NOX4-deficient mice, authors demonstrated that these animals were resistant to fibrosis due to the abrogation of TGF-β-induced apoptosis in epithelial cells. Prevention of apoptosis impaired fibrosis development, although inflammation was comparable to wild-type. A similar situation may occur in liver fibrosis, where engulfment of apoptotic bodies by HSC contributes to induce their activation [7]. Indeed, hepatocyte apoptosis not only would facilitate fibrosis through blocking liver regeneration, but it could play an active role. In this line of evidence, inhibiting apoptosis decreased the liver profibrogenic response [7,42]. Additionally to the crucial role of NOX4 in TGF-β-induced cell death, recent results indicate that it may be also required for apoptosis induced by other stimuli in liver cells, such as FasL and TNF-α/actinomycin D [32].

Finally, the finding that NOX4 is induced during the progression of a HCV disease reinforces the hypothesis of a role for NOX4 in human liver fibrosis. The magnitude of NOX4 up-regulation is higher than that observed for its co-partner NOX2 and, interestingly, we could not find any significant change in the expression of NOX1. NOX4 induction is observed at early stages of the disease when increases of TGF-β1 and 2 are not significant yet. This could be mediated by release of inflammatory signals that, indeed, up-regulate NOX4 in hepatocytes [31]. Further-more, different reports support that HCV induces a persistent elevation and increased nuclear localization of NOX4 in *in vitro* assays in hepatocytes, a process that was TGF-β-dependent [43,44]. Collectively, all these data provide evidences to propose that HCV-induced NOX4 may contribute to ROS production and may be related to HCV-induced liver disease. Results presented in this manuscript support that NOX4 could play an essential role inducing activation of stellate cells and apoptosis of hepatocytes under these conditions of human disease, contributing to the development of liver fibrosis.

Development of first-in-class series of NOX4 inhibitors for the potential treatment of fibrotic diseases, cardiovascular and metabolic syndromes is in progress [45]. Liver fibrosis might be considered for future clinical trials with these drugs. Likewise, ROS and NOX4 induced by TGF-β have proved to be therapeutic targets of polyenylphosphatidylcholine in the suppres-sion of human stellate cell activation [46]. Since NOX4 is mainly expressed in hepatocytes and HSC [8], according to the results presented in this manuscript, NOX4 inhibitors would specifically prevent HSC activation and hepatocytes cell death, without altering the role of other NOXes, such as NOX2, which might play defense function in Kupffer cells. In advanced stages of the disease, NOX4 inhibitors might be able to reverse the fibrotic phenotype acting on MFBs. Furthermore, and not less important, we demonstrate that silencing NOX4 prevents fibrogenesis but has no effect on TGF-β-mediated Smads phosphorylation. Indeed, the use of pharmacological drugs targeting NOX4 expression/activation would inhibit fibrogenesis without blocking other beneficial effects of TGF-β, such as growth inhibition in the epithelial cells, which prevents initiation of a pre-neoplastic stage.

In summary, here we show that NOX4 expression is elevated in the livers of experimental in vivo models of liver fibrosis and in patients with chronic HCV-derived infection, increasing along the fibrosis degree. NOX4, downstream TGF-β pathway, would play a role in the acquisition and maintenance of the MFB phenotype, as well as in mediating death of hepatocytes, which provokes inflammation and facilitates extracellular matrix deposit.

Supporting Information

Figure S1   Fibrosis development in Mdr2$^{-/-}$/p19$^{ARF-/-}$ mice. Representative histological sections of livers from control or 2 or 7 weeks-old Mdr2$^{-/-}$/p19$^{ARF-/-}$ mice. H&E, trichrome C staining and immunohistochemistru of F4/80, α-SMA, E-cadherin (E-cad) or vimentin (Vim) are shown.

Figure S2   Fibrosis development in Stat3^{Δhc}/Mdr2$^{-/-}$ mice. Representative histological sections of livers from control or 2 or 7 weeks-old Stat3^{Δhc}/Mdr2$^{-/-}$ mice. H&E, trichrome C staining and immunohistochemistru of F4/80, α-SMA, E-cadherin (E-cad) or vimentin (Vim) are shown.

Figure S3   TGF-β pathway is activated in Mdr2$^{-/-}$/p19$^{ARF-/-}$ and Stat3^{Δhc}/Mdr2$^{-/-}$ mice. Immunohisto-chemistry analysis of TGF-β, phospho-Smad2 or Smad7 in Mdr2$^{-/-}$/p19$^{ARF-/-}$ (**A**) and Stat3^{Δhc}/Mdr2$^{-/-}$ mice (**B**).

Figure S4   NOX4 expression in hepatocytes correlates with activation of caspase-3 in fibrotic tissues from Mdr2$^{-/-}$/p19$^{ARF-/-}$ mice. Immunohistochemistry analysis of NOX4 and the active form (cleaved) of caspase-3 in: hepatocytes around the vascular (up) or fibrotic (bottom) areas (**A**); two serial sections showing coincidence in the expression of both proteins in the same cells (**B**).

Figure S5   NOX4 expression is increased concomitant with fibrosis development in CCl$_4$ injection. Liver samples were collected and processed for immunohistochemical analysis. Representative results for NOX4, cleaved caspase-3 and Ki67 are shown.

Figure S6   Additional information to Figure 4. Expression of the different proteins analyzed in the Western blot of Figure 4A in HSC cells cultures for 24, 48 and 72 h in the absence of treatments (**A**). Quantitation of the intensity of the bands through densitometric analysis, relative to loading (β-actin) is shown above each band. A similar quantification approach for Western blot in Figure 4A is shown in **B**.

Figure S7   Role of NOX4 knock-down with specific siRNA on the expression of NOX4, NOX2 and NOX1 in HSC (A) and MFB (B). p19$^{ARF-/-}$ HSC cells (**A**) and Mdr2$^{-/-}$/p19$^{ARF-/-}$ MFB (**B**) were transfected with either an unsilencing siRNA (uns. siRNA) or a specific siRNA for NOX4 (NOX4 siRNA) as described in Figs. 4 and 5, respectively. In the case of HSC (**A**), cells were either not treated or treated with TGF-β (2 ng/ml), as indicated in the figure. Data shown correspond to the real-time PCR analysis of the mRNA levels of NOX4, NOX2 and NOX1, which were calculated relative to 18S expression. In order to compare the expression level among the different isoforms, we gave an arbitrary value of 1 to NOX4 expression under basal conditions in both HSC (**A**) and MFB (**B**), and all the data are referred to this value. Mean ± S.E.M. is shown and the specific value of the mean detailed above each bar.

Figure S8   Role of antioxidants (GEE and BHA) or a NADPH oxidase inhibitor (DPI) on the effects of TGF-β on ROS production and apoptosis in hepatocytes (A and B, respectively) and activation of HSC (C). Cells were pre-incubated during 30 min with 1 μM DPI, 2 mM GEE or 200 μM BHA, as indicated in each figure, before adding 2 ng/ml of TGF-β. The same concentrations of the agents were maintained during all the TGF-β treatment. **A.** After 3 h of treatment in hepatocytes, intracellular content of ROS was analyzed through fluorimetric assay as detailed in the Materials and Methods section. Data represent the mean ± S.E.M. of 3 independent experiments in triplicate and are referred to the value in untreated cells (100%). **B.** After 16 h of treatment in hepatocytes, proteins were collected for caspase-3 analysis. Data represent the mean ± S.E.M. of 3 independent experiments in duplicate and are expressed as arbitrary units per hour and per microgram of protein. **C.** After 48 h of treatment in HSC, RNA was collected for analysis of expression by RT-PCR of the genes detailed in the figure. A representative experiment out of 3 is shown.

Table S1 Mouse primer sequences used for semiquantitative PCR.

Table S2 Mouse and human primer sequences used for quantitative real-time PCR.

Acknowledgments

We acknowledge the encouraging advices of Dr. Victor Thannickal (University of Alabama at Birmingham, USA) and the excellent technical support of Esther Bertran, Greta Ripoll and Judit Lopez. We also thank Dr. Valeria Poli for providing the floxed Stat3 mice. We dedicate this manuscript to the memory of Dr. Nelson Fausto, Professor of Pathology and Senior Advisor to the Dean of the School of Medicine and former Chairman of the Department of Pathology at the University of Washington Medical School, died last April. We enthusiastically acknowledge his continuous help for the development of our research line, his inspiration, his advices and his friendship.

Author Contributions

Conceived and designed the experiments: PS WM IF. Performed the experiments: PS JM EC-M CR HH. Analyzed the data: PS CR CMF-R WM IF. Contributed reagents/materials/analysis tools: CMF-R FP RE. Wrote the paper: PS IF.

References

1. Brenner DA (2009) Molecular pathogenesis of liver fibrosis. Trans Am Clin Climatol Assoc 120: 361–368.
2. Matsuzaki K (2009) Modulation of TGF-beta signaling during progression of chronic liver diseases. Front Biosci 14: 2923–2934.
3. Proell V, Carmona-Cuenca I, Murillo MM, Huber H, Fabregat I, et al. (2007) TGF-beta dependent regulation of oxygen radicals during transdifferentiation of activated hepatic stellate cells to myofibroblastoid cells. Comp Hepatol 6: 1.
4. Sanchez A, Alvarez AM, Benito M, Fabregat I (1996) Apoptosis induced by transforming growth factor-beta in fetal hepatocyte primary cultures: involvement of reactive oxygen intermediates. J Biol Chem 271: 7416–7422.
5. De Minicis S, Seki E, Paik YH, Osterreicher CH, Kodama Y, et al. (2010) Role and cellular source of nicotinamide adenine dinucleotide phosphate oxidase in hepatic fibrosis. Hepatology 52: 1420–1430.
6. Aram G, Potter JJ, Liu X, Wang L, Torbenson MS, et al. (2009) Deficiency of nicotinamide adenine dinucleotide phosphate, reduced form oxidase enhances hepatocellular injury but attenuates fibrosis after chronic carbon tetrachloride administration. Hepatology 49: 911–919.
7. Jiang JX, Venugopal S, Serizawa N, Chen X, Scott F, et al. (2010) Reduced nicotinamide adenine dinucleotide phosphate oxidase 2 plays a key role in stellate cell activation and liver fibrogenesis in vivo. Gastroenterology 139: 1375–1384.
8. Paik YH, Iwaisako K, Seki E, Inokuchi S, Schnabl B, et al. (2011) The nicotinamide adenine dinucleotide phosphate oxidase (NOX) homologues NOX1 and NOX2/gp91(phox) mediate hepatic fibrosis in mice. Hepatology 53: 1730–1741.
9. Carmona-Cuenca I, Roncero C, Sancho P, Caja L, Fausto N, et al. (2008) Upregulation of the NADPH oxidase NOX4 by TGF-beta in hepatocytes is required for its pro-apoptotic activity. J Hepatol 49: 965–976.
10. Barnes JL, Gorin Y (2011) Myofibroblast differentiation during fibrosis: role of NAD(P)H oxidases. Kidney Int 79: 944–956.
11. Hecker L, Vittal R, Jones T, Jagirdar R, Luckhardt TR, et al. (2009) NADPH oxidase-4 mediates myofibroblast activation and fibrogenic responses to lung injury. Nat Med 15: 1077–1081.
12. Cucoranu I, Clempus R, Dikalova A, Phelan PJ, Ariyan S, et al. (2005) NAD(P)H oxidase 4 mediates transforming growth factor-beta1-induced differentiation of cardiac fibroblasts into myofibroblasts. Circ Res 97: 900–907.
13. Bondi CD, Manickam N, Lee DY, Block K, Gorin Y, et al. (2010) NAD(P)H oxidase mediates TGF-beta1-induced activation of kidney myofibroblasts. J Am Soc Nephrol 21: 93–102.
14. Sampson N, Koziel R, Zenzmaier C, Bubendorf L, Plas E, et al. (2011) ROS signaling by NOX4 drives fibroblast-to-myofibroblast differentiation in the diseased prostatic stroma. Mol Endocrinol 25: 503–515.
15. van Zijl F, Mair M, Csiszar A, Schneller D, Zulehner G, et al. (2009) Hepatic tumor-stroma crosstalk guides epithelial to mesenchymal transition at the tumor edge. Oncogene 28: 4022–4033.
16. Baghdasaryan A, Claudel T, Kosters A, Gumhold J, Silbert D, et al. Curcumin improves sclerosing cholangitis in Mdr2−/− mice by inhibition of cholangiocyte inflammatory response and portal myofibroblast proliferation. Gut 59: 521–530.
17. Barikbin R, Neureiter D, Wirth J, Erhardt A, Schwinge D, et al. Induction of heme oxygenase 1 prevents progression of liver fibrosis in Mdr2 knockout mice. Hepatology 55:553–562.
18. Mair M, Zollner G, Schneller D, Musteanu M, Fickert P, et al. (2010) Signal transducer and activator of transcription 3 protects from liver injury and fibrosis in a mouse model of sclerosing cholangitis. Gastroenterology 138: 2499–2508.
19. Proell V, Mikula M, Fuchs E, Mikulits W (2005) The plasticity of p19 ARF null hepatic stellate cells and the dynamics of activation. Biochim Biophys Acta 1744: 76–87.
20. Gonzalez-Rodriguez A, Clampit JE, Escribano O, Benito M, Rondinone CM, et al. (2007) Developmental switch from prolonged insulin action to increased insulin sensitivity in protein tyrosine phosphatase 1B-deficient hepatocytes. Endocrinology 148: 594–608.
21. Caja L, Ortiz C, Bertran E, Murillo MM, Miro-Obradors MJ, et al. (2007) Differential intracellular signalling induced by TGF-beta in rat adult hepatocytes and hepatoma cells: implications in liver carcinogenesis. Cell Signal 19: 683–694.
22. Sancho P, Bertran E, Caja L, Carmona-Cuenca I, Murillo MM, et al. (2009) The inhibition of the epidermal growth factor (EGF) pathway enhances TGF-beta-induced apoptosis in rat hepatoma cells through inducing oxidative stress coincident with a change in the expression pattern of the NADPH oxidases (NOX) isoforms. Biochim Biophys Acta 1793: 253–263.
23. Murillo MM, Carmona-Cuenca I, Del Castillo G, Ortiz A, Roncero C, et al. (2007) Activation of NADPH oxidase by transforming growth factor-beta in hepatocytes mediates up-regulation of epidermal growth factor receptor ligands through a nuclear factor-kappaB-dependent mechanism. Biochem J 405: 251–259.
24. Fickert P, Fuchsbichler A, Wagner M, Zollner G, Kaser A, et al. (2004) Regurgitation of bile acids from leaky bile ducts causes sclerosing cholangitis in Mdr2 (Abcb4) knockout mice. Gastroenterology 127: 261–274.
25. Valdes F, Alvarez AM, Locascio A, Vega S, Herrera B, et al. (2002) The epithelial mesenchymal transition confers resistance to the apoptotic effects of transforming growth factor Beta in fetal rat hepatocytes. Mol Cancer Res 1: 68–78.
26. de Andrade JA, Thannickal VJ (2009) Innovative approaches to the therapy of fibrosis. Curr Opin Rheumatol 21: 649–655.
27. Abhilash PA, Harikrishnan R, Indira M (2012) Ascorbic acid supplementation down-regulates the alcohol induced oxidative stress, hepatic stellate cell activation, cytotoxicity and mRNA levels of selected fibrotic genes in guinea pigs. Free Radic Res 46: 204–213.
28. Foo NP, Lin SH, Lee YH, Wu MJ, Wang YJ (2011) alpha-Lipoic acid inhibits liver fibrosis through the attenuation of ROS-triggered signaling in hepatic stellate cells activated by PDGF and TGF-beta. Toxicology 282: 39–46.
29. Cui W, Matsuno K, Iwata K, Ibi M, Matsumoto M, et al. (2011) NOX1/nicotinamide adenine dinucleotide phosphate, reduced form (NADPH) oxidase promotes proliferation of stellate cells and aggravates liver fibrosis induced by bile duct ligation. Hepatology 54: 949–958.
30. Jiang JX, Venugopal S, Serizawa N, Chen X, Scott F, et al. (2010) Reduced nicotinamide adenine dinucleotide phosphate oxidase 2 plays a key role in stellate cell activation and liver fibrogenesis in vivo. Gastroenterology 139: 1375–1384.
31. Sancho P, Martin-Sanz P, Fabregat I (2011) Reciprocal regulation of NADPH oxidases and the cyclooxygenase-2 pathway. Free Radic Biol Med 51: 1789–1798.
32. Jiang JX, Chen X, Serizawa N, Szyndralewicz C, Page P, et al. (2012) Liver fibrosis and hepatocyte apoptosis are attenuated by GKT137831, a novel NOX4/NOX1 inhibitor in vivo. Free Radic Biol Med 53:289–296.
33. Povero D, Busletta C, Novo E, di Bonzo LV, Cannito S, et al. (2010) Liver fibrosis: a dynamic and potentially reversible process. Histol Histopathol 25: 1075–1091.
34. Amara N, Goven D, Prost F, Muloway R, Crestani B, et al. NOX4/NADPH oxidase expression is increased in pulmonary fibroblasts from patients with idiopathic pulmonary fibrosis and mediates TGFbeta1-induced fibroblast differentiation into myofibroblasts. Thorax 65: 733–738.
35. Martin-Garrido A, Brown DI, Lyle AN, Dikalova A, Seidel-Rogol B, et al. NADPH oxidase 4 mediates TGF-beta-induced smooth muscle alpha-actin via p38MAPK and serum response factor. Free Radic Biol Med 50: 354–362.
36. Caja L, Bertran E, Campbell J, Fausto N, Fabregat I (2011) The transforming growth factor-beta (TGF-beta) mediates acquisition of a mesenchymal stem cell-like phenotype in human liver cells. J Cell Physiol 226: 1214–1223.
37. Wells RG (2011) The epithelial-to-mesenchymal transition in liver fibrosis: here today, gone tomorrow? Hepatology 51: 737–740.
38. Franco DL, Mainez J, Vega S, Sancho P, Murillo MM, et al. (2010) Snail1 suppresses TGF-beta-induced apoptosis and is sufficient to trigger EMT in hepatocytes. J Cell Sci 123: 3467–3477.

39. Rowe RG, Lin Y, Shimizu-Hirota R, Hanada S, Neilson EG, et al. (2011) Hepatocyte-derived Snail1 propagates liver fibrosis progression. Mol Cell Biol 31: 2392–2403.

40. Dooley S, Hamzavi J, Ciuclan L, Godoy P, Ilkavets I, et al. (2008) Hepatocyte-specific Smad7 expression attenuates TGF-beta-mediated fibrogenesis and protects against liver damage. Gastroenterology 135: 642–659.

41. Carnesecchi S, Deffert C, Donati Y, Basset O, Hinz B, et al. (2011) A key role for NOX4 in epithelial cell death during development of lung fibrosis. Antioxid Redox Signal 15: 607–619.

42. Mitchell C, Robin MA, Mayeuf A, Mahrouf-Yorgov M, Mansouri A, et al. (2009) Protection against hepatocyte mitochondrial dysfunction delays fibrosis progression in mice. Am J Pathol 175: 1929–1937.

43. Boudreau HE, Emerson SU, Korzeniowska A, Jendrysik MA, Leto TL (2009) Hepatitis C virus (HCV) proteins induce NADPH oxidase 4 expression in a transforming growth factor beta-dependent manner: a new contributor to HCV-induced oxidative stress. J Virol 83: 12934–12946.

44. de Mochel NS, Seronello S, Wang SH, Ito C, Zheng JX, et al. (2010) Hepatocyte NAD(P)H oxidases as an endogenous source of reactive oxygen species during hepatitis C virus infection. Hepatology 52: 47–59.

45. Laleu B, Gaggini F, Orchard M, Fioraso-Cartier L, Cagnon L, et al. (2010) First in class, potent, and orally bioavailable NADPH oxidase isoform 4 (Nox4) inhibitors for the treatment of idiopathic pulmonary fibrosis. J Med Chem 53: 7715–7730.

46. Ikeda R, Ishii K, Hoshikawa Y, Azumi J, Arakaki Y, et al. (2011) Reactive oxygen species and NADPH oxidase 4 induced by transforming growth factor beta1 are the therapeutic targets of polyenylphosphatidylcholine in the suppression of human hepatic stellate cell activation. Inflamm Res 60: 597–604.

9

Lack of the Matricellular Protein SPARC (Secreted Protein, Acidic and Rich in Cysteine) Attenuates Liver Fibrogenesis in Mice

Catalina Atorrasagasti[1], Estanislao Peixoto[1,9], Jorge B. Aquino[1,2,9], Néstor Kippes[1], Mariana Malvicini[1], Laura Alaniz[1,2], Mariana Garcia[1,2], Flavia Piccioni[1], Esteban J. Fiore[1], Juan Bayo[1], Ramón Bataller[3], Elizabeth Guruceaga[4], Fernando Corrales[4], Osvaldo Podhajcer[5,2], Guillermo Mazzolini[1,2]*

1 Gene Therapy Laboratory, School of Medicine, Austral University. Derqui-Pilar, Buenos Aires, Argentina, 2 CONICET (Consejo Nacional de Investigaciones Científicas y Técnicas), Buenos Aires, Argentina, 3 Department of Medicine and Nutrition, University of North Carolina, Chapel Hill, North Carolina, United States of America, 4 Centro de Investigación Médica Aplicada, Universidad de Navarra, Pamplona, España, 5 Gene Therapy Laboratory, Fundación Instituto Leloir, Buenos Aires, Argentina

Abstract

Introduction: Secreted Protein, Acidic and Rich in Cysteine (SPARC) is a matricellular protein involved in many biological processes and found over-expressed in cirrhotic livers. By mean of a genetic approach we herein provide evidence from different *in vivo* liver disease models suggesting a profibrogenic role for SPARC.

Methods: Two *in vivo* models of liver fibrosis, based on TAA administration and bile duct ligation, were developed on SPARC wild-type (SPARC$^{+/+}$) and knock-out (SPARC$^{-/-}$) mice. Hepatic SPARC expression was analyzed by qPCR. Fibrosis was assessed by Sirius Red staining, and the maturation state of collagen fibers was analyzed using polarized light. Necroinflammatory activity was evaluated by applying the Knodell score and liver inflammatory infiltration was characterized by immunohistochemistry. Hepatic stellate cell activation was assessed by α-SMA immunohistochemistry. In addition, pro-fibrogenic genes and inflammatory cytokines were measured by qPCR and/or ELISA. Liver gene expression profile was analyzed in SPARC$^{-/-}$ and SPARC$^{+/+}$ mice using Affymetrix Mouse Gene ST 1.0 array.

Results: SPARC expression was found induced in fibrotic livers of mouse and human. SPARC$^{-/-}$ mice showed a reduction in the degree of inflammation, mainly CD4+ cells, and fibrosis. Consistently, collagen deposits and mRNA expression levels were decreased in SPARC$^{-/-}$ mice when compared to SPARC$^{+/+}$ mice; in addition, MMP-2 expression was increased in SPARC$^{-/-}$ mice. A reduction in the number of activated myofibroblasts was observed. Moreover, TGF-β1 expression levels were down-regulated in the liver as well as in the serum of TAA-treated knock-out animals. Ingenuity Pathway Analysis (IPA) analysis suggested several gene networks which might involve protective mechanisms of SPARC deficiency against liver fibrogenesis and a better established machinery to repair DNA and detoxify from external chemical stimuli.

Conclusions: Overall our data suggest that SPARC plays a significant role in liver fibrogenesis. Interventions to inhibit SPARC expression are suggested as promising approaches for liver fibrosis treatment.

Editor: Wing-Kin Syn, Institute of Hepatology, Foundation for Liver Research, United Kingdom

Funding: This work was supported by grants from Austral University, Agencia Nacional de Promoción Científica y Tecnológica (PICT-2006-1882, PICT-2005-34788, PICT 2007-00736, PICTO-CRUP 2005-31179, PICT 2008-00123), CTE-06 and AECI 2008, FIMA and the "UTE project CIMA", grants Plan Nacional SAF2011-29312 and PIB2010AR-00474 from Ministerio de Ciencia e Innovación to FJC, and ISCIII-RETIC RD06/0020 to FJC. The funders had no role in study design, data collection and analysis, decision to publish, or preparation of the manuscript.

Competing Interests: The authors have declared that no competing interests exist.

* E-mail: gmazzoli@cas.austral.edu.ar

⑨ These authors contributed equally to this work.

Introduction

Secreted protein, acidic and rich in cysteine (SPARC), also called osteonectin or BM-40, is a secreted multifunctional extracellular matrix (ECM)-associated protein involved in a number of biological processes [1,2]. Among other functions, SPARC plays a major role in the wound healing response to injury and tissue remodeling [1]. Regarding mechanisms likely therein involved, locally produced SPARC was found to stimulate collagen deposition, inflammatory cells recruitment, TGF-β1 production, mesenchymal cell proliferation and ECM proteins synthesis, in the context of kidney, skin and/or lung fibrogenesis [3,4], while no studies were performed on liver fibrosis models. Due to its biological properties, SPARC was proposed as a therapeutic target to prevent fibrosis in chronic inflammatory and profibrogenic conditions [5].

Although SPARC is constitutively expressed in the liver under non-pathological conditions [6], it was found upregulated in fibrotic-related liver diseases such as cirrhosis [7,8] and hepatocellular carcinoma [9,10,11]. During liver fibrogenesis, SPARC was found overexpressed in activated hepatic stellate (HSCs) and in endothelial cells [6,7]. These findings suggest that SPARC may have a prominent role in liver fibrogenesis; moreover, we have recently demonstrated that a forced transitory reduction in SPARC expression levels by an adenovirus encoding an antisense specific for SPARC mRNA (AdasSPARC) attenuates fibrosis development in an *in vivo* experimental rat model [5].

During liver fibrogenesis TGF-β1 expression is induced. This cytokine plays a key role in the activation of HSCs and in the development of hepatic fibrosis [12]. Thus, different molecular strategies have been explored to block/reduce TGF-β1 mediated mechanisms including gene transfer of truncated TGF-β1 receptor type II or administration of a soluble TGF-β1 type II receptor, [13,14]. Interestingly, a positive feedback between SPARC and TGF-β1 has been previously reported [3,15].

To further elucidate the role of SPARC in hepatic fibrogenesis, we have herein used different *in vivo* disease models, i.e. involving either hepatotoxicity or biliary duct obstruction, in SPARC genetically deficient mice. Liver fibrosis development was found markedly attenuated in SPARC$^{-/-}$ when compared to SPARC$^{+/+}$ mice. Our data suggest that SPARC plays a major role in the pathogenesis of liver fibrosis, through myofibroblast recruitment/activation and induction of TGF-β1 expression. Additionally, microarray analyses likely involve DNA protective and repair mechanisms. Overall these results give further support to new therapeutic approaches based on SPARC expression inhibition for the treatment of patients with chronic liver diseases.

Materials and Methods

Animals and Experimental Design

Male C57BL/6x129SvJ (The Jackson Laboratory, Bar Harbor, Maine, USA) SPARC$^{+/+}$ and SPARC$^{-/-}$ mice (2–3 months-old) were used. In a hepatotoxic model, animals were administered intraperitoneally (i.p.) with 200 mg/kg of thioacetamide (TAA) (Sigma, St Louis, MO), 3 times a week as described previously [16,17]. Animals were sacrificed at 2 and 10 weeks after TAA application onset and blood and liver samples were obtained. In a cholestasis model, mice were subjected to bile duct ligation (BDL) or sham-operation or they were left untreated. For surgeries, animals were anesthetized with sodium pentobarbital. A midline laparotomy was performed and the common bile duct was doubly ligated with 4–0 silk. Sham operation procedure was similar but without ligating the bile duct. Animals were sacrificed at 7 days after surgery and blood and liver samples were obtained. All experimental procedures were performed according to the "Guide for the Care and Use of Laboratory Animals" published by the U.S. National Research Council (National Academy Press, Washington, D.C. 1996) and approved by the School of Medicine, Austral University (Permission number: FBA002).

Human Liver Specimens

A total of 7 liver biopsies, from 2 non-cirrhotic and 5 cirrhotic subjects were used in real-time polymerase chain reaction studies. Cirrhosis etiology was diverse (primary biliary cirrhosis, biliary atresia, hepatitis C virus (HCV) infection, hemochromatosis and cryptogenic; patients #1 to #5). All participants gave their written informed consent to the study, which was approved by the Institutional Ethics Committee and by the Ministry of Health of Buenos Aires State (Permission number: 2919/179/2011).

Reverse Transcription-polymerase Chain Reaction (RT-PCR)

Liver tissue was homogenized and total RNA was extracted by using Trizol Reagent (Sigma-Aldrich Co., St. Louis, MO). Total RNA (2 μg) was reverse transcribed with 200 U of SuperScript II Reverse Transcriptase (Invitrogen, Carlsbad, CA) using 500 ng of Oligo (dT) primers. cDNAs were subjected to real-time polymerase chain reaction (qPCR) (Stratagene Mx3005p, Stratagene, La Jolla, CA, USA). For qPCR of mouse samples the mRNA levels of SPARC, alpha 2-type I collagen (COL1A2), matrix metalloproteinase-2 (MMP-2) and transforming growth factor-β1 (TGF-β1) were quantified by SYBR® Green (Invitrogen), using the following primers: SPARC sense (5′-CCACACGTTTCTTTGAGACC-3′); SPARC antisense (5′-GATGTCCTGCTCCTTGATGC-3′), COL1A2, 5′-CCTACATGGACCAGCAGACTG -3 (forward), 5′- GGAGGTCTTGGTGGTTTTGTA -3′ (reverse), TGF-β1 5′-CCACTCGCTTCTTTGAGACC-3′ (forward), 5′-TAGTG-GAAGTGGGTGGGGAC-3′ (reverse) and MMP-2 5′-CTCA-GATCCGTGGTGAGAT -3 (forward), 5′-AGGCTGGT-CAGTGGCTTGG-3′ (reverse). For qPCR of human samples, the following primers were used: SPARC, 5′-AAACCGAAGAG-GAGGTGGTG-3′ (forward), 5′-GCAAAGAAGTGGCAG-GAAGA-3′ (reverse). All PCR amplifications were carried out using a cycle of 95°C for 10 min and 40 cycles under the following parameters: 95°C for 30 sec, corresponding melting temperature for 30 sec, 72°C for 1 min. At the end of the PCR reaction, the temperature was increased from 60°C to 95°C at a rate of 2°C/min, and the fluorescence was measured every 15 sec to construct the melting curve. Values were normalized to levels of glyceraldehyde-3-phosphate dehydrogenase (GAPDH; used as housekeeping) transcript (forward 5′-CATCTCTGCCCCCTCTGCTG -3′; reverse 5′-GCCTGCTTCACCACCTTCTTG-3′). Data were processed by the ΔΔCt method. The relative amount of the PCR product amplified from untreated cells was set as 1. A non-template control (NTC) was run in every assay, and all determinations were performed in triplicate in two or three separated experiments.

Pathology, Immunofluorescence and Immunohistochemistry Studies

Some harvested livers were immersed in 10% phosphate-buffered formalin. Fixed tissue was embedded in paraffin, sectioned (5 μm) and hematoxylin-eosin (H&E), Masson-trichrome or Sirius red stained, or used for immunohistochemical analysis of α-SMA expression. The Knodell score was used to grade the severity of the necroinflammatory process and fibrosis [18]. Assessments were blinded performed by an experienced pathologist. For CD4 immunohistochemistry, tissue was embedded in OCT, cryostat sectioned and fixed for 15 min in alcoholic formalin. In brief, after tissue dehydration endogenous peroxidase was blocked with 3% H_2O_2 in 95% ethanol. Thereafter, sections were subsequently blocked for endogenous biotin and avidin (Blocking kit, Vector Laboratories Inc.) and sections were incubated with the primary antibody anti-CD4 (1:75, 0.2% BSA in PBS) overnight. After being washed in phosphate-buffered saline, slides were incubated with peroxidase-linked biotinylated goat anti-mouse secondary antibody (1:100, Vector Laboratories Inc.) for 2 h, washed and further incubated with AB complex at RT. They were then washed twice with PBS and twice with 0.1 M acetate buffer before incubation with a solution of 3.3-diaminobenzidine (DAB; Sigma), ammonium nickel sulfate and H_2O_2 until signal was developed.

For immunofluorescence SPARC analysis, mice were perfused with 4% paraformaldehyde and liver tissue was dissected out, post-fixed for 90 minutes and subsequently placed in 10 and 20% sucrose. For SPARC immunofluorescence assay, samples were embedded in OCT and cryostat sectioned (12 μm). After a 1 hour incubation in blockage buffer (5% normal donkey serum -Jackson ImmunoResearch, PA, USA), 1% BSA, 0.3% Triton-X in 1×PBS; room temperature), tissue was incubated with a rat anti-SPARC monoclonal antibody (1:150, 0.1% BSA, 0.3% Triton-X, 0.02% sodium azide in PBS; overnight, 4°C; R&D, MN, USA), together with either rabbit anti-mouse α-SMA (1:75; ab5694, Abcam, MA, USA) or rabbit anti-Von Willebrand factor (vWF; 1:215; Sigma, MO, USA) polyclonal antibodies. After extensive washing, tissue was incubated with Cy3-conjugated donkey anti-rat IgG and FITC-conjugated donkey anti-rabbit IgG secondary antibodies (1:450; 1% BSA in PBS, 2 hours, room temperature; Jackson ImmunoResearch). Images were captured using a Nikon C1 laser confocal microscope.

For chromogenic immunohistochemical analysis and quantification of α-SMA expression, sections were deparaffinized, rehydrated and heated with buffer citrate (pH = 6) in a microwave protocol. Endogenous peroxidase was blocked with 3% H_2O_2 in 95% ethanol. Thereafter, sections were subsequently blocked for endogenous biotin and avidin (Blocking kit, Vector Laboratories Inc.), and for unspecific binding of the primary antibody (1% BSA-PBS). Tissue was then incubated with the rabbit anti-mouse α-SMA polyclonal antibody (1:100; Abcam). After extensive washing, slides were incubated with peroxidase-linked biotinylated goat anti-rabbit secondary antibodies for 2 h, washed and further incubated with AB complex at RT. They were then washed twice with PBS and twice with 0.1 M acetate buffer before incubation with a solution of 3.3-diaminobenzidine (DAB; Sigma), ammonium nickel sulfate and H_2O_2 until signal was developed. Primary antibody incubation was omitted in control slides, only rendering a faint staining (not shown). Quantitative analysis of α-SMA immunostained area was performed by computerized morphometric analysis (CMA). About 80 light microscope images (200X) per specimen were captured and analyzed using a color threshold detection system developed in ImageJ software (NIH, USA). Results were expressed as percentage of positive area.

Quantification of Hepatic Collagen Content, Collagen Fibers Maturation and Hyaluronan Deposition

Quantitative analysis of collagen content was performed by CMA on samples stained with Sirius red. For this purpose, randomly sampled two hundred light microscope images (200X) per liver specimen, excepting large centrilobular veins and large portal tracts (≥150 μm) were analyzed. About 80 light microscope images (200X) per specimen were captured and analyzed using a color threshold detection system developed in ImageJ (National Institutes of Health). Values are expressed as percentage of positive area. To assess the degree of packaging of collagen fibers and their maturation state, liver sections were examined with polarized light microscopy using an Olympus BX60 microscope (Olympus, Tokyo, Japan). Hyaluronan staining was performed as previously described [19,20].

ELISA Assay of TGF-β1

Total TGF-β1 serum levels after 10 weeks of TAA treatment were measured by ELISA (R&D systems, Minneapolis, MN, USA), following manufacturer recommendations. To convert all latent TGF-β1 to the active form, samples were pretreated with 1 M HCl for 15 min at room temperature. Finally, the reaction was stopped, by 1 M NaOH neutralization, and the optical density of each well was determined at 540 or 570 nm.

Microarray Data Analysis

Samples were processed following Affymetrix recommendations and cRNA was hybridized to the Affymetrix Mouse Gene ST 1.0 array. Both background correction and normalization were done using RMA (Robust Multichip Average) algorithm [21]. Then, a filtering process was performed to eliminate low expression probe sets. Applying the criterion of an expression value greater than 64 in 2 samples for each experimental condition, 18187 probesets were selected for statistical analysis. R and Bioconductor were used for preprocessing and statistical analysis. LIMMA (Linear Models for Microarray Data) [22,23] was used to find out the probe sets that showed significant differential expression between experimental conditions. Genes were selected as significant using a criteria of p-value <0.01.

Functional and Pathway Analysis

Functional enrichment analysis of Gene Ontology (GO) categories was carried out using standard hypergeometric test [24]. The biological knowledge extraction was complemented through the use of Ingenuity Pathway Analysis (Ingenuity Systems, www.ingenuity.com), which database includes manually curated and fully traceable data derived from literature sources.

Transaminases Measurement

Serum alanine (ALT) and aspartate (ALT) transaminases were measured using an ARCHITECT® (Abbott) autoanalyzer.

Migration Assay

SPARC$^{+/+}$ and SPARC$^{-/-}$ mice were sacrificed, spleen were excised, and single cell suspensions were prepared. Cell suspension were treated with RBC lysis buffer (0.15 mol/L NH_4Cl, 1 mmol/L $KHCO_3$, 0.1 mmol/L Na_2EDTA) and washed with PBS 1% bovine serum albumin. Then, cells were plated in a plastic petri dish for 15 min and finally counted and subjected to migration assay. Migratory capacity to rCCL19 (Peprotech) was assayed using a 48-Transwell microchemotaxis Boyden Chamber unit (Neuroprobe, Inc.). In brief, splenocytes (20,000 cells/well) were placed in the upper chamber of the Transwell unit, which was separated from the lower chamber by 8 μm pore polycarbonate filters (Nucleopore membrane, Neuroprobe). rCCL19 (10 ng/μl) was placed in the lower chamber of the Transwell unit. All the system units were incubated for 2 h at 37°C in a 5% CO_2 humidified atmosphere. After that, the membrane was carefully removed and cells on the upper side of the membrane were scraped off with a blade. Cells attached to the lower side of the membrane were fixed in 2% formaldehyde, and the membranes from the microchemotaxis Boyden Chamber unit were stained with 40.6 diamidino-2-phenylindole dihydrochloride (DAPI, Sigma-Aldrich). Cells were counted using fluorescent-field microscopy and a 10x objective lens: the images captured in three representative visual fields were analyzed using CellProfiler software (www.cellprofiler.com), and the mean number of cells/field (SEM was calculated).

Statistical Analysis

Data are expressed as mean ± SEM when appropriate. Statistical analysis was performed using Student's t test or Mann-Whitney, according to value data distribution. Differences were considered to be significant when p<0.05.

Results

Expression of SPARC during Liver Fibrogenesis

We first investigated whether SPARC expression levels may be upregulated in the liver of cirrhotic patients. To address this issue, liver biopsies taken from cirrhotic and non-cirrhotic patients were processed for qPCR studies. A significant upregulation in SPARC expression levels was observed in cirrhotic samples when compared to non-fibrotic ones (Figure 1A). These data suggest a possible role for SPARC in liver fibrogenesis.

We next asked whether or not SPARC expression could be similarly induced in different *in vivo* models developed in SPARC$^{+/+}$ mice. To address whether SPARC expression levels may change during liver fibrogenesis, samples were processed for qPCR studies. SPARC was found to be induced after 2 weeks of TAA treatment and its expression levels remained similar after 10 weeks of treatment, as well as in mice subjected to BDL (Figure 1B). While in non-treated animals SPARC expression was undetectable (Figure 2 B and E), after 10 weeks of TAA treatment, SPARC was additionally expressed in fibrous septae as well as in parenchymal areas, surrounding sinusoids (Figure 2H and K). SPARC was found to be expressed by α-SMA$^+$ myofibroblast cells, mainly within fibrous septae (Figure 2G–I). In addition, SPARC was also found to be expressed by vWF$^+$ endothelial cells (Figure 2J–and L). A similar expression pattern was observed in the liver of mice subjected to BDL. SPARC was expressed by α-SMA$^+$ myofibroblast cells mainly in the portal areas, but most of the expression was observed in endothelial cells (Figure 2M–R). From these results we can conclude that SPARC is overexpressed in the liver of cirrhotic patients and of mice exposed to different stimuli inducing fibrogenesis.

Decreased Liver Fibrosis and Necroinflammation in SPARC Deficient Mice

We next decided to investigate whether SPARC deficiency may influence liver fibrogenesis and processes therein involved. With this aim, two types of liver fibrosis *in vivo* models were applied to SPARC$^{-/-}$ and in SPARC$^{+/+}$ mice: chronic TAA application and bile duct ligation. After 10 weeks of TAA administration, SPARC$^{+/+}$ livers showed extensive appearance of portal-portal and central-portal fibrous septae, regenerative nodules, and distortion of liver architecture (Figures 3). However, a marked reduction in the amount of fibrous septae and of regenerative nodules was found in TAA-treated SPARC$^{-/-}$ animals (Figure 3A–F). Similar results were observed in animals subjected to BDL at 7 days post-surgery: while SPARC$^{+/+}$ mice developed prominent fibrous expansions in periportal areas, they were almost absent in SPARC$^{-/-}$ animals (Figure 3G–J).

Chronic liver injury and fibrogenesis are intimately linked to hepatocyte death and inflammation. To further study whether SPARC deficiency may induce changes in these mechanisms during liver fibrogenesis, these features were analyzed by an expert pathologist. A significant reduction in the periportal or periseptal interface hepatitis, focal necrosis and portal inflammation were observed in TAA-treated SPARC$^{-/-}$ when compared to TAA-treated SPARC$^{+/+}$ mice (Figure 3A–F and Table 1). All these differences contributed to the significant reduction in the Knodell score, frequently used to evaluate necroinflammatory activity, obtained from SPARC deficient fibrotic liver sections when compared to wild type fibrotic control tissue (Table 1). Similar results were obtained in BDL SPARC$^{-/-}$ mice although the amount of portal inflammation was similar in comparison with SPARC$^{+/+}$ mice.

The present study has shown that there was a significant increase in aspartate transaminase (AST) and alanine transaminase (ALT) levels in SPARC$^{+/+}$ BDL mice in comparison with BDL SPARC$^{-/-}$. No significant differences were observed in SPARC$^{+/+}$ and SPARC$^{-/-}$ mice in TAA groups (Figure 3K) suggesting that the inflammatory stimuli generated by TAA intoxication is strong during the first weeks of administration and correlates with elevated levels of transaminases but not at week 10, when the fibrotic changes predominate over necrosis of hepatocytes.

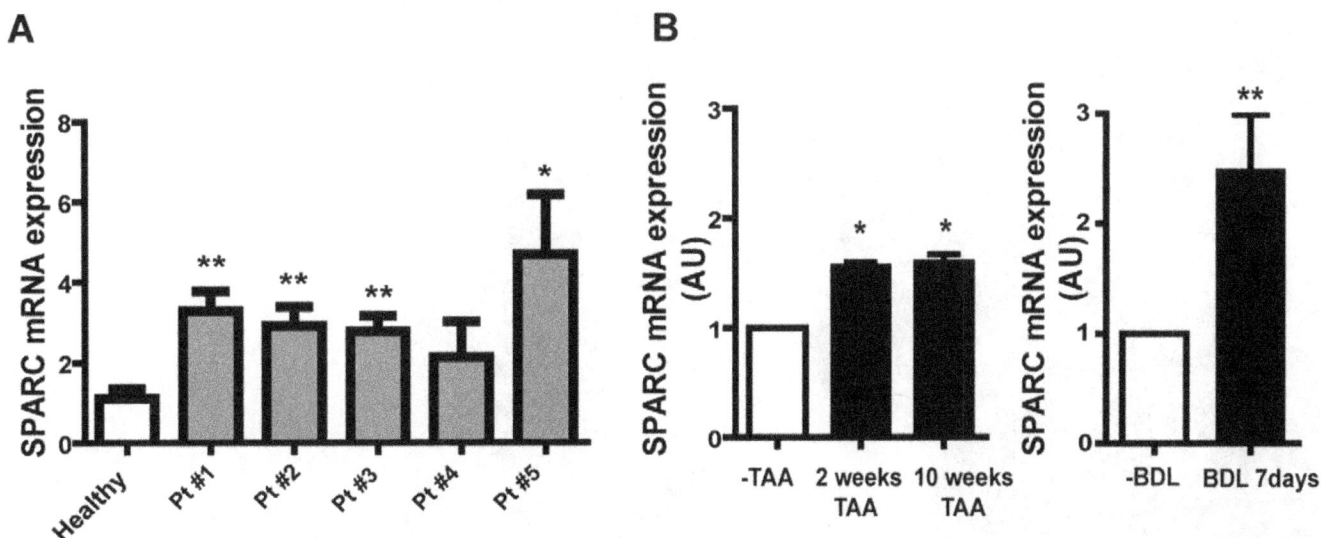

Figure 1. Induction of SPARC mRNA expression during liver fibrogenesis. (A) Quantitative data showing differences in SPARC mRNA expression levels in human cirrhotic (Pt#1 to Pt#5) with fibrosis degree F4 and non-cirrhotic liver samples as measured by qPCR. *p<0.05, **p<0.01 compared with healthy liver samples. Mann-Whitney test. (B) qPCR analyses of liver samples from TAA and BDL mice. Complementary DNA was synthesized and was subjected to qPCR for the expression of SPARC transcripts. The relative amount of the PCR product (AU, arbitrary units) amplified from control liver samples was set at 1. *p<0.05 versus control (−TAA), **p<0.01 versus control (−BDL), Mann-Whitney test.

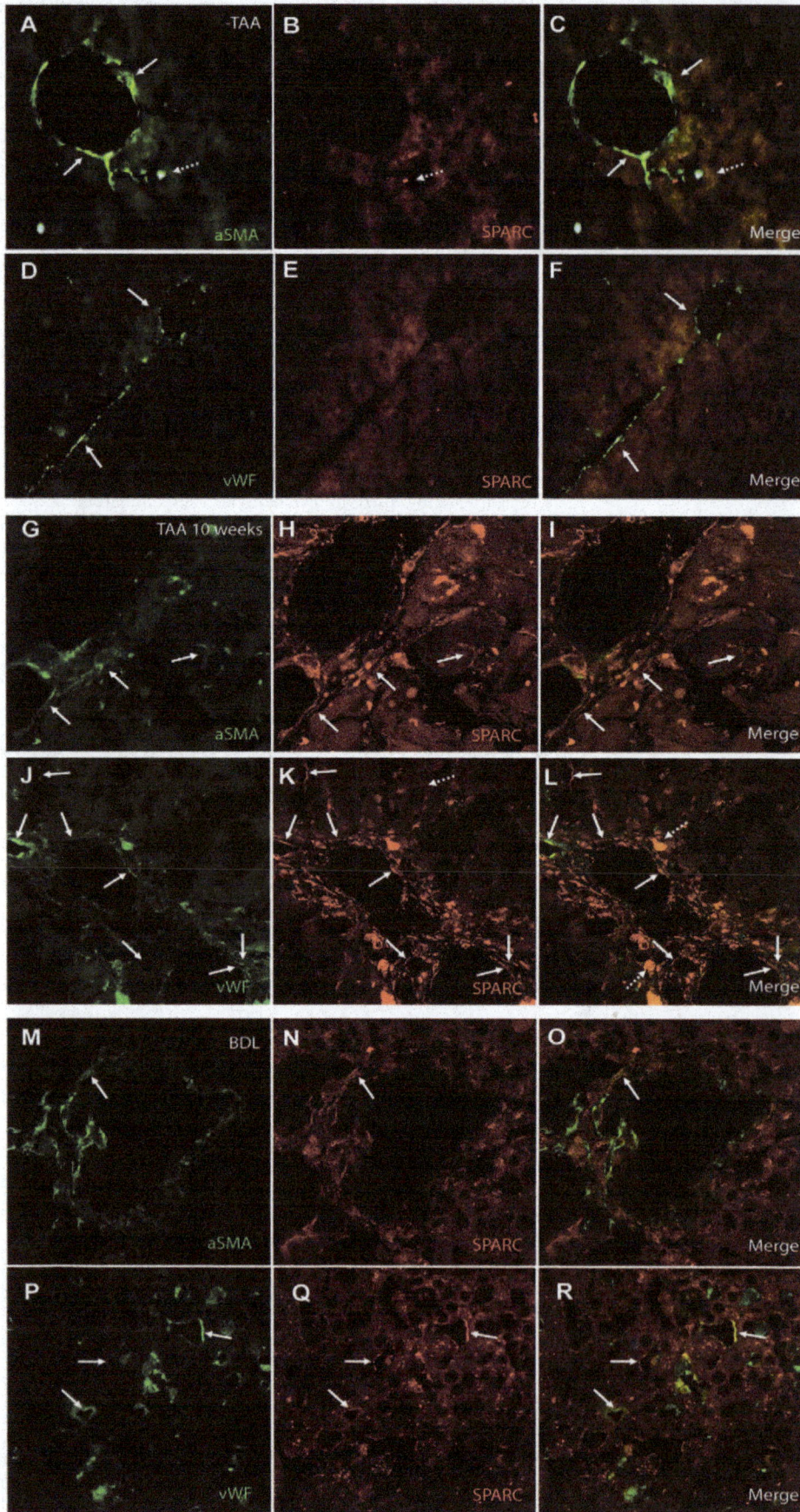

Figure 2. Patterns of SPARC expression during liver fibrogenesis. (A–F) Representative images taken from SPARC[+/+] mice liver sections stained for SPARC (B, E; red) and SMA (A; green) or vWF (D; green) and merge of both images (C, F). (G–L). Representative images taken from 10 weeks TAA-treated SPARC[+/+] mice liver sections (n =4–6) stained for SPARC (H, K; red) and SMA (G; green) or vWF (J; green). Co-localization of SPARC and SMA (I) or SPARC and vWF (L). (M–R) Representative images taken from 7 days BDL SPARC[+/+] mice liver stained for SPARC (N, Q; red) and SMA (M; green) or vWF (P; green). Arrows: co-expression of the two markers; dotted arrows: autofluorescence due to hepatic ceroid-laden macrophages. Original magnification 400X (A–F) or 1000X (G–R).

In order to characterize the profile of immune cells in the hepatic inflammatory infiltrate we performed immunohistochemistry for CD4+ T cells and observed that the amount of CD4+ cells was greatly decreased in SPARC[−/−] mice (Figure 4 A–D). Migration ability towards rCCL19 chemokine was explored in splenocytes derived from SPARC[−/−] and SPARC[+/+] mice in vitro. We observed a reduced migration in SPARC[−/−] mice in response to CCL19 after 2 h of incubation (Figure 4E). Flow cytometry analysis of splenocytes showed similar expression of CCR7 receptor (not shown). In agreement with the microarrays results showing a decreased expression of CCL19 in SPARC[−/−] mice (Table 2), qPCR assay confirmed down-regulation of the transcript (Figure S2).

SPARC Deficient Mice Showed a Decreased Collagen Deposition

In order to quantify liver content of collagen, the ECM protein most abundantly accumulated in fibrous septae, tissue sections from 10 weeks TAA-treated animals were Sirius red stained and morphometric analysis was thereafter performed. A significant reduction in Sirius red[+] area was found in SPARC[−/−] when compared to SPARC[+/+] mice (Figure 5A–B). Consistently, α2(I) collagen mRNA expression levels were significantly reduced in SPARC deficient when compared to wild-type animals (3.31 ± 0.64 vs. 6.48 ± 0.95; SPARC[−/−] vs. SPARC[+/+]) (Figure 5C). Matrix metalloproteinases (MMPs) are known to be involved in ECM regulation. We observed that hepatic MMP-2 expression was significantly increased in SPARC[−/−] TAA-treated mice in comparison with SPARC[+/+] (8.15 ± 0.42 vs. 3.25 ± 0.64, respectively) (Figure 5D).

In accordance with previous results, Sirius red staining on liver tissue and morphometric analysis obtained from BDL SPARC[−/−] mice showed a remarkable decrease in the appearance of collagen deposits when compared with similarly treated control animals. While very little Sirius red staining was observed in SPARC deficient mice, abundant collagen deposits were found within fibrous expansions in periportal areas as well as in liver parenchyma of SPARC[+/+] mice (Figure 5E–F). Consistent with Sirius red staining, α2(I) collagen mRNA expression levels were significantly reduced in SPARC deficient when compared to wild-type animals (6.03 ± 0.67 vs. 10.86 ± 1.08; SPARC[−/−] vs. SPARC[+/+]).

SPARC Deficiency Results in Immature Collagen Fibers Appearance and Packaging in Fibrotic Livers and in a Decrease Deposition of Hyaluronic Acid

In SPARC[−/−], both TAA and BDL resulted in Sirius red stained fibers which in most cases could not be observed under polarized light due to their reduce thickness and immature state: in this setting they turned into green which make very difficult to distinguish them from the overall tissue (Figure 6). On the other hand, most of Sirius red stained collagen fibers observed in TAA and BDL SPARC[+/+] mice could be also observed under polarized light, due to their increase in thickness and in maturation state: in this case they became orange to red in color after applying this procedure.

Hyaluronic acid accumulation in the liver is considered a sign of advanced liver fibrogenesis [25]. Consistent with previous results, TAA-treated SPARC[+/+] mice livers showed significant deposition of hyaluronan within fibrous septae while it was almost absent in TAA-treated SPARC[−/−] animals (Figure S1).

Reduced Number of Activated Myofibroblasts in Fibrotic Livers from SPARC[−/−] Mice

Liver fibrogenesis is characterized by trans-differentiation of different cells into myofibroblasts, including HSCs. HSC-derived myofibroblasts are known to upregulate their α-SMA expression levels during the activation process. In order to address whether either the number of myofibroblasts in fibrous septae and/or the activation state of myofibroblasts might be affected by SPARC deficiency, liver tissue obtained from TAA-treated and BDL mice was immunostained with α-SMA. A significant reduction in the α-SMA[+] immunostained area was found in TAA-treated SPARC[−/−] when compared to TAA-treated SPARC[+/+] mice (0.11 ± 0.01 vs. 0.45 ± 0.02, respectively) (Figure 7A–F and 7I) and in SPARC[−/−] subjected to BDL compared to SPARC[+/+] mice (0.1 ± 0.03 vs. 0.7 ± 0.19, respectively) (Figure 7G–H and 7I). These results suggest that a reduction in the number of activated myofibroblasts is likely involved in the inhibition of liver fibrogenesis found in SPARC deficient mice.

Downregulation of TGF-β1 Hepatic Expression and Systemic Levels in TAA Treated SPARC Deficient Mice

SPARC is known to be involved in a positive autocrine feedback loop with TGF-β1, a fibrogenic cytokine with a crucial role in liver fibrosis. In order to analyze whether SPARC deficiency may cause downregulation of TGF-β1 expression, its mRNA expression levels in fibrotic liver from 10 weeks TAA-treated and BDL mice were measured by qPCR. A significant decrease in the expression of this cytokine was found in SPARC deficient mice when compared to control (Figure 7J). To further confirm these results, serum levels of TGF-β1 were measured by ELISA. Significant lower levels of TGF-β1 were found in samples obtained from 10 weeks TAA-treated SPARC[−/−] when compared to those from TAA-treated SPARC[+/+] mice (Figure 7K). These results suggest that anti-fibrotic effects of SPARC deficiency are likely partially mediated by downregulation of TGF-β1 expression levels.

Microarray Analyses Show Changes in Gene Expression Profile in Naïve SPARC Deficient Mice

In order to explore whether lack of SPARC expression might influence liver gene expression profile in late fibrogenic processes, cDNA expression arrays were performed and analyzed (Affymetrix Mouse Gene ST 1.0 array). To analyze a possible involvement of basal physiological conditions ("background" effects) in the liver of SPARC deficient or wild-type mice which might partially explain the differences observed in liver fibrosis models, we have first compared gene expression profiles among samples of untreated animals. The genes responsible for basal effect should be found up- or down- regulated.

A total of 139 upregulated genes (124 known genes and 15 unknown cDNAs or ESTs) and 155 downregulated genes (138

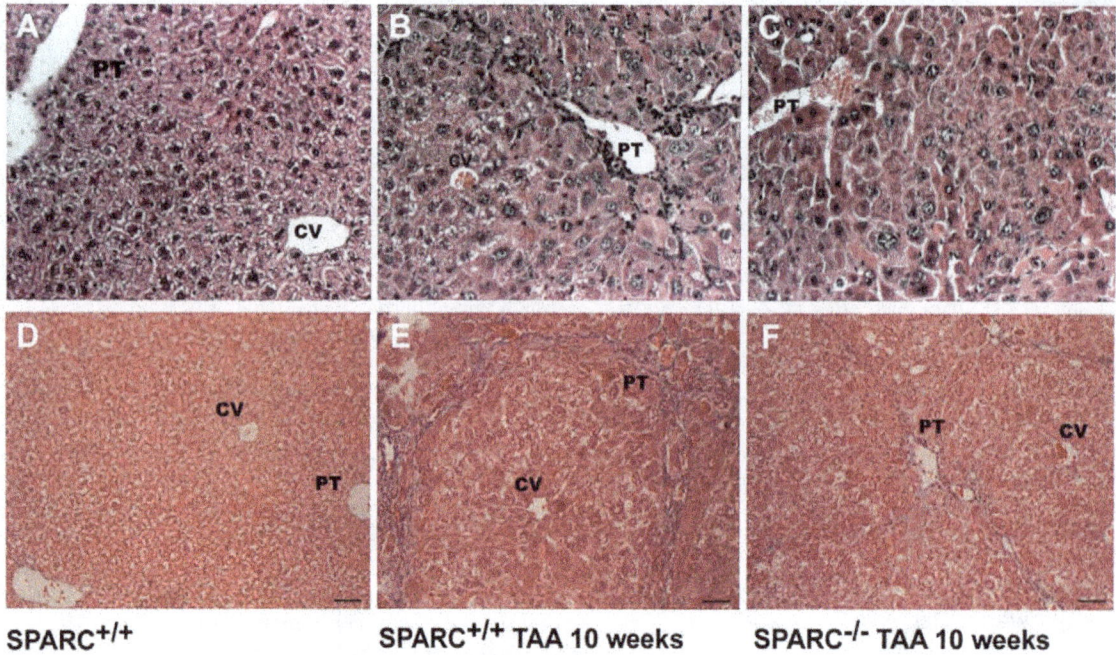

SPARC$^{+/+}$ SPARC$^{+/+}$ TAA 10 weeks   SPARC$^{-/-}$ TAA 10 weeks

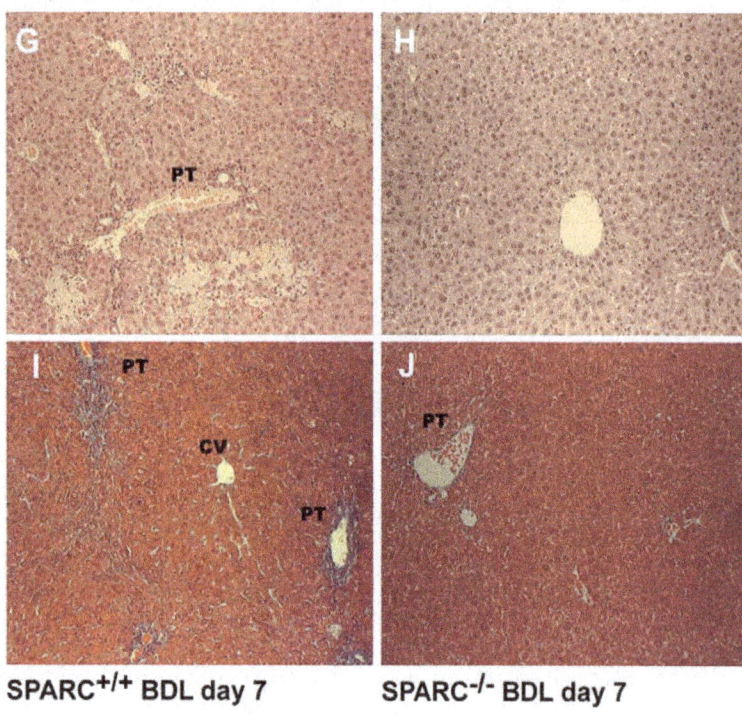

SPARC$^{+/+}$ BDL day 7   SPARC$^{-/-}$ BDL day 7

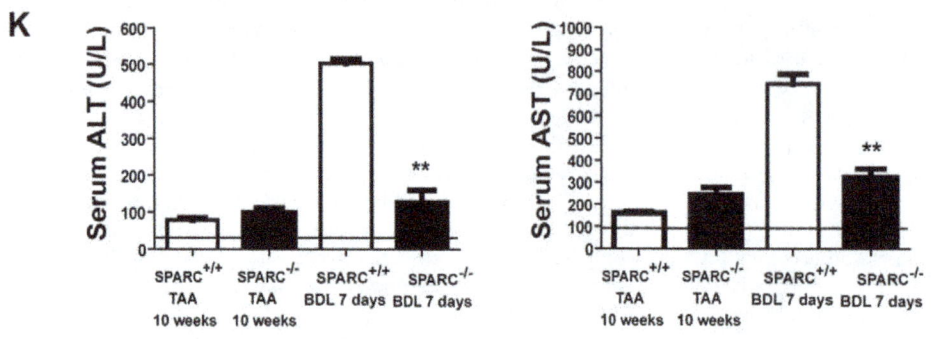

Figure 3. Reduced liver damage in SPARC deficient mice. (A–F) Representative photomicrographs of liver sections from untreated SPARC[+/+] (A) or 10 weeks TAA-treated SPARC[+/+] or SPARC[−/−] mice (n = 6–8), stained with H&E (A–C) or Masson's trichrome (D–F). (G–J) Representative photomicrographs of liver sections from SPARC[+/+] and SPARC[−/−] mice subjected to BDL, stained with H&E (G–H) or Masson's trichrome (I–J). Original magnification 200X. PT, portal tract; CV, central vein. (K) Serum ALT and AST levels were measured at the indicated time in TAA-treated and BDL mice. Dotted lines, upper normal limited. **p<0.05 versus treated SPARC[+/+].

known genes and 17 unknown cDNAs or ESTs) were obtained (Table S1). To analyze microarray data, three strategies were followed. Lists of the 10 top upregulated or downregulated gene lists (Table 2) and gene-interactions networks were performed (Ingenuity) (Figure 8), and modified genes were classified in ontological categories (GO, gene ontology) (Table S2). The analyses of the top up- or down- regulated showed relevant candidate genes in SPARC[−/−] mice compared to SPARC[+/+] mice. It is worth to noting that LOXL4, an important protein involved in the regulation of extracellular matrix components [26], was found increased while USP2, previously involved in triggering hepatocyte apoptosis and CCL19, related with inflammation and fibrogenesis [27,28], were down-regulated in SPARC[−/−] untreated liver tissues when compared to SPARC[+/+] mice, likely suggesting an initial condition of liver cells which would make them less susceptible to death and compatible with a subsequent reduction in fibrosis development.

Ingenuity Pathway Analysis (IPA) analyses (p<0.01) suggested several gene networks which likely involve protective mechanisms of SPARC deficiency against liver fibrogenesis. The network with the highest score and biological significance was chosen (Figure 8A). In this model, lack of SPARC expression was found related to Sox9 expression. Thus, Sox9 (sex determining region Y-box 9) and CDH1 (Cadherin-1 or E-cadherin; with a gene expression activity regulated by and known to be able to bind to Sox9) were found up-regulated in the liver of SPARC[−/−] mice. In addition, other genes showing increased expression levels in these mice within the same gene interaction network were cldn1 (claudin 1), secretase gamma, aph1b (anterior pharynx defective 1b homolog), pag1 (phosphoprotein associated with glycosphingolipid microdomains 1), mpzl1 (myelin protein zero-like 1) and agk (acylglycerol kinase). In addition, lack of SPARC expression was found related to a down-regulation in PCGF2 (polycomb group ring finger), a factor that maintains repression of genes related to tumorigenesis and cell cycle [29]. In turn, PCGF2 likely interacts with UBE2U (ubiquitin-conjugating enzyme E2U), involved in ubiquitination, found upregulated in SPARC[−/−] mice. Consistently, other proteins able to interact with UBE2U, such as two members of the TRIM (tripartite motif-containing) family and MID2 (midline 2), were also found upregulated upon SPARC deficiency.

Interestingly, the GO analysis revealed statistically enriched ontological categories including those related in chromatin remodeling, cAMP signaling or cell cycle regulation. A complete list of all genes included in each GO category is given as supplementary information. Overall our data suggest that the liver of SPARC deficient animals have a gene expression profile which likely makes them less susceptible to develop liver fibrosis.

Microarray Analyses Show Changes in Gene Expression Pattern in Advanced Liver Fibrogenesis due to SPARC Deficiency

To uncover new protective mechanisms involved in the observed reduction in the degree of liver fibrosis observed in SPARC deficient mice, cDNA expression array analyses were performed comparing liver tissue samples obtained from SPARC[−/−] and SPARC[+/+] mice after 10 weeks of TAA administration. A total of 492 genes showed a p<0.01 (281 upregulated and 211 downregulated genes) in SPARC[−/−] mice. Top up-regulated and down-regulated genes are shown in Table 2. They include upregulation of CLDN4 (Claudin 4), a component of the tight junction strands, and downregulation of CIDEC (cell death-inducing DNA fragmentation factor-α-like effector C), a potent apoptosis inducer [30]. Interestingly, canonical pathway and biological functions identified by IPA showed a large group of upregulated genes associated with DNA repair and detoxification. Remarkably a large group of interacting genes were found upregulated (Figure 8B) in the context of SPARC deficiency including at the center of the network those encoding ATM (ataxia telangiectasia-mutated) kinase [31] and the transcription factors BRCA (breast cancer) 1 [32], BRCA2 [33] and BARD1 (BRCA1-associated RING domain) [34] and including effector genes such as topbp1 (topoisomerase (DNA) II binding protein 1) [31], rrm1 (ribonucleotide reductase M1) [35], brip1 (BRCA1 interacting protein C-terminal helicase 1) [36], pole1 (polymerase (DNA directed), epsilon, catalytic subunit) and 2 (polymerase (DNA directed), epsilon 2, accessory subunit) [37], msh2 (mutS homolog 2, colon cancer, nonpolyposis type 1 (E. coli) [38], mbd4 (methyl-CpG binding domain protein 4) [39], blm (Bloom syndrome, RecQ helicase-like) [38], fancb (Fanconi anemia, complementation group B) [40], rfc4 (replication factor C (activator 1) 4) [37],

Table 1. Severity of necroinflamatory activity and fibrosis in SPARC[+/+] and SPARC[−/−] mice after 10 weeks of TAA treatment (n = 6–8) or in SPARC[+/+] and SPARC[−/−] BDL mice (n = 5–6).

	SPARC[+/+] TAA 10 weeks	SPARC[−/−] TAA 10 weeks	SPARC[+/+] BDL 7 days	SPARC[−/−] BDL 7 days
Periportal or Periseptal Interface hepatitis	2.7±0.5	1.3±0.4*	1.6±0.5	0.62±0.2
Focal (spotty) lytic necrosis, focal necrosis, apoptosis and focal inflammation	4±1.4	2.3±0.5*	3.5±0.3	0.75±0.25*
Portal inflammation	2.5±0.6	1.16±0.9*	2±0.0	1.5±0.3
Fibrosis	3.7±0.5	2.5±0.5*	2.6±0.2	0.5±0.0*
Knodell score	13.25±1.2	7.33±1.5*	9.75±0.5	3.25±0.3*

*p<0.05.

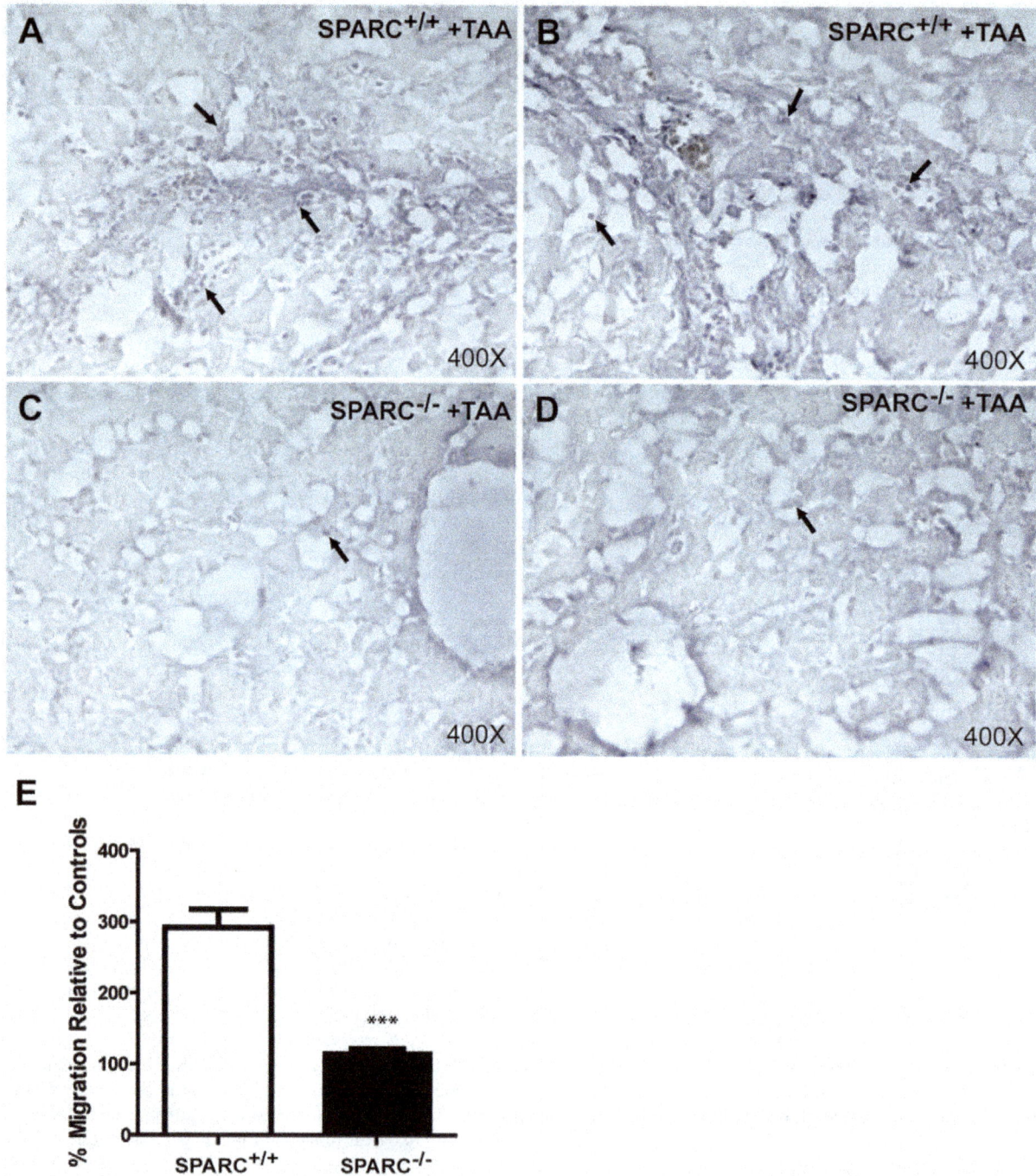

Figure 4. Reduced hepatic inflammatory infiltration and migratory capacity in SPARC deficient mice. Photomicrographs of representative liver sections from TAA-treated animals. SPARC$^{+/+}$ mice showed an increased CD4^{+} cells infiltration in hepatic parenchyma, especially around portal tracts (A,B); while in TAA-treated SPARC$^{-/-}$ mice CD4^{+} cells are scarce and located near the sinusoids (C,D). Arrows indicate CD4^{+} cells. Original magnification 400X. (E) Migratory response of splenocytes towards CCL19 chemokine. Percentage of cells that migrated relative to respective controls for SPARC$^{+/+}$ and SPARC$^{-/-}$ splenocytes (n = 3 replicates) in a Boyden Chamber system. Splenocytes were placed into the upper well, separated from the lower by a 5-μm porosity membrane. The bottom well contained either DMEM or DMEM with 10 ng/μl rCCL19 and cells were allowed to migrate during 2 h. ***p < 0.001, Mann Whitney test.

chaf1A (chromatin assembly factor 1, subunit A (p150) and B (chromatin assembly factor 1, subunit B (p60)) [41], Hist1H3A (histone cluster 1, H3a) and hat1 (histone acetyltransferase 1) [42]. Consistently, E2F, able to induce gene expression of many transcriptional factors and effectors in DNA repair and stability pathways including some of the most relevant ones mentioned

above [43], was found upregulated at the center of the second most relevant IPA gene network map, as well as other related functional proteins such as PCNA (proliferating cell nuclear antigen), MCM2 (minichromosome maintenance deficient 2 mitotin), MCM3, MCM4 (minichromosome maintenance deficient 4 homolog), MCM6, MCM7, RPA2 (replication protein A2),

Table 2. IPA® top molecules which were significantly alters in SPARC$^{-/-}$ versus SPARC$^{+/+}$ mice and those modified in SPARC$^{-/-}$ versus SPARC$^{+/+}$ 10 weeks TAA treated mice.

IPA® Top Molecules. Background

Fold change up-regulated

	Gene ID	Exponential Value
NIPAL1	NM_001081205	1,975
ACCN5	NM_021370	1,608
PIK3C2G	NM_207683	1,561
LOXL4	NM_001164311	1,514
SLC34A2	NM_011402	1,232
C17orf78	NM_001037932	1,230
UBE2U	NM_001033773	1,171
NDRG1	NM_008681	1,118
THEM5	NM_025416	1,117
FOXQ1	NM_008239	1,102

Fold change down-regulated

	Gene ID	Exponential Value
SPARC	NM_009242	−4,051
C1orf51	BC132471	−2,245
USP2	NM_198092	−1,994
CCL19	NM_011888	−1,544
TSKU	NM_001168541	−1,508
CABYR	NM_027687	−1,338
PPIH	NM_001110130	−1,335
PER2	NM_011066	−1,120
P2RY2	NM_008773	−0,984
SYDE2	NM_001166064	−0,892

IPA® Top Molecules. Ten Weeks of TAA Treatment

Fold change up-regulated

	Gene ID	Exponential Value
NPY	NM_023456	2,092
CYP1A1	NM_009992	2,053
1600029D21Rik	NM_029639	2,028
Sprr1a	NM_009264	1,615
SLC7A11	NM_011990	1,498
CLDN4	NM_009903	1,487
ARG2 (includes EG:11847)	NM_009705	1,471
MCM6	NM_008567	1,449
TMC5	NM_001105252	1,358
TMEM45A	NM_019631	1,287

Fold change down-regulated

	Gene ID	Exponential Value
SPARC	NM_009242	−4,517
UBLCP1	NM_024475	−2,273
CIDEC	NM_178373	−1,723

Table 2. Cont.

IPA® Top Molecules. Background

Fold change up-regulated

	Gene ID	Exponential Value
AKR1C3	NM_134066	−1,659
ACOT2	NM_134188	−1,637
CHRNA2	NM_144803	−1,223
SLC22A5	NM_011396	−1,097
CYP8B1	NM_010012	−1,022
CPT1B	NM_009948	−1,002
LYVE1	NM_053247	−0,965

PRIM1 (DNA primase, p49 subunit), PRIM2 (A primase, p58 subunit), CDT1 (chromatin licensing and DNA replication factor 1) and ASF1B (ASF1 anti-silencing function 1 homolog B); not shown). It is worth noting that the first and most significant gene network model showed an upregulation of ABCC4 (ATP-binding cassette sub-family C member 4), a key ABC transporter involved in the removal of chemicals, xenobiotics and products of oxidative stress [44], and the downregulation of TRIM25 (tripartite motif-containing 25) [45] and CTSF (cathepsin F) [46] involved in protein degradation processes.

Discussion

SPARC expression is known to be induced during liver fibrogenesis in different species. In mouse, SPARC upregulation has only been reported in a schistosomiasis model of liver fibrosis [6]. In this work, we confirmed this result in two additional models of this disease caused by different etiologies: hepatotoxicity mediated by chronic TAA intoxication, and cholestasis induced by BDL. In addition, we provide new evidence, based on a genetic *in vivo* model, showing that SPARC, expressed by HSC and endothelial cells, is involved in liver fibrogenesis. Moreover, our data support that SPARC plays a major role in key pathogenic events related to the fibrogenic process such as hepatocyte necrosis, inflammation and recruitment/activation of myofibroblasts as well as in the induction of the profibrogenic cytokine TGF-β1. These findings are consistent with previous reports, based on studies performed with other tissues, showing SPARC involvement in proinflammatory and profibrogenic mechanisms [47,48]. Our gene expression profile analyses suggest that SPARC upregulation in the fibrotic liver might induce deficiencies in DNA repair mechanisms likely resulting in enhanced liver cell death and subsequent increased ECM deposition as a consequence of scar formation process. Overall, our data strongly support that SPARC plays a prominent profibrogenic role in the context of chronic liver injures, providing new clues to understand mechanisms therein involved. Although gene targeting is a powerful tool for the study of a disease on a uniform genetic background, the gene knockout approach must be used with caution, particularly in interpretations of the phenotypes that are obtained in liver biology, where many genes have pleiotropic functions.

Myofibroblasts do normally accumulate in the parenchyma close to liver injured areas. Many of them most likely derive from resident HSCs, the main source of fibrillar collagen and the major targets of anti-fibrotic therapies [49]. By mean of immunohisto-

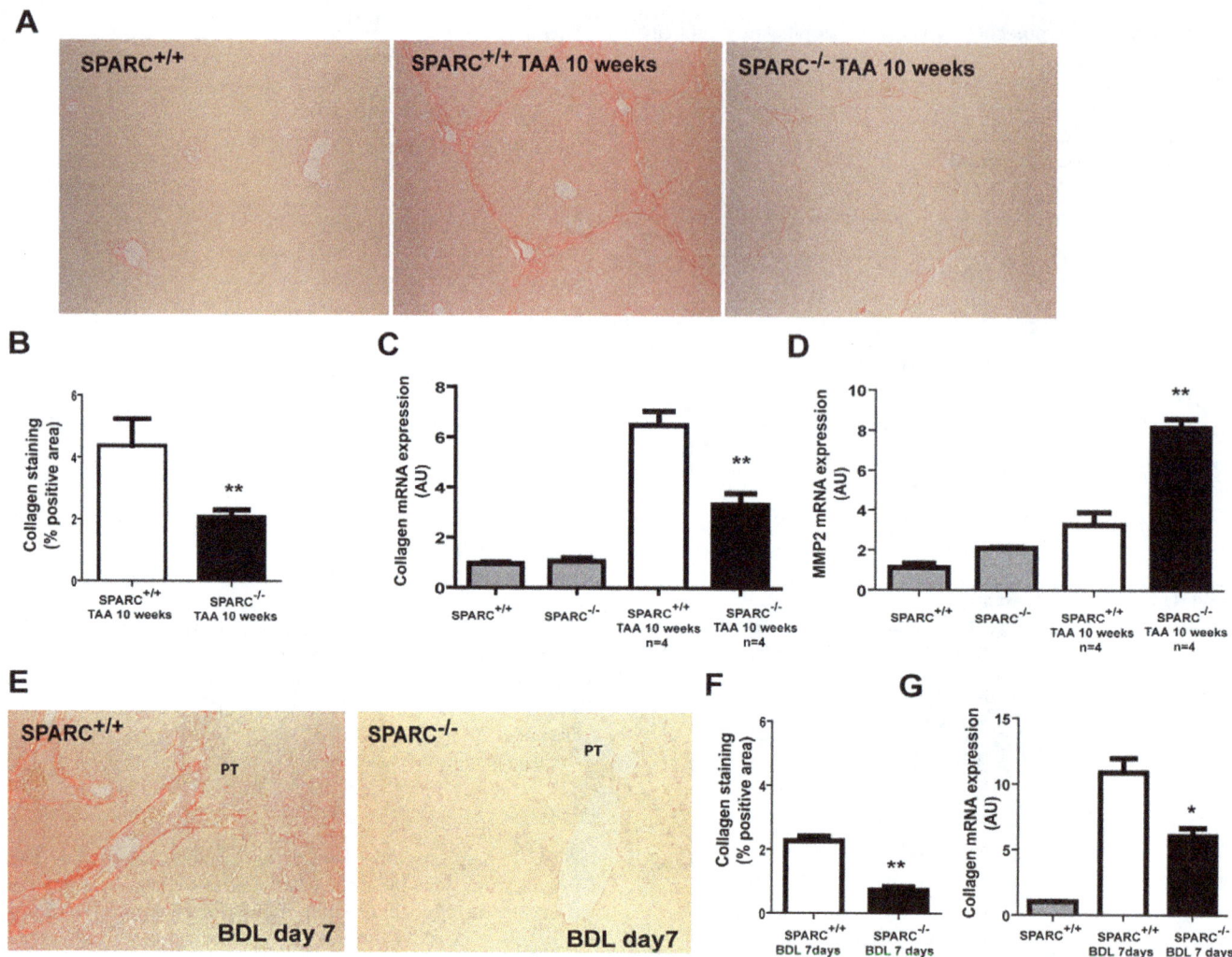

Figure 5. Reduced liver fibrosis in SPARC deficient mice. (A) Representative photomicrographs of liver sections stained with picrosirius red. SPARC$^{+/+}$ mice show staining limited to periportal areas (left panel), while liver sections from TAA-treated SPARC$^{+/+}$ mice exhibits marked portal fibrosis and portal-portal bridges (central panel) and those from TAA-treated SPARC$^{-/-}$ mice present weak fibrotic response (right panel). (B) Morphometric quantification of Sirius red stained area showing a significant attenuation of the fibrotic process in TAA-treated SPARC$^{-/-}$ mice when compared to treated wild-type mice. **$p < 0.01$, Mann-Whitney test. (C–D) Quantitative data from qPCR analysis of collagen (COL1A2) and MMP-2 mRNA expression. *$p < 0.05$, **$p < 0.01$ versus SPARC$^{+/+}$ TAA 10 weeks, Mann-Whitney test. (E) Representative pictures taken from liver sections of from SPARC$^{+/+}$ or SPARC$^{-/-}$ mice, at 7 days after BDL. Original magnification 200X. PT, portal tract; CV, central vein. (F) Morphometric quantification of Sirius red stained area showing a significant attenuation of the fibrotic process in SPARC$^{-/-}$ mice at day 7 after BDL when compared to wild-type mice. **$p < 0.01$, Mann-Whitney test. (G) qPCR analysis of collagen mRNA expression in SPARC$^{+/+}$ and SPARC$^{-/-}$ mice subjected to BDL. *$p < 0.05$, versus BDL SPARC$^{+/+}$ Mann-Whitney test.

chemical studies, a decrease in the number of α-SMA$^+$ myofibroblasts was observed in fibrotic livers of SPARC deficient mice. This finding is consistent with our recently published data showing that specific SPARC knock-down in activated HSCs reduces their migratory ability as well as their activation state [50]. Thus, the induction of SPARC expression in activated HSCs likely promotes their accumulation in chronically injured liver areas further aggravating the pathologic state. Whether SPARC may or not participate in the activation/proliferation of other non-parenchymal cells such as Kupffer, endothelial or biliary epithelial cells in response to chronic injury is unknown and merits further investigation.

In addition, recent studies demonstrated that SPARC is able to exert potent stimulatory effects on TGF-β1 expression in cultured HSCs [5], skin and lung fibroblasts, and mesangial cells [4,15,51]. In agreement with this, it is worth noting that in these studies

lower levels of TGF-β1 were found in fibrotic livers and in serum samples from TAA-treated SPARC deficient mice when compared to wild-type counterparts. Therefore, and in the context of fibrotic diseases, these data further emphasizes the prevailing hypothesis of TGF-β1 expression being dependent on local SPARC expression levels. Based on the abundant literature related to the function of TGF-β1 in fibrogenesis [52] we hypothesize that this mechanism likely explain most of the observed phenotype.

Collagen fibrillar formation is a critical step in fibrogenesis and SPARC is a well-known collagen-binding matricellular protein with a reported role in type I collagen packaging. Thus by mean of in vitro studies, Rentz et al. have shown that collagen I produced by SPARC$^{-/-}$ cells was not efficiently incorporated into detergent-insoluble fractions [53]. In agreement with this, we herein show that fibrotic livers obtained from SPARC deficient mice contain thin, dispersed and predominantly immature collagen fibers while

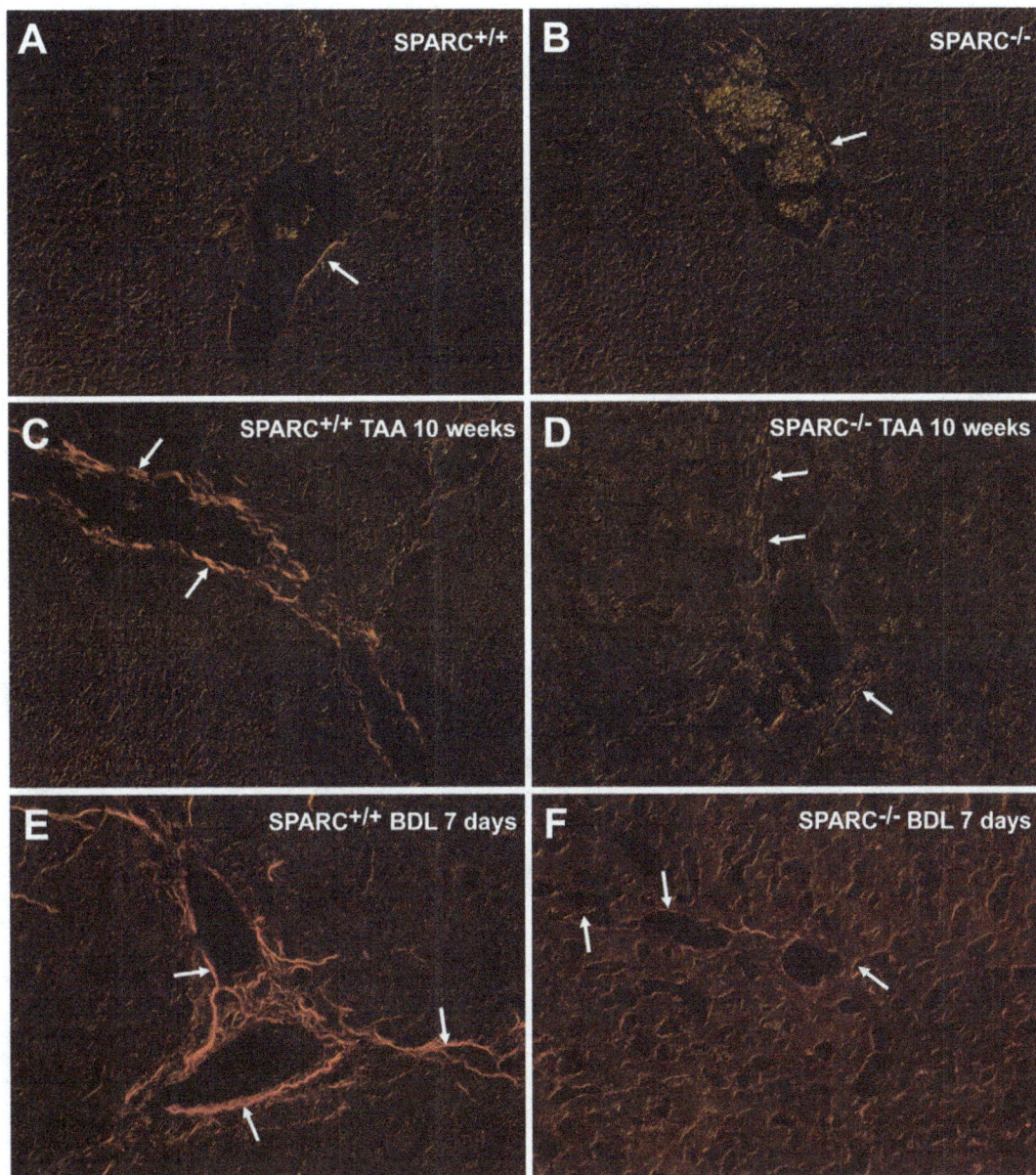

Figure 6. Reduced maturation of SPARC$^{-/-}$ collagen fiber deposits. Representative pictures showing picrosirius red stained liver sections obtained from SPARC$^{+/+}$ (A,C,E) or SPARC$^{-/-}$ (B,D,F) mice (n =6–8) observed under polarized light. Animals were left untreated (A,B), or were TAA-treated during 10 weeks (C,D) or subjected to BDL (E, F). Note the predominant mature and compacted nature of collagen fibers in wild-type treated mice and their immature and thin appearance in SPARC$^{-/-}$ animals. Original magnification 400X.

they were thick, highly compacted and mature in those from SPARC$^{+/+}$ animals. Therefore, our data are consistent with previous reports on SPARC function in the context of collagen fiber maturation and compaction [54]. Little information is available on the role of SPARC in human liver fibrosis: we (herein) and others [7] showed that SPARC is overexpressed in the liver of cirrhotic patients. Nevertheless, these new data obtained from a mouse genetic model, using different *in vivo* disease models, are consistent with a profibrogenic role of SPARC in the context of chronic liver disease. Moreover, SPARC is shown to likely mediate key events in liver fibrogenesis such as liver inflammation, induction of TGF-β1 expression levels and the accumulation of active myofibroblasts.

Matrix metalloproteinase-2 (MMP-2), a type IV collagenase, is upregulated in chronic liver disease and is considered a profibrotic factor [55]. However, recent evidence in *in vivo* animal models revealed that MMP-2 deficiency is associated with increased hepatic collagen type I expression and fibrogenesis [56]. In agreement with these results, we observed that MMP-2 messenger RNA was increased at week 10 of TAA treatment in SPARC$^{-/-}$ mice. In addition, our microarray analysis also demonstrated that MMP-2 is significantly increased in SPARC$^{-/-}$ TAA-treated mice (not shown), suggesting that this effect may be involved, at least in part, in the protective effect of SPARC knock-down on liver fibrogenesis.

In an effort to identify changes in gene expression profile, which could explain the observed protective mechanisms against TAA

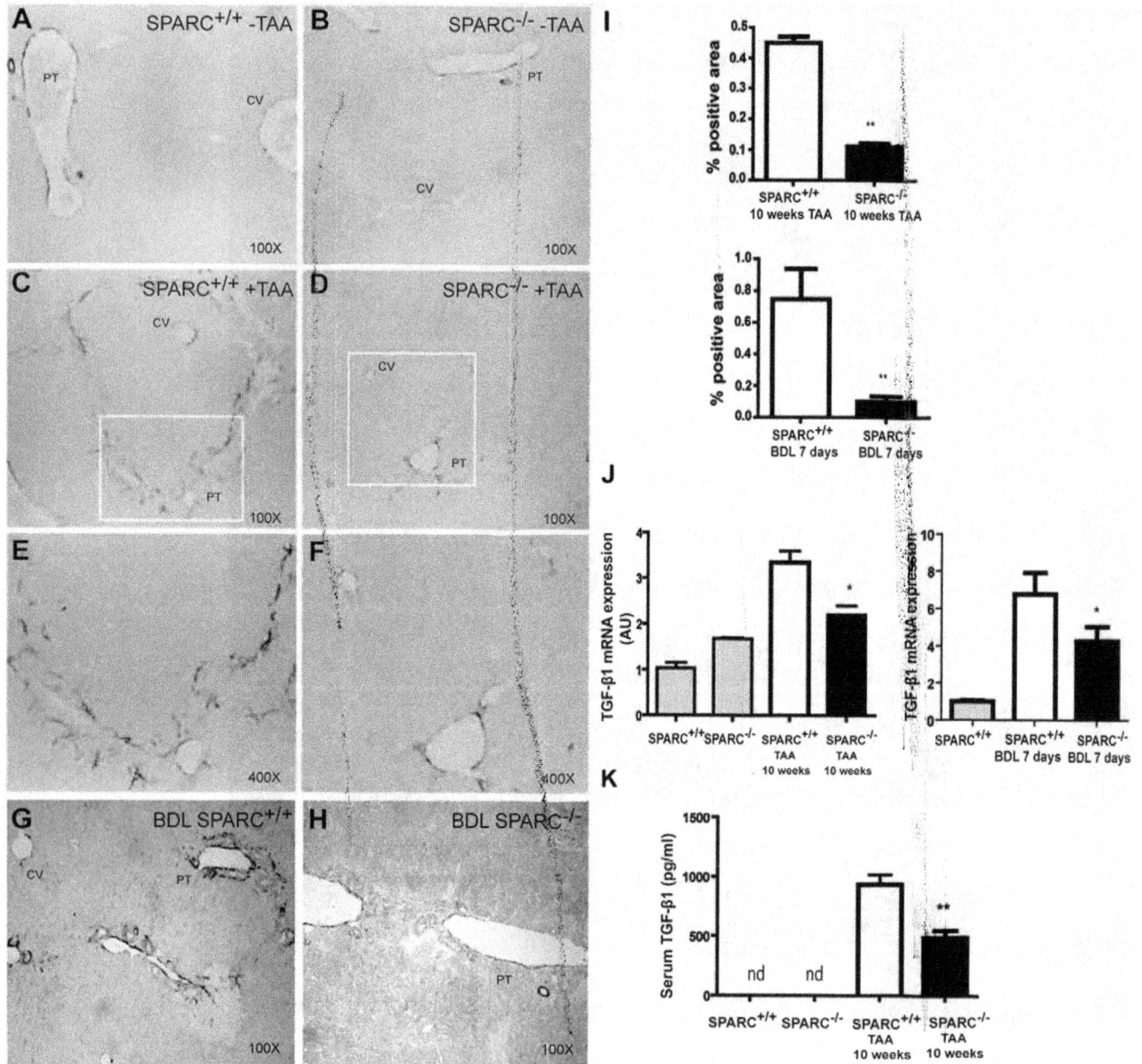

Figure 7. Reduction in the number of active myofibroblasts and in liver and serum TGF-β1 levels in SPARC deficient fibrotic mice.
(A–H) Representative pictures taken from liver sections of untreated SPARC$^{+/+}$ and SPARC$^{-/-}$ (A,B), 10 weeks TAA treated SPARC$^{+/+}$ (C,E) andSPARC$^{-/-}$ (D,F), or BDL SPARC$^{+/+}$ (G) and SPARC$^{-/-}$ (H) mice immunostained for α-SMA. (E,F) are higher magnification images from box areas in C,D respectively. (I) Quantitative data of densitometric analyses of αSMA immunostained area from TAA-treated and BDL SPARC$^{-/-}$ or SPARC$^{+/+}$ mice. **p<0.01, Mann-Whitney test. (J) Quantitative data of TGF-β1 mRNA levels obtained by qPCR analysis from 10 weeks TAA-treated and BDL SPARC$^{+/+}$ or SPARC$^{-/-}$ mice (n =6–8). Data are expressed as relative values to those of wild-type mice without treatment. *p<0.05, SPARC$^{+/+}$ treated vs SPARC$^{-/-}$ treated. Mann-Whitney test. (K) Serum levels of TGF-β1 were measured after 10 weeks of TAA treatment. nd, non-detectable. **p<0.01, Mann-Whitney test.

damage in SPARC$^{-/-}$ mice in an established model of liver fibrosis, microarray analyses were performed. A number of genes were narrowed down; nevertheless, a number of candidates showed a significant difference in expression when comparing SPARC knockout and wild-type mice. Our overall results suggest that the reduction in liver fibrogenesis observed in SPARC deficient mice seems to be the result of a sum of several mechanisms rather than the effect of changes in a small group of specific genes. Accordingly to this, we chose the approach of

comparing ingenuity networks rather than analyzing changes in individual gene expression.

Interestingly, the list of top modified genes in untreated mice showed differential regulation of certain gene categories which might partially explain a protective status against any insult as a result of SPARC deficiency: the specific involvement of several of these genes in liver pathologies will be analyzed in our future research. A candidate gene would be LOXL4, a target of TGF-β1 [26] found to cause reduction in TGFβ1-mediated cell motility of

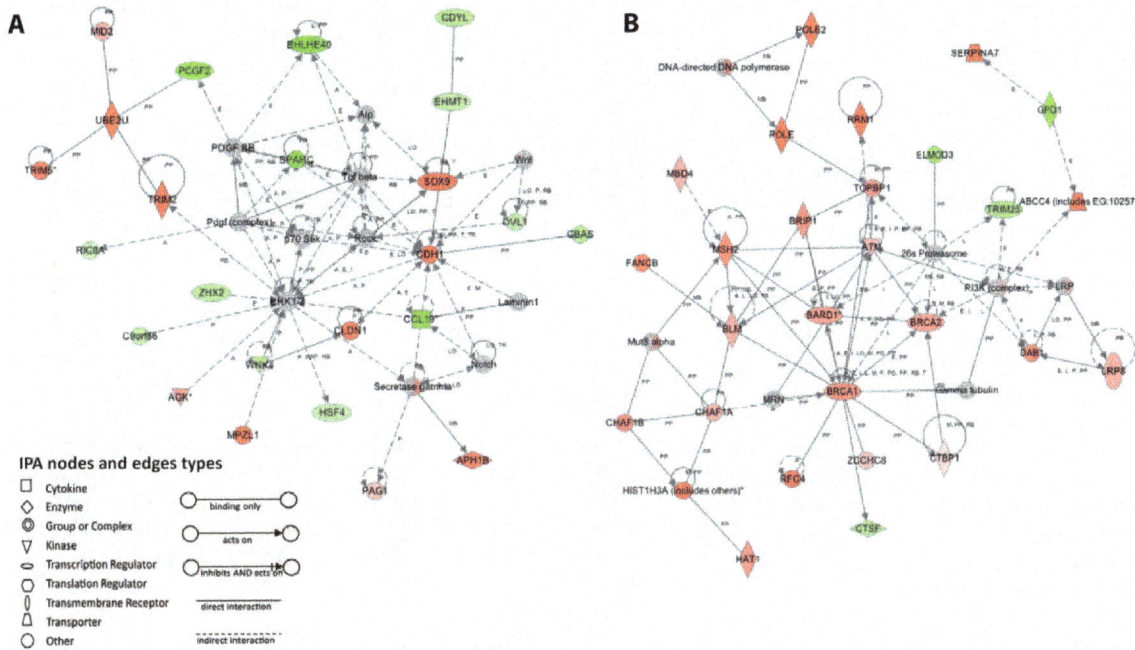

Figure 8. The top network of differentially expressed genes. The networks are presented as graphical displays where genes appear as nodes and the molecular relationships are represented by lines. Up-regulated and down-regulated genes in SPARC$^{-/-}$ mice are shown as red spot or green spot, respectively. The top network of differentially expressed genes in SPARC$^{-/-}$ versus SPARC$^{+/+}$ mice (A) or SPARC$^{-/-}$ after 10 weeks of TAA treatment versus SPARC$^{+/+}$ TAA treated mice (B), as identified by IPA analysis. Intensity of the red or green color shows the level of gene expression. Gray represents a gene found which is related to the others but did not meet the cutoff criteria. A Activation, E Expression (includes metabolism/synthesis for chemicals), I Inhibition, L Proteolysis (includes degradation for Chemicals), LO Localization, M Biochemical Modification, MB Group/complex Membership, P Phosphorylation/Dephosphorylation, PD Protein-DNA binding, PP Protein-Protein binding, RB Regulation of Binding,T Transcription,TR Translocation.

hepatoma cells. In addition, USP2 was found down-regulated in SPARC$^{-/-}$ mice likely rendering hepatocytes less susceptible to TNF-mediated apoptosis [57]. Another top down-regulated gene was CCL19, a chemokine known to attract dendritic cells and lymphocytes [58,59,60] which might be involved in the reduction of inflammation observed in SPARC deficient mice after TAA treatment. However, no significant differences were observed in CCL19 gene expression at week 10 of TAA administration leading us to speculate that low expression levels of CCL19 in null mice at the beginning of the injury with TAA could be critical for the subsequent generation of inflammation, necrosis of hepatocytes and fibrogenesis. The magnitude of inflammatory infiltrates was markedly reduced in SPARC$^{-/-}$ mice, especially CD4$^+$ cells, and the decreased migratory capacity of their splenocytes towards CCL19 chemokine *in vitro* leading us to speculate that the decreased fibrosis observed in these animals could be mediated, at least in part, by lessening of an inflammatory effect. This observation was not confirmed in BDL model. These results are in agreement with Rempel *et al.* who consider that that SPARC$^{-/-}$ mice have an impaired immune system [61].

Furthermore, CCL19 receptor is expressed in HSCs and its activation was previously shown to induce its migration capacity [62] a relevant feature involved in liver fibrogenesis [63]. Upon TAA long-term treatment, CIDEC, a known potent inducer of apoptosis [30,64], is among the top down-regulated genes in SPARC deficient mice, likely cross-linking altered metabolism with programmed cell death in the TAA-induced fibrosis model.

Using the IPA tool we were able to find highly significant networks and pathways likely involved in the described functional phenotype. In fact, naïve SPARC$^{-/-}$ and SPARC$^{+/+}$ mice seem to significantly differ in their gene expression profiles. As previously discussed, a positive feedback between SPARC and TGF-β1 was experimentally established; in addition, it is speculated that SPARC might regulate the signaling pathway induced by TGF-β1 [65]. Our best IPA gene network model showed that SPARC depletion was associated with an increased in SOX9 expression levels, likely mediated by TGF-β1 signaling pathway. SOX9 is a transcription factor involved in liver development, shown to contribute to hepatic physiology preservation [66]. However, a previous work suggested that SOX9 has a role as a transcriptional regulator in fibrogenesis promoting extracellular matrix deposition [67].

Additionally, the shown network establishes a relationship with CDYL and EHMT1 genes, codifying for histone methylases and acetylases likely involved in SOX9 gene regulatory function. Furthermore, in our network model SOX9 is shown to interact and to induce E-cadherin gene expression, also found upregulated in the liver of naïve SPARC deficient mice. E-cadherin is an important epithelial cell-cell adhesion protein considered as a marker of non-activated HSCs [68]. Claudin 1, a tight junction protein, is another adhesion protein also found overexpressed in SPARC null mice and known to interact and mutually activate each other with E-cadherin. Tight junctions are confined to epithelial cells, forming continuous belts around cells and serving as a physical barrier to regulate transport through the paracellular space. Another important event shown in the gene network model is the decrease of CCL19 in SPARC$^{-/-}$ mice, likely involved in the observed reduction in lymphocyte recruitment and process of liver inflammation which normally characterizes liver fibrosis as previously discussed. In turn, the decrease in CCL19 gene activity is related with several transcriptional repressor and stress response factors (such as HSF4, ZHX2), linked to ERK1/2 pathway, also found down-regulated. SPARC$^{-/-}$ mice have an increased in secretase gamma (protease complex) and its protein complex partner APH1B, as well as PAG1 (a protein shown to be phosphorylated by secretase gamma), likely involving Notch signaling pathway-related changes. Secretase gamma and PAG1 might be also involved in the regulation of T cell activation. Overall our results support the concept of basal conditions in the context of SPARC deficiency making the liver less susceptible to external insults such as those causing liver fibrosis.

In addition to the influence of a basal phenotype condition, the results of pathway analyses on samples obtained from TAA treated animals suggest that SPARC deficient mice have a more intact or better established machinery to repair DNA or detoxify the body from external chemical stimuli as suggested by the remarkable upregulation in genes such as ATM, BRCA1, BRCA2 and BARD1. ATM is a sensor of DNA damage and phosphorylates p53 (tumor suppressor, which can activate apoptosis and arrest the cell cycle if DNA damage is not resolved) [69]. Additionally, ATM knockout affects cell survival and liver regeneration [70]. Consistently, BRCA1 complexed with BARD1 has tumor suppression properties and is involved on protein ubiquitination for degradation. Moreover, it needs to form a complex with BRCA2, also herein upregulated, to repair damaged DNA. It is reported that TGFβ1/Smad3 counteracts BRCA1-mediated DNA repair [71] and expression [72]. Our results on upregulation in BRCA1 as well as in its related partners and effectors involved in DNA repair are consistent with the decreased in TGF-β1 levels found in our study. Via PI3K, ATM likely up-regulates ABCC4, a key ABC transporter involved in the removal of chemicals, xenobiotics and products of oxidative stress, as well as the efflux of GSH and bile salts through the basolateral membrane of hepatocytes [73]. Exported GSH may be mediating protection against oxidative damage in the tissue. It was previously reported that the expression and localization of this transporter in centrilobular hepatocytes was increase in mice receiving hepato-toxic doses of acetaminophen or CCl$_4$ [74], which correlates with protection against further doses of acetaminophen [75]. Therefore, upregulation in the expression of ATM and of its related BCRA transcriptional factor complex components as well as of their specific effectors suggest the establishment of a more efficient machinery mounted to repair DNA defects likely resulting in less susceptibility to liver cell apoptosis. Such mechanisms together to detoxifying activities mediated by ABCC4 might explain the reduction in liver damage and subsequent fibrosis observed in SPARC deficient mice.

In summary, we herein show that SPARC depletion in a mouse genetic model results in protection against liver fibrosis development. Mechanisms therein involved are complex and likely act at different levels and through diverse processes implicated in fibrogenesis. Thus, our new evidences implicate reduction in the

extent of liver inflammation, in TGF-β1 expression levels (a master molecule involved in the ECM deposition) and in the activation status of HSCs, and an increase in MMP2 expression. In addition, they suggest the establishment of a transcriptional activation of the DNA repair machinery making liver cells less susceptible to apoptosis thus likely preventing liver damage. Overall, giving the complexity of advanced liver fibrosis it is believed that therapeutic avenues need also to act at different parallel mechanisms to be efficient in ameliorating disease mechanisms. These studies further support a beneficial effect of SPARC downregulation and suggest that this might be a good candidate for an *in vivo* approach using gene therapy tools (e.g. long-term expression vectors) for future antifibrotic therapeutic actions.

Supporting Information

Figure S1   SPARC deficiency shows decrease deposition of hyaluronic acid. Representative pictures taken from liver sections of TAA untreated (A, B) or 10 weeks TAA treated SPARC$^{+/+}$ (C) or SPARC$^{-/-}$ (D) mice stained for hyaluronic acid (n = 6–8). Original magnification 100X. PT, portal tract; CV, central vein.

Figure S2   qPCR analysis for selected microarray genes. mRNA expression levels in liver samples of SPARC$^{+/+}$ and SPARC$^{-/-}$ mice, untreated or treated 10 weeks with TAA, of: (A) CCL19, (B) Brca1, (C) ABCC4F, (D) Cldn1, (E) ATMF, (F) Cdh1, (G) Bard1. Values were normalized to levels of GAPDH transcript. Error bars represent SD values. p values are presented in the figure.

Table S1   List of the significantly upregulated and downregulated genes between SPARC$^{-/-}$ and SPARC$^{+/+}$, 6 weeks TAA treated SPARC$^{+/+}$ and TAA treated SPARC$^{-/-}$, 10 weeks TAA treated SPARC$^{+/+}$ and TAA treated SPARC$^{-/-}$.

Table S2   List of the significantly modified gene classified by ontological categories.

Acknowledgments

We would like to thank Soledad Arregui, Guillermo Gastón and Juan Politti for expert technical assistance, and Dr. Alejandra Camino, for advice.

Author Contributions

Conceived and designed the experiments: GM JA CA. Performed the experiments: CA EP NK MM LA MG FC EG EF JB GM FP. Analyzed the data: GM RB OP FC. Wrote the paper: CA JA EP GM.

References

1. Bradshaw AD, Sage EH (2001) SPARC, a matricellular protein that functions in cellular differentiation and tissue response to injury. J Clin Invest 107: 1049–1054.

2. Brekken RA, Sage EH (2000) SPARC, a matricellular protein: at the crossroads of cell-matrix. Matrix Biol 19: 569–580.

3. Francki A, Bradshaw AD, Bassuk JA, Howe CC, Couser WG, et al. (1999) SPARC regulates the expression of collagen type I and transforming growth factor-beta1 in mesangial cells. J Biol Chem 274: 32145–32152.

4. Wang JC, Lai S, Guo X, Zhang X, de Crombrugghe B, et al. (2010) Attenuation of fibrosis in vitro and in vivo with SPARC siRNA. Arthritis Res Ther 12: R60.

5. Camino AM, Atorrasagasti C, Maccio D, Prada F, Salvatierra E, et al. (2008) Adenovirus-mediated inhibition of SPARC attenuates liver fibrosis in rats. J Gene Med 10: 993–1004.

6. Frizell E, Liu SL, Abraham A, Ozaki I, Eghbali M, et al. (1995) Expression of SPARC in normal and fibrotic livers. Hepatology 21: 847–854.

7. Blazejewski S, Le Bail B, Boussarie L, Blanc JF, Malaval L, et al. (1997) Osteonectin (SPARC) expression in human liver and in cultured human liver myofibroblasts. Am J Pathol 151: 651–657.

8. Lamireau T, Le Bail B, Boussarie L, Fabre M, Vergnes P, et al. (1999) Expression of collagens type I and IV, osteonectin and transforming growth factor beta-1 (TGFbeta1) in biliary atresia and paucity of intrahepatic bile ducts during infancy. J Hepatol 31: 248–255.

9. Le Bail B, Faouzi S, Boussarie L, Guirouilh J, Blanc JF, et al. (1999) Osteonectin/SPARC is overexpressed in human hepatocellular carcinoma. J Pathol 189: 46–52.

10. Goldenberg D, Ayesh S, Schneider T, Pappo O, Jurim O, et al. (2002) Analysis of differentially expressed genes in hepatocellular carcinoma using cDNA arrays. Mol Carcinog 33: 113–124.

11. Lau CP, Poon RT, Cheung ST, Yu WC, Fan ST (2006) SPARC and Hevin expression correlate with tumour angiogenesis in hepatocellular carcinoma. J Pathol 210: 459–468.

12. Gressner AM, Weiskirchen R (2006) Modern pathogenetic concepts of liver fibrosis suggest stellate cells and TGF-beta as major players and therapeutic targets. J Cell Mol Med 10: 76–99.

13. George J, Roulot D, Koteliansky VE, Bissell DM (1999) In vivo inhibition of rat stellate cell activation by soluble transforming growth factor beta type II receptor: a potential new therapy for hepatic fibrosis. Proc Natl Acad Sci U S A 96: 12719–12724.

14. Qi Z, Atsuchi N, Ooshima A, Takeshita A, Ueno H (1999) Blockade of type beta transforming growth factor signaling prevents liver fibrosis and dysfunction in the rat. Proc Natl Acad Sci U S A 96: 2345–2349.

15. Wrana JL, Overall CM, Sodek J (1991) Regulation of the expression of a secreted acidic protein rich in cysteine (SPARC) in human fibroblasts by transforming growth factor beta. Comparison of transcriptional and post-transcriptional control with fibronectin and type I collagen. Eur J Biochem 197: 519–528.

16. Muller A, Machnik F, Zimmermann T, Schubert H (1988) Thioacetamide-induced cirrhosis-like liver lesions in rats–usefulness and reliability of this animal model. Exp Pathol 34: 229–236.

17. Oren R, Dotan I, Papa M, Marravi Y, Aeed H, et al. (1996) Inhibition of experimentally induced cirrhosis in rats by hypothyroidism. Hepatology 24: 419–423.

18. Knodell RG, Ishak KG, Black WC, Chen TS, Craig R, et al. (1981) Formulation and application of a numerical scoring system for assessing histological activity in asymptomatic chronic active hepatitis. Hepatology 1: 431–435.

19. Jameson JM, Cauvi G, Sharp LL, Witherden DA, Havran WL (2005) Gammadelta T cell-induced hyaluronan production by epithelial cells regulates inflammation. J Exp Med 201: 1269–1279.

20. Piccioni F, Malvicini M, Garcia MG, Rodriguez A, Atorrasagasti C, et al. (2012) Antitumor effects of hyaluronic acid inhibitor 4-methylumbelliferone in an orthotopic hepatocellular carcinoma model in mice. Glycobiology 22: 400–410.

21. Irizarry RA, Bolstad BM, Collin F, Cope LM, Hobbs B, et al. (2003) Summaries of Affymetrix GeneChip probe level data. Nucleic Acids Res 31: e15.

22. Smyth GK (2004) Linear models and empirical bayes methods for assessing differential expression in microarray experiments. Stat Appl Genet Mol Biol 3: Article3.

23. Gentleman R (2005) Bioinformatics and computational biology solutions using R and Bioconductor: Springer Verlag.

24. Draghici S, Drăghici S (2003) Data analysis tools for DNA microarrays: CRC Press.

25. George J, Tsutsumi M, Takase S (2004) Expression of hyaluronic acid in N-nitrosodimethylamine induced hepatic fibrosis in rats. Int J Biochem Cell Biol 36: 307–319.

26. Kim DJ, Lee DC, Yang SJ, Lee JJ, Bae EM, et al. (2008) Lysyl oxidase like 4, a novel target gene of TGF-beta1 signaling, can negatively regulate TGF-beta1-induced cell motility in PLC/PRF/5 hepatoma cells. Biochem Biophys Res Commun 373: 521–527.

27. Grant AJ, Goddard S, Ahmed-Choudhury J, Reynolds G, Jackson DG, et al. (2002) Hepatic expression of secondary lymphoid chemokine (CCL21) promotes the development of portal-associated lymphoid tissue in chronic inflammatory liver disease. Am J Pathol 160: 1445–1455.

28. Marra F (2002) Chemokines in liver inflammation and fibrosis. Front Biosci 7: d1899–1914.

29. Kanno M, Hasegawa M, Ishida A, Isono K, Taniguchi M (1995) mel-18, a Polycomb group-related mammalian gene, encodes a transcriptional negative regulator with tumor suppressive activity. EMBO J 14: 5672–5678.

30. Tang X, Xing Z, Tang H, Liang L, Zhao M (2011) Human cell-death-inducing DFF45-like effector C induces apoptosis via caspase-8. Acta Biochim Biophys Sin (Shanghai) 43: 779–786.

31. Sancar A, Lindsey-Boltz LA, Unsal-Kacmaz K, Linn S (2004) Molecular mechanisms of mammalian DNA repair and the DNA damage checkpoints. Annu Rev Biochem 73: 39–85.

32. Moynahan ME, Chiu JW, Koller BH, Jasin M (1999) Brca1 controls homology-directed DNA repair. Mol Cell 4: 511–518.

33. Patel KJ, Yu VP, Lee H, Corcoran A, Thistlethwaite FC, et al. (1998) Involvement of Brca2 in DNA repair. Mol Cell 1: 347–357.

34. Boulton SJ, Martin JS, Polanowska J, Hill DE, Gartner A, et al. (2004) BRCA1/BARD1 orthologs required for DNA repair in Caenorhabditis elegans. Curr Biol 14: 33–39.

35. Zheng Z, Chen T, Li X, Haura E, Sharma A, et al. (2007) DNA synthesis and repair genes RRM1 and ERCC1 in lung cancer. N Engl J Med 356: 800–808.

36. Bridge WL, Vandenberg CJ, Franklin RJ, Hiom K (2005) The BRIP1 helicase functions independently of BRCA1 in the Fanconi anemia pathway for DNA crosslink repair. Nat Genet 37: 953–957.

37. Ronen A, Glickman BW (2001) Human DNA repair genes. Environ Mol Mutagen 37: 241–283.

38. Wang Y, Cortez D, Yazdi P, Neff N, Elledge SJ, et al. (2000) BASC, a super complex of BRCA1-associated proteins involved in the recognition and repair of aberrant DNA structures. Genes Dev 14: 927–939.

39. Riccio A, Aaltonen LA, Godwin AK, Loukola A, Percesepe A, et al. (1999) The DNA repair gene MBD4 (MED1) is mutated in human carcinomas with microsatellite instability. Nat Genet 23: 266–268.

40. Wood RD, Mitchell M, Sgouros J, Lindahl T (2001) Human DNA repair genes. Science 291: 1284–1289.

41. Bensimon A, Schmidt A, Ziv Y, Elkon R, Wang SY, et al. (2010) ATM-dependent and -independent dynamics of the nuclear phosphoproteome after DNA damage. Sci Signal 3: rs3.

42. Qin S, Parthun MR (2002) Histone H3 and the histone acetyltransferase Hat1p contribute to DNA double-strand break repair. Mol Cell Biol 22: 8353–8365.

43. Bracken AP, Ciro M, Cocito A, Helin K (2004) E2F target genes: unraveling the biology. Trends Biochem Sci 29: 409–417.

44. Nakata K, Tanaka Y, Nakano T, Adachi T, Tanaka H, et al. (2006) Nuclear receptor-mediated transcriptional regulation in Phase I, II, and III xenobiotic metabolizing systems. Drug Metab Pharmacokinet 21: 437–457.

45. Meroni G, Diez-Roux G (2005) TRIM/RBCC, a novel class of 'single protein RING finger' E3 ubiquitin ligases. Bioessays 27: 1147–1157.

46. Santamaria I, Velasco G, Pendas AM, Paz A, Lopez-Otin C (1999) Molecular cloning and structural and functional characterization of human cathepsin F, a new cysteine proteinase of the papain family with a long propeptide domain. J Biol Chem 274: 13800–13809.

47. Socha MJ, Manhiani M, Said N, Imig JD, Motamed K (2007) Secreted protein acidic and rich in cysteine deficiency ameliorates renal inflammation and fibrosis in angiotensin hypertension. Am J Pathol 171: 1104–1112.

48. Strandjord TP, Madtes DK, Weiss DJ, Sage EH (1999) Collagen accumulation is decreased in SPARC-null mice with bleomycin-induced pulmonary fibrosis. Am J Physiol 277: L628–635.

49. Kisseleva T, Brenner DA (2008) Mechanisms of fibrogenesis. Exp Biol Med (Maywood) 233: 109–122.

50. Atorrasagasti C, Aquino JB, Hofman L, Alaniz L, Malvicini M, et al. (2011) SPARC down-regulation attenuates the profibrogenic response of hepatic stellate cells induced by TGF-{beta}1 and PDGF. Am J Physiol Gastrointest Liver Physiol.

51. Bradshaw AD, Francki A, Motamed K, Howe C, Sage EH (1999) Primary mesenchymal cells isolated from SPARC-null mice exhibit altered morphology and rates of proliferation. Mol Biol Cell 10: 1569–1579.

52. Gressner AM, Weiskirchen R, Breitkopf K, Dooley S (2002) Roles of TGF-beta in hepatic fibrosis. Front Biosci 7: d793–807.

53. Rentz TJ, Poobalarahi F, Bornstein P, Sage EH, Bradshaw AD (2007) SPARC regulates processing of procollagen I and collagen fibrillogenesis in dermal fibroblasts. J Biol Chem 282: 22062–22071.

54. Bradshaw AD, Baicu CF, Rentz TJ, Van Laer AO, Bonnema DD, et al. (2010) Age-dependent alterations in fibrillar collagen content and myocardial diastolic function: role of SPARC in post-synthetic procollagen processing. Am J Physiol Heart Circ Physiol 298: H614–622.

55. Benyon RC, Hovell CJ, Da Gaca M, Jones EH, Iredale JP, et al. (1999) Progelatinase A is produced and activated by rat hepatic stellate cells and promotes their proliferation. Hepatology 30: 977–986.

56. Radbill BD, Gupta R, Ramirez MC, DiFeo A, Martignetti JA, et al. (2011) Loss of matrix metalloproteinase-2 amplifies murine toxin-induced liver fibrosis by upregulating collagen I expression. Dig Dis Sci 56: 406–416.

57. Haimerl F, Erhardt A, Sass G, Tiegs G (2009) Down-regulation of the de-ubiquitinating enzyme ubiquitin-specific protease 2 contributes to tumor necrosis factor-alpha-induced hepatocyte survival. J Biol Chem 284: 495–504.

58. Robbiani DF, Finch RA, Jager D, Muller WA, Sartorelli AC, et al. (2000) The leukotriene C(4) transporter MRP1 regulates CCL19 (MIP-3beta, ELC)-dependent mobilization of dendritic cells to lymph nodes. Cell 103: 757–768.

59. Reif K, Ekland EH, Ohl L, Nakano H, Lipp M, et al. (2002) Balanced responsiveness to chemoattractants from adjacent zones determines B-cell position. Nature 416: 94–99.

60. Bromley SK, Thomas SY, Luster AD (2005) Chemokine receptor CCR7 guides T cell exit from peripheral tissues and entry into afferent lymphatics. Nat Immunol 6: 895–901.

61. Rempel SA, Hawley RC, Gutierrez JA, Mouzon E, Bobbitt KR, et al. (2007) Splenic and immune alterations of the Sparc-null mouse accompany a lack of immune response. Genes Immun 8: 262–274.

62. Sahin H, Trautwein C, Wasmuth HE (2010) Functional role of chemokines in liver disease models. Nat Rev Gastroenterol Hepatol 7: 682–690.

63. Atorrasagasti C, Aquino JB, Hofman L, Alaniz L, Malvicini M, et al. (2011) SPARC downregulation attenuates the profibrogenic response of hepatic stellate cells induced by TGF-beta1 and PDGF. Am J Physiol Gastrointest Liver Physiol 300: G739–748.

64. Yonezawa T, Kurata R, Kimura M, Inoko H (2011) Which CIDE are you on? Apoptosis and energy metabolism. Mol Biosyst 7: 91–100.

65. Francki A, McClure TD, Brekken RA, Motamed K, Murri C, et al. (2004) SPARC regulates TGF-beta1-dependent signaling in primary glomerular mesangial cells. J Cell Biochem 91: 915–925.

66. Furuyama K, Kawaguchi Y, Akiyama H, Horiguchi M, Kodama S, et al. (2011) Continuous cell supply from a Sox9-expressing progenitor zone in adult liver, exocrine pancreas and intestine. Nat Genet 43: 34–41.

67. Hanley KP, Oakley F, Sugden S, Wilson DI, Mann DA, et al. (2008) Ectopic SOX9 mediates extracellular matrix deposition characteristic of organ fibrosis. J Biol Chem 283: 14063–14071.
68. Lim YS, Lee HC, Lee HS (2007) Switch of cadherin expression from E- to N-type during the activation of rat hepatic stellate cells. Histochem Cell Biol 127: 149–160.
69. May P, May E (1999) Twenty years of p53 research: structural and functional aspects of the p53 protein. Oncogene 18: 7621–7636.
70. Lu S, Shen KC, Wang Y, Brooks SC, Wang YA (2005) Impaired hepatocyte survival and liver regeneration in Atm-deficient mice. Hum Mol Genet 14: 3019–3025.
71. Dubrovska A, Kanamoto T, Lomnytska M, Heldin CH, Volodko N, et al. (2005) TGFbeta1/Smad3 counteracts BRCA1-dependent repair of DNA damage. Oncogene 24: 2289–2297.
72. Satterwhite DJ, Matsunami N, White RL (2000) TGF-beta1 inhibits BRCA1 expression through a pathway that requires pRb. Biochem Biophys Res Commun 276: 686–692.
73. Rius M, Nies AT, Hummel-Eisenbeiss J, Jedlitschky G, Keppler D (2003) Cotransport of reduced glutathione with bile salts by MRP4 (ABCC4) localized to the basolateral hepatocyte membrane. Hepatology 38: 374–384.
74. Aleksunes LM, Scheffer GL, Jakowski AB, Pruimboom-Brees IM, Manautou JE (2006) Coordinated expression of multidrug resistance-associated proteins (Mrps) in mouse liver during toxicant-induced injury. Toxicol Sci 89: 370–379.
75. Aleksunes LM, Campion SN, Goedken MJ, Manautou JE (2008) Acquired resistance to acetaminophen hepatotoxicity is associated with induction of multidrug resistance-associated protein 4 (Mrp4) in proliferating hepatocytes. Toxicol Sci 104: 261–273.

10

Asiatic Acid Inhibits Liver Fibrosis by Blocking TGF-beta/Smad Signaling *In Vivo* and *In Vitro*

Li-xia Tang[1], Rui-hua He[1], Guang Yang[1], Jia-ju Tan[1], Li Zhou[2], Xiao-ming Meng[3], Xiao Ru Huang[3], Hui Yao Lan[3]*

1 Institute of Medical Research, The First People's Hospital of Foshan, Foshan, Guangdong, China, 2 Department of Medicine, West China Hospital of Sichuan University, Chengdu, China, 3 Li Ka Shing Institute of Health Sciences and Department of Medicine and Therapeutics, The Chinese University of Hong Kong, Hong Kong, China

Abstract

Liver fibrosis is a major cause of liver failure, but treatment remains ineffective. In the present study, we investigated the mechanisms and anti-hepatofibrotic activities of asiatic acid (AA) in a rat model of liver fibrosis induced by carbon tetrachloride (CCl₄) and *in vitro* in TGF-beta1-stimulated rat hepatic stellate cell line (HSC-T6). Treatment with AA significantly attenuated CCl₄-induced liver fibrosis and functional impairment in a dosage-dependent manner, including blockade of the activation of HSC as determined by inhibiting *de novo* alpha smooth muscle actin (a-SMA) and collagen matrix expression, and an increase in ALT and AST (all p<0.01). The hepatoprotective effects of AA on fibrosis were associated with upregulation of hepatic Smad7, an inhibitor of TGF-beta signaling, thereby blocking upregulation of TGF-beta1 and CTGF and the activation of TGF-beta/Smad signaling. The anti-fibrosis activity and mechanisms of AA were further detected *in vitro* in HSC-T6. Addition of AA significantly induced Smad7 expression by HSC-T6 cells, thereby inhibiting TGF-beta1-induced Smad2/3 activation, myofibroblast transformation, and collagen matrix expression in a dosage-dependent manner. In contrast, knockdown of Smad7 in HSC-T6 cells prevented AA-induced inhibition of HSC-T6 cell activation and fibrosis in response to TGF-beta1, revealing an essential role for Smad7 in AA-induced anti-fibrotic activities during liver fibrosis *in vivo* and *in vitro*. In conclusion, AA may be a novel therapeutic agent for liver fibrosis. Induction of Smad7-dependent inhibition of TGF-beta/Smad-mediated fibrogenesis may be a central mechanism by which AA protects liver from injury.

Editor: Kwan Man, The University of Hong Kong, Hong Kong

Funding: This work was supported by grants from Guangdong Medical Research Foundation (A2007627 to GY and 2008225 to LXT) and Research Grant Council of Hong Kong (RGC CUHK5/CRF/09, GRF 768207 and 767508 to HYL). The funders had no role in study design, data collection and analysis, decision to publish, or preparation of the manuscript.

Competing Interests: The authors have declared that no competing interests exist.

* E-mail: hylan@cuhk.edu.hk

Introduction

Liver fibrosis represents the final common pathway of virtually all chronic liver diseases. It is characterized by the excessive accumulation of extracellular matrix (ECM) and activated hepatic stellate cells (HSC) that are undergoing myofibroblast transition identified by *de novo* a-SMA expression [1,2]. Although a significant progress has been made in our understanding of hepatic fibrosis, treatment for liver fibrosis remains ineffective. Therefore, there is an urgent need for searching and developing antifibrotic strategies which can prevent, halt or reverse hepatic fibrosis.

In hepatic fibrosis, the excessive ECM, including collagen type I and III, is produced by activated mesenchymal cells which resemble myofibroblasts derived from quiescent HSC, periportal or perivenular fibroblasts, circulating fibrocytes, and bone marrow cells [1,2]. Increasing evidence shows that TGF-beta1 is a key mediator in the process of liver fibrosis [3,4]. The finding of increased HSCl activation and liver fibrosis in mice with tetracycline-regulated TGF-beta1 expression in the liver provides a direct evidence for a critical role of TGF-beta1 in hepatic fibrosis [5]. It is now clear that after binding to its receptors, TGF-beta1 activates its downstream signaling pathway, Smad 2 and Smad3,

to mediate fibrosis, which is negatively regulated by Smad7, an inhibitor of TGF-beta signaling, via the ubiquitin-proteasome degradation mechanism [6,7]. In the context of liver fibrosis, Smad3 is pathogenic because mice null for Smad3 are protected against dimethylnitrosamine-induced hepatic fibrosis [8]. In contrast, Smad7 is protective since deletion of Smad7 promotes, but overexpression of Smad7 protects against HSC activation and hepatic fibrosis in vitro and in vivo [9–11]. The inhibitory role of Smad7 in fibrosis is also found in chronic kidney disease [12]. We detected that disruption of Smad7 gene promotes renal fibrosis in a mouse model of obstructive nephropathy [13]. In contrast, overexpression of Smad7 is capable of inhibiting TGF-beta1 and angiotensin II-induced fibrosis in vitro [14,15] and in a number of disease models including diabetic nephropathy [16–18]. However, it is also known that TGF-beta1 is an anti-inflammatory cytokine. Thus, therapies with general blockade of TGF-beta1 may risk in enhancing the inflammatory response, which has largely limited the development of anti-TGF-beta therapy clinically. Nevertheless, the better understanding of the mechanisms of TGF-beta/Smad signaling in diseases associated with fibrosis may be a critical step towards the development of novel and specific anti-fibrosis drugs.

Asiatic acid (AA) is one of the triterpenoid components found in *Centella asiatica* [19]. Many studies have shown that AA has a variety of pharmacological effects on anti-inflammation [20,21], antioxidation [22], anti-tumor [23,24], neuroprotection [25,26], and wound healing [27,28]. In particular, AA has been shown to be a hepatoprotective agent. A number of studies demonstrated that AA can protect liver from injury via mechanisms underlying anti-mitochondrial stress and cellular antioxidant system in cultured hepatocytes and Kupffer cells, and in a mouse model induced by D-galactosamine and lipopolysaccharides [29–31]. It has been also reported that AA is capable of inhibiting collagen matrix production by HSC and keloid fibroblasts by blocking the autocrine effect of TGF-beta1 in vitro [32,33], however, the role and mechanisms by which AA inhibits liver fibrosis remain largely unknown. Therefore, the present study investigated the therapeutic effect and mechanisms of AA in a rat model of CCl_4-induced liver fibrosis and in vitro in TGF-beta1-stimulated rat HSC-T6 cell line.

Methods

Asiatic Acid

Purified nature product of AA (95%) was obtained from Changzhou Natural Product Inc (Guangxi, China) and was used

for in vivo treatment as described below, while the HPLC-purified AA (Sigma-Aldrich, St. Louis, MO) was used for in vitro studies.

Animal Model of CCl_4-Induced Liver Fibrosis and Asiatic Acid Treatment

Male Sprague-Dawley (SD) rats (6–8 weeks of age, 180–200 g) were obtained from the Guangdong Medical Laboratory Animal Center, fed with a standard laboratory diet and tap water in a temperature- and humidity-controlled animal house under 12-h light–dark cycles. Forty rats were divided randomly into five groups (n = 8 for each group) including: 1) normal control, 2) disease control, and 3) three AA treatment groups at doses of 0.5 mg/kg, 2 mg/kg, and 8 mg/kg, respectively. In addition, one group of normal 6 rats was treated with a dose of 8 mg/kg of AA as AA toxicity control. Except the normal control groups, all animals were treated with intra-peritoneal injection of 2 ml/kg of CCl_4 (diluted in 20% peanut oil) twice per week for 6 weeks to induce liver fibrosis. For those received the AA treatment, animals were given with three different doses of AA (0.5, 2, and 8 mg/kg) suspended in a 1.5% methyl cellulose (MC) mixture by oral gavage daily for the 6 week-period, while rats from disease control group

A. Histology

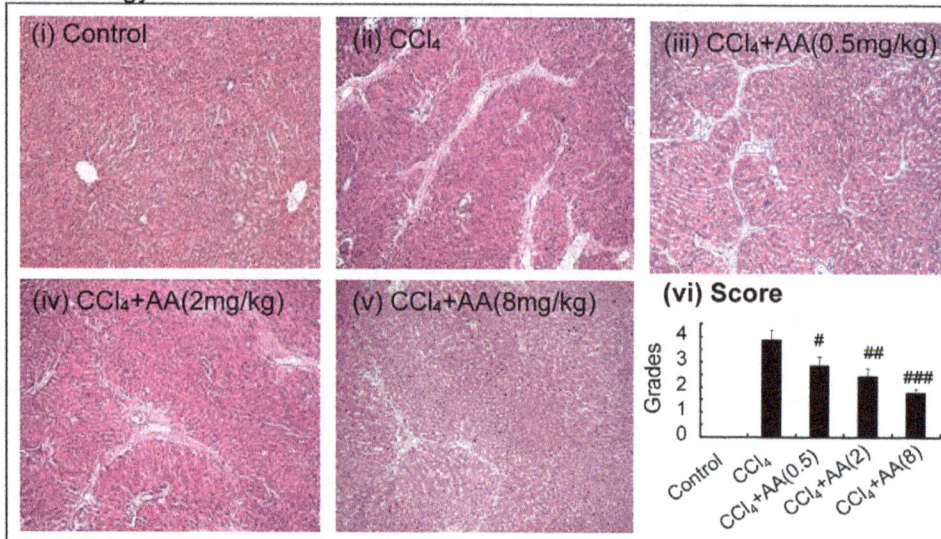

B. Liver Function

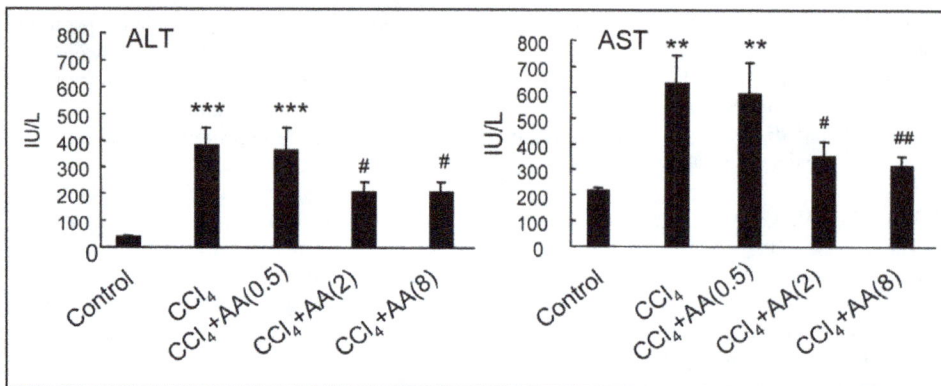

Figure 1. AA treatment attenuates CCl_4-induced liver damage and functional impairment in a dosage-dependent manner in rats.
A. Histology (H&E). **B.** Liver function. Data represent mean ± SEM for groups of 8 animals. **p<0.01, *** p<0.001 versus normal control; #p<0.05, ##p<0.01, ###p<0.001 versus CCl_4-induced disease control. Magnification: ×100.

were treated with equivalent volumes of the MC mixture solution without AA. Normal control animals were also received the same volumes of peanut oil equivalent to the CCl₄-treated animals. To

exclude the toxicity of AA *in vivo*, one group of normal 6 rats was treated with a dose of 8 mg/kg of AA following the same experimental protocol of AA treatment. At the end of the sixth

A. Collagen I expression

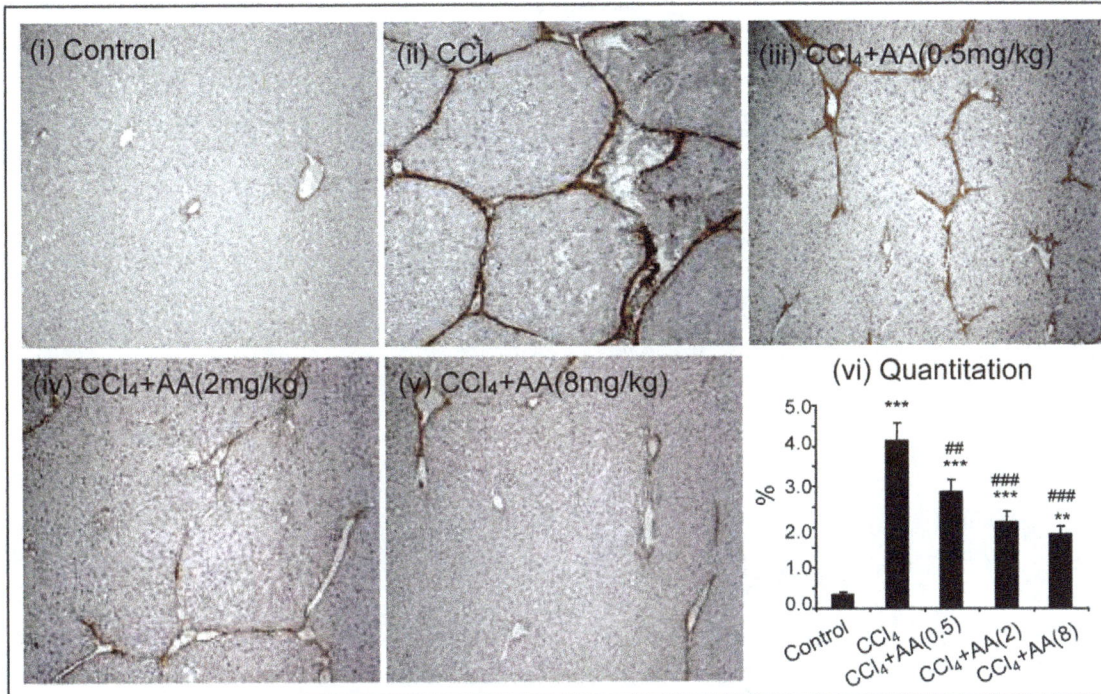

B. Collagen III expression

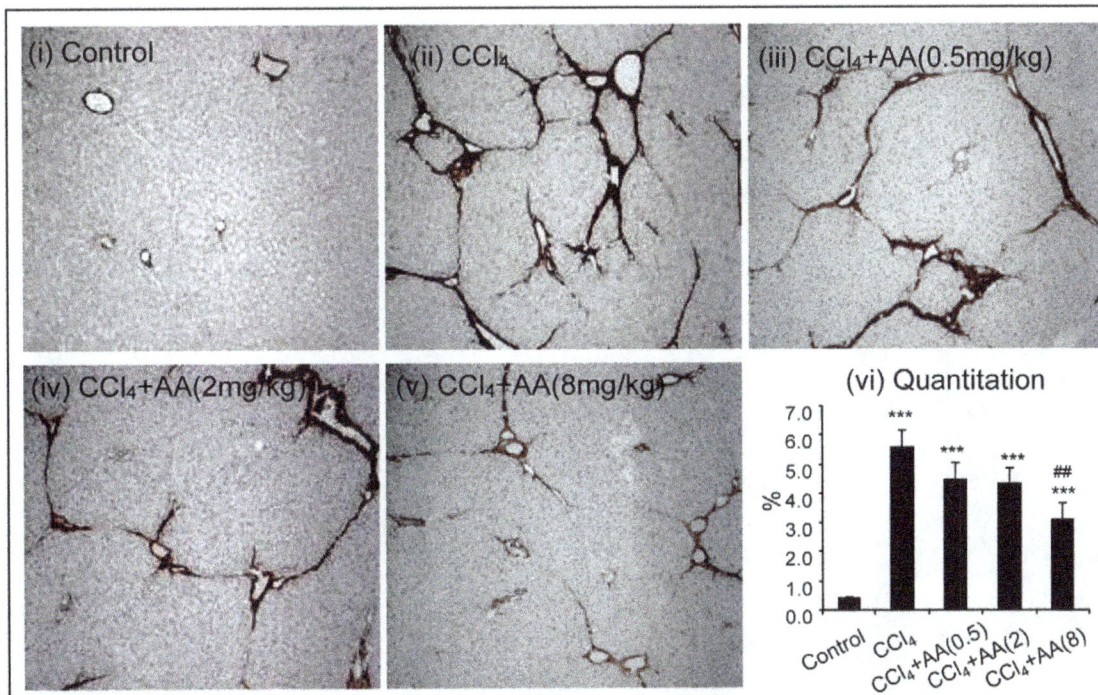

Figure 2. Immunohistochemistry detects that AA treatment attenuates CCl₄-induced liver fibrosis in a dosage-dependent manner in rats. A. Collagen I expression. **B.** Collagen III expression. Data represent mean ± SEM for groups of 8 animals. **p<0.01, *** p<0.001 versus normal control; ##p<0.01, ###p<0.001 versus CCl₄-induced disease control. Magnification: ×100.

week, all of rats were sacrificed under anesthesia with 3% sodium pentobarbital (45 mg/kg, ip). Blood samples and liver specimens were obtained for analyses of liver functions, mRNA and protein expression of fibrotic indexes by real-time reverse transcription polymerase chain reaction (RT-PCR), Western blot, histology, and immunohistochemistry. All experimental procedures were approved by the Animal Experimental Committee at the First People's Hospital of Foshan (A0331).

Liver Function Test

Serum alanine transaminase (ALT) and aspartate transaminase (AST) activities, markers for hepatotoxicity, were detected with an

automatic analyzer (Olympus, Japan) at the Department of Chemical Pathology.

Histopathology and Immunohistochemistry

Changes in liver morphology were examined in methyl Carnoy's fixed, paraffin-embedded tissue sections (3 micrometer) stained with hematoxylin and eosin. The histopathological scores of fibrosis were evaluated following the published criteria [34]: 0) normal liver; 1) an increase in collagen matrix accumulation without the formation of septa (small stellate expansions of the portal fields); 2) formation of incomplete septa from the portal tract to the central vein (septa that do not interconnect with each other);

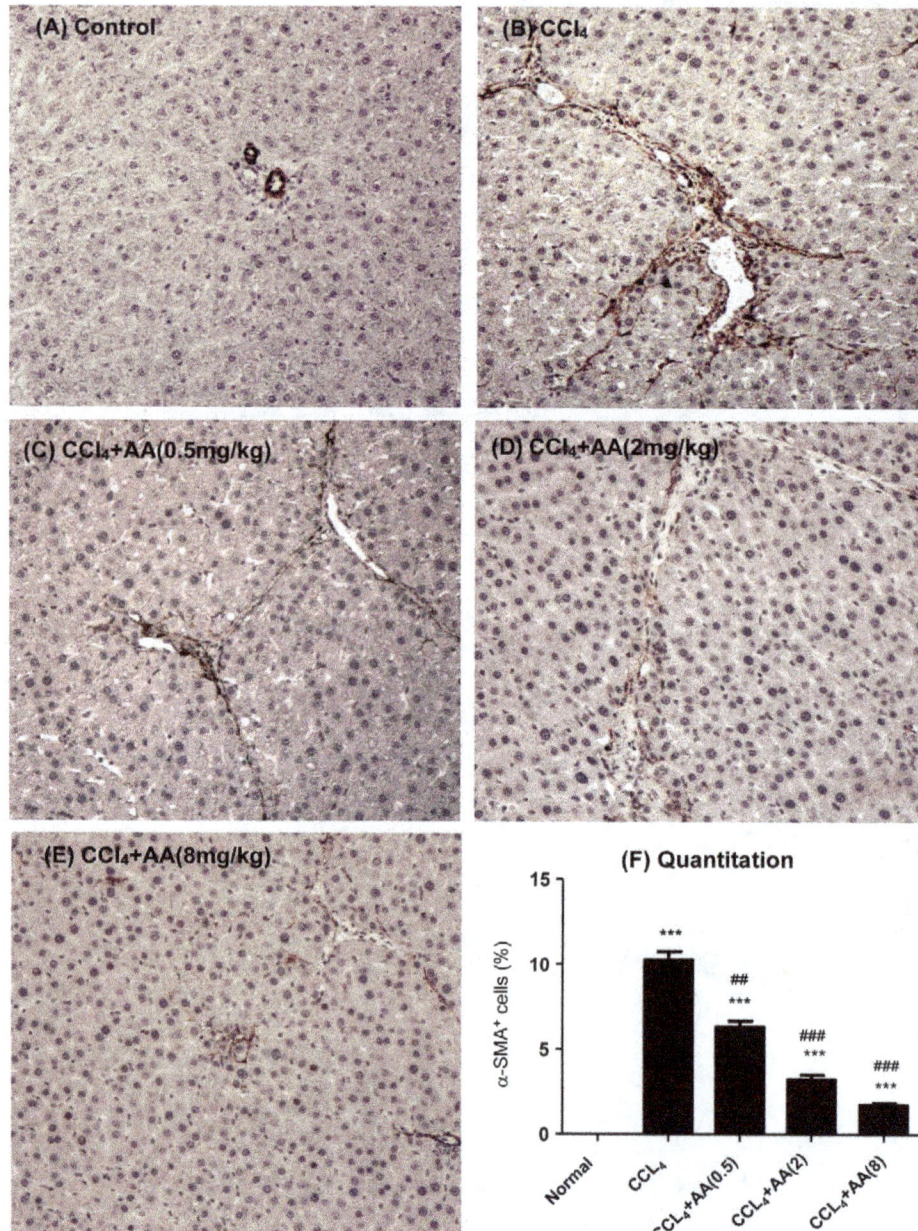

Figure 3. Immunohistochemistry detects that AA treatment attenuates CCl$_4$-induced activation of HSC in a dosage-dependent manner in rats. Activation of HSC was determined by a-SMA+ myofibroblast transition. **A.** Representative picture from a control rat treated with 20% peanut oil. **B.** Representative picture from a rat treated with CCl$_4$. **C–E.** Representative pictures from CCl$_4$-treated rats received AA in a dosage-dependent manner. **F.** Quantitation of a-SMA+ cells. Data represent mean ± SEM for groups of 8 animals. *** p<0.001 versus normal control; ##p<0.01, ###p<0.001 versus CCl$_4$-induced disease rats. Magnification: ×200.

3) complete but thin septa interconnecting with each other to divide the parenchyma into separate fragments; 4) same as grade 3, except for the presence of thick septa (complete cirrhosis).

Immunohistochemistry was performed in paraffin sections using the microwaved-based antigen retrieval method as described previously [35]. Antibodies used in this study included: rabbit polyclonal antibodies to collagen I, III (Southern Tech, Birmingham, AL), and a-SMA (Sigma, St. Louis, MO). An irrelevant isotype rabbit IgG was used as a negative control. The stained sections were developed with diaminobenzidine to produce brown products and counterstained with hematoxylin.

Quantitation of immunostaining was carried out on coded slides as previously described [13,18]. Expression of collagen I, III, and a-SMA in the liver cross-sections was determined using the quantitative Image Analysis System (AxioVision 4, Carl Zeiss, Jena, Germany). Briefly, 10 fields (×20) were randomly selected from each section and positive signals within the section were highlighted, measured, and expressed as percent positive area of the entire liver tissues examined.

Cell culture

The HSC-T6 cell line was gifted by Professor SL Friedman (Liver Disease Research Center of San Francisco General Hospital, CA, USA). HSC-T6 cells were routinely cultured in DMEM (Gibco, USA) supplemented with 10% heat-inactivated fetal bovine serum (FBS).

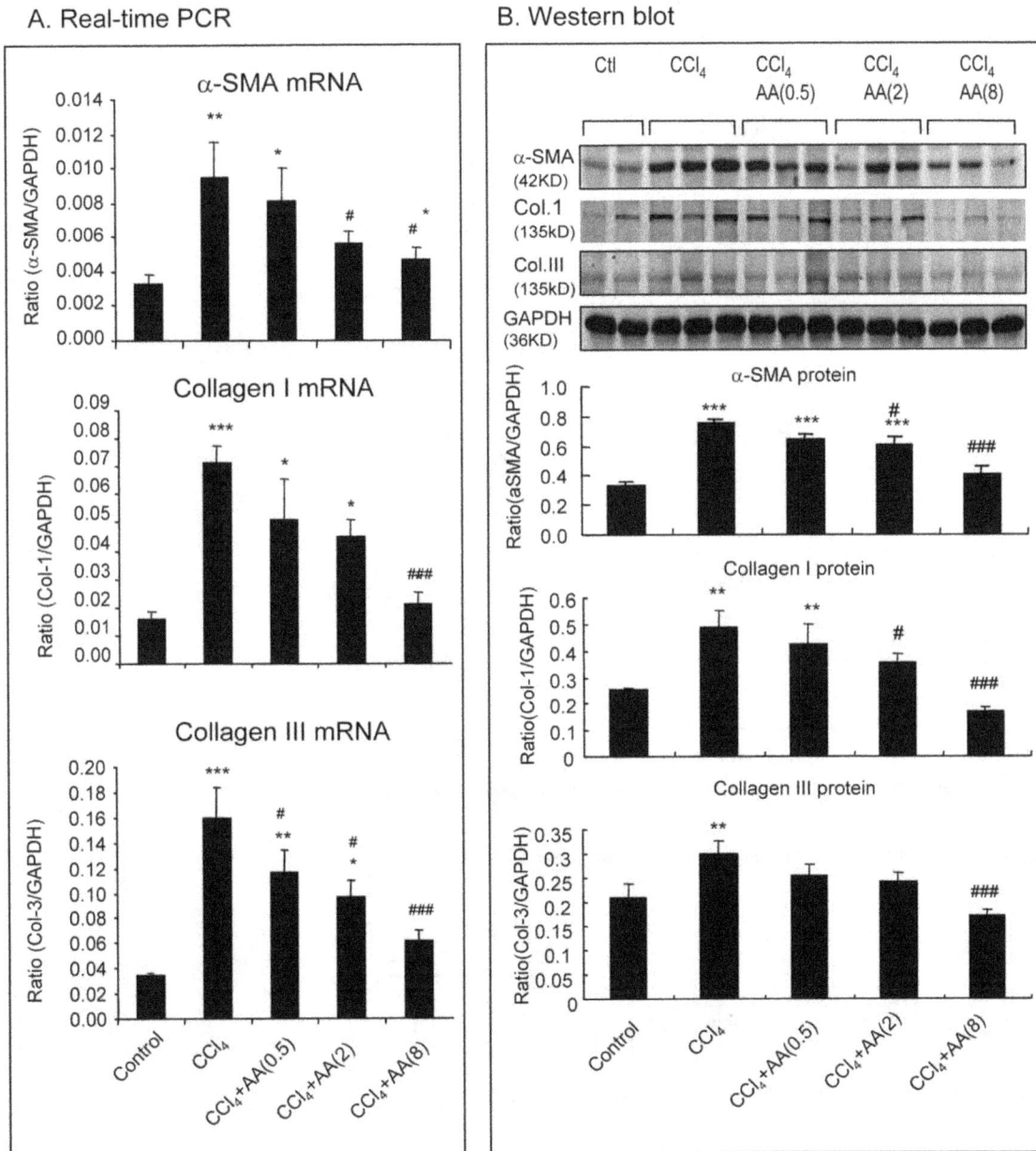

Figure 4. Real-time PCR and Western blot analysis show that AA treatment blocks CCl₄-induced liver fibrosis in a dosage-dependent manner in rats. A. Real-time PCR for a-SMA, collagen type I and III mRNA expression. **B.** Western blot analysis for a-SMA, collagen type I and III protein expression. Data represent mean ± SEM for groups of 8 animals. *p<0.05, **p<0.01, *** p<0.001 versus normal control; #p<0.05, ###p<0.001 versus CCl₄-induced disease control.

We first determined the safe dosages of AA for the study, HSC-T6 cells were cultured at a density of 5×10^4 cells/mL in 100 uL DMEM containing 0.2% FBS in 96-well microplates and AA or DMSO as control in various dosages (0.0, 2.5, 5.0, 10.0, 20.0, 30.0, 40.0, 60.0, and 80.0 micro molar) was added to the culture for 24 h. A dosage-dependent cytotoxicity of AA was measured by 3-(4, 5-dimethylthiazol-2-yl)-2, 5-diphenyl tetrazolium bromide (MTT) assay kit (Sigma-Aldrich) and lactate dehydrogenase (LDH) release kit (Sigma-Aldrich) following the manufacturer instructions. The extent of cytotoxicity and the IC_{50} of AA were calculated using the results of both MTT and LDH assays.

To determine the optimal dose of TGF-beta1 on collagen matrix expression, HSC-T6 cells were treated with TGF-beta1 (R&D System) at dosages of 0.0, 0.1, 0.5, 1.0, 2.0, and 5.0 ng/ml for various time of 0, 1, 3, 6, 12, 24 h. TGF-beta1-induced collagen I and III expression was determined at the mRNA level by real-time PCR and at the protein level by Western blot analysis.

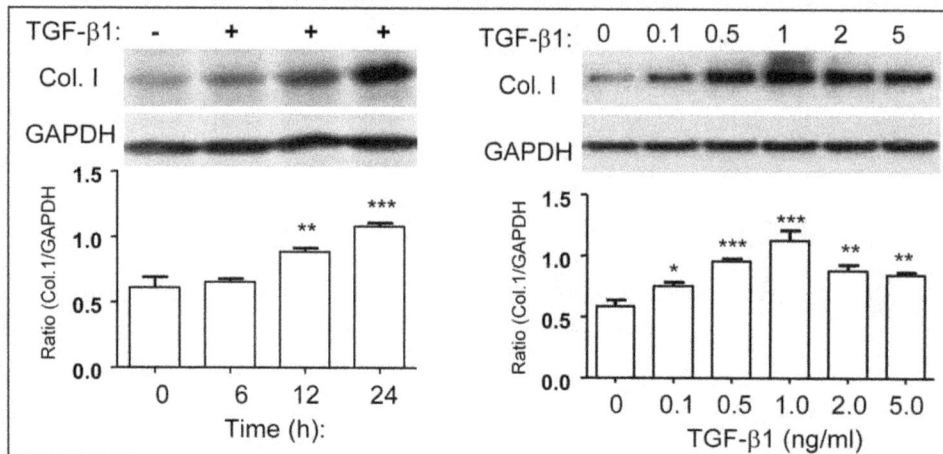

To investigate the inhibitory effect and mechanism of AA on TGF-beta1-mediated fibrosis, HSC-T6 cells were pre-treated with AA at dosages of 0, 5, 10, 20, 30 micro molar for over night, followed by addition of an optimal dose of TGF-beta1 (1 ng/ml) for various time periods for examination of phospho-Smad2/3 and expression of Smad7, collagen I, and a-SMA by real-time and Western blot analysis as described below.

To confirm the protective role of AA in TGF-beta1-induced fibrosis in HSC-T6 cells *via* induction of Smad7, a stable HSC-T6 cell line with Smad7 knockdown was established. In brief, Smad7 siRNA was cloned into the P-super1 plasmid and transfected into HSC-T6 cells with lipofectamine 2000 following the manufacturer's protocol (Invitrogen). The cells were then selected with G418

Figure 5. TGF-beta1 induces collagen I and a-SMA expression by HSC-T6 cells *in vitro*. A. Real-time PCR show that TGF-beta1 (1 ng/ml) induces collagen I and a-SMA mRNA expression in a time and dosage-dependent manner. B. Western blot analysis for a time (TGF-beta1 1 ng/ml) and dosage (24 h)-dependent effects of TGF-beta1 on collagen I expression. Data represent mean ± SEM for at least 3 independent experiments. *p<0.05, **p<0.01, ***p<0.001 versus medium control.

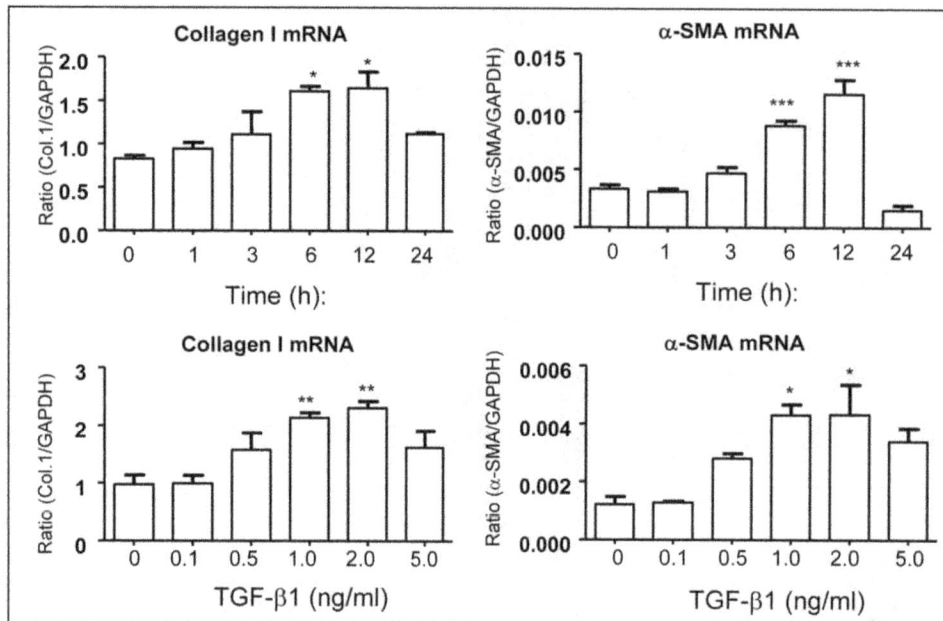

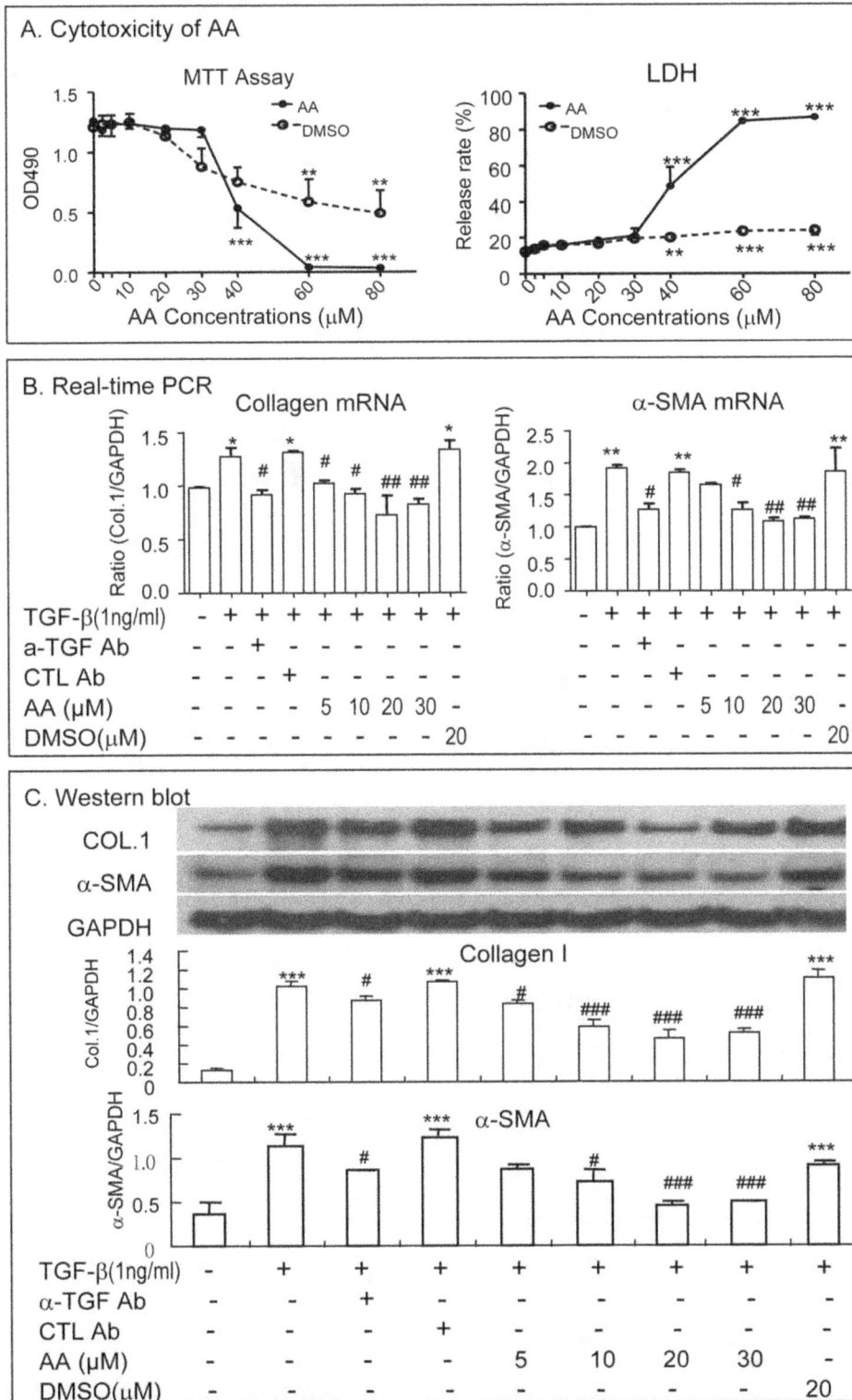

Figure 6. AA inhibits TGF-beta1-induced collagen I and a-SMA expression by HSC-T6 cells in a dosage-dependent manner *in vitro.*
A. Dose-dependent effects of AA on cytotoxicity of HSC-T6 cells by MTT and LDH release assays. **B and C.** Real-time PCR and Western blot analysis for a dosage-dependent inhibitory effect of AA on collagen type I and a-SMA expression. Data represent mean ± SEM for at least 3 independent experiments. *p<0.05, **p<0.01, ***p<0.001 versus medium control; #p<0.05, ##p<0.01, ###p<0.001 versus TGF-beta1-treated, isotype control antibody-treated (CTL Ab), or DMSO-treated cells.

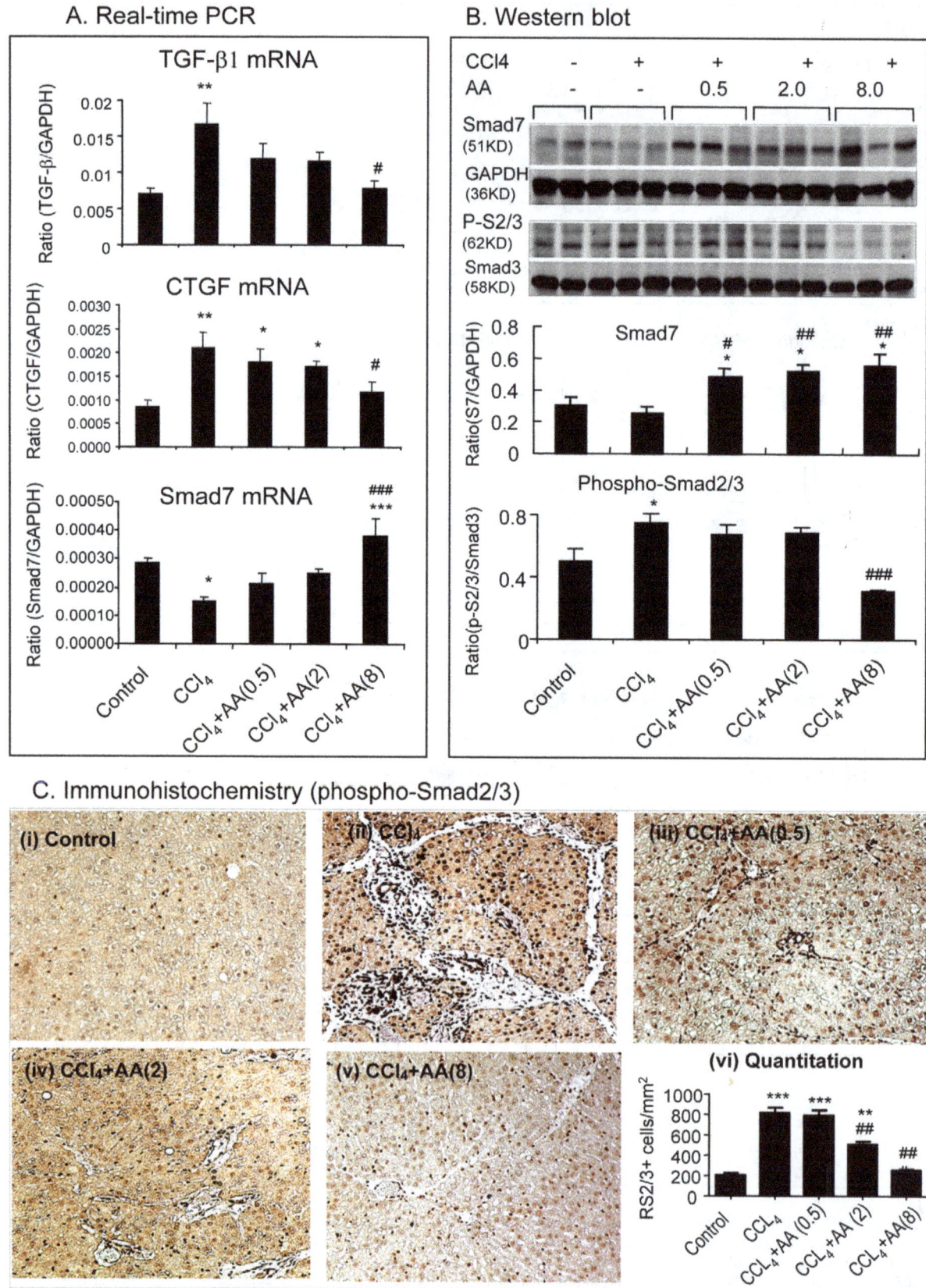

Figure 7. AA treatment upregulates hepatic Smad7, but blocks expression of TGF-beta1 and CTGF and activation of Smad2/3 in CCl₄-induced liver disease in rats. A. Real-time PCR analysis of TGF-beta1, CTGF, and Smad7 mRNA expression. **B.** Western blot analysis for levels of phospho-Smad2/3 and Smad7 protein expression. **C.** Immunohistochemistry for nuclear location of phospho-Smad2/3. Data represent mean ± SEM for groups of 8 animals. *p<0.05, **p<0.01, ***p<0.001 versus normal control; #p<0.05, ##p<0.01, ###p<0.001 versus CCl₄-induced disease control. Magnification: ×200 (C).

in 100 mg/ml for one month and maintained in 50 mg/ml of G418. A stable HSC-T6 cell line transfected with P-super1 empty plasmid only was used as control.

Real-time Reverse Transcription Polymerase Chain Reaction (RT-PCR)

Total RNA was extracted from frozen liver samples or cultured cells using the RNeasy Mini Kit (Qiagen Inc)following the manufacturer's protocol. mRNA expression of collagen I, collagen III, a-SMA, TGF-beta1, CTGF, Smad7, and GAPDH was detected by quantitative real time PCR using an Opticon 2 DNA Engine Real Time PCR Detection (MJ Research Inc., Waltham, MA) as previously described [13,16,17]. The expression levels of all the transcripts were normalized to that of the housekeeping gene GAPDH in the same tissue.

Western Blot Analysis

Proteins extracted from either liver tissues or cultured HSC were analyzed by Western blotting as previously described [13,16,17]. Antibodies used in this study included: collagen I, collagen III (Southern Biotech), α-SMA(Sigma, St. Louis, MO), Smad7, phospho-Smad2/3 (Santa Cruz Biotechnology Inc., Santa Cruz, CA), GAPDH (Chemicon Inc., Temecula, CA), and IRDyeTM800 conjugated secondary antibodies (Rockland Immunochemical Inc., Gilbertsville, PA). Signals were scanned and visualized by Odyssey Infrared Imaging System (LiCor Inc., Lincoln, NE). The ratio of the protein interested was subjected to GAPDH and was densitometrically analyzed by Image J software (NIH, Bethsda, MD).

Statistical Analyses

All data are expressed as mean $\pm$ SEM. The differences between multiple groups were evaluated by a one-way analysis of variances (ANOVA), followed by Newman-Keuls Post Test using Prism 4.0 Program (GraphPad Software, Inc. San Diego, CA).

Results

Asiatic Acid Treatment Inhibits CCl4-Induced Liver Functional and Histological Damage

Administration of CCl_4 for 6 weeks caused a moderate to severe liver injury as demonstrated by the development of severe liver damage with thick fibrotic septa and pseudolobular formation (Fig. 1Aii, vi). Serologically, levels of ALT and AST were also highly significantly elevated in disease control rats when compared to normal control rats (Fig. 1B). In contrast, treatment with AA resulted in attenuation of both histological and functional injury in a dosage-dependent manner, being significant at doses of 2 and 8 mg/kg (Fig. 1A iii–vi and B). Normal rats treated with AA (8 mg/kg) exhibited normal histological and serological changes similar to the normal control rats (data not shown).

Asiatic Acid Treatment Attenuates CCl4-Induced Liver Fibrosis in vivo

We next examined the therapeutic effect of AA on liver fibrosis. As shown in Figure 2 , immunohistochemistry detected that compared to normal control rats, CCl_4-treatment caused a remarkable collagen I and III accumulation in the liver (Fig. 2A and B, i–ii). In contrast, treatment with AA reduced hepatic collagen matrix accumulation in a dosage-dependent manner (Fig. 2 A and B, iii–v), which was confirmed by quantitative analysis (Fig. 2A and B, vi). Importantly, treatment with AA on protection of liver from CCl_4-induced fibrosis was associated with

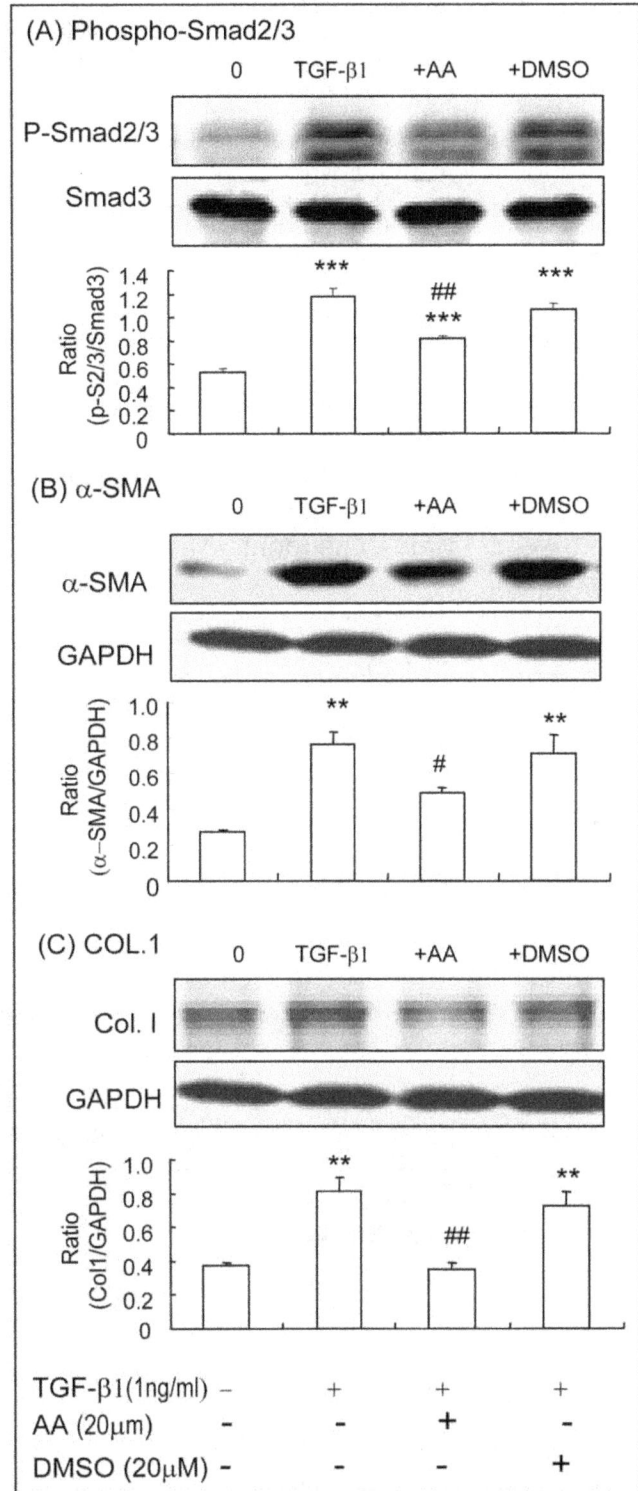

Figure 8. AA blocks TGF-beta1-induced phosphorylation of Smad2/3, a-SMA, and collagen matrix production by HSC-T6 cells in vitro. Western blot analysis detects that HSC-T6 cells pretreated with AA (20 uM) for overnight blocks TGF-beta1 (1 ng/ml)-induced Smad2/3 phosphorylation at 30 mins (**A**) and upregulation of α-SMA and collagen I expression at 24 h (**B,C**). Data represent mean $\pm$ SEM for at least 3 independent experiments. **p<0.01, ***p<0.001 versus medium control; #p<0.05, ##p<0.01 versus TGF-beta1-treated or DMSO-treated cells.

inhibition of HSC activation as determined by blockade of a-SMA+ myofibroblast transition. As shown in Figure 3, addition of AA was capable of blocking a-SMA+ cell accumulation along the fibrotic septa in a dosage-dependent manner.

The inhibitory effect of AA on liver fibrosis was also demonstrated by at the mRNA levels by real-time PCR. As shown in Figure 4(A), CCl4-induced upregulation of a-SMA and collagen type I and III mRNA was significantly attenuated in those treated with AA in a dose-dependent manner. These findings were also evidenced by Western blot analysis (Fig. 4B).

Asiatic Acid Inhibits TGF-beta1-Induced HSC Activation of Collagen Matrix Expression by HSC-T6 Cells *in Vitro*

Because TGF-beta1 has been long considered as a key mediator in the pathogenesis of liver fibrosis [1–4], we examined if AA is able to inhibit the fibrotic effects of TGF-beta1 on ECM expression in a well-characterized HSC-T6 cells. We first determined an optimal dose of TGF-beta1 in fibrosis response on HSC-T6 cells. As shown in Figure 5, both real-time PCR and Western blot analyses detected that addition of TGF-beta1 induced collagen I and a-SMA mRNA and protein expression in a time- and dosage-dependent manner, being an optimal dose of TGF-beta1 at 1 ng/ml with the peaked time for mRNA expression at 6 h and protein expression at 24 h.

We then determined the safe dose of AA without causing cytotoxicity for the *in vitro* study in HCS-T6 cells. As shown in Figure 6(A), AA at doses over 40 micro molar (uM) caused a significant cytotoxicity on HSC-T6 by inhibiting HSC-T6 cell proliferation (MTT assay) and increasing LDH release. In contrast, there was not detectable cytotoxicity when doses of AA

(A) AA induces Smad7 mRNA expression in a time and dose-dependent manner

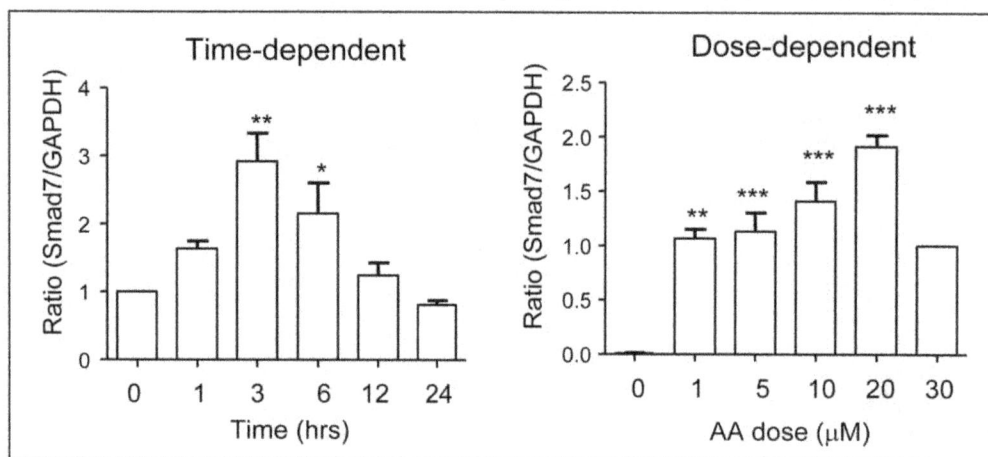

(B) AA induces Smad7 protein expression in a time and dose-dependent manner

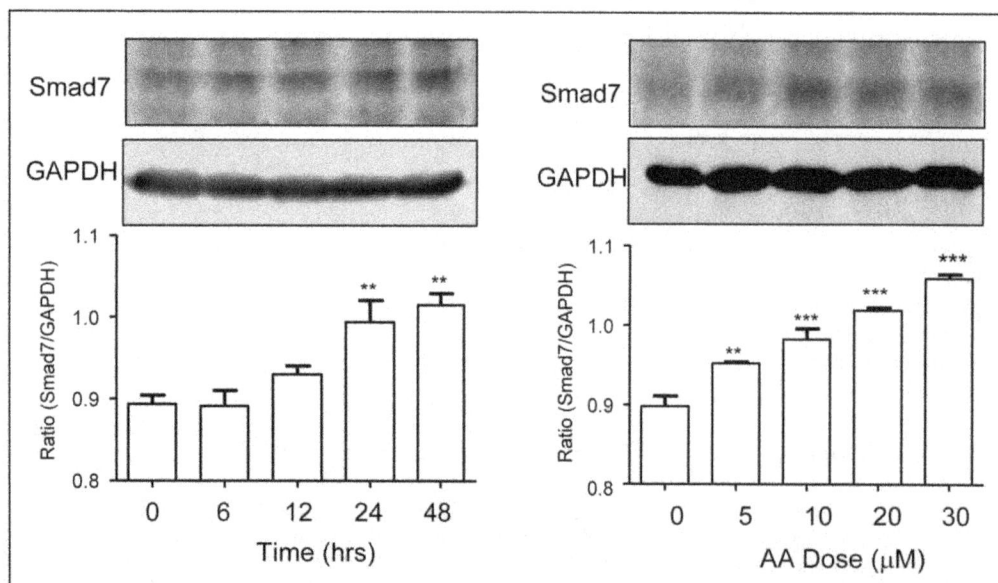

Figure 9. AA induces Smad7 expression by HSC-T6 cells in a time and dosage-dependent manner *in vitro.* **A.** Real-time PCR. **B.** Western blots. Results show that addition of AA induces Smad7 mRNA and protein expression in a time (at a dose of 20 uM) and dosage (3 h for mRNA and 24 h for protein)-dependent manner. Data represent mean ± SEM for at least 3 independent experiments. *p<0.05, **p<0.01, ***p<0.001 versus medium control.

were at and below 30 μM. Thus, safe doses of AA (0, 5, 10 20, 30 uM) were used for studying the inhibitory effect of AA on TGF-beta1 (1 ng/ml)-induced HSC activation and ECM production *in vitro*. As shown in Figure 6(B,C), real-time PCR demonstrated that addition of AA significantly inhibited TGF-beta1-inudced collagen I and a-SMA mRNA expression in a dosage-dependent manner, being an optimal dose at 20-30 uM (Fig. 6B). Similar results were also observed at the protein levels as demonstrated by Western blot analysis (Fig. 6C).

Upregulation of Hepatic Smad7, thereby inhibiting TGF-beta/Smad signaling, Is a Key Mechanism by Which Asiatic Acid Attenuates hepatic fibrosis *in vivo* and *in vitro*

Since TGF-beta/Smad signaling is a key pathway leading to liver fibrosis [8–11], we then investigated the mechanisms by which AA attenuates CCl_4-induced liver fibrosis by examining the TGF-beta/Smad signaling pathway. As shown in Figure 7, compared to normal control rats, CCl_4-induced liver fibrosis was associated with a marked upregulation of TGF-beta1 and CTGF mRNA (Fig. 7A), which was associated with a marked activation of Smad2/3 as identified by higher levels of phospho-Smad2/3 and its nuclear translocation (Fig.7B,C), and a fall of hepatic Smad7 (Fig. 7A and B). In contrast, diseased rats treated with AA significantly reduced TGF-beta and CTGF mRNA expression and blocked activation of Smad2/3 in a dosage-dependent manner (Fig. 7). Importantly, the inhibitory effect of AA on TGF-beta/Smad signaling was associated with a marked upregulation of hepatic Smad7 as demonstrated at the mRNA level by real-time PCR and at the protein level by Western blot analysis (Fig. 7 A and B).

The mechanism of AA-induced upregulation of hepatic Smad7 to inhibit CCl_4-induced liver fibrosis was further investigated in vitro by knocking down Smad7 in HSC-T6 cells. Western blot analysis detected that addition of AA, but not DMSO, was capable of blocking TGF-beta1-induced phosphorylation of Smad2/3 and α-SMA and collagen I expression by HSC-T6 cells (Fig.8). The inhibitory effect of AA in TGF-beta/Smad-mediated hepatic fibrosis was associated with upregulation of Smad7 as demonstrated by the findings that AA alone was able to induce Smad7 mRNA and protein in a time and dosage-dependent manner (Fig. 9 A and B). To further examine the hypothesis that AA induces Smad7 to inhibit TGF-beta1-mediated hepatic fibrosis, Smad7 gene was knocked down from HSC-T6 cells by siRNA technique. As shown in Figure 10, knockdown of Smad7 from HSC-T6 cells was able to prevent the inhibitory effect of AA on TGF-beta1-induced collagen I and a-SMA expression.

Discussion

Although it is now well accepted that TGF-beta/Smad signaling is a major pathway leading to end-stage liver failure featuring with cirrhosis, treatments for hepatic fibrosis remain non-specific and ineffective. In this study, we reported here that AA, a natural product from *Centella asiatica*, may be a novel therapeutic agent for liver fibrosis. Administration of AA significantly inhibited CCl_4-induced activation of HSC and liver fibrosis and largely improved liver functional injury in a dosage-dependent manner in rats. In addition, we also found that addition of AA was able to block TGF-beta1-induced HSC activation such as a-SMA+ myofibroblast transition and collagen matrix expression in a rat HSC-T6 cell line. More importantly, upregulation of hepatic Smad7, thereby blocking TGF-beta/Smad signaling, may be the underlying mechanism by which AA attenuated CCl_4-induced liver

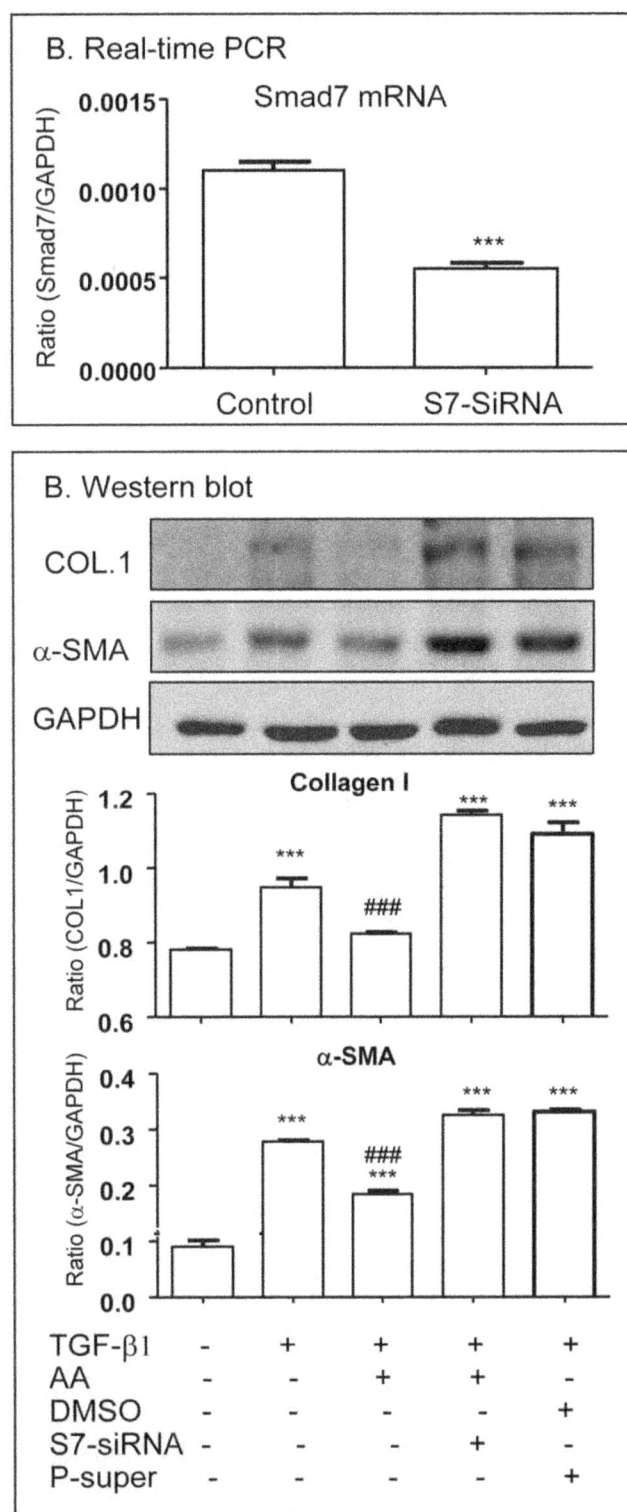

Figure 10. Knockdown of Smad7 from HSC-T6 cells prevents the inhibitory effect of AA on TGF-beta1-induced hepatic fibrosis *in vitro*. A. Real-time PCR shows reduction of Smad7 mRNA by siRNA technique. **B.** Western blot analysis detects that knockdown of Smad7 from HSC-T6 cells results in a loss of AA (20 uM)-induced inhibition of TGF-beta1 (1 ng/ml)-mediated collagen I and a-SMA expression at 24 h. Data represent mean ± SEM for at least 3 independent experiments. *p<0.05, **p<0.01, ***p<0.001 versus control; ###p<0.001 versus TGF-beta1, DMSO, and control vector (P-super)-treated cells.

fibrosis *in vivo* and TGF-beta1-stimulated HSC activation and ECM production *in vitro*.

In the context of liver fibrosis, TGF-beta1 is a key mediator to activate HSCs to transform into a-SMA+ myofibroblast-like cells, a cell type producing ECM during fibrogenesis [2–5]. It has been shown that AA derivatives are able to inhibit ECM production by HSC and keloid fibroblasts by blocking the autocrine effect of TGF-beta1 *in vitro* [32,33]. The present study added new information that AA was capable of blocking exogenous TGF-beta1-induced myofibroblast transition and collagen I matrix expression by HSC, suggesting that AA may counter-regulate the profibrotic effect of TGF-beta1 in liver fibrosis. This was further confirmed *in vivo* in a rat model of CCl4-induced hepatic fibrosis in which treatment with AA significantly attenuated CCl4-induced liver fibrosis and functional injury. All these findings demonstrated that AA may be a novel and effective therapeutic agent for hepatofibrosis.

A novel and significant finding in the present study was the identification that AA-induced upregulation of hepatic Smad7, thereby inhibiting TGF-beta/Smad signaling, was a mechanism by which AA inhibits CCl4 or TGF-beta1-induced HSC activation and liver fibrosis *in vivo* and *in vitro*. Indeed, activation of TGF-beta/Smad signaling is a key mechanism of liver fibrosis in both experimental and human chronic liver diseases [2–4]. The functional importance of TGF-beta/Smad signaling in liver fibrosis has been demonstrated by the finding that disruption of Smad3 protects against dimethylnitrosamine-induced hepatic fibrosis [8]. In contrast, deletion of Smad7, an inhibitor of TGF-beta/Smad signaling, enhances CCl4-induced liver damage and fibrosis in mice [9]. In the present study, CCl4-induced liver fibrosis was associated with a marked activation of Smad2/3 but a

loss of Smad7, suggesting that the imbalance between Smad2/3 and Smad7 signaling could be important in the pathogenesis of liver fibrosis. This is confirmed by the recent studies that overexpression of Smad7 in the liver attenuates TGF-beta/Smad signaling and protects against HSC activation and liver fibrogenesis in CCl4-induced mouse and rat models [10,11]. Although the mechanisms of TGF-beta/Smad-mediated liver fibrosis are well understood, the development of therapeutic drugs directly targeting this pathway remains unexplored. The present study identified that treatment with AA was able to induce hepatic Smad7, thereby blocking TGF-beta/Smad signaling and fibrosis in a rat model of CCl4-induced liver fibrosis and in TGF-beta1-activated HSC *in vitro*. These results suggest that induction of Smad7, thereby restoring the balance of TGF-beta/Smad signaling, may be a central mechanism by which AA inhibits liver fibrosis *in vivo* and *in vitro*. This was supported by the finding that knockdown of Smad7 was able to protect against HSC from TGF-beta1-induced activation and fibrosis *in vitro*.

In summary, the present study demonstrates that AA may be a novel therapeutic agent for liver fibrosis. Induction of hepatic Smad7, thereby inhibiting activation of TGF-beta/Smad signaling, may be an underlying mechanism by which AA protects against chronic liver disease associated with fibrosis.

Author Contributions

Conceived and designed the experiments: HYL J-JT GY. Performed the experiments: L-XT R-HH XRH LZ X-MM. Analyzed the data: L-XT R-HH XRH LZ X-MM. Contributed reagents/materials/analysis tools: XRH. Wrote the paper: L-XT HYL.

References

1. Bataller R, Brenner DA (2005) Liver fibrosis. J Clin Invest 115: 209–218.
2. Friedman SL (2008) Mechanisms of Hepatic Fibrogenesis. Gastroenterology 134: 1655–1669.
3. Inagaki Y, Okazaki I (2007) Emerging insights into transforming growth factor beta Smad signal in hepatic fibrogenesis. Gut 56: 284–292.
4. Meindl-Beinker NM, Dooley S (2008) Transforming growth factor-β and hepatocyte transdifferentiation in liver fbrogenesis. J Gastroenterol Hepatol 23 (Suppl): S122–127.
5. Ueberham E, Löw R, Ueberham U, Schönig K, Bujard H, et al. (2003) Conditional tetracycline-regulated expression of TGF-beta1 in liver of transgenic mice leads to reversible intermediary fibrosis. Hepatology 37: 1067–1078.
6. Derynck R, Zhang YE (2003) Smad-dependent and Smad-independent pathways in TGF-beta family signalling. Nature 425: 577–584.
7. Kavsak P, Rasmussen RK, Causing CG, Bonni S, Zhu H, et al. (2000) Smad7 binds to Smurf2 to form an E3 ubiquitin ligase that targets the TGF-beta receptor for degradation. Mol Cell 6: 1365–1375.
8. Latella G, Vetuschi A, Sferra R, Catitti V, D'Angelo A, et al. (2009) Targeted disruption of Smad3 confers resistance to the development of dimethylnitrosamine-induced hepatic fibrosis in mice. Liver Int 29: 997–1009.
9. Hamzavi J, Ehnert S, Godoy P, Ciuclan L, Weng H, et al. (2008) Disruption of the Smad7 gene enhances CCl4-dependent liver damage and fibrogenesis in mice. J Cell Mol Med 12: 2130–2144.
10. Dooley S, Hamzavi J, Breitkopf K, Godoy P, Ilkavets I, et al. (2003) Smad7 prevents activation of hepatic stellate cells and liver fbrosis in rats. Gastroenterology 125: 178–191.
11. Dooley S, Hamzavi J, Ciuclan L, Godoy P, Ilkavets I, et al. (2008) Hepatocyte-specific Smad7 expression attenuates TGF-beta-mediated fibrogenesis and protects against liver damage. Gastroenterology 135: 642–659.
12. Lan HY (2008) Smad7 as a therapeutic agent for chronic kidney diseases. Front Biosci 13: 4984–4992.
13. Chung AC, Huang XR, Zhou L, Heuchel R, Lai KN, et al. (2009) Disruption of the Smad7 gene promotes renal fibrosis and inflammation in unilateral ureteral obstruction (UUO) in mice. Nephrol Dial Transplant 24: 1443–1454.
14. Li JH, Zhu HJ, Huang XR, Lai KN, Johnson RJ, et al. (2002) Smad7 inhibits fibrotic effect of TGF-beta on renal tubular epithelial cells by blocking Smad2 activation. J Am Soc Nephrol 13: 1464–72.
15. Yang F, Chung AC, Huang XR, Lan HY (2009) Angiotensin II induces connective tissue growth factor and collagen I expression via transforming growth factor-beta-dependent and -independent Smad pathways: the role of Smad3. Hypertension 54: 877–884.
16. Lan HY, Mu W, Tomita N, Li JH, Zhu HJ, et al. (2003) Inhibition of renal fibrosis by gene transfer of inducible Smad7 using ultrasound-microbubble system in rat UUO model. J Am Soc Nephrol 14: 1535–1548.
17. Hou CC, Wang W, Huang XR, Fu P, Chen TH, et al. (2005) Ultrasound-microbubble-mediated gene transfer of inducible Smad7 blocks transforming growth factor-beta signaling and fibrosis in rat remnant kidney. Am J Pathol 166: 761–771.
18. Chen H, Huang XR, Wang W, Li J, Heuchel RL, et al. (2011) The Protective Role of Smad7 in Diabetic Kidney Disease: Mechanism and Therapeutic Potential. Diabetes 60: 590–601.
19. Schaneberg BT, Mikell JR, Bedir E, Khan IA (2003) An improved HPLC method for quantitative determination of six triterpenes in Centella asiatica extracts and commercial products. Pharmazie 58: 381–384.
20. Yun KJ, Kim JY, Kim JB, Lee KW, Jeong SY, et al. (2008) Inhibition of LPS-induced NO and PGE2 production by asiatic acid via NF-kappa B inactivation in RAW 264.7 macrophages: possible involvement of the IKK and MAPK pathways. Int Immunopharmacol 8: 431–441.
21. Won JH, Shin JS, Park HJ, Jung HJ, Koh DJ, et al. (2010) Anti-inflammatory effects of madecassic acid via the suppression of NF-kappaB pathway in LPS-induced RAW 264.7 macrophage cells. Planta Med 76: 251–257.
22. Pittella F, Dutra RC, Junior DD, Lopes MT, Barbosa NR (2009) Antioxidant and cytotoxic activities of Centella asiatica (L) Urb. Int J Mol Sci 10: 3713–3721.
23. Hsu YL, Kuo PL, Lin LT (2005) Asiatic Acid, a Triterpene, Induces Apoptosis and Cell Cycle Arrest through Activation of Extracellular Signal-Regulated Kinase and p38 Mitogen-Activated Protein Kinase Pathways in Human Breast Cancer Cells. J Pharmacol Exp Ther 313: 333–344.
24. Park BC, Bosire KO, Lee ES, Lee YS, Kim JA (2005) Asiatic acid induces apoptosis in SK-MEL-2 human melanoma cells. Cancer Lett 218: 81–90.
25. Krishnamurthy RG, Senut MC, Zemke D, Min J, Frenkel MB, et al. (2009) Asiatic acid, a pentacyclic triterpene from Centella asiatica, is neuroprotective in a mouse model of focal cerebral ischemia. J Neurosci Res 87: 2541–2550.
26. Soumyanath A, Zhong YP, Gold SA, Yu X, Koop DR, et al. (2005) Centella asiatica accelerates nerve regeneration upon oral administration and contains multiple active fractions increasing neurite elongation in-vitro. J Pharm Pharmacol 57: 1221–1229.
27. Cheng CL, Guo JS, Luk J, Koo MWL (2004) The healing effects of Centella extract and asiaticoside on acetic acid induced gastric ulcers in rats. Life Sci 74: 2237–2249.

28. Kimura Y, Sumiyoshi M, Samukawa K-I, Satake N, Sakanaka M (2008) Facilitating action of asiaticoside at low doses on burn wound repair and its mechanism. Eur J Pharmacol 584: 415–423.

29. Gao J, Chen J, Tang X, Pan L, Fang F, et al. (2006) Mechanism underlying mitochondrial protection of asiatic acid against hepatotoxicity in mice. J Pharm Pharmacol 58: 227–233.

30. Ma K, Zhang Y, Zhou D, Lou Y (2009) Protective effects of asiatic acid against D-galactosamine/lipopolysaccharide-induced hepatotoxicity in hepatocytes and kupffer cells co-cultured system via redox-regulated leukotriene C4 synthase expression pathway. Eur J Pharmacol 603: 98–107.

31. Lee MK, Kim SH, Yang H, Lim DY, Ryu JH, et al. (2009) Asiatic acid derivatives protect primary cultures of rat hepatocytes against carbon tetrachloride-induced injury via the cellular antioxidant system. Nat Prod Commun 4: 765–768.

32. Dong MS, Jung SH, Kim HJ, Kim JR, Zhao LX, et al. (2004) Structure-related cytotoxicity and anti-hepatofibric effect of asiatic acid derivatives in rat hepatic stellate cell-line, HSC-T6. Arch Pharm Res 27: 512–517.

33. Tang B, Zhu B, Liang Y, Bi L, Hu Z, et al. (2011) Asiaticoside suppresses collagen expression and TGF-beta/Smad signaling through inducing Smad7 and inhibiting TGF-betaRI and TGF-betaRII in keloid fibroblasts. Arch Dermatol Res 303: 563–572.

34. Ruwart MJ, Wilkinson KF, Rush BD, Vidmar TJ, Peters KM, et al. (1989) The integrated value of serum procollagen III peptide over time predicts hepatic hydroxyproline content and stainable collagen in a model of dietary cirrhosis in the rat. Hepatology 10: 801–806.

35. Lan HY, Mu W, Nikolic-Paterson DJ, Atkins RC (1995) A novel, simple, reliable, and sensitive method for multiple immunoenzyme staining: use of microwave oven heating to block antibody crossreactivity and retrieve antigens. J Histochem Cytochem 43: 97–102.

11

Functional Contribution of Elevated Circulating and Hepatic Non-Classical CD14$^+$CD16$^+$ Monocytes to Inflammation and Human Liver Fibrosis

Henning W. Zimmermann[1], Sebastian Seidler[1], Jacob Nattermann[2], Nikolaus Gassler[3], Claus Hellerbrand[4], Alma Zernecke[5], Jens J. W. Tischendorf[1], Tom Luedde[1], Ralf Weiskirchen[6], Christian Trautwein[1], Frank Tacke[1]*

1 Department of Medicine III, University Hospital Aachen, Aachen, Germany, 2 Department of Medicine I, University of Bonn, Bonn, Germany, 3 Institute of Pathology, University Hospital Aachen, Aachen, Germany, 4 Department of Medicine I, University of Regensburg, Regensburg, Germany, 5 Institute for Molecular Cardiovascular Research, University Hospital Aachen, Aachen, Germany, 6 Institute of Clinical Chemistry and Pathobiochemistry, University Hospital Aachen, Aachen, Germany

Abstract

Background: Monocyte-derived macrophages critically perpetuate inflammatory responses after liver injury as a prerequisite for organ fibrosis. Experimental murine models identified an essential role for the CCR2-dependent infiltration of classical Gr1/Ly6C$^+$ monocytes in hepatic fibrosis. Moreover, the monocyte-related chemokine receptors CCR1 and CCR5 were recently recognized as important fibrosis modulators in mice. In humans, monocytes consist of classical CD14$^+$CD16$^-$ and non-classical CD14$^+$CD16$^+$ cells. We aimed at investigating the relevance of monocyte subpopulations for human liver fibrosis, and hypothesized that 'non-classical' monocytes critically exert inflammatory as well as profibrogenic functions in patients during liver disease progression.

Methodology/Principal Findings: We analyzed circulating monocyte subsets from freshly drawn blood samples of 226 patients with chronic liver disease (CLD) and 184 healthy controls by FACS analysis. Circulating monocytes were significantly expanded in CLD-patients compared to controls with a marked increase of the non-classical CD14$^+$CD16$^+$ subset that showed an activated phenotype in patients and correlated with proinflammatory cytokines and clinical progression. Correspondingly, CD14$^+$CD16$^+$ macrophages massively accumulated in fibrotic/cirrhotic livers, as evidenced by immunofluorescence and FACS. Ligands of monocyte-related chemokine receptors CCR2, CCR1 and CCR5 were expressed at higher levels in fibrotic and cirrhotic livers, while CCL3 and CCL4 were also systemically elevated in CLD-patients. Isolated monocyte/macrophage subpopulations were functionally characterized regarding cytokine/chemokine expression and interactions with primary human hepatic stellate cells (HSC) *in vitro*. CD14$^+$CD16$^+$ monocytes released abundant proinflammatory cytokines. Furthermore, CD14$^+$CD16$^+$, but not CD14$^+$CD16$^-$ monocytes could directly activate collagen-producing HSC.

Conclusions/Significance: Our data demonstrate the expansion of CD14$^+$CD16$^+$ monocytes in the circulation and liver of CLD-patients upon disease progression and suggest their functional contribution to the perpetuation of intrahepatic inflammation and profibrogenic HSC activation in liver cirrhosis. The modulation of monocyte-subset recruitment into the liver via chemokines/chemokine receptors and their subsequent differentiation may represent promising approaches for therapeutic interventions in human liver fibrosis.

Editor: Patricia T. Bozza, Fundaçao Oswaldo Cruz, Brazil

Funding: This work was supported by the German Research Foundation (DFG Ta434/2-1 to F.T., DFG SFB/TRR 57), by the START-Program and the Interdisciplinary Centre for Clinical Research (IZKF) within the Faculty of Medicine at the RWTH Aachen University (to H.W.Z and F.T.). The funders had no role in study design, data collection and analysis, decision to publish, or preparation of the manuscript.

Competing Interests: The authors have declared that no competing interests exist.

* E-mail: frank.tacke@gmx.net

Introduction

Sustained inflammation is a common characteristic of chronic liver injury in mice and men and induces the development of liver fibrosis [1,2]. Monocytes are circulating blood leukocytes that play important roles in the pathogenesis of inflammatory disorders, because they serve as precursors for tissue macrophages and dendritic cells [3]. Over recent years, several studies have emphasized the crucial role of infiltrating monocytes for the progression of liver fibrosis in experimental mouse models [4,5,6,7,8,9]. It has become clear that the macrophage compartment of the liver, traditionally called 'Kupffer cells', is constantly replenished to a significant extent by blood monocytes [4,10] and is greatly augmented by a vast number of infiltrating monocytes upon acute or chronic liver injury [6,11]. During fibrosis progression in mice, monocyte-derived macrophages release cytokines perpetuating chronic inflammation as well as directly activate hepatic stellate cells (HSC), resulting in their proliferation and transdifferentiation into collagen-producing myofibroblasts [5,6,9]. Independent studies highlighted the importance of the chemokine receptor CCR2 and its cognate ligand monocyte-chemoattractant protein 1 (MCP-1/CCL2) for monocyte recruitment during experimental hepatic fibrosis [5,6,7,8]. Moreover, CCR1 and CCR5, receptors for the chemokines CCL3/MIP1α, CCL4/MIP1β and CCL5/RANTES, promote liver fibrosis in mice [11].

Human and mouse blood each contain two main monocyte subsets, which can be distinguished by high or low Gr1 (Ly6C) expression ('Gr1^{hi} or Gr1^{lo} monocytes') in mice [12]. We demonstrated previously that only Gr1^{hi} monocytes are massively recruited into the murine liver upon toxic injury dependent on CCR2-mediated bone marrow egress, constituting an up to 10-fold increase in CD11b$^+$F4/80$^+$ intrahepatic macrophages. During chronic liver damage, Gr1^{hi} monocyte-derived cells differentiate into iNOS-producing macrophages exerting proinflammatory and profibrogenic actions [6]. At present it is unclear how these findings from mouse models precisely relate to liver diseases in humans. It is well established that the number of macrophages increases during chronic liver injury and fibrogenesis [4], but detailed phenotypic characterizations of human intrahepatic monocyte-derived cells are lacking at present. Mouse Gr1^{hi} monocytes are believed to resemble the human CD14$^+$CD16$^-$, and Gr1^{lo} the human CD14$^+$CD16$^+$ subset [12]. This assumption is based on similar expression patterns of activation markers, adhesion molecules and chemokine receptors. Namely, CCR1 and CCR2 are more highly expressed on CD14$^+$CD16$^-$ human and Gr1^{hi} mouse monocytes, whereas CCR5 is elevated on CD14$^+$CD16$^+$ human and Gr1^{lo} mouse monocytes [12,13,14]. It is believed that CD14$^+$CD16$^+$ monocytes originate from CD14$^+$CD16$^-$ cells and represent the more mature/differentiated monocyte subset [12].

However, some discrepancies between murine and human monocyte subpopulations have not been convincingly resolved at present. For instance, Gr1^{hi} monocytes constitute about 50% of murine monocytes, while CD14$^+$CD16$^-$ cells represent about 90–95% of human monocytes [12]. In mice, Gr1^{hi} monocytes are often named 'inflammatory monocytes' due to their preferential recruitment to sites of inflammation and their proinflammatory differentiation potential, whereas in humans the CD14$^+$CD16$^+$ subset has long been considered to constitute 'inflammatory monocytes', because it is found upregulated in many inflammatory disorders and has the potential to release high amounts of proinflammatory cytokines upon stimulation *in vitro* [3,15]. In patients with liver cirrhosis, both increased peripheral CD14$^+$CD16$^-$ and CD14$^+$CD16$^+$ monocytes have been reported from small clinical studies [16,17].

As the interference with monocyte subset infiltration, differentiation and activation may represent interesting novel targets for future therapeutic approaches in liver fibrosis [4], we aimed at defining the functional contributions of monocyte subpopulations to liver fibrogenesis in humans. Our study, comprising 226 patients with chronic liver diseases (CLD) at various stages of fibrosis/cirrhosis from different disease etiologies and 184 controls, demonstrates that circulating monocytes increase during disease progression, specifically the CD14$^+$CD16$^+$ subset. Correspondingly, CD14$^+$CD16$^+$ monocytes/macrophages massively accumulate in the fibrotic/cirrhotic liver. Monocyte-related chemokine pathways are differentially activated in the liver and circulation of patients with liver disease. Functionally, CD14$^+$CD16$^+$ monocytes likely perpetuate intrahepatic inflammation via secretion of proinflammatory cytokines, but also directly activate profibrogenic HSC.

Results

Blood monocytes increase in patients with chronic liver disease, are associated with disease progression and shift towards the 'non-classical' CD16$^+$ monocyte subset

Recent reports from experimental liver injury in mouse models demonstrated an important functional role of the inflammatory Ly6C^{hi} (Gr1^{hi}) monocyte subset for the progression of liver fibrosis, because the chemokine-driven accumulation of these monocyte-derived intrahepatic macrophages crucially perpetuates hepatic inflammation and can promote activation of hepatic stellate cells (HSC) as the main collagen-producing cells in the liver [6,18]. In order to translate these findings from animal models into human pathogenesis, we subjected peripheral blood of 226 patients with chronic liver diseases (CLD) and 184 healthy controls to immediate FACS analysis. CLD patients had significantly higher circulating monocytes than controls, both as relative contribution to WBC (p = 0.002) as well as in absolute cell counts (p = 0.002, Fig. 1A–C, Table 1). Increasing monocyte numbers were associated with disease progression, specifically with the progression from non-cirrhotic to cirrhotic disease (Fig. 1A–C, Table 1). Patients with end-stage cirrhosis (Child C) showed higher blood monocytes than early stages of liver cirrhosis (p = 0.001, Fig. 1C). Moreover, there were inverse correlations between monocyte counts and parameters indicating the hepatic biosynthetic capacity, such as serum albumin (r = −0.305, p<0.001), prothrombin time (r = −0.310, p<0.001) or pseudocholinesterase activity (r = −0.324, p<0.001), and positive correlations to serological fibrosis markers, e.g. pro-collagen-III-peptide (r = 0.432, p<0.001) and hyaluronic acid (r = 0.241, p = 0.001, Fig. 1D, Table 2). Higher blood monocytes were also found in patients with clinical complications of CLD, such as icterus, encephalopathy, ascites or esophageal varices (data not shown). However, in patients with established liver cirrhosis, monocyte counts were not indicative of clinical complications (not shown).

In humans, the 'classical' CD14$^+$CD16$^-$ monocytes share many characteristics with murine Gr1^{hi} (Ly6C^{hi}) monocytes, whereas 'non-classical' CD14$^+$CD16$^+$ cells are considered counterparts of murine Gr1^{lo} (Ly6C^{lo}) monocytes [13]. The CD14$^+$CD16$^+$ subset has long been thought to constitute 'inflammatory monocytes' in humans [12]. Strikingly, we observed a strong shift towards the CD14$^+$CD16$^+$ monocyte subset in CLD patients, especially in patients with established cirrhosis (Fig. 2A–B). The increase in absolute numbers of both subsets, however, did not reach statistical significance (Fig. S1). The relative abundance of CD14$^+$CD16$^+$ monocytes was correlated with inflammatory cytokines and parameters indicative of disease progression, while CD14$^+$CD16$^-$ monocytes showed inverse correlations to these markers (Table 2), indicating a contribution of CD14$^+$CD16$^+$ monocytes to the chronic inflammatory state of patients with CLD and cirrhosis. Of note, we could not observe any differences in monocyte counts or monocyte subsets between the different underlying etiologies of CLD (data not shown), suggesting that the quantitative and qualitative changes in the monocyte compartment represent a rather uniform response during CLD progression and fibrogenesis. However, patients with liver cirrhosis and hepatocellular carcinoma (HCC) even displayed significantly higher CD14$^+$CD16$^+$ monocytes than cirrhotic patients without HCC (p = 0.008, Fig. 2C).

A striking feature of the two major monocyte subpopulations is their differential expression of the MHC-II molecule HLA-DR [13], because CD14$^+$CD16$^+$ express HLA-DR much stronger than the CD14$^+$CD16$^-$ cells (Fig. 2D). In CLD patients, HLA-DR expression is significantly upregulated on CD14$^+$CD16$^+$ mono-

A

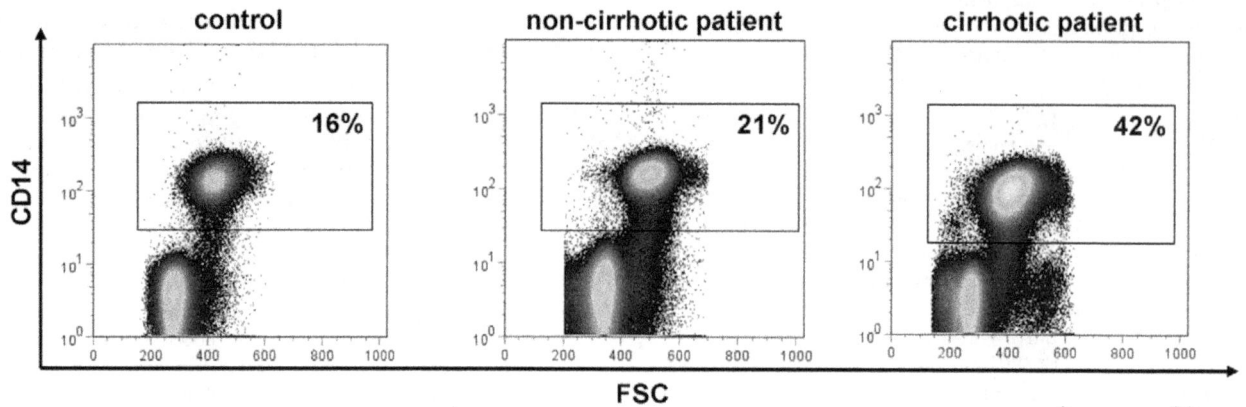

B

*p<0.05; **p<0.001

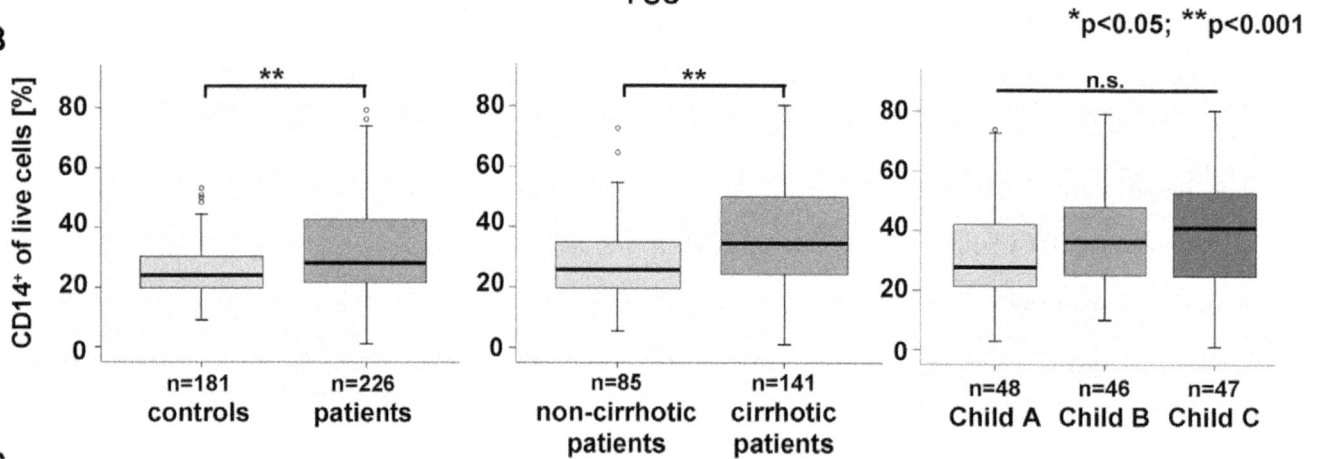

C

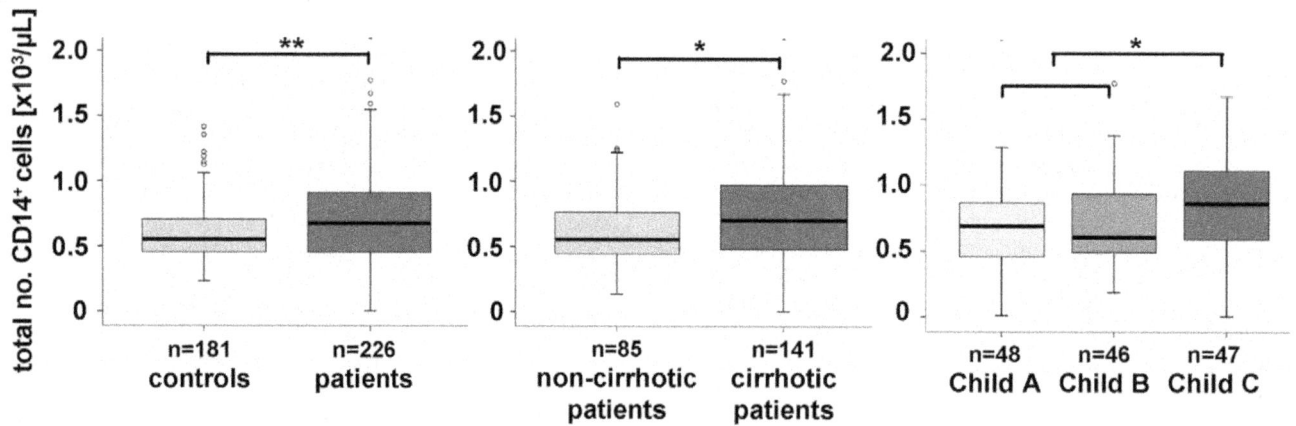

D

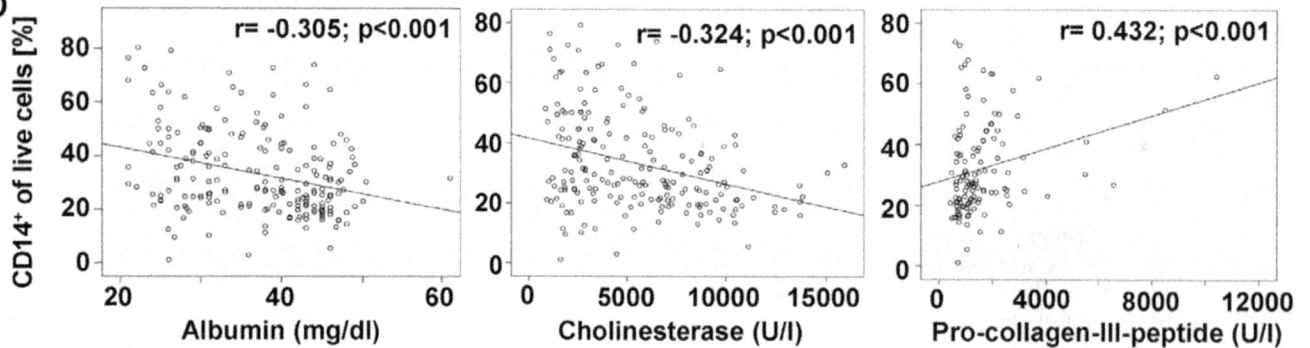

Figure 1. Blood monocytes increase in patients with chronic liver disease and are associated with disease progression. (A) Monocytes are defined by CD14 staining of PBMC (representative FACS plots shown). (B+C) Relative proportion of monocytes (CD14$^+$) (B) and absolute monocyte numbers (C). (D) Association of circulating monocytes with laboratory parameters in CLD patients. *p<0.05, **p<0.001.

cytes (p = 0.027, Fig. 2D and Fig. S2), thereby indicating a markedly enhanced activation and maturation status. This results in a significant increase in the ratio of HLA-DR expression between both subsets in CLD patients and especially in those with liver cirrhosis (p<0.001, Fig. 2E). Collectively, these data demonstrate a substantial shift of circulating monocytes towards the 'non-classical' monocyte subset that is associated with inflammation, fibrosis and disease progression in CLD patients.

Intrahepatic CD16$^+$ macrophages predominantly increase during liver fibrosis progression

It is well established that the number of macrophages increases during chronic liver injury and fibrogenesis [4], but the phenotype of intrahepatic monocyte-derived cells remains poorly defined. Thus, we tested whether CD14$^+$CD16$^-$ and CD14$^+$CD16$^+$ monocyte/macrophage subpopulations are also present within the liver. In fact, conventional histology already identified mononuclear infiltrates in the portal regions of cirrhotic versus normal liver (Fig. 3A), and immunohistochemical co-staining for CD14 and CD16 was established to classify the intrahepatic monocytes/macrophages (Fig. 3B). We observed a significant increase of CD14$^+$CD16$^+$ cells in cirrhosis (p = 0.02 compared to F2–F3 fibrosis, p = 0.001 compared to F0–F1), which account for approximately 50% of the total intrahepatic monocytes/macro-

phages in cirrhotic, but only for about 10% in non-cirrhotic livers, and mostly explain the total increase in hepatic macrophages in cirrhosis (Fig. 3C). A similar trend was noticed when early stages of fibrosis (scored F0 and F1 by a blinded pathologist) were compared to progressive (F2–F3) and cirrhotic (F4) disease (Fig. 3D).

We next aimed to characterize these intrahepatic macrophage subpopulations further and to establish the relationship between intrahepatic and peripheral blood monocyte/macrophage subsets. Unlike in peripheral blood (Fig. 2A), FACS analysis from freshly obtained liver biopsies (n>30) revealed the existence of three CD14$^+$ intrahepatic monocyte/macrophage populations (Fig. 4A) that could be defined as CD14 high-expressing cells (CD14^{hi}CD16$^-$), CD14 low-expressing cells and CD14/CD16 double-positive macrophages (CD14$^+$CD16$^+$). Characteristically, CD14^{hi}CD16$^-$ hepatic cells expressed low HLA-DR and low DC-SIGN (CD209), similar to peripheral CD14$^+$CD16$^-$ monocytes. In contrast, the intrahepatic CD14$^+$CD16$^+$ cells expressed high HLA-DR and some DC-SIGN (CD209), similar to peripheral CD14$^+$CD16$^+$ monocytes (Fig. 4A). In addition, we found CD14^{lo} cells which are negative for CD16, HLA-DR and DC-SIGN, hence likely representing sessile hepatic macrophages (classical Kupffer cells).

In order to further substantiate these observations, intrahepatic macrophage subsets were directly compared to peripheral blood

Table 1. Characteristics of the patient cohort.

	Healthy controls	All patients	Stages of liver cirrhosis			
			No cirrh.	Child A	Child B	Child C
n	184	226	85	48	46	47
Sex (male/female) n	109/75	142/84	53/32	26/22	26/20	37/10
Age yrs	43 (16–68)	53 (17–82)	43 (17–73)	63 (30–82)	60 (28–77)	53 (21–81)
Liver disease etiology n	n.a.					
Viral hepatitis		89	49	19	15	6
Biliary/autoimmune		27	15	7	3	2
Alcohol		65	5	14	17	29
Other origin		45	16	8	11	10
Clinical complications n	n.a.					
Esophageal varices		85	0	21	29	35
Ascites		80	1	7	31	41
HCC		23	0	9	8	6
WBC x10^3/µl	5.9 (1.7–11.6)	6.1 (1.4–28.8)	5.8 (2.2–14.3)	6.3 (2.0–22.3)	5.3 (1.8–16.3)	6.85 (1.4–28.8)
Total monocytes x10^3/µl	0.55 (0.23–1.42)	0.68 (0.01–2.72)	0.60 (0.14–1.59)	0.69 (0.01–2.62)	0.61 (0.19–2.72)	0.86 (0.01–1.67)
CD14$^+$CD16$^-$ monocytes %	92.4 (78.2–97.9)	90.0 (72.1–98.7)	90.7 (78.2–98.7)	89.5 (72.1–97.6)	90.6 (77.2–97.1)	88.4 (77.1–98.7)
CD14$^+$CD16$^-$ monocytes x10^3/µl	0.50 (0.2–1.31)	0.61 (0.01–2.55)	0.54 (0.12–1.57)	0.59 (0.01–2.55)	0.57 (0.17–2.54)	0.74 (0.01–1.47)
CD14$^+$CD16$^+$ monocytes %	7.5 (2.1–21.9)	9.9 (1.1–27.4)	9.3 (1.1–21.7)	10.7 (2.5–27.4)	9.4 (2.9–23.0)	11.2 (1.3–22.9)
CD14$^+$CD16$^+$ monocytes x10^3/µl	0.04 (0.01–0.14)	0.06 (<0.01–0.5)	0.05 (0.01–0.17)	0.05 (<0.01–0.28)	0.06 (0.02–0.5)	0.09 (<0.01–0.38)
Serum MCP-1 pg/ml [CCL2]	88.3 (<1.3–237.0)	102.8 (<1.3–24794)	115.8 (16.8–365.2)	116.7 (17.2–24794)	90.3 (<1.3–904.8)	56.0 (<1.3–1484.5)
Serum MIP1α pg/ml [CCL3]	<1.3 (<1.3–2.8)	3.0 (<1.3–183.3)	2.2 (<1.3–60)	3.9 (<1.3–60)	4.5 (1.8–66.3)	3.4 (<1.3–183.3)
Serum MIP1(pg/ml [CCL4]	30.6 (<1.3–62.5)	47.2 (<1.3–443.9)	47.0 (<1.3–139.5)	53.7 (20.3–249.5)	46.7 (8.8–443.9)	41.6 (9.3–443.5)

For quantitative variables, the median is given with the range in parenthesis. n.a., not applicable; HCC, hepatocellular carcinoma; WBC, white blood cell count. For chemokine serum concentrations, alternative names are given in square brackets.

Table 2. Correlation analysis.

	total monocytes		CD14⁺CD16⁻ monocytes		CD14⁺CD16⁺ monocytes	
	R	p	r	p	r	p
Clinical scores						
Child-Pugh (points)	0.188	0.038	-	n.s.	-	n.s.
MELD	0.190	0.031	-	n.s.	-	n.s.
Liver function						
Bilirubin total	0.242	0.000	−0.202	0.004	0.174	0.013
Bilirubin conjugated	0.235	0.001	−0.218	0.002	-	n.s.
Albumin	−0.305	<0.001	−0.179	0.011	-	n.s.
PCHE	−0.324	<0.001	0.176	0.013	−0.174	0.014
Prothrombin time (%)	−0.310	<0.001	-	n.s.	−0.223	0.001
INR	0.264	<0.001	-	n.s.	0.167	0.016
Factor V	−0.172	0.023	-	n.s.	-	n.s.
Fibrosis markers						
Procollagen-III-peptide	0.432	<0.001	−0.315	<0.001	0.307	<0.001
Hyaluronic acid	0.241	0.001	-	n.s.	-	n.s.
Inflammatory cytokines & chemokines						
IL6	0.261	<0.001	-	n.s.	-	n.s.
TNFα	0.389	<0.001	−0.252	0.001	0.243	0.002
MCP-1 (CCL2)	-	n.s.	-	n.s.	0.261	0.002
MIP1β (CCL4)	-	n.s.	-	n.s.	0.150	0.043
MIG (CXCL9)	-	n.s.	−0.265	0.002	-	n.s.
IP-10 (CXCL10)	0.212	0.018	−0.244	0.006	0.169	0.002
Hematology						
Total WBC	0.282	<0.001	-	n.s.	-	n.s.
Lymphocyte count	−0.635	<0.001	-	n.s.	-	n.s.
Platelets	-	n.s.	-	n.s.	−0.186	0.007
Hemoglobin	-	n.s.	0.161	0.020	-	n.s.

Correlation analysis (Spearman rank correlation test) between total monocytes, the relative abundance of CD14⁺CD16⁻ or CD14⁺CD16⁺ monocytes and clinical scores, serum markers of liver function, inflammatory cytokine and chemokine serum concentrations and other blood counts are given in the table. Only significant results are shown. MELD, model of end stage liver disease; PCHE, pseudocholinesterase; INR, international normalized ratio; IL, interleukin; WBC, white blood cell count; n.s., not significant.

monocyte subpopulations in representative patients. Despite the principal similarities between intrahepatic CD14⁺CD16⁺ and circulating CD14⁺CD16⁺ cells, intrahepatic CD16⁺ macrophages showed up-regulated HLA-DR, DC-SIGN and (moderately) CD56 expression in comparison to their blood counterparts (Fig. 4B), thereby indicating intrahepatic maturation of this macrophage population. The CD14^hiCD16⁻ cells, on the other hand, express similar levels of HLA-DR as circulating CD14⁺CD16⁻ monocytes, but differ by displaying higher levels of the differentiation markers DC-SIGN and CD56 (Fig. 4B). Interestingly, HLA-DR expression appeared down-regulated on CD14⁺CD16⁺ intrahepatic macrophages in patients with advanced compared to early or absent fibrosis, while DC-SIGN was up-regulated, further indicating an activated (pro-inflammatory) state of this macrophage subpopulation in advanced fibrosis (Fig. 4B).

Activation of monocyte-related chemokine pathways in chronic liver disease

Our data demonstrate the distinct accumulation of CD16⁺ monocytes in the liver during fibrosis progression, prompting us to

study possible chemokine pathways that are activated in CLD and could mediate monocyte subset infiltration. In experimental murine models, the chemokine receptors CCR2, CCR1 or CCR5 that are differentially expressed on monocyte subsets have been implicated in hepatic fibrosis progression [6,8,11]. In humans, CCR2 is primarily expressed on CD14⁺CD16⁻ monocytes, whereas CD14⁺CD16⁺ monocytes express higher levels of CCR5 on their surface; CCR1 is expressed on both subsets, with moderately higher levels on CD14⁺CD16⁻ monocytes [13,19,20]. Gene expression analysis from whole liver tissue at different stages of fibrosis progression demonstrated a clear up-regulation of intrahepatic ccr2 (F0-1 compared to F4 fibrosis, p = 0.021), ccr5 (F0-1 compared to F4 fibrosis, p<0.0001) and ccr1 (F0-1 compared to F4 fibrosis, p = 0.0008) in fibrosis (Fig. 5A), which matches well with the observed accumulation of monocytes in the fibrotic/cirrhotic liver (Fig. 3). As not only monocytes/macrophages, but also other immune cell subsets or non-parenchymal liver cells may express these chemokine receptors [2], we performed FACS analyses from fresh liver samples after biopsy and surgical resection. CCR2 expression was primarily found on hepatic monocytes/macrophages (defined as CD14⁺ cells) and (at lower

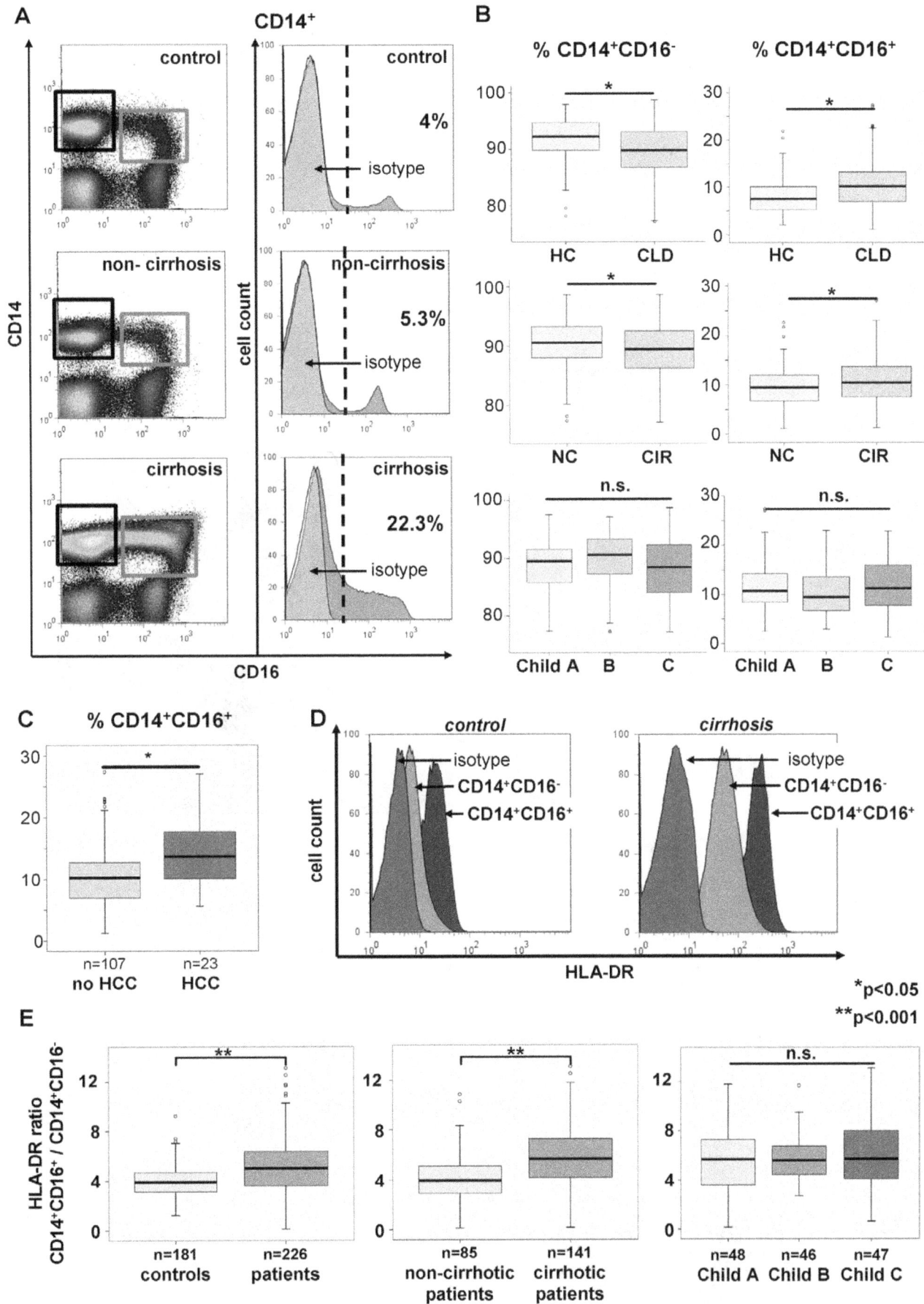

Figure 2. Relative increase of CD14$^+$CD16$^+$ blood monocytes and more activated phenotype in patients with liver cirrhosis. (A) Representative FACS plots displaying an increase of CD14$^+$CD16$^+$ monocytes (black gate: CD14$^+$CD16$^-$, grey gate: CD14$^+$CD16$^+$) among PBMC in patients with cirrhosis compared to healthy controls and non-cirrhotic patients (left). The histograms show the relative distribution of CD16 expression on CD14$^+$ cells (right; grey: isotype control). (B) Statistical analysis of monocyte subsets. HC, healthy controls (n = 181); CLD, patients (n = 226); NC, non-cirrhotic (n = 85); CIR, cirrhotic (n = 141). (C) Patients with liver cirrhosis and hepatocellular carcinoma (HCC) have significantly (p = 0.008) higher CD16$^+$ monocytes than cirrhotics without HCC. (D) Representative FACS staining for HLA-DR on monocyte subsets. (E) Ratio of HLA-DR expression on CD16$^+$ vs. CD16$^-$ monocytes. *p<0.05, **p<0.001.

levels) on intrahepatic NKT-, but not NK- or T-cells (Fig. 5B). CCR1 was expressed at high levels by almost all CD14$^+$ cells, but also by subsets of T-, NK- and NKT-cells (Fig. 5B). CCR5 expression was primarily found on T-cells and subsets of NK- and NKT-cells, but hepatic monocytes/macrophages also express CCR5 at variable levels (Fig. 5B).

In line, hepatic mRNA expression of the chemokines *ccl2* (F0-1 compared to F4 fibrosis, p = 0.0088) and *ccl5* (F0-1 compared to F4 fibrosis, p<0.0001), but not of *ccl3*, was strongly up-regulated in fibrosis (Fig. 5C). Moreover, the serum concentrations of the CCR1/CCR5 ligands MIP1α (CCL3) and MIP1β (CCL4), but

not of the CCR2 ligand MCP-1 (CCL2), were significantly increased in CLD patients (Fig. 5D), suggesting additional systemic actions of these chemokines.

Given the expression of CCR2, CCR1 and CCR5 by hepatic monocytes/macrophages, the local upregulation of *ccl2* and *ccl5* in the whole liver and the systemic elevation of CCL3 (healthy controls compared to CLD patients, p = 0.0387) and CCL4 (healthy controls compared to CLD patients, p = 0.0064) in the circulation, we speculated that peripheral blood monocytes in patients might regulate their chemokine receptor expression, rendering them more prone to accumulate in the diseased liver.

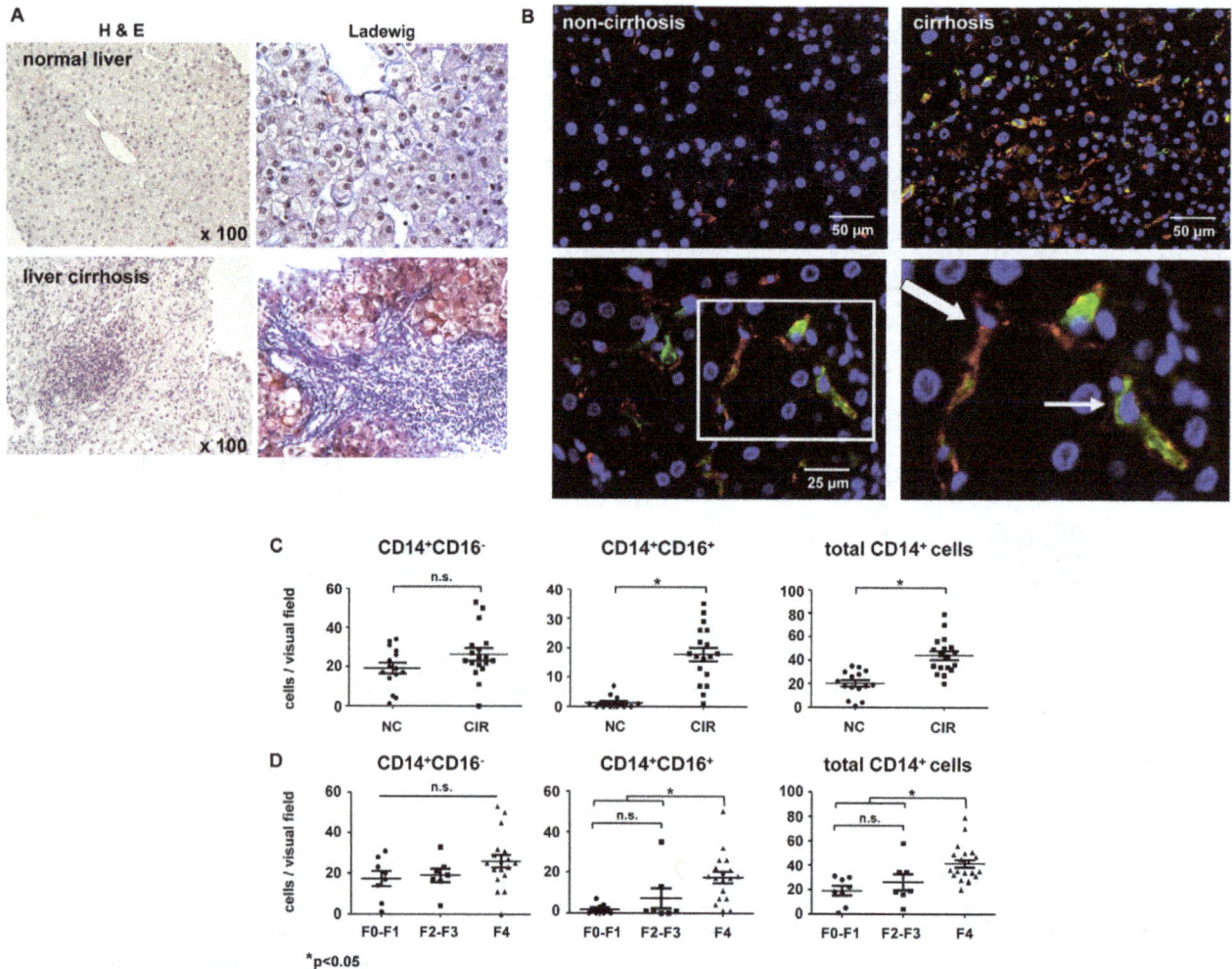

Figure 3. Intrahepatic CD16$^+$ macrophages predominantly increase during liver fibrosis progression. (A) Representative examples of biopsies from normal liver (upper panel) and cirrhotic liver (lower panel) show mononuclear inflammatory infiltrates in fibrotic periportal regions (left: H&E staining, right: Ladewig staining, in which collagen stains blue). (B) Immunofluoresecent co-staining for CD14 (red) and CD16 (green) identifies CD14$^+$CD16$^-$ and CD14$^+$CD16$^+$ macrophages in human liver tissue (blue: nuclei counterstained with DAPI). Bold arrow, CD14$^+$CD16$^-$ macrophage; thin arrow, CD14$^+$CD16$^+$ macrophage. (C+D) Semiquantative analysis of CD14$^+$CD16$^-$, CD14$^+$CD16$^+$ and total CD14$^+$ intrahepatic cells. *p<0.05, **p<0.001.

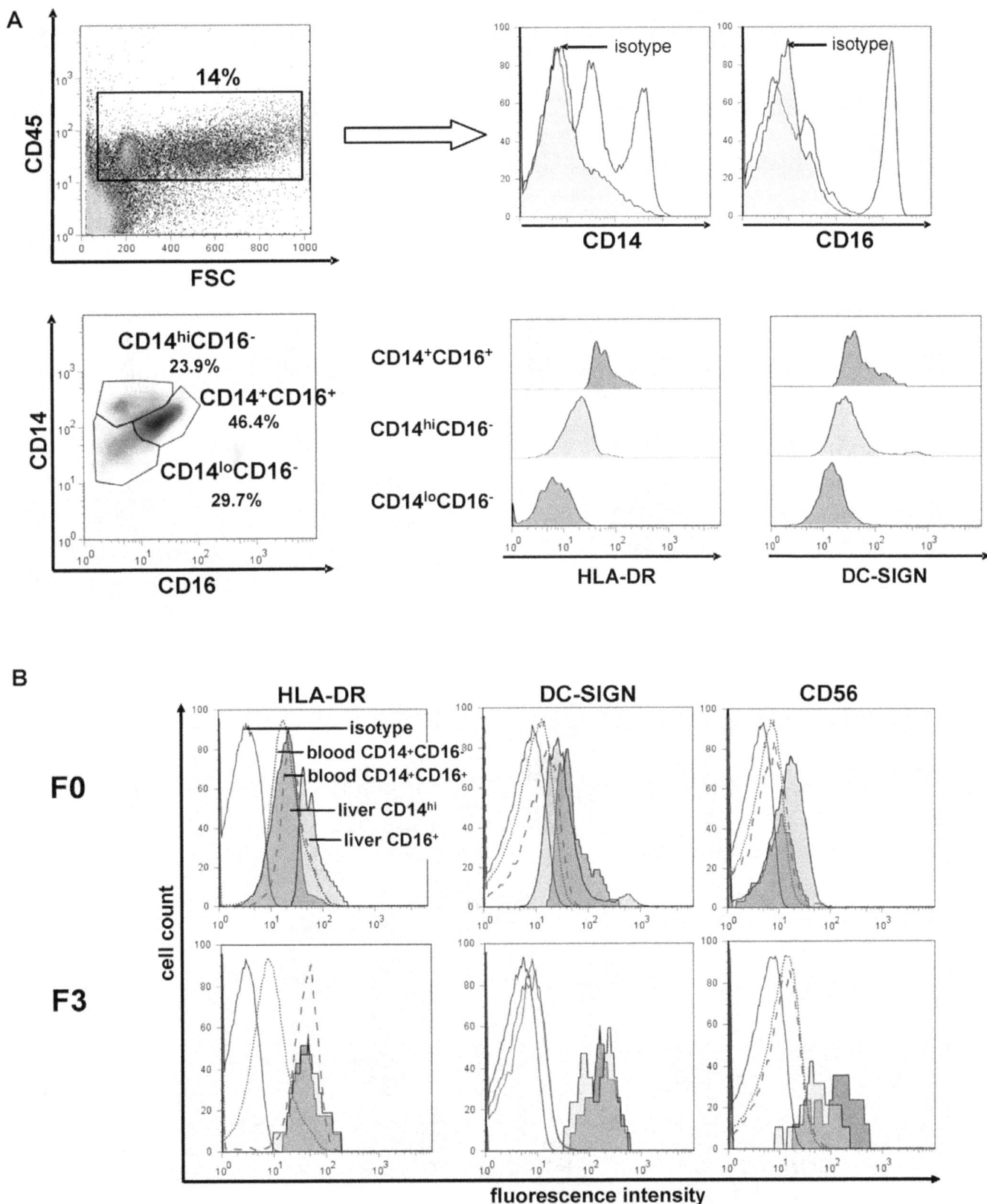

Figure 4. Intrahepatic macrophages consist of different subpopulations mirroring blood monocyte subsets. (A) FACS analysis of intrahepatic monocytes/macrophages, based on >30 fresh liver biopsies. Representative plots are displayed. Among the CD45+ intrahepatic leukocytes, three different populations of intrahepatic CD14+ macrophages can be distinguished based on CD14 and CD16 expression that also differ characteristically in HLA-DR and DC-SIGN expression. (B) Expression levels of monocyte/macrophage activation and differentiation markers were compared in the same patients between blood CD14+CD16− monocytes (dotted line) and liver CD14hiCD16− macrophages (dark grey) as well as

CD14+CD16+ monocytes (dashed line) and liver CD14+CD16+ macrophages (light grey); representative analyses from patients with a F0 fibrosis (no fibrosis, upper panel) and a F3 fibrosis (advanced fibrosis, lower panel) are shown. Isotype control, black line. Blood was drawn at the time of liver biopsy, and blood/liver samples were run with the same FACS settings at the same time.

We therefore isolated circulating monocytes by CD14-microbeads via MACS methodology from patients (n = 113) and healthy controls (n = 32) at purities greater than 95% (not shown). Monocytic $ccr1$ (p = 0.031 for healthy controls compared to CLD patients), but not $ccr2$ or $ccr5$, expression was increased on peripheral monocytes in patients (Fig. 6A), possibly in response to elevated serum levels of CCL3 and CCL4. With respect to monocyte subsets, CCR2 was predominantly expressed on CD14+CD16− monocytes (Fig. 6B). On a protein level, CCR2 surface expression was modestly down-regulated on

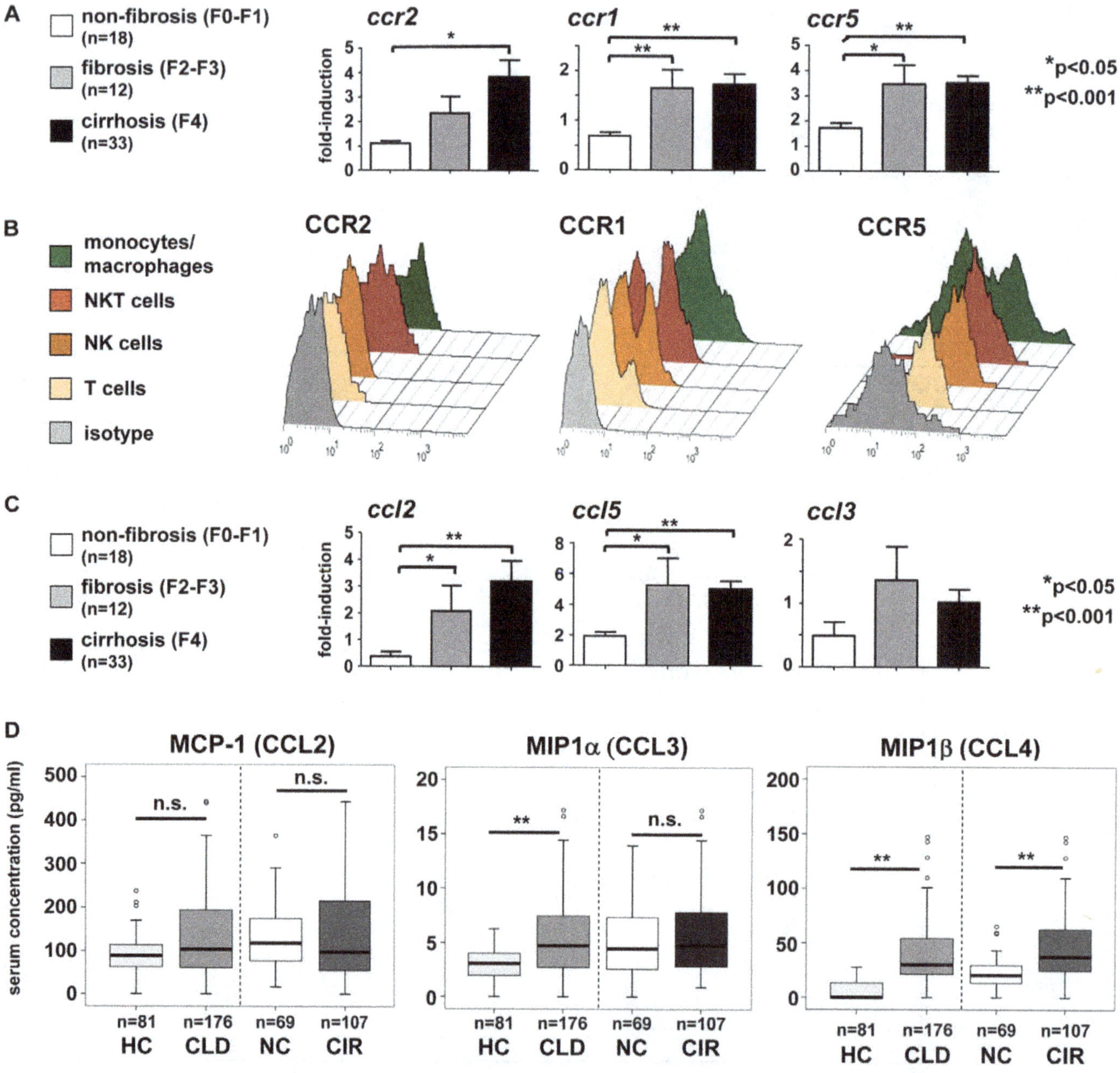

Figure 5. Activation of monocyte-related chemokine pathways and of monocytic chemokine receptors in chronic liver disease. (A) Intrahepatic gene expression levels of chemokine receptors. (B) Expression of CCR2, CCR1 and CCR5 was assessed by FACS on monocytes/macrophages (CD14+, green), T- (CD3+CD56−, light orange), NK- (CD3−CD56+, dark orange) and NKT-cells (CD3+CD56+, red) from freshly isolated liver tissue. Representative histograms are shown, isotype control in grey. (C) Intrahepatic gene expression levels of chemokines. (D) Serum concentrations of monocyte-related chemokines in patients with chronic liver diseases and healthy controls. Abbreviations are: HC, healthy control; CLD, chronic liver disease; NC, no cirrhosis; CIR, cirrhosis. *p<0.05, **p<0.001.

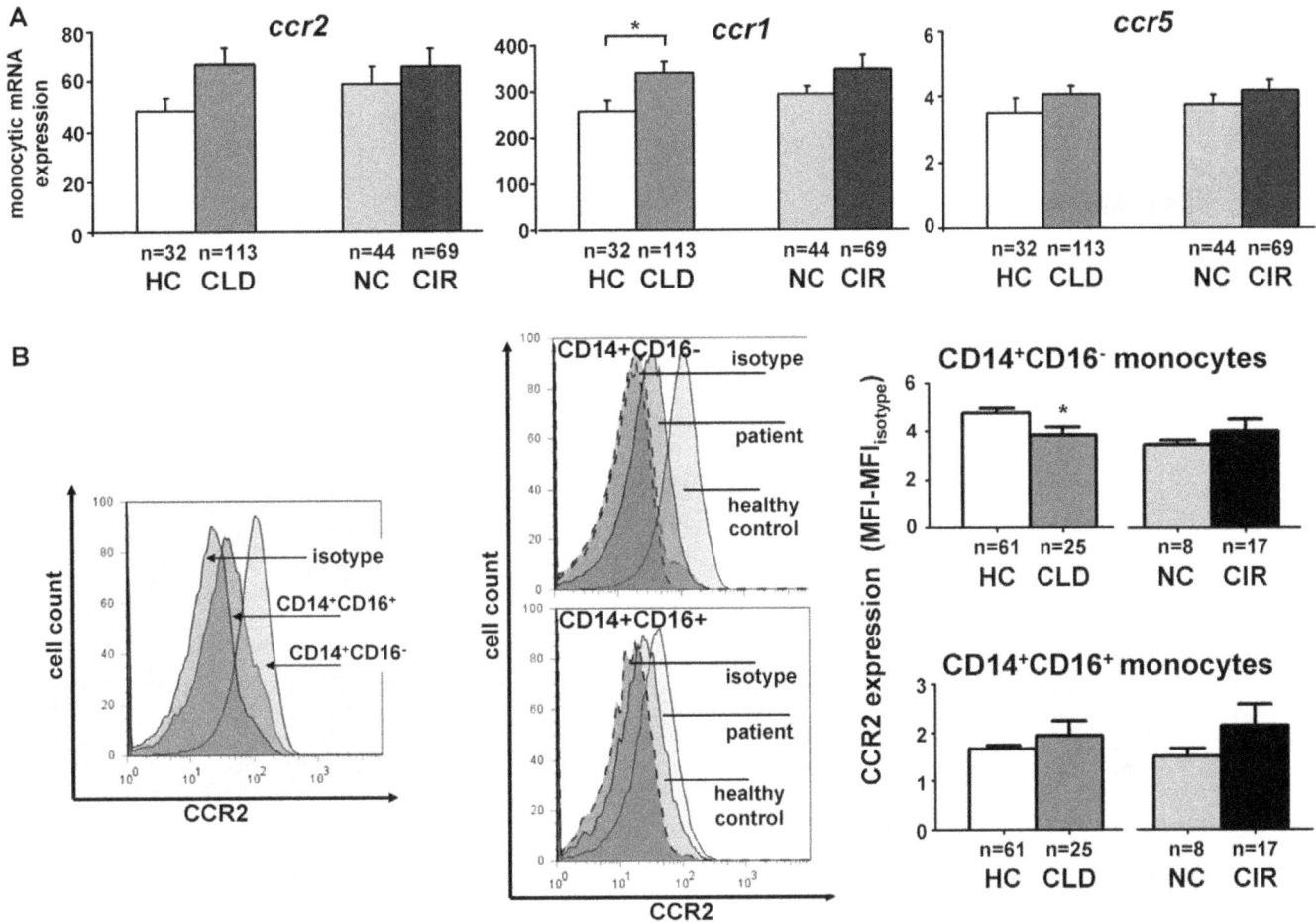

Figure 6. Regulation of chemokine receptors on circulating monocytes in chronic liver disease. (A) Monocytic chemokine receptor gene expression by real-time PCR after purification of circulating monocytes by CD14 microbeads (MACS). (B) CCR2 expression (MFI, mean fluorescence intensity) on blood monocyte subsets by FACS. Abbreviations are: HC, healthy control; CLD, chronic liver disease; NC, no cirrhosis; CIR, cirrhosis. Representative histograms are shown, comparing either CCR2 expression levels between both monocyte subsets as well as between healthy controls and CLD patients on the two monocyte subpopulations in peripheral blood. *p<0.05, **p<0.001.

CD14$^+$CD16$^-$ monocytes of patients as compared to healthy controls, but not on CD14$^+$CD16$^+$ cells (Fig. 6B). Within the liver, CD14^{hi}CD16$^-$ macrophages expressed CCR2 at similar (high) levels as circulating CD14$^+$CD16$^-$ monocytes; liver CD14$^+$CD16$^+$ macrophages, in contrast, displayed lower levels than CD14^{hi}CD16$^-$ macrophages, but higher CCR2 expression than blood CD14$^+$CD16$^+$ monocytes, suggesting that the CD14$^+$CD16$^+$ subset up-regulated CCR2 intrahepatically (detailed data not shown). These results collectively revealed that monocyte-related chemokines targeting CCR2 and CCR1/CCR5 are up-regulated in the intra- and extrahepatic compartment of CLD patients.

Functionality of monocytes in liver cirrhosis and differential cytokine and chemokine secretion by monocyte subsets

Although we consistently found more circulating monocytes in CLD patients and a close association with disease progression (Fig. 1, Table 2), it remained unclear if these monocytes were fully functionally active. It had been speculated before that monocyte activation might be impaired in liver cirrhosis, contributing to a so-called "immune-paralysis" in those patients [21,22]. We therefore cultured isolated circulating monocytes from patients

with advanced liver cirrhosis (Child B/C, n = 16) and matched healthy controls (n = 20) in media supplemented with autologous serum and assessed the secretion of proinflammatory cytokines and chemokines after LPS stimulation. Monocytes from healthy volunteers secreted high amounts of proinflammatory cytokines (TNFα, IL6, IL1β) and chemokines (MCP-1, MIP1α, MIP1β) upon stimulation with LPS (Fig. 7A–B). The chemokine MIG was not significantly induced by LPS. Monocytes isolated from patients with advanced cirrhosis did not differ with respect to any of the cytokines or chemokines analyzed at baseline or after LPS stimulation (Fig. 7A–B), suggesting that circulating monocytes in CLD patients preserved overall their normal capacity to secrete pro- or anti-inflammatory mediators.

Given the marked preferential intrahepatic accumulation of CD14$^+$CD16$^+$ monocytes in liver cirrhosis (Fig. 3), we next aimed to define the likely function of this subset in the pathogenesis of chronic liver inflammation and fibrosis. CD14$^+$CD16$^-$ and CD14$^+$CD16$^+$ monocytes were isolated by MACS methodology, and cytokine/chemokine secretion was measured after five days of culture without additional stimulation. Due to ethical considerations (large blood volume required for subset isolation) and based on the identical cytokine secretion of total monocytes upon stimulation (Fig. 7A–B), monocyte subpopulations were only isolated from healthy volun-

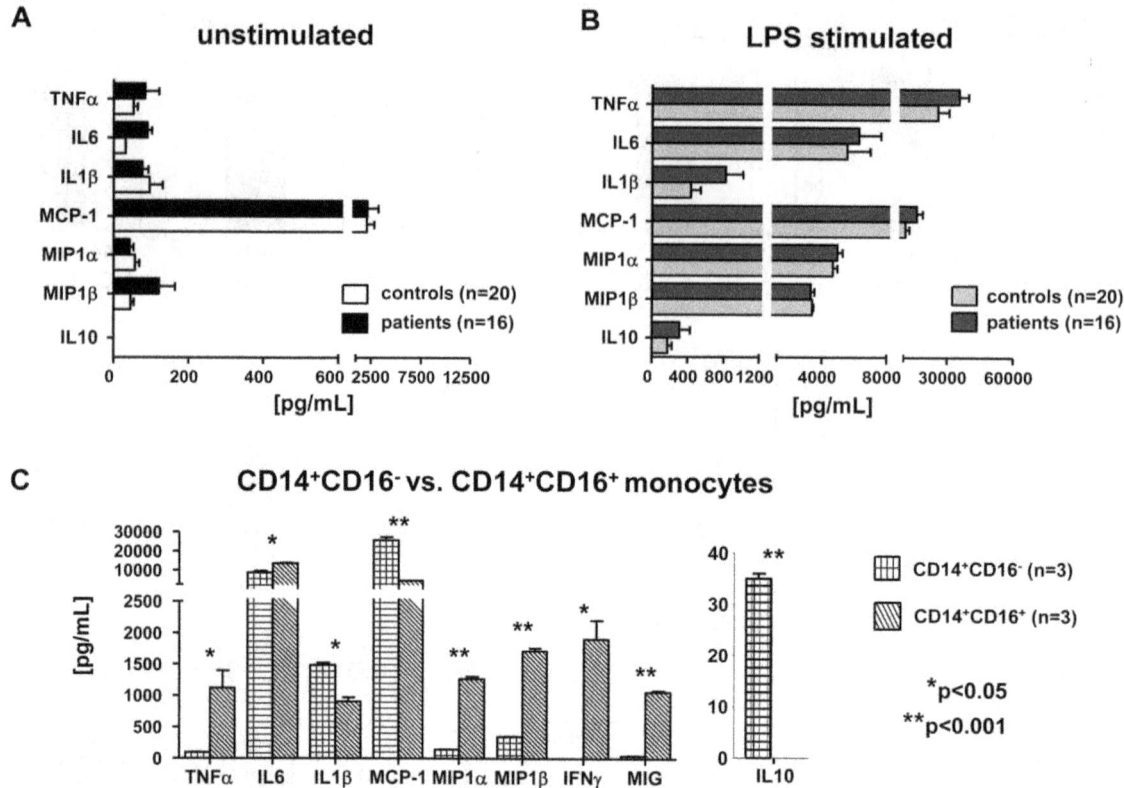

Figure 7. Monocytes are functionally active in liver cirrhosis with a differential release of distinct cytokines/chemokines by monocyte subsets. (A+B) Cytokine/chemokine release of monocyte-derived macrophages (2 days in culture) without stimulation (A) and after stimulation with 1 mg/ml LPS (B). (C) Cytokine/chemokine release of purified monocyte subsets after 5 days of culture without stimulation. *p<0.05, **p<0.001.

teers. Strikingly, CD14+CD16+ monocytes were the major producers of TNFα, IL6 (CD14+CD16+ vs. CD14+CD16−, p = 0.038), IFNγ (CD14+CD16+ vs. CD14+CD16−, p = 0.0242), MIP1α (CD14+CD16+ vs. CD14+CD16−, p = 0.0011) and MIP1β (Fig. 7C), indicating that they primarily perpetuate inflammatory processes by releasing proinflammatory cyto- and chemokines. This conclusion is corroborated by correlations between circulating CD14+CD16+ monocyte counts and proinflammatory serum cytokine levels (e.g., TNFα, MIP1β) in CLD patients (Table 2).

CD14+CD16− monocytes, on the other hand, were the main producers of MCP-1 (CD14+CD16+ vs. CD14+CD16−, p = 0.0068), in line with observations that MCP-1 can stimulate MCP-1 expression via CCR2 binding in an autocrine manner [23]. Moreover, CD14+CD16−, but not CD14+CD16+ monocytes were capable of producing the antiinflammatory cytokine IL10 (Fig. 7C). Collectively, these data imply that the CD14+CD16+ monocytes that accumulate in the fibrotic/cirrhotic liver are important sources of proinflammatory mediators thereby perpetuating the chronic inflammation in the liver.

CD16+ monocytes directly activate hepatic stellate cells

Monocyte-derived macrophages can activate HSC and hence are potent inductors of liver fibrosis [18]. In murine models of hepatic fibrosis, Gr1+ monocytes ('classical monocytes') can directly activate HSC in a TGFβ-dependent manner [6]. We therefore assessed possible effects of human monocyte subpopulations on HSC by co-culturing either subset with primary HSC isolated from explanted human livers of three independent donors (Fig. 8A). The experimental set-up was validated by stimulating

primary HSC by recombinant TGFβ, which resulted in significant up-regulation of col1A mRNA, but not of Acta2; expression of Acta2 could therefore be used as a house-keeping gene for HSC (not shown). In the co-culture experiments CD14+CD16+ monocytes, but not CD14+CD16− monocytes significantly up-regulated collagen gene expression in HSC (CD14+CD16+ vs. CD14+CD16−, p = 0.0243) (Fig. 8B). It could be excluded that CD14+CD16+ monocytes directly differentiated into collagen-producing fibrocytes in vitro [24], because cultures of monocyte subsets by itself did not result in detectable collagen mRNA within five days (not shown). Of note, also the mixed population of lymphocytes induced HSC activation, highlighting that not only macrophages, but also NK, NKT and T cell subsets may interact with HSC during fibrosis development [2]. The activation of HSC by CD14+CD16+ monocytes could be partially blocked by anti-TGFβ antibodies (Fig. 8B). These data indicate that 'non-classical' CD14+CD16+ monocytes not only provide proinflammatory cytokines, but also exert direct fibrogenic actions on HSC.

Moreover, co-culture with HSC in turn differentially affected the expression of chemokine receptors and activation markers of monocyte subsets. CCR2 and DC-SIGN were strongly induced upon co-culture with HSC only on CD14+CD16+ monocytes (CCR2 expression at d0 compared to d5, p = 0.0147; DC-SIGN expression at d0 compared to d5, p = 0.0004) (Fig. 8C), indicating that the increase of ccr2 mRNA transcripts in whole liver (Fig. 5A) might be partially attributed to up-regulated expression by CD16+ monocyte-derived macrophages. In contrast, HLA-DR was down-regulated in response to co-culture with HSC in both monocyte subsets (Fig. 8C). These observations emphasize that monocytes/

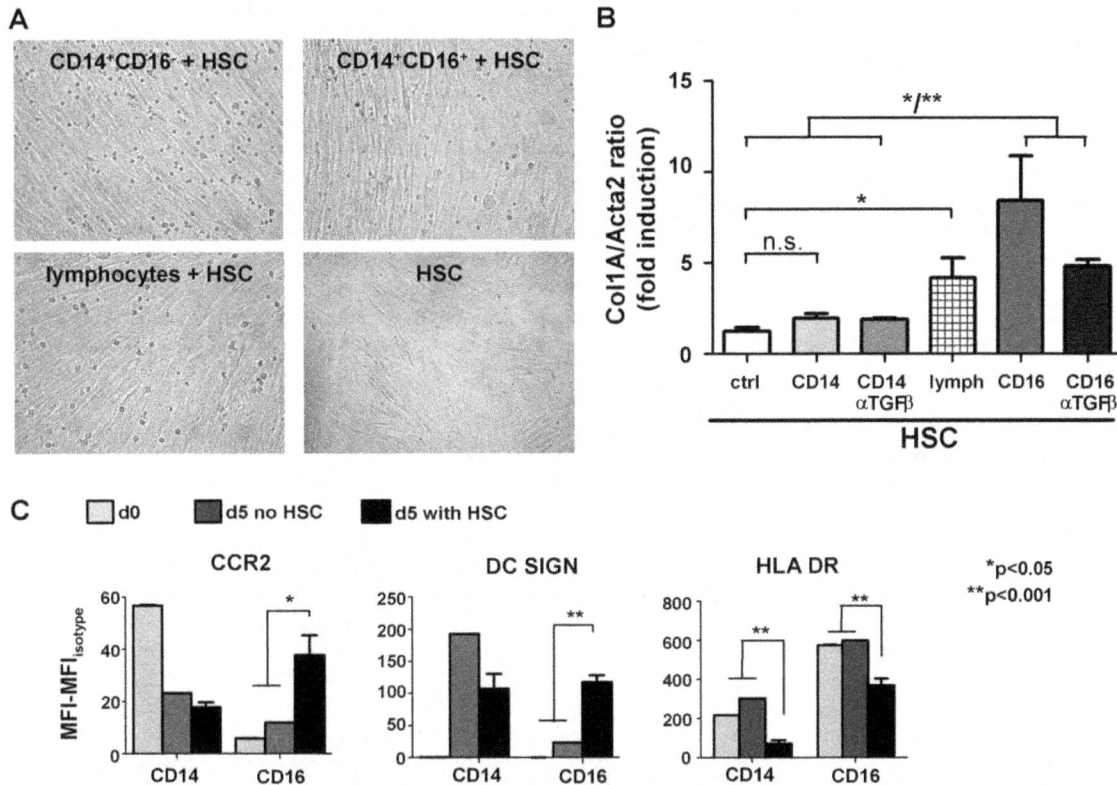

Figure 8. CD14$^+$CD16$^+$, but not CD14$^+$CD16$^-$ monocytes directly activate hepatic stellate cells. (A) Primary human HSC were isolated and co-cultured for 5 days with CD14$^+$CD16$^-$, CD14$^+$CD16$^+$ monocytes or lymphocytes. No morphological differences were noted on HSC in these conditions. (B) HSC activation was determined by *collagen-1A (col1A)* mRNA expression, normalized to the 'HSC-house keeping gene' *Acta2*. (C) Expression of surface molecules by FACS (MFI, mean fluorescence intensity) on CD14$^+$CD16$^-$ (CD14) and CD14$^+$CD16$^+$ (CD16) monocytes/macrophages at day 0, and after 5 days in culture or co-culture with HSC. All results derived from three independent experiments. *p<0.05, **p<0.001.

macrophages distinctly interact with other cellular components of the hepatic microenvironment.

Discussion

Accumulating evidence from murine models indicated that monocyte infiltration into the liver is a major pathogenic factor for chronic hepatic inflammation and fibrosis [5,6,7,8]. In this study, we demonstrate that monocytes increase in the circulation as well as in the liver of patients during progression of chronic liver disease, and that this is associated with a shift towards the 'non-classical' subset of CD14$^+$CD16$^+$ monocytes. These CD14$^+$CD16$^+$ cells have an activated phenotype and produce high amounts of pro-inflammatory cytokines and chemokines upon differentiation. Given the assumption that CD14$^+$CD16$^+$ monocytes would resemble Gr1^{lo} cells in mice, our findings reveal a considerable discrepancy from mouse models, because fibrosis induction and progression in mice is accompanied by Gr1^{hi} monocytosis in peripheral blood and infiltration of Gr1^{hi} monocytes into the injured liver [6,7]. One obvious difference between murine models and the human diseased liver is the strikingly dissimilar time-course of fibrosis development. Whereas experimental murine fibrosis is analyzed at three or six weeks after induction, e.g. by biliary duct ligation or carbon tetrachloride injection, human fibrosis and cirrhosis usually develops over decades of chronic injury and inflammation. Human cirrhosis is thereby a more advanced disease with respect to collagen deposition, tissue reorganization and myofibroblast activation than even 8-weeks-

murine fibrosis models [25]. In this respect, it is important to point out that the most prominent enrichment of these non-classical CD14$^+$CD16$^+$ monocytes in peripheral blood and in the liver was observed in patients with liver cirrhosis, in contrast to the similar levels observed between healthy volunteers and CLD patients at early stages of liver fibrosis. This suggests that the proposed pro-inflammatory and profibrogenic actions of CD14$^+$CD16$^+$ monocytes/macrophages are most relevant at advanced fibrosis or cirrhosis, possibly explaining different observations between human cirrhosis and experimental mouse models.

The assumption that CD14$^+$CD16$^+$ human monocytes are equivalents of murine Gr1^{lo} monocytes is primarily based on conserved gene and protein profiles between these subsets [13], but not on functional assays. In fact, murine Gr1^{hi} monocyte-derived cells in inflammatory conditions and human CD14$^+$CD16$^+$-derived macrophages share important functional properties, particularly the expression of pro-inflammatory cytokines such as TNFα or nitric oxide [3,26]. Our study revealed correlations between CD14$^+$CD16$^+$ monocytes and pro-inflammatory cytokines/chemokines in patients as well as a preferential secretion of pro-inflammatory cytokines by this subset, suggesting that the increase of CD14$^+$CD16$^+$ monocytes in patients with liver cirrhosis as the 'inflammatory monocyte subset' thereby mirrors the increase of Gr1^{hi} monocytes in murine models.

This raised the question if similar chemokine-pathways are activated in human liver diseases as in murine experimental models, given the substantial differences in chemokine receptor expression between murine Gr1^{hi} and human CD14$^+$CD16$^+$

monocytes [12]. Several recent independent animal studies defined an important function of CCR2 and MCP-1/CCL2 for hepatic fibrosis [5,6,7,8]. In analogy to these findings, upregulated intrahepatic MCP-1 expression has been described during human hepatic fibrogenesis, predominantly by HSC, biliary epithelial cells and macrophages, and directly correlated with the number of hepatic macrophages in a small group of 15 patients [27]. We confirmed these observations in our large cohort, as ccl2 and also ccr2 mRNA transcripts were significantly increased in cirrhotic livers. However, unlike in mice where MCP-1 is thought to promote the exit of Gr1[hi] monocytes from the bone marrow into the circulation [6,28], systemic levels of MCP-1 were not significantly regulated in liver disease patients in comparison to healthy controls. Moreover, CCR2 expression was moderately lower in CD14[+]CD16[−] monocytes of patients compared to controls and slightly increased in CD14[+]CD16[+] monocytes. This might possibly indicate distinct local functions of CCR2/MCP-1 interactions in the liver during fibrosis progression, likely not limited to CCR2[hi]-expressing CD14[+]CD16[−], but also on CD14[+]CD16[+] monocytes. This hypothesis is corroborated by the fact that CD14[+]CD16[+], but not CD14[+]CD16[−] monocytes strongly upregulate CCR2 expression upon co-culture with HSC. In-vitro-experiments suggested that MCP-1 may activate the expression of profibrogenic genes such as TGFβ or pro-α1 chain of type I collagen in monocyte-derived macrophages by an MCP-1/CCR2-dependent amplification loop [23], indicating that local intrahepatic MCP-1 may fulfil other functions in addition to regulating monocyte recruitment in liver cirrhosis.

On the other hand, CCR1- and CCR5-related chemokines might contribute to monocyte recruitment. It is well established that HSC express CCL5/RANTES upon activation [29,30]. We found a clear induction of intrahepatic ccl5 expression, confirming a smaller prior study including 15 patients [11], alongside elevated serum CCL3/MIP1α, CCL4/MIP1β and CCL5/RANTES (not shown) concentrations in patients versus controls. Moreover, monocytic ccr1 expression, but not ccr5, was increased in patients. These data demonstrate that monocyte-related chemokine pathways targeting CCR2, CCR1 and CCR5 are activated in patients with liver cirrhosis, likely regulating recruitment (CCR1, CCR5, CCR2) and local differentiation/activation (CCR2) of monocyte subsets in patients with chronic liver diseases. However, it is important to note that CCR1 and CCR5 expression is not restricted to monocyte/macrophages, but also found on other immune cells subsets within the, namely T-, NK- and NKT-cell populations [2,31]. Both CCR1 and CCR5 have also been described on other non-parenchymal liver cells, including resting and activated HSC [11,30]. Therefore, elevation of circulating or intrahepatic CCL3-CCL5 chemokines likely not only influences monocyte/macrophage recruitment, but also other cell populations in the diseased liver.

In patients with liver cirrhosis, intrahepatic monocytes/ macrophages are significantly increased [4], and our analysis revealed that this can be mainly attributed to a selective accumulation of CD14[+]CD16[+] monocytes/macrophages in the cirrhotic liver. Cells of the monocytic lineage are important elements of the hepatic inflammation, because these cells can phagocytize foreign material, present antigen to T cells, and produce a host of cytokines, including TNFα, IL1 and IL6 [4]. Dissecting the diverse functional capacities of both monocyte subsets in vitro confirmed that the CD14[+]CD16[+] monocyte subset is the main producer of pro-inflammatory cytokines and chemokines such as TNFα, IL6, IFNγ, MIP1α and MIP1β, while CD14[+]CD16[−] monocytes readily secrete more MCP-1, IL1β and IL10 [12]. Moreover, in line with experiments co-culturing murine

Gr1[hi] monocytes and murine HSC [6], CD14[+]CD16[+] monocytes were also able to directly activate primary human HSC upon co-culture. These data indicate that non-classical CD14[+]CD16[+] monocytes are crucial regulators in the pathogenesis of CLD in humans by secreting an abundance of cytokines perpetuating chronic inflammatory processes within the liver and by directly activating HSC that in turn can secrete multiple chemokines for monocyte recruitment [18]. Our study furthermore suggests that the modulation of monocyte-subset recruitment into the liver and subsequent differentiation in the inflamed hepatic environment may represent possible novel approaches for interventions targeting proinflammatory and profibrogenic actions of either monocyte subset in chronic liver diseases and liver fibrosis.

Methods

Patients and controls

The study protocol was approved by the local ethics committee (ethics committee of University Hospital Aachen, RWTH Aachen), and written informed consent was obtained from each patient. The study was conducted according to the principles expressed in the Declaration of Helsinki. Inclusion criteria were either any CLD with a predisposition to liver fibrosis or an already established liver fibrosis/cirrhosis of any origin. Established cirrhosis (in contrast to non-cirrhotic CLD) was defined, if imaging (ultrasound, CT or MRI scan), biopsy or laparoscopy indicated liver cirrhosis or if cirrhosis-related complications were present. Patients with established liver cirrhosis were staged according to Child-Pugh's criteria [32]. Patients with acute liver failure or acute hepatitis B or C were not included. Exclusion criteria were conditions known to directly affect monocyte subset distributions in humans, specifically ongoing bacterial infections (procalcitonin concentration above normal value [<0.5 μg/L]), HIV-infection, systemic steroid medication (prednisolone >7.5 mg/d or equivalent doses) and malignant tumor(s) except hepatocellular or cholangiocellular carcinoma. Furthermore, patients were excluded in case of systemic inflammatory response syndrome (SIRS) or sepsis criteria [33]. The etiologies of liver diseases comprised viral hepatitis (n = 89, 39.4%; HBV n = 38, HCV n = 51), biliary or autoimmune disease (n = 27, 11.9%; autoimmune hepatitis n = 10, primary biliary cirrhosis n = 8, primary sclerosing cholangitis n = 9), alcoholic liver disease (n = 65, 28.7%) and other liver diseases (n = 45, 20%, e.g. non-alcoholic steatohepatitis n = 7, hemochromatosis n = 4, cryptogenic n = 23). Grading and staging of liver samples (biopsies and explants) were performed according to Desmet-Scheuer score by one experienced pathologist, who was fully blinded to any experimental data [34].

As a control group, 181 healthy volunteers were recruited from the local blood transfusion institute that had normal aminotransferase activities, no history of liver disease or alcohol abuse and tested negative for HBV, HCV and HIV infections.

FACS analysis of circulating monocyte subsets and intrahepatic macrophages

Fresh blood samples were collected by venipuncture in the morning in EDTA separator tubes from all patients and controls and promptly applied to PBMC isolation by Ficoll density gradient, using LSM-1077 (PAA, Pasching, Austria) and standard protocols [13]. After blocking nonspecific binding, the following monoclonal antibodies and appropriate isotype controls were used: CD14, CD16, CD56, HLA-DR, CD3, CD4, CD8, CD56, CD209/DC-SIGN, CD19 and CD45 (all BD, Heidelberg, Germany); CCR2, CCR1, CCR5 (R&D Systems, Minneapolis, MN). Flow cytometric analysis was performed on a FACS-Canto-

II (BD), data were analysed by FlowJo software (TreeStar, Ashland, OR). In order to exclude that difference in cell isolation procedures for FACS analysis influences cell counts, absolute numbers for circulating cells were calculated using the relative values from FACS and automated WBC counts without the PMN fraction. Cell surface marker expression was quantified by determining mean fluorescence intensity minus the respective isotype control ('MFI-MFI$_{isotype}$'). For flow cytometric characterization of intrahepatic monocytes, a small piece of fresh liver biopsy cylinders was minced in PBS and digested with collagenase type IV (Worthington, Lakewood, NJ) for 30 min at 37°C, and subjected to staining for FACS [6].

Monocyte separation, RNA isolation and gene expression analysis

After isolation of PBMC by density gradient, total monocytes were purified using CD14-microbeads and MACS separation technique (Miltenyi, Bergisch Gladbach, Germany). FACS analysis confirmed a purity of >95%. RNA was isolated from purified blood monocytes by pegGOLD (peqLab, Erlangen, Germany), and complementary DNA was generated from 1 µg RNA (Roche, Mannheim, Germany). Quantitative real-time PCR was performed using SYBR Green Reagent (Invitrogen, Karlsruhe, Germany). β-actin values were used to normalize gene expression. Gene expression was either expressed by fold induction or arbitrary relative expression [14]. Primer sequences are available upon request. RNA and gene expression analyses from liver tissue, cell-culture and co-culture experiments were performed analogously.

Immunofluorescence analysis of intrahepatic monocyte subsets

After deparaffinization and rehydration, slides were boiled in citrate buffer, and blocking solution (Vector Labs, Burlingame, CA) was applied. Rabbit anti-human CD14 antibody (HPA001887; Sigma), mouse anti-human CD16 (clone 2H7; MBL), or appropriate isotype control antibodies (Santa Cruz Biotechnology, Santa Cruz, CA) were detected by secondary anti-rabbit Cy-3 and anti-mouse-FITC-antibodies (Jackson ImmunoResearch, West Grove, PA). Cell nuclei were counterstained with DAPI (Vectashield, Vector Labs). Slides were then analysed by fluorescence microscopy (Zeiss, Jena, Germany). Ten bright fields per slide were randomly chosen for quantitative analysis. The investigator was blinded to the stage of fibrosis or experimental data.

In vitro stimulation of monocytes

After isolation of PBMC by density gradient, 1×10^6 cells/ml were resolved in 2 ml RPMI (Invitrogen) containing 1% penicillin-streptomycin (PAA) and 1.5% autologous serum and allowed to adhere for 35 min in a Petri dish. Non-adherent cells were discarded. Cells were then cultured for 24 h in 2 ml RPMI (5% autologous serum, 1% penicillin-streptomycin), followed by stimulation with 1 mg/ml LPS (Sigma, Hamburg, Germany) and additional incubation for 24 h.

Cytokine/chemokine expression of human monocyte subsets ex vivo

PBMC of three different healthy donors were isolated by density gradient. CD14$^+$CD16$^-$ and CD14$^+$CD16$^+$ monocytes were selectively purified by MACS methodology using 'Monocyte-isolation-Kit-II' and 'CD16$^+$-monocytes-isolation-kit', respectively (Miltenyi). Lymphocytes serving as control cells were isolated from PBMC after depletion of monocytes with anti-CD14 microbeads.

Purity >90% was confirmed by FACS analysis. Cells were cultured in RPMI containing 10% BSA and 1% penicillin-streptomycin (PAA) for 5 days.

Cytokine and chemokine detection

The release of cytokines/chemokines in human serum or in culture medium supernatant was measured using FlowCytomix (Bender Medsystems, Austria, Vienna). Measurements were performed in duplicates at 50 µL sample volume. Serum concentrations of MCP-1, MIP1α and MIP1β were assessed by Cytometric Bead Assay (BD) according to the manufacturer's instructions.

Co-culture of monocyte subsets with primary human stellate cells

Human liver tissue was obtained from patients undergoing partial liver resection for metastatic liver tumors of colorectal cancer. Experimental procedures were performed according to guidelines of the local ethics committee with patient's informed consent. Primary human HSC were isolated using EGTA/collagenase perfusion and pronase incubation as described previously [35,36]. HSC were separated from other non-parenchymal liver cells by arabinogalactan gradient ultracentrifugation, yielding HSC that were more than 90% pure and viable. 8×10^4 HSC were seeded on uncoated plastic dishes and cultured in DMEM supplemented with 10% FCS and 100 IU/ml penicillin-streptomycin. Growth medium was changed daily for the first 4 days in culture, then every other day thereafter [37].

Monocytes of three different healthy donors were pooled, and monocyte subsets were isolated as described above. After 7 days in pre-culture primary human HSC were co-cultured for 5 days with either CD14$^+$CD16$^-$, CD14$^+$CD16$^+$ or lymphocytes (each 8×10^5 cells/plate). As a positive control, HSC were stimulated with 5 ng/mL recombinant human TGFβ (R&D systems). Col1A and Acta2 were found to be exclusively expressed in HSC (and not in PMBC, monocytes/macrophages or lymphocytes), and col1A, but not Acta2, was induced in HSC by recombinant TGFβ. Therefore, col1A mRNA was normalized to Acta2 expression, in order to be able to evaluate HSC activation in cultures with mixed cell populations. In some co-culture assays, 2 ng/ml polyclonal anti-human TGFβ-Ab (sc-146; Santa Cruz) was applied [6].

Statistical analysis

Due to the skewed distribution of most parameters assessed in patients, data are presented as median, minimum and maximum. Differences between two groups were assessed by Mann-Whitney-U-test, multiple comparisons between more than two groups by Kruskal-Wallis-ANOVA and Mann-Whitney-U-test for post hoc analysis (SPSS, Chicago, IL). Box plot graphics illustrate comparisons between subgroups, displaying a statistical summary of median, quartiles, range and extreme values. The whiskers extend from the minimum to the maximum value excluding outside (open circle) and far out (asterisk) values which are shown as separate points. Correlations between variables were assessed by Spearman rank correlation test (SPSS).

For the ex vivo and in vitro experiments, bar graphs represent the mean and the standard error of the mean (SEM). Statistical comparisons between groups were performed using Mann-Whitney-U-test (GraphPad Prism). P-values <0.05 were considered statistical significant.

Supporting Information

Figure S1 Absolute numbers of circulating monocyte subsets do not differ between liver disease patients and healthy controls:

Statistical analysis reveals no significant shifts in absolute numbers of CD14+CD16- and CD14+CD16+ monocytes comparing healthy controls (n = 181) with chronic liver disease patients (n = 226) or non-cirrhotic (n = 85) with cirrhotic (n = 141) patients. No significant alterations are observed between the Child's stages of cirrhosis either (Child A, n = 48; B, n = 46; C, n = 47). Box plots are displayed, where the bold black line indicates the median per group, the box represents 50% of the values, and horizontal lines show minimum and maximum values of the calculated non-outlier values; open circles indicate outlier values.

Figure S2 Increased HLA-DR expression on CD14+CD16+ monocytes in chronic liver disease: Statistical analysis reveals an increase in HLA-DR expression (mean fluorescence intensity, MFI) on CD14+CD16+ monocytes, but not on CD14+CD16- monocytes comparing healthy controls (n = 181) with chronic liver disease patients (n = 226) or non-cirrhotic (n = 85) with cirrhotic (n = 141) patients. No significant alterations are observed between the Child's stages of cirrhosis (Child A, n = 48; B, n = 46; C, n = 47). Box plots are displayed, where the bold black line indicates the median per group, the box represents 50% of the values, and horizontal lines show minimum and maximum values of the calculated non-outlier values; open circles indicate outlier values. Significant differences (U-test) are marked by *p<0.05.

Acknowledgments

The authors thank Ms. Aline Müller for excellent technical assistance.

Author Contributions

Conceived and designed the experiments: HWZ CT FT. Performed the experiments: HWZ SS NG. Analyzed the data: HWZ SS TL FT. Contributed reagents/materials/analysis tools: JN NG CH AZ JJWT TL RW CT FT. Wrote the paper: HWZ FT.

References

1. Iredale JP (2007) Models of liver fibrosis: exploring the dynamic nature of inflammation and repair in a solid organ. J Clin Invest 117: 539–548.
2. Karlmark KR, Wasmuth HE, Trautwein C, Tacke F (2008) Chemokine-directed immune cell infiltration in acute and chronic liver disease. Expert Rev Gastroenterol Hepatol 2: 233–242.
3. Auffray C, Sieweke MH, Geissmann F (2009) Blood monocytes: development, heterogeneity, and relationship with dendritic cells. Annu Rev Immunol 27: 669–692.
4. Heymann F, Trautwein C, Tacke F (2009) Monocytes and macrophages as cellular targets in liver fibrosis. Inflamm Allergy Drug Targets 8: 307–318.
5. Imamura M, Ogawa T, Sasaguri Y, Chayama K, Ueno H (2005) Suppression of macrophage infiltration inhibits activation of hepatic stellate cells and liver fibrogenesis in rats. Gastroenterology 128: 138–146.
6. Karlmark KR, Weiskirchen R, Zimmermann HW, Gassler N, Ginhoux F, et al. (2009) Hepatic recruitment of the inflammatory Gr1+ monocyte subset upon liver injury promotes hepatic fibrosis. Hepatology 50: 261–274.
7. Mitchell C, Couton D, Couty JP, Anson M, Crain AM, et al. (2009) Dual role of CCR2 in the constitution and the resolution of liver fibrosis in mice. Am J Pathol 174: 1766–1775.
8. Seki E, de Minicis S, Inokuchi S, Taura K, Miyai K, et al. (2009) CCR2 promotes hepatic fibrosis in mice. Hepatology 50: 185–197.
9. Duffield JS, Forbes SJ, Constandinou CM, Clay S, Partolina M, et al. (2005) Selective depletion of macrophages reveals distinct, opposing roles during liver injury and repair. J Clin Invest 115: 56–65.
10. Klein I, Cornejo JC, Polakos NK, John B, Wuensch SA, et al. (2007) Kupffer cell heterogeneity: functional properties of bone marrow derived and sessile hepatic macrophages. Blood 110: 4077–4085.
11. Seki E, De Minicis S, Gwak GY, Kluwe J, Inokuchi S, et al. (2009) CCR1 and CCR5 promote hepatic fibrosis in mice. J Clin Invest 119: 1858–1870.
12. Tacke F, Randolph GJ (2006) Migratory fate and differentiation of blood monocyte subsets. Immunobiology 211: 609–618.
13. Ingersoll MA, Spanbroek R, Lottaz C, Gautier EL, Frankenberger M, et al. (2010) Comparison of gene expression profiles between human and mouse monocyte subsets. Blood 115: e10–19.
14. Tacke F, Alvarez D, Kaplan TJ, Jakubzick C, Spanbroek R, et al. (2007) Monocyte subsets differentially employ CCR2, CCR5, and CX3CR1 to accumulate within atherosclerotic plaques. J Clin Invest 117: 185–194.
15. Ziegler-Heitbrock L (2007) The CD14+ CD16+ blood monocytes: their role in infection and inflammation. J Leukoc Biol 81: 584–592.
16. Leicester KL, Olynyk JK, Brunt EM, Britton RS, Bacon BR (2006) Differential findings for CD14-positive hepatic monocytes/macrophages in primary biliary cirrhosis, chronic hepatitis C and nonalcoholic steatohepatitis. Liver Int 26: 559–565.
17. Panasiuk A, Zak J, Kasprzycka E, Janicka K, Prokopowicz D (2005) Blood platelet and monocyte activations and relation to stages of liver cirrhosis. World J Gastroenterol 11: 2754–2758.
18. Seki E, De Minicis S, Osterreicher CH, Kluwe J, Osawa Y, et al. (2007) TLR4 enhances TGF-beta signaling and hepatic fibrosis. Nat Med 13: 1324–1332.
19. Geissmann F, Jung S, Littman DR (2003) Blood monocytes consist of two principal subsets with distinct migratory properties. Immunity 19: 71–82.
20. Gordon S, Taylor PR (2005) Monocyte and macrophage heterogeneity. Nat Rev Immunol 5: 953–964.
21. Lin CY, Tsai IF, Ho YP, Huang CT, Lin YC, et al. (2007) Endotoxemia contributes to the immune paralysis in patients with cirrhosis. J Hepatol 46: 816–826.
22. Wasmuth HE, Kunz D, Yagmur E, Timmer-Stranghoner A, Vidacek D, et al. (2005) Patients with acute on chronic liver failure display "sepsis-like" immune paralysis. J Hepatol 42: 195–201.
23. Sakai N, Wada T, Furuichi K, Shimizu K, Kokubo S, et al. (2006) MCP-1/CCR2-dependent loop for fibrogenesis in human peripheral CD14-positive monocytes. J Leukoc Biol 79: 555–563.
24. Roderfeld M, Rath T, Voswinckel R, Dierkes C, Dietrich H, et al. (2010) Bone marrow transplantation demonstrates medullar origin of CD34+ fibrocytes and ameliorates hepatic fibrosis in Abcb4-/- mice. Hepatology 51: 267–276.
25. Weiler-Normann C, Herkel J, Lohse AW (2007) Mouse models of liver fibrosis. Z Gastroenterol 45: 43–50.
26. Serbina NV, Salazar-Mather TP, Biron CA, Kuziel WA, Pamer EG (2003) TNF/iNOS-producing dendritic cells mediate innate immune defense against bacterial infection. Immunity 19: 59–70.
27. Marra F, DeFranco R, Grappone C, Milani S, Pastacaldi S, et al. (1998) Increased expression of monocyte chemotactic protein-1 during active hepatic fibrogenesis: correlation with monocyte infiltration. Am J Pathol 152: 423–430.
28. Tsou CL, Peters W, Si Y, Slaymaker S, Aslanian AM, et al. (2007) Critical roles for CCR2 and MCP-3 in monocyte mobilization from bone marrow and recruitment to inflammatory sites. J Clin Invest 117: 902–909.
29. De Minicis S, Seki E, Uchinami H, Kluwe J, Zhang Y, et al. (2007) Gene expression profiles during hepatic stellate cell activation in culture and in vivo. Gastroenterology 132: 1937–1946.
30. Schwabe RF, Bataller R, Brenner DA (2003) Human hepatic stellate cells express CCR5 and RANTES to induce proliferation and migration. Am J Physiol Gastrointest Liver Physiol 285: G949–958.
31. Ajuebor MN, Wondimu Z, Hogaboam CM, Le T, Proudfoot AE, et al. (2007) CCR5 deficiency drives enhanced natural killer cell trafficking to and activation within the liver in murine T cell-mediated hepatitis. Am J Pathol 170: 1975–1988.
32. Tacke F, Brabant G, Kruck E, Horn R, Schoffski P, et al. (2003) Ghrelin in chronic liver disease. J Hepatol 38: 447–454.
33. Koch A, Gressner OA, Sanson E, Tacke F, Trautwein C (2009) Serum resistin levels in critically ill patients are associated with inflammation, organ dysfunction and metabolism and may predict survival of non-septic patients. Crit Care 13: R95.
34. Desmet VJ, Gerber M, Hoofnagle JH, Manns M, Scheuer PJ (1994) Classification of chronic hepatitis: diagnosis, grading and staging. Hepatology 19: 1513–1520.
35. Muhlbauer M, Bosserhoff AK, Hartmann A, Thasler WE, Weiss TS, et al. (2003) A novel MCP-1 gene polymorphism is associated with hepatic MCP-1 expression and severity of HCV-related liver disease. Gastroenterology 125: 1085–1093.
36. Hellerbrand, Wang SC, Tsukamoto H, Brenner DA, Rippe RA (1996) Expression of intracellular adhesion molecule 1 by activated hepatic stellate cells. Hepatology 24: 670–676.
37. Tacke F, Gabele E, Bataille F, Schwabe RF, Hellerbrand C, et al. (2007) Bone morphogenetic protein 7 is elevated in patients with chronic liver disease and exerts fibrogenic effects on human hepatic stellate cells. Dig Dis Sci 52: 3404–3415.

12

TGF-β and TGF-β/Smad Signaling in the Interactions between *Echinococcus multilocularis* and its Hosts

Junhua Wang[1,2⑨], Chuanshan Zhang[1⑨], Xufa Wei[1], Oleg Blagosklonov[2,3], Guodong Lv[1], Xiaomei Lu[1], Georges Mantion[3], Dominique A. Vuitton[3], Hao Wen[1]*, Renyong Lin[1]*

1 State Key Lab Incubation Base of Xinjiang Major Diseases Research (2010DS890294) and Xinjiang Key Laboratory of Echinococcosis, First Affiliated Hospital of Xinjiang Medical University, Urumqi, Xinjiang, China, 2 Department of Nuclear Medicine, University of Franche-Comté and Jean Minjoz University Hospital, Besançon, Franche-Comté, France, 3 WHO-Collaborating Centre for the Prevention and Treatment of Human Echinococcosis, University of Franche-Comté and University Hospital, Besançon, Franche-Comté, France

Abstract

Alveolar echinococcosis (AE) is characterized by the development of irreversible fibrosis and of immune tolerance towards *Echinococcus multilocularis* (E. multilocularis). Very little is known on the presence of transforming growth factor-β (TGF-β) and other components of TGF-β/Smad pathway in the liver, and on their possible influence on fibrosis, over the various stages of infection. Using Western Blot, qRT-PCR and immunohistochemistry, we measured the levels of TGF-β1, TGF-β receptors, and down-stream Smads activation, as well as fibrosis marker expression in both a murine AE model from day 2 to 360 post-infection (p.i.) and in AE patients. TGF-β1, its receptors, and down-stream Smads were markedly expressed in the periparasitic infiltrate and also in the hepatocytes, close to and distant from AE lesions. Fibrosis was significant at 180 days p.i. in the periparasitic infiltrate and was also present in the liver parenchyma, even distant from the lesions. Over the time course after infection TGF-β1 expression was correlated with CD4/CD8 T-cell ratio long described as a hallmark of AE severity. The time course of the various actors of the TGF-β/Smad system in the *in vivo* mouse model as well as down-regulation of Smad7 in liver areas close to the lesions in human cases highly suggest that TGF-β plays an important role in AE both in immune tolerance against the parasite and in liver fibrosis.

Editor: Valli De Re, Centro di Riferimento Oncologico, IRCCS National Cancer Institute, Italy

Funding: This work was supported by the Xinjiang Young Scientist Foundation (2010211B19), the Program for Changjiang Scholars and Innovative Research Team in Universities (IRT1181), NSFC Grant Projects (30960342, 81260452, 81260252), and Xinjiang Key-Lab Projects (XJDX0202-2009-03). The funders had no role in study design, data collection and analysis, decision to publish, or preparation of the manuscript.

Competing Interests: The authors have declared that no competing interests exist.

* E-mail: renyongl@yahoo.com.cn (RL); Dr.wenhao@163.com (HW)

⑨ These authors contributed equally to this work.

Introduction

Alveolar echinococcosis (AE) is a rare, but severe zoonotic helminthic disease due to the proliferation of the larval stage of cestode *Echinococcus multilocularis* (E. multilocularis) [1]. In humans, accidental intermediate hosts, the severity of this disease results from both a continuous asexual proliferation of the metacestode and an intense inflammatory granulomatous infiltration around the parasite which causes pathological damages in the liver. The lesions act like a slow-growing liver cancer, progressively invading the neighboring tissues and organs. Granulomas around the parasitic vesicles, extensive fibrosis, and necrosis are the characteristic pathological findings [2]. Studies performed in the 1980s–1990s showed that dense and irreversible fibrosis composed of thick concentric bundles of heavily cross-linked type I and type III collagens surrounded the parasitic vesicles, and that α-smooth muscle actin (α-SMA)-expressing myofibroblasts (MFB) derived from the hepatic stellate cells (HSC) could play an important role in fibrosis development [3–7]. The diffusion of the fibrotic process even far from the parasitic lesions strongly suggested that cytokines produced in the periparasitic area could be involved in collagen synthesis, locally in the lesions and also in the liver distant from the

lesions; it was also suggested that cytokines might be involved in the cross-linking of the collagen bundles. Little evidence, however, has been given until now on how *E. multilocularis* metacestode interacts with its host to promote fibrosis and especially on the nature and role of cytokines in fibrosis development in AE.

TGF-β is a major regulator of the immune responses, inducing and maintaining T-regulatory cells, reducing cytotoxic effector immune response and balancing the tolerogenic and immunogenic forces at play in various physiological states and chronic diseases, such as fetus growth and survival during gestation [8], cancer [9], chronic inflammatory diseases [10], or chronic and allergic respiratory diseases [11]. In these conditions, this polypeptide also regulates a variety of cell events involved in tissue regeneration and fibrosis. Similarly, its role has been recognized both to induce and maintain immune tolerance towards parasites and to induce fibrosis in several examples of helminth infection [12]. However, opposite to the recognized role of Interleukin-10 [12,13], little is known about TGF-β involvement in the pathophysiology of larval echinococcosis. Only preliminary studies are available in AE: Zhang et al. [14] showed that TGF-β was expressed in most lymphocytes of the periparasitic infiltrate in liver biopsies from AE patients. It was suggested that TGF-β may play a role in maintaining host tolerance against *E. multilocularis* growth by preventing T-cell cytotoxicity against the parasite [14]. In cystic echinococcosis (CE), immunostaining of TGF-β has also been shown at the periphery of hydatid cysts in the liver of patients [15]; and another study confirmed a progressive increase in the expression of mRNA of TGF-β in the liver of *E. granulosus*-infected BALB/c mice [16]. There is abundant evidence that TGF-β1, besides its role in immune tolerance, is an extremely potent inducer of the synthesis of procollagen and other extra-cellular matrix (ECM) components [17,18], and has an essential role in the pathogenesis of liver fibrosis. The major signaling pathway for all TGF-β members is activated through ligand binding to a cell-surface receptor complex of type I and type II serine–threonine kinases receptors; and a group of intracellular signaling intermediates known as Smads is then phosphorylated. Phosphorylated Smads translocate to the nucleus where they function as transcription factors, initiating target gene transcription [19]. Smad4 is apparently common to all ligand-specific Smad pathways, and is a central mediator in TGF-β superfamily signaling [20]. Smad7, which is induced by TGF-β itself, forms part of an inhibitory feedback loop by binding to the intracellular domain of the activated TGF-β RI [21–24]. Because Smad7 is responsible for the fine-tuning of TGF-β signals [25], an aberrant expression of Smad7 might disrupt the balanced activity of TGF-β under physiological and pathophysiological conditions. However, although it may be crucial in the host-parasite interactions (Fig. 1), the relationship between the TGF-β/Smad pathway, and especially Smad7 expression, and clinical and/or pathological features of AE in experimental models as well as in humans has never been addressed.

The aims of this study were 1) to delineate the location of TGF-β and components of the TGF-β pathway in the periparasitic immune cells and in hepatocytes, close to and distant from the lesions in the liver; 2) to better understand the functioning of the TGF-β/Smad pathway, and its possible relationship with the development of liver fibrosis in the parasite's hosts; 3) to further explore how TGF-β was secreted and regulated. For this purpose, and to get a comprehensive appraisal of TGF-β secretion and of its role in *E. multilocularis* infection, experimental AE in a mouse model of liver-targeted secondary AE [4] allowed us to study the time course of TGF-β expression as well as the dynamics of TGF-β signaling-related components, TGF-β RI, TGF-β RII, pSmad 2/3, Smad4 and Smad7, and to correlate them with the time course of the periparasitic infiltration by T-cell subpopulations, and to biochemical indicators of liver fibrosis, such as α-smooth muscle actin (α-SMA), and collagens I (COL I), and III (COL III). We also studied TGF-β and TGF-β signaling-related components in the liver of AE patients both at the protein and mRNA levels, in order to assess the situation at the late stage of infection in resistant hosts where immune tolerance and development of fibrosis are combined.

Results

Pathological Examination of the Livers Infected with *E. multilocularis*

In experimental mice, at the very early stage (2 and 8 days p.i.), in the surrounding of the metacestode injection site, lipid accumulation was observed in some hepatocytes (focal steatosis), and lymphocytes infiltrated the portal areas. No obvious change was found in the distant liver. From day 30 to day 90 after infection, at the periphery of the lesion, fibroblasts and inflammatory cells proliferated and an obvious increase of liver fibrosis was observed at the periphery of the lesion. There was no change

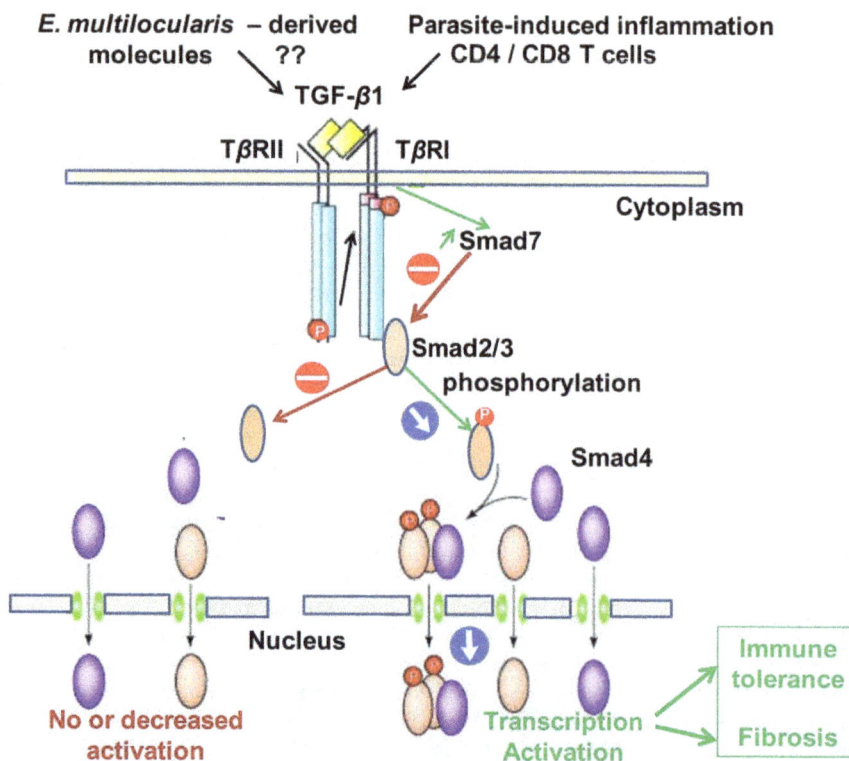

Figure 1. The TGF-β/Smad pathway; hypothesis for its involvement in the host-parasite relationship in *E. multilocularis* infection.

in the areas distant from the lesion, except fibroblast and Kupffer cell proliferation, and an increased presence of lymphocytes in portal spaces. From day 180 to day 360, the typical granulomatous and fibrous periparasitic infiltrate of AE was fully established; in the liver, degenerating hepatocytes with atrophy and necrosis, as well as fibrous tissue development were observed in the areas immediately surrounding the granulomatous host response. Both fibroblasts and Kupffer cells proliferated in areas distant from the lesion. Mice in the control group at the same time-points showed normal hepatic histology (data not shown; available from reference [26]).

In AE patients, the liver lesions were similar to those observed in experimental mice at day 180 after infection, with the typical granulomatous and fibrous reaction surrounding parasite vesicles either active or degenerating. In the liver areas distant from the lesions, there was Kupffer cell proliferation, and lymphocytes infiltrated the portal areas. In the liver areas immediately surrounding the lesions, a few hepatocytes showed degeneration (data not shown).

Expression of α-SMA, and Collagen I, III in the Livers Infected with E. multilocularis

In experimental mice, in the liver of control animals α-SMA expression was present in the cytoplasm of smooth muscle cells, i.e. restricted to the walls of most of the portal and central veins while there was nearly no staining in the liver parenchyma (Fig. 2). 180 days after E. multilocularis infection, α-SMA positive score was higher in infected than in control mice; distribution of α-SMA positive cells was diffuse in the liver parenchyma, suggesting a myofibroblastic differentiation of stellate cells in the liver (Fig. 3A).

In AE patients, in the liver areas close to lesions, there was a strong α-SMA immunostaining present in the ECM and α-SMA expression scores were significantly higher in the areas close to lesions compared to those distant from lesions (Fig. 2 and 3F).

In experimental mice, there was a marked difference between E. multilocularis-infected mice and control mice with regard to the nature and location of collagens in the liver. At all time-points, strong staining for Collagen I and III was present in the peri-parasitic granuloma as concentric bundles extending from the laminated layer of the parasitic vesicles to the border of the normal liver (Fig. 2). Collagen III was also present as dotted lines between the cells at the outer part of the granulomatous infiltrate and, occasionally, in the cytoplasm of round cells in the sinusoids of the surrounding liver (Fig. 2).

In AE patients, in the liver areas close to lesions, there was a strong Collagen I and III immunostaining in the ECM. Expression scores of Collagen I and Collagen III were significantly higher in the areas close to lesions compared to those distant from lesions (Fig. 3F).

Infiltration by CD4+ and CD8+ T Cells in the Periparasitic Area in E.multilocularis-infected Mice

As the experimental model of AE allowed us to study the correlation, if any, between T lymphocyte infiltration in the liver and TGF-β expression over the time course of infection, CD4 and CD8 immunostaining was performed in the liver of mice; this was not performed in the liver of AE patients, since the time course could not be assessed. There was nearly no infiltration by CD4+ T cells nor by CD8+ T cells in the control groups whenever the time point after sham injection of saline in the liver (Fig. 2). In the periparasitic infiltrate surrounding the metacestode, in experimental infected mice, CD4+ T cells were present from day 60 to day 360. CD4 positive scores ranged from 0.6 to 3.7 and reached

the peak point at day 90 (Fig. 3D). Infiltration by CD8+ T cells was expressed by scores which ranged from 2.3 to 5.4 and reached the peak point later than CD4+ T cells, at day 360 (Fig. 3E).

Expression of TGF-β1 in the Livers Infected with E. multilocularis

Protein expression of TGF-β1. In experimental mice, a strong immunostaining for TGF-β1 was observed in the periparasitic infiltrate in most of areas with inflammatory granulomas from 30 days to 360 days p.i. In the liver area close to the parasitic lesions, a faint expression of TGF-β1 was observed in the endothelial cells at day 30; a marked expression was observed in endothelial cells of the hepatic sinusoids and in fibroblasts at day 60, as well as in endothelial cells of the hepatic sinusoids and in hepatocytes close to the parasitic lesions from 90 days to 360 days p.i. In the liver distant from the parasitic lesions, a faint staining for TGF-β1 was observed in the endothelial cells of hepatic sinusoids from 30 to 90 days p.i.; there was a moderate staining in endothelial cells of hepatic sinusoids from 180 to 360 days p.i., while a faint staining was observed in the hepatocytes from 90 and 360 days p.i. (Fig. 4 and 5A). An increased TGF-β1 expression measured using Western Blot in the liver of experimental infected mice was observed from day 2 (0.9-fold) to day 360 (3.2-fold); it peaked at day 180 (8.2-fold) after infection with E. multilocularis, then decreased to lower levels, albeit higher than in control mice until the end of follow-up; difference between experimental and control mice was significant at day 90, 180, 270 and 360 ($P<0.05$).

In AE patients, as observed in the mouse model, a strong immunostaining for TGF-β1 was observed in most lymphocytes and macrophages in the periparasitic infiltrate, as well as in Kupffer cells, fibroblasts, and endothelial cells in hepatic sinusoids, especially around the granulomas, and in infiltrating immune cells of portal spaces (Fig. 4). In the non-infiltrated liver, faint staining with anti-TGF-β1 antibodies was observed in hepatocytes, even in those observed in areas distant from the parasitic lesions (Fig. 4). Percentage of TGF-β1 positive cells was higher in areas close to than distant from lesions (Fig. 6A), with an intensity gradient from the periparasitic areas to the distant liver, since TGF-β1 staining appeared stronger close to the granulomatous reaction (Fig. 4). Western Blot measurements of TGF-β1 also showed that protein levels of the cytokine were significantly higher in the liver tissue close to lesions than in that distant from lesions (Fig. 6B and C) ($P<0.05$).

Correlation with T cell subpopulations and fibrosis markers. TGF-β1 expression in the periparasitic infiltrate was highly positively correlated with CD4/CD8 ratio (r = 0.818) but not correlated with either CD4+ or CD8+ T cell scores, taken independently (Table 1).

Spearman correlation coefficients indicated a positive correlation between TGF-β1 expression and α-SMA, Collagen I, and Collagen III expression scores (r = 0.628, $P = 0.009$; r = 0.836, $P<0.001$; r = 0.781, $P<0.001$ respectively) in the livers from day 90 to day 360 p.i. in experimental mice under study (Table 2). There was also a positive correlation between TGF-β1 expression and α-SMA, Collagen I, and Collagen III expression scores (r = 0.620, $P = 0.001$; r = 0.498, $P = 0.013$; r = 0.655, $P = 0.001$ respectively) in the livers from the 16 patients with AE under study (Table 3).

RNA expression of TGF-β1. In experimental mice, real-time RT-PCR showed an increase in TGF-β1 mRNA expression from day 8 to the end of follow-up, with a peak at day 180 after infection. TGF-β1 mRNA expression increased from 0.57-fold at day 2 to 5.37-fold at day 180 (Fig. 5D) compared to control mice. There was a significant difference between E. multilocularis infected

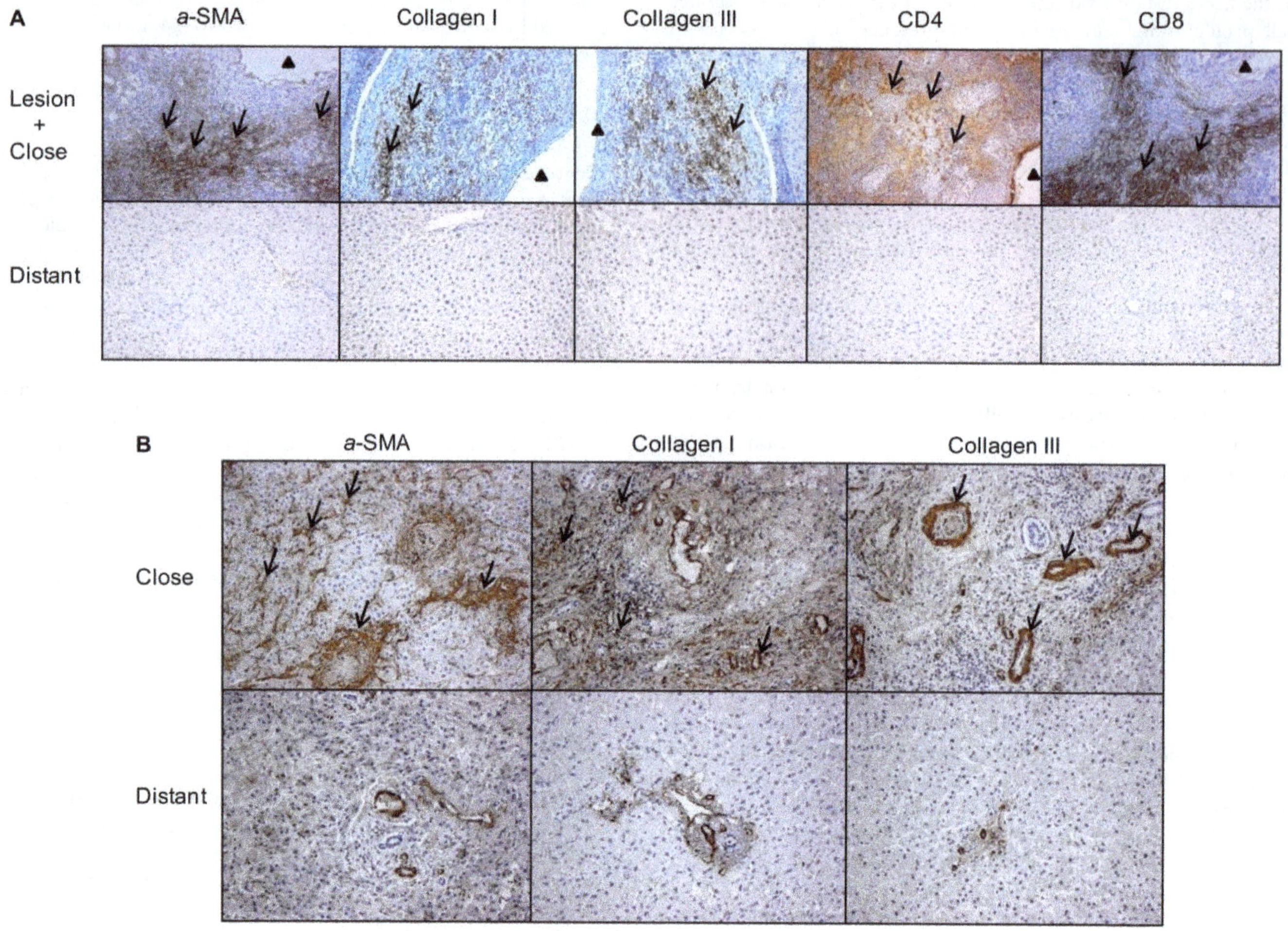

Figure 2. Immuno-histochemical expression of fibrosis markers in *E. multilocularis*-**infected livers of experimental mice and AE patients, and of the periparasitic infiltration by CD4⁺ T and CD8⁺ T lymphocytes in the liver of experimental mice (arrow).** A: In experimental mice. α-SMA: expression at day 8, in the cytoplasm of smooth muscle cells, hepatic stellate cells and myofibroblasts in the liver parenchyma; collagen I: expression at day 360, in the peri-parasitic granuloma as concentric bundles extending from the laminated layer of the parasitic vesicles to the border of the normal liver; collagen III: expression at day 360, in the peri-parasitic granuloma as concentric bundles extending from the laminated layer of the parasitic vesicles to the border of the normal liver, also present as dotted lines between the cells at the outer part of the granulomatous infiltrate and, occasionally, in the cytoplasm of round cells in the sinusoids of the surrounding liver; CD4⁺ T cells: expression at day 90, in the periparasitic infiltrate surrounding the metacestode; CD8⁺ T cells: expression at day 180, in the periparasitic infiltrate surrounding the metacestode. B: In AE patients. α-SMA: expressed in the extracellular matrix; collagen I expressed both in the extracellular matrix and hepatocytes; collagen III expressed in the extracellular matrix and hepatocytes. The arrowheads indicate the parasitic lesions in the liver of infected mice and human patients. Final magnification: 200×. 'Lesion': *E. multilocularis* metacestode and surrounding immune infiltrate; 'Close': liver parenchyma close to *E. multilocularis* lesion; 'Distant': liver parenchyma distant from *E. multilocularis* lesion.

and control group at the time points of 60-, 90- and 180-days p.i. ($P<0.05$).

In AE patients, real-time RT-PCR showed that TGF-β1 mRNA expression was significantly higher in the liver tissue close to lesions compared to that distant from lesions (Fig. 6D) ($P<0.05$).

Expression of TGF-β RI and RII in the Livers Infected with *E. multilocularis*

Protein expression of TGF-β RI and RII. In experimental mice, TGF-β RI immunostaining was observed in the cytoplasm of lymphocytes and macrophages in the periparasitic infiltrate, and in most of the hepatocytes, fibroblasts, and endothelial cells in the liver close to the periparasitic infiltrate; no positive staining was observed in the control liver sections (Fig. 4). Positive cells ranged from 0.25% to 20.5% and reached a peak at day 60 p.i. In the liver distant from the parasitic lesions, a

very faint staining for TGF-β RI was observed in the endothelial cells of hepatic sinusoids from 30 to 90 days p.i., a faint staining was observed in the hepatocytes from 60 to 360 days p.i. and in endothelial cells of hepatic sinusoids from 180 to 360 days p.i. (Fig. 7A). There was a significant difference between *E. multilocularis*-infected and control groups, close to lesion and distant from lesion at all time-points since day 30 ($P<0.05$, Fig. 7A). However, Western Blot results could not show a significant difference in the protein levels of TGF-β RI and TGF-β RII in infected versus control mice during the whole time course of *E. multilocularis* infection. TGF-β RII immunostaining was observed in the same cells as TGF-β RI in infected mice (Fig. 4). Positive cells ranged from 4.0% to 15.0% and reached a peak at day 60. There was a significant difference between *E. multilocularis* infected and control groups,

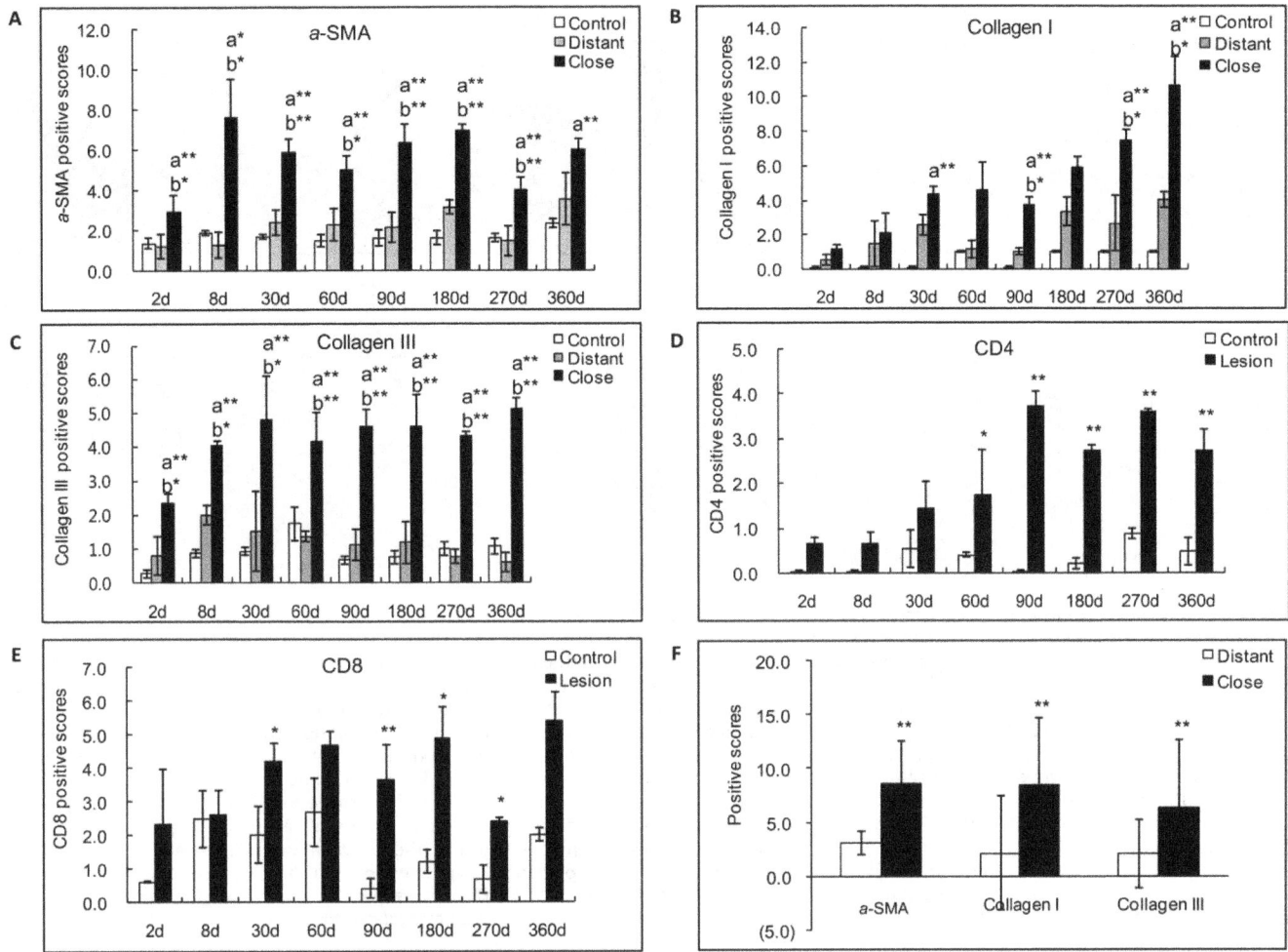

Figure 3. Semiquantitative expression of fibrosis markers in _E. multilocularis_-infected liver in experimental mice and in AE patients. Score for each marker expression was calculated from quantitative analysis of the histo-immunostaining using both staining intensity and the percentage of cells stained at a specific range of intensities (arrow) (see Materials and Methods section). A: Course of α-SMA expression in _E. multilocularis_-infected mice. B: Course of collagen I expression in _E. multilocularis_-infected mice; C: Course of collagen III expression in _E. multilocularis_-infected mice; D: Course of CD4+ T cell infiltration in _E. multilocularis_-infected mice; E: Course of CD8+ T cell infiltration in _E. multilocularis_-infected mice; F: Expression of fibrosis markers in the liver of AE patients. a: close versus control; b: close versus distant. *P<0.05; **P<0.01. 'Control', non-infected mice; 'Lesion': _E. multilocularis_ metacestode and surrounding immune infiltrate; 'Close': liver parenchyma close to _E. multilocularis_ lesion; 'Distant': liver parenchyma distant from _E. multilocularis_ lesion.

close to lesion and distant from lesion at all time-points (P<0.05, Fig. 7A).

In AE patients, expression of TGF-β RI differed markedly between patients and taking all 16 patients into account, there was no significant difference between the positive cells for TGF-β RI in areas close to and distant from lesions (Fig. 6A). Similarly, Western Blot results showed that TGF-β RI protein levels were not different in the liver tissue close to lesions compared to that distant from lesions (Fig. 6B and C). There was no significant difference either between the expression of TGF-β RII in areas close to and distant from lesions (Fig. 6B and C). However, compared with the areas distant from the parasitic lesions, the areas close to lesions displayed a stronger staining for TGF-β RII protein both at the cell membrane and in the cytoplasm (Fig. 4). Western Blot results showed that TGF-β RII protein levels were significantly elevated in the liver tissue close to lesions compared to that distant from lesions (Fig. 6B and C).

mRNA expression of TGF-β RI and RII. In experimental mice, an increased TGF-β RI mRNA expression was observed in

infected mice at day 60 to day 180, which peaked at day180. _E.multilocularis_ infection increased TGF-β RI mRNA expression from 0.43-fold at day 8 to 3.48-fold at day 180 (Fig. 7D). There was a significant difference between _E. multilocularis_ infected and control groups at day 270 p.i. (P<0.05); however at that time, mRNA expression was lower in infected mice, despite a marked increase in the expression of the receptor as measured by immunostaining. Increased TGF-β RII mRNA expression was observed from day 30 to 90 and peaked at day 60 after infection. _E.multilocularis_ infection increased TGF-β RII mRNA expression from 0.70-fold at 8 days to 2.52-fold at 60 days (Fig. 7D). The difference between _E. multilocularis_-infected and control mice was significant at day 60 and 90 (P<0.05).

In AE patients, there were no significant differences in TGF-β RI as well as TGF-β RII mRNA levels measured by real-time RT-PCR in the liver close to and distant from the lesions (Fig. 6D).

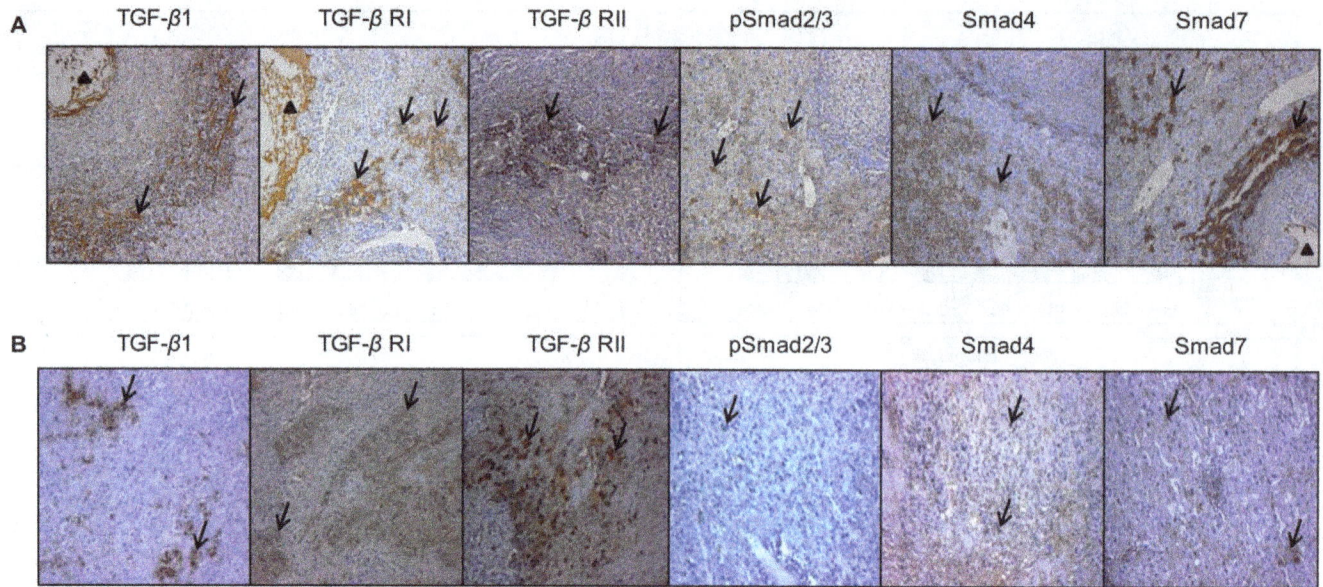

Figure 4. Immunohistochemical expression of the various components of the TGF-_β_/Smad pathway in the _E. multilocularis_-infected liver in experimental mice and in AE patients. A: In experimental mice. Expression of the various components of the TGF-_β_/Smad pathway at their peak of expression in the liver. TGF-_β_1: expression at day 90, in most of the immune cells in most of areas with inflammatory granulomas, in the cytoplasm of hepatocytes, endothelial cells of the hepatic sinusoids and fibroblasts; TGF-_β_ RI and RII: expression at day 60, in the cytoplasm of lymphocytes and macrophages in the periparasitic infiltrate and in most of the hepatocytes, fibroblasts, and endothelial cells close to the periparasitic infiltrate; pSmad2/3: expression at day 30, in both the cytoplasm and nuclear of the hepatocytes; Smad4: expression at day 60, in both the cytoplasm and nuclear of the hepatocytes; Smad7: expression at day 90, in the cytoplasm of the hepatocytes. B: In AE patients. Specimen 'Close' was taken close to the parasitic lesions (0.5 cm from the macroscopic changes due to the metacestode/granuloma lesion), and Specimen 'Distant' was taken in the liver distant from the lesions (the non-diseased lobe of the liver whenever possible, or at least at 10 cm from the lesion). TGF-_β_1: expressed in most of the immune cells in most of areas with inflammatory granulomas, in the cytoplasm of hepatocytes, endothelial cells of the hepatic sinusoids and fibroblasts; TGF-_β_ RI and RII: expressed in the cytoplasm of lymphocytes and macrophages in the periparasitic infiltrate and in most of the hepatocytes, fibroblasts, and endothelial cells close to the periparasitic infiltrate; pSmad2/3: expressed in both the cytoplasm and nuclear of the hepatocytes; Smad4: expressed in both the cytoplasm and nuclear of the hepatocytes; Smad7: expressed in the cytoplasm of the hepatocytes. The arrowheads indicate the parasitic lesions in the liver of infected mice and human patients. Final magnification: 200×.

Phosphorylation of Smad2/3 and Expression of Smad4 in the Livers Infection with _E. multilocularis_

Protein expression of phosphorylated Smad 2/3. In experimental mice, pSmad2/3 was most usually expressed in the cytoplasm of the hepatocytes; very little nuclear expression was observed. In infected mice, immunostaining displayed a patchy distribution, and strong staining was observed in those hepatocytes which were close to the periparasitic infiltrate (Fig. 4). Conversely, no or a faint staining was observed in the liver distant from the parasitic lesions and in the liver from control mice. The positive cells of pSmad 2/3 ranged from 0.15% to 8.2% in the liver close to lesion, and reached a peak at day 30 and day 60 after infection. There was a significant difference between _E. multilocularis_ infected and control groups, close to lesion and distant from lesion at day 30, 60, 90 and 180 ($P<0.05$, Fig. 8A). Western Blot measurements showed that there was no difference either in the phosphorylation of Smad2/3 protein in the areas close to lesions compared to those distant from lesions (Fig. 8B and C).

In AE patients, immunostaining of pSmad2/3 displayed a patchy distribution (Fig. 4), however non-related to the lobular structure of the liver and/or to the distance to the parasitic lesions. There was no significant difference between the positive cells of pSmad2/3 in areas close to and distant from lesions (Fig. 6A). Western Blot measurements showed that there was no difference either in the phosphorylation of Smad2/3 protein in the areas close to lesions compared to those distant from lesions (Fig. 6B and C).

mRNA expression of Smad2 and 3. In experimental mice, increased Smad2 and Smad3 mRNA expression was observed from day 30 to day 90. Smad2 mRNA expression peaked at day 90 and ranged from 0.8-fold at day 2 to 4.4-fold at day 90 (Fig. 8D). There was a significant difference between _E. multilocularis_ infected and control groups at day 30 ($P<0.05$). Smad3 mRNA expression peaked at day 60 and ranged from 2.6-fold at day 60 days to 0.5-fold at day 360 (Fig. 8D). There was a significant difference of between _E. multilocularis_ infected and control groups at day 60 ($P<0.05$).

In AE patients, there were no significant differences in Smad2 mRNA levels measured by real-time RT-PCR (Fig. 6D). However, mRNA levels of Smad3 were significantly higher in tissue samples close to lesions compared to those distant from lesions (Fig. 6D).

Protein expression of Smad4. In experimental mice, immunohistochemical study of Smad4 protein revealed higher cytoplasmic and nuclear staining of hepatocytes in areas close to lesions compared with areas distant from lesions. Distribution of Smad4 expression was similar to that of pSmad2/3 in its location, but more diffuse (Fig. 4). Positive cells for Smad4 ranged from 0.2% to 18.0% in the liver close to lesion, and reached a peak at day 60 p.i. There was a significant difference between _E. multilocularis_-infected and control groups, close to lesion and distant from lesion at day 30, 60, 90, 180, and 270 ($P<0.05$, Fig.9A). However, Western Blot analysis of Smad4 expression did not show any difference between infected and control mice, as well as

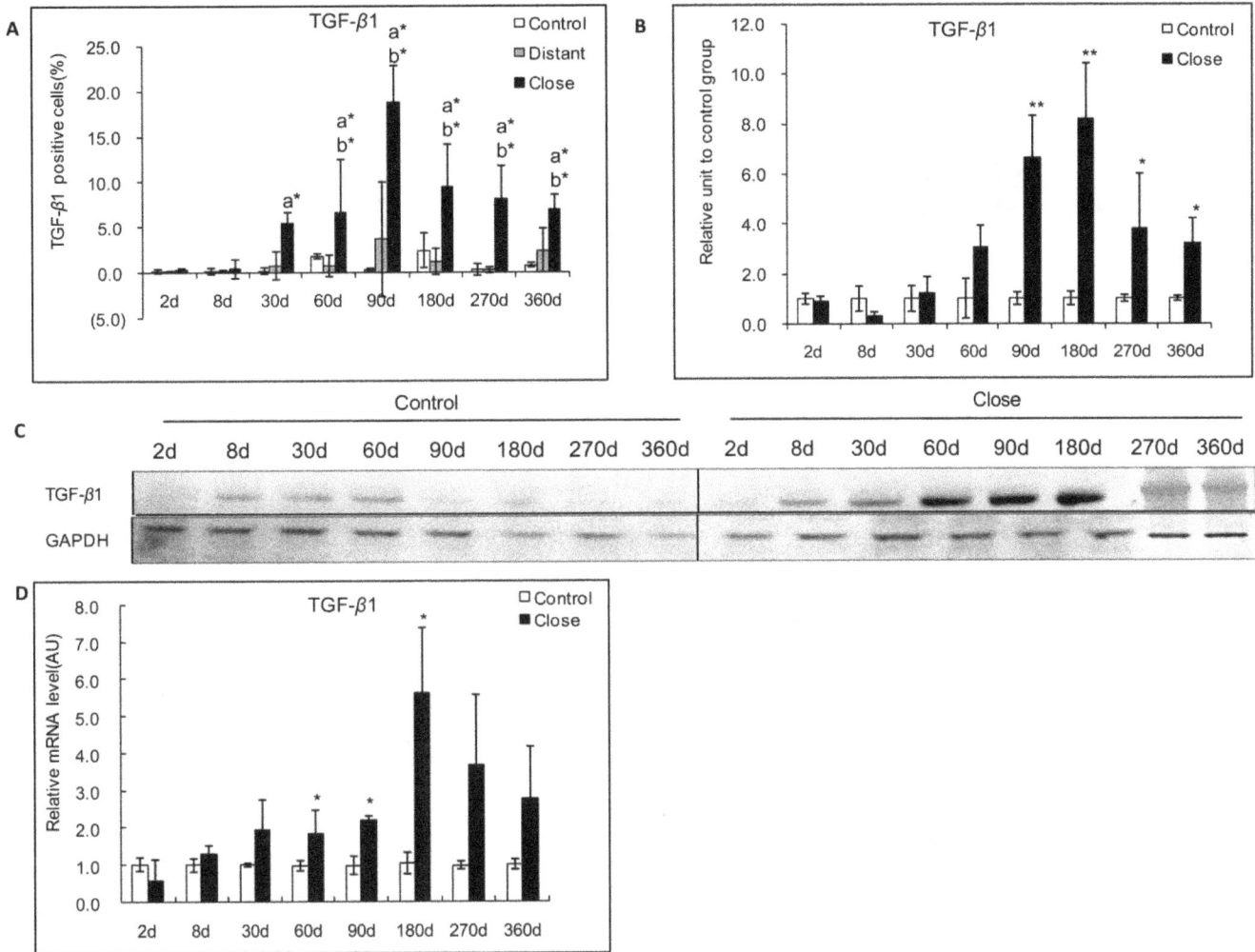

Figure 5. Course of TGF-β1 expression in the liver of experimental mice during E. multilocularis infection. A: Course of TGF-β1 expression observed by immune-staining in the liver from E. multilocularis infected mice, calculated as the percent of positive cells to the total number of counted cells (see Materials and Methods section). B: Relative amount of TGF-β1 calculated from semi-quantitative analysis of the Western Blot using densitometry. C: Representative example of the course of TGF-β1 protein measured by Western Blot. D: Course of TGF-β1 mRNA expression measured by real time RT-PCR. a: 'close' versus 'control'; b: 'close' versus 'distant'. *$P<0.05$; **$P<0.01$. 'Control', non-infected mice; 'Lesion': E. multilocularis metacestode and surrounding immune infiltrate; 'Close': liver parenchyma close to E. multilocularis lesion; 'Distant': liver parenchyma distant from E. multilocularis lesion. AU: arbitrary units; GAPDH: glyceraldehyde-3-phosphate dehydrogenase.

between the liver close to and distant from the lesions, all over the time course (Fig. 9B and C).

In AE patients, immunohistochemical staining for Smad4 protein in the liver revealed cytoplasmic and nuclear staining of hepatocytes, with a homogenous distribution among cells; positive cells were higher in the areas close to lesions compared with those distant to lesions. Intensity of nuclear staining of Smad4 protein was noticeably higher in the areas close to the lesions (Fig. 4). Western Blot results also confirmed that Smad4 protein levels were significantly higher in the liver parenchyma close to lesions compared to that distant from lesions (Fig. 6B and C).

mRNA expression of Smad4. In experimental mice, increased Smad4 mRNA expression was observed from day 30 to day 90. Smad4 mRNA expression peaked at day 90 and ranged from 0.6-fold at day 8 to 1.9-fold at day 90 (Fig. 9D). There was a significant difference between E. multilocularis infected and control mice at day 90 ($P<0.05$).

In AE patients, the "lesions to periphery gradient" observed for the protein expression was also demonstrated at the mRNA level,

as measured by real-time RT-PCR, with higher expression close to the lesions (Fig. 6D).

Expression of Smad 7 in the Livers Infected with E. multilocularis

Protein expression of Smad7. In experimental mice, Smad7 immunostaining was mostly present in the cytoplasm of the hepatocytes, with a varying intensity throughout the liver, higher in the areas close to the lesion than in those distant from the lesion (Fig. 4). A faint staining was observed in the hepatocytes from 30 to 360 days in the areas distant from the lesion and in the control group (Fig. 10A). Smad7 positive cells in the hepatic cells ranged from 0.40% to 9.45% and reached a peak at 90 days. There was a significant difference between E. multilocularis infected and control groups, close to lesion and distant from lesion at 60 days, 90 days, 180 days and 270 days p.i. ($P<0.05$, Fig. 10A). Western Blot results showed that there was no change in Smad7 expression between E. multilocularis infected and control mice

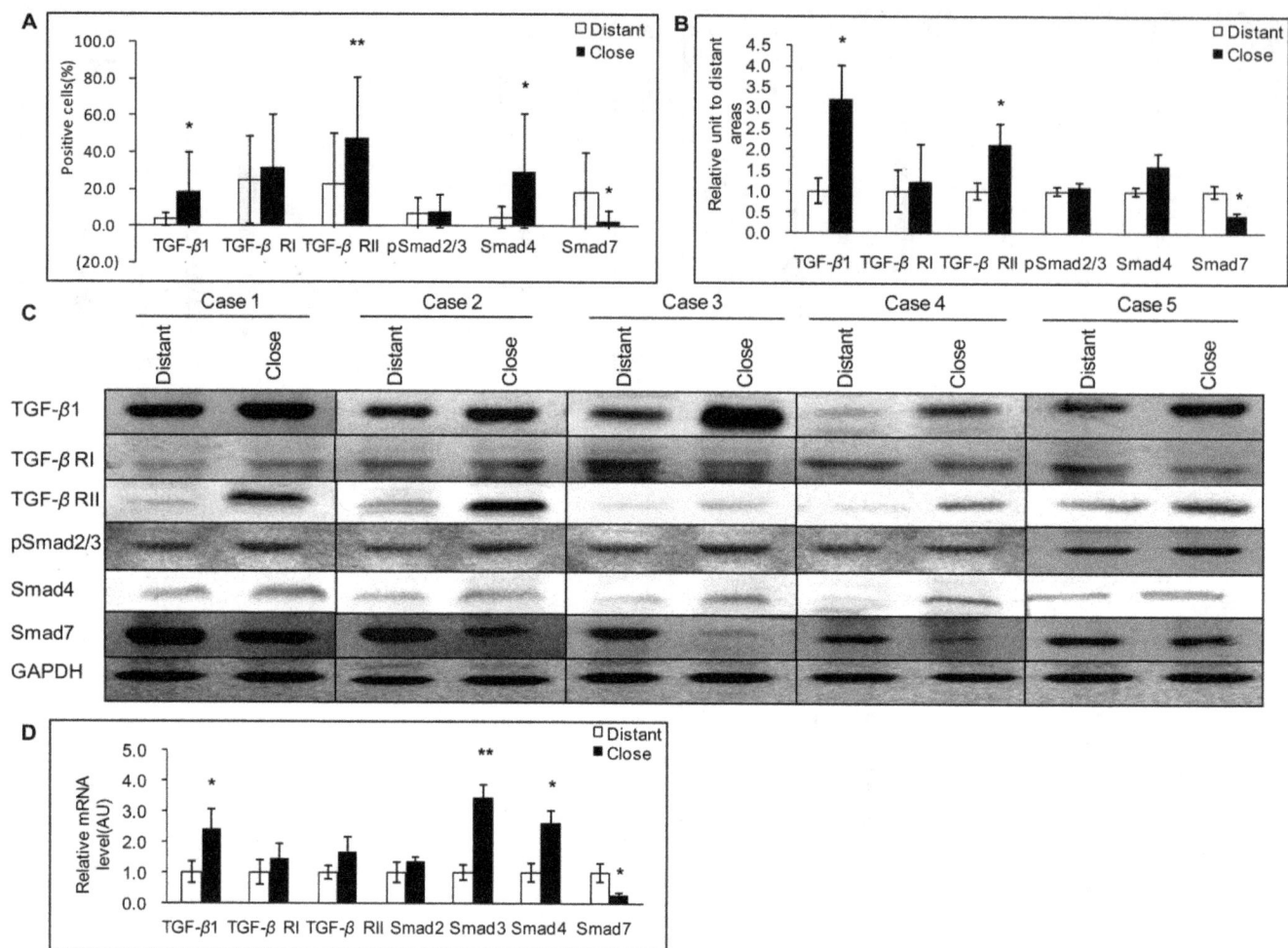

Figure 6. Expression of the various components of the TGF-β1/Smad pathway in the liver of AE patients. A: Expression of TGF-β1/ Smads calculated as the percent of positive cells to the total number of counted cells after immunostaining (see Materials and Methods section). B: Relative amount of TGF-β1/Smads calculated from semi-quantitative analysis of the Western Blot using densitometry. C: Representative examples of Western Blot analyses performed on lysates from liver samples with antibodies that recognize TGF-β1, TGF-β RI, TGF-β RII, phosphorylated (p-) Smad2/3, Smad4 and Smad7. D: TGF-β1/Smads mRNA expression measured by real time RT-PCR. *P<0.05 versus control, **P<0.01 versus control. 'Distant': distant from lesion; 'Close': close to lesion; AU: arbitrary units; GAPH: glyceraldehyde-3-phosphate dehydrogenase.

during the whole time course of *E. multilocularis* infection (Fig. 10B and C).

In AE patients, Smad7 immunostaining was mostly present in the cytoplasm of the hepatocytes, with a varying intensity throughout the liver. Opposite to the decreasing gradient from the lesions to the distant parenchyma observed with most of the other components, the expression scores of Smad7 expression were

lower in the areas close to lesions than in those distant from the lesions (Fig. 4B). Western Blot results also showed that Smad7

Table 1. Results of the correlation analysis between TGF-β1 and CD4/CD8, CD4, CD8 positive cells in murine AE (from the histo-immunochemistry analysis).

		CD4/CD8	CD4	CD8
TGF-β1	Spearman's rho	0.818*	0.639	−0.118
	Sig.	0.013	0.088	0.780
	N	8	8	8

Note: *P<0.05.

Table 2. Results of the correlation analysis between TGF-β1, Smad7 and liver fibrosis markers in murine AE (from the histo-immunochemistry analysis).

		α-SMA	Collagen I	Collagen III
TGF-β1	Spearman's rho	0.628**	0.836**	0.781**
	Sig.	0.009	P< 0.001	P< 0.001
	N	8	8	8
Smad7	Spearman's rho	−0.600	−0.853**	−0.316*
	Sig.	0.400	P< 0.001	0.684
	N	8	8	8

Note: *P<0.05,
**P<0.01.

Table 3. Results of the correlation analysis between TGF-β1, Smad7 and liver fibrosis markers in human AE (from the histo-immunochemistry analysis).

		α-SMA	Collagen I	Collagen III
TGF-β1	Spearman's rho	0.620**	0.498**	0.655**
	Sig.	0.001	0.013	0.001
	N	16	16	16
Smad7	Spearman's rho	−0.569**	−0.313	−0.463*
	Sig.	0.004	0.136	0.023
	N	16	16	16

Note: *P<0.05,
**P<0.01.

protein levels were significantly lower in the liver parenchyma close to lesions compared to that distant from lesions (Fig. 6B and C).

Correlation with T cell subpopulations and fibrosis markers. Spearman correlation coefficients indicated a negative correlation between Smad7 expression and α-SMA, Collagen I, and Collagen III expression scores which was significant for Collagen I and Collagen III (r = −0.853, P<0.01; and r = −0.316, P<0.05 respectively) in the livers from day 90 to day 360 p.i. in experimental mice under study (Table 2). There was also a negative correlation between Smad7 expression and α-SMA, Collagen I, and Collagen III expression scores, which was significant for α-SMA and Collagen III (r = −0.569, P=0.01; and r = −0.463, P=0.05, respectively) in the livers from the 16 patients with AE under study (Table 3).

mRNA expression of Smad7. In experimental mice, Smad7 mRNA expression was significantly higher in E. multilocularis-infected than in control mice at day 30 (P<0.01) (Fig. 10D).

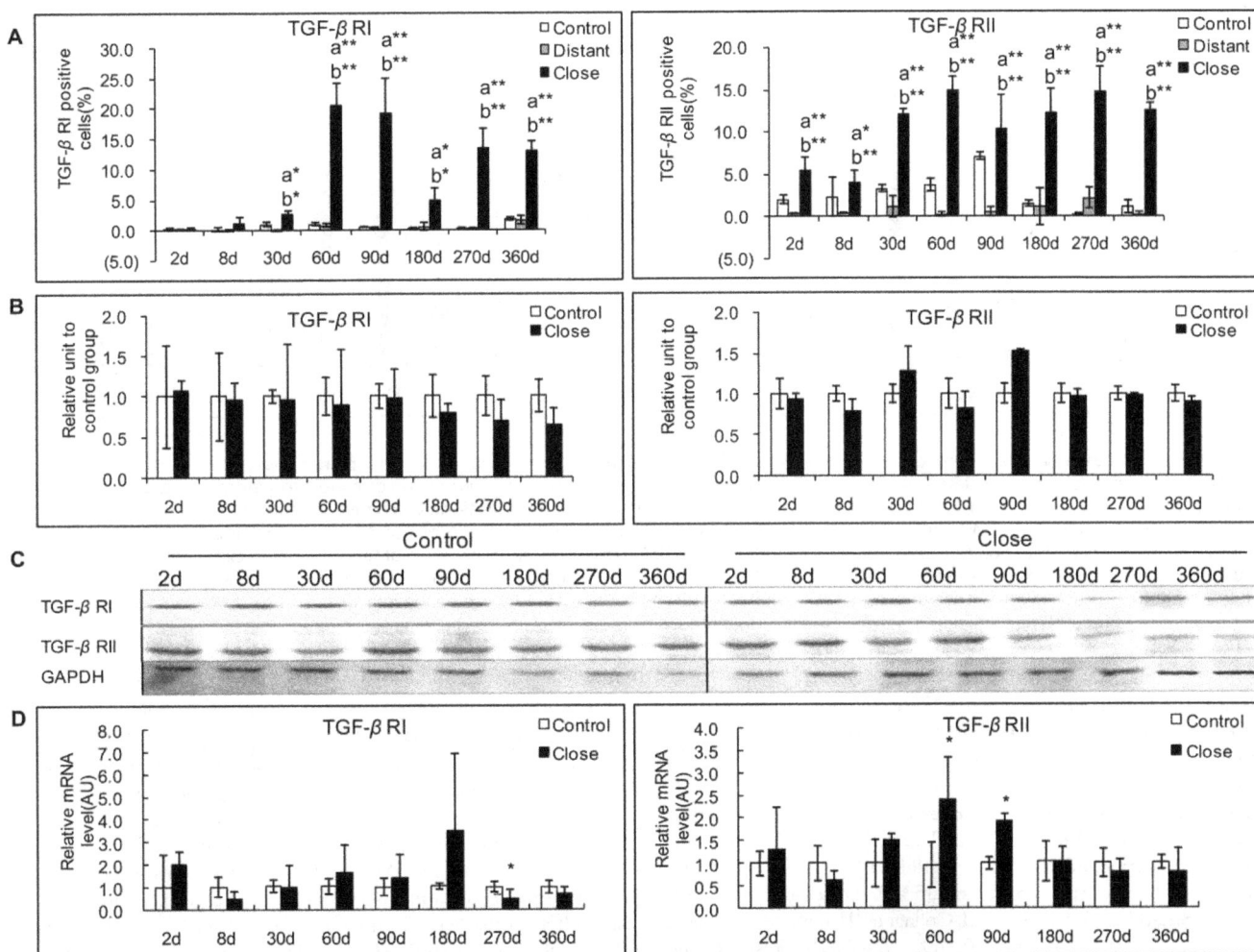

Figure 7. Course of TGF-β1 receptors (TGF-β RI and TGF-β RII) expression in the liver of mice during *E. multilocularis* infection in experimental mice. A: Course of TGF-β RI and RII expression observed by immune-staining in the liver from *E. multilocularis* infected mice compared to control mice, calculated as the percent of positive cells to the total number of counted cells (see Materials and Methods section). B: Relative amount of TGF-β RI and RII calculated from semi-quantitative analysis of the Western Blot using densitometry. C: Representative example of the course of TGF-β RI and RII protein measured by Western Blot in experimental mice. D: Course of TGF-β RI and RII mRNA expression measured by real time RT-PCR in experimental mice. a: 'close' versus 'control'; b: 'close' versus 'distant'. *P<0.05; **P<0.01. 'Control', non-infected mice; 'Lesion': *E. multilocularis* metacestode and surrounding immune infiltrate; 'Close': liver parenchyma close to *E. multilocularis* lesion; 'Distant': liver parenchyma distant from *E. multilocularis* lesion. AU: arbitrary units; GAPDH: glyceraldehyde-3-phosphate dehydrogenase.

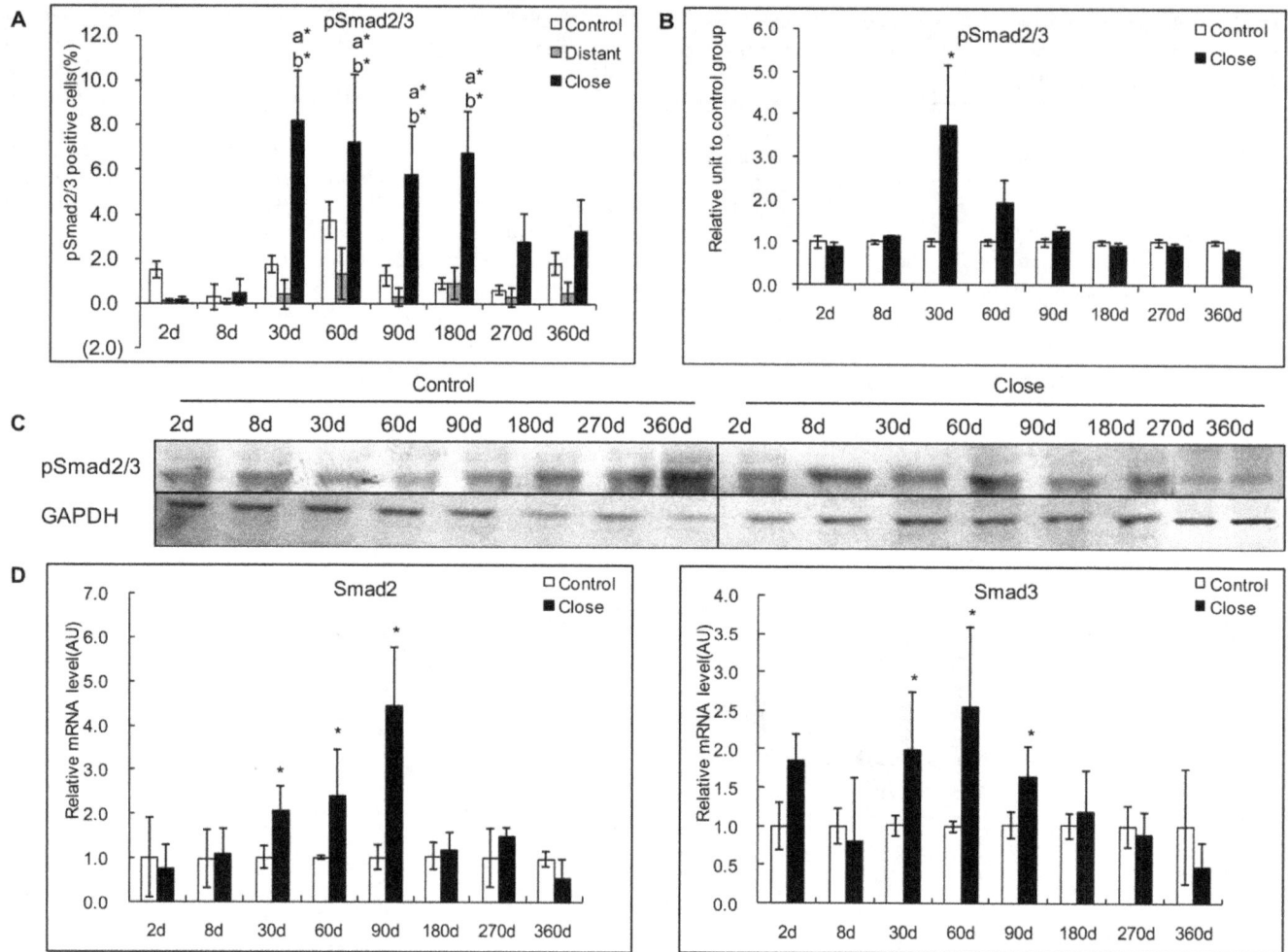

Figure 8. Course of pSmad2/3 expression in the liver of mice during *E. multilocularis* infection in experimental mice. A: Course of pSmad2/3 expression observed by immune-staining in the liver from *E. multilocularis* infected mice compared to control mice, calculated as the percent of positive cells to the total number of counted cells (see Materials and Methods section). B: Relative amount of pSmad2/3 calculated from semi-quantitative analysis of the Western blot using densitometry. C: Representative example of the course of pSmad2/3 protein measured by Western Blot in experimental mice. D: Course of Smad2 and Smad3 mRNA expression measured by real time RT-PCR in experimental mice. a: 'close' versus 'control'; b: 'close' versus 'distant'. *$P<0.05$; **$P<0.01$. 'Control', non-infected mice; 'Lesion': *E. multilocularis* metacestode and surrounding immune infiltrate; 'Close': liver parenchyma close to *E. multilocularis* lesion; 'Distant': liver parenchyma distant from *E. multilocularis* lesion. AU: arbitrary units; GAPDH: glyceraldehyde-3-phosphate dehydrogenase.

In AE patients, lower Smad7 mRNA levels close to the lesions, as measured by real-time RT-PCR, further confirmed the reverse gradient from the lesions to the periphery observed at the protein level (Fig. 6D).

Correlation with fibrosis markers. There was a significant negative correlation between Smad7 and Collagen I expression scores in experimental mice under study ($r = -0.853$, $P<0.001$) (Table 2). There was also a significant negative correlation between Smad7 and α-SMA and Collagen III expression scores ($r = -0.569$, $P=0.004$; $r = -0.463$, $P=0.023$ respectively) (Table 3) in the liver of the 16 AE patients under study.

Discussion

Despite the major potential role attributed to TGF-β in the tolerance and the fibrosis processes in AE, only one study until now reported that TGF-β was expressed in the periparasitic infiltrate in liver biopsies from a patient with AE [14]; however, quantified expression of TGF-β protein and mRNA was never

studied, and neither the presence of TGF-β receptors nor that of components of the TGF-β metabolic pathway were ever looked for in *E. multilocularis*-infected livers. In the present study, both in humans and in the longitudinal study of experimental *E. multilocularis* infection model, we confirmed that TGF-β and members of its pathway were actually present in *E. multilocularis*-infected livers (Fig. 11). We could show the expression of TGF-β in most lymphocytes and macrophages of the periparasitic infiltrate as well as in the liver parenchyma, even distant from the parasitic lesion. Phenotypic study of cells within the periparasitic granuloma also confirmed that CD4[+] T cells represented the major population of T cells at the beginning of the infection and that this sub-population was progressively replaced by CD8[+] T cells [9], and this change of CD4/CD8 ratios could contribute to maintain TGF-β1 secretion. TGF-β receptors were also expressed at the membrane of most cells in the periparasitic infiltrate and in the liver parenchyma from early to late stage post *E. multilocularis* infection. Expression of the receptors suggested that the markedly

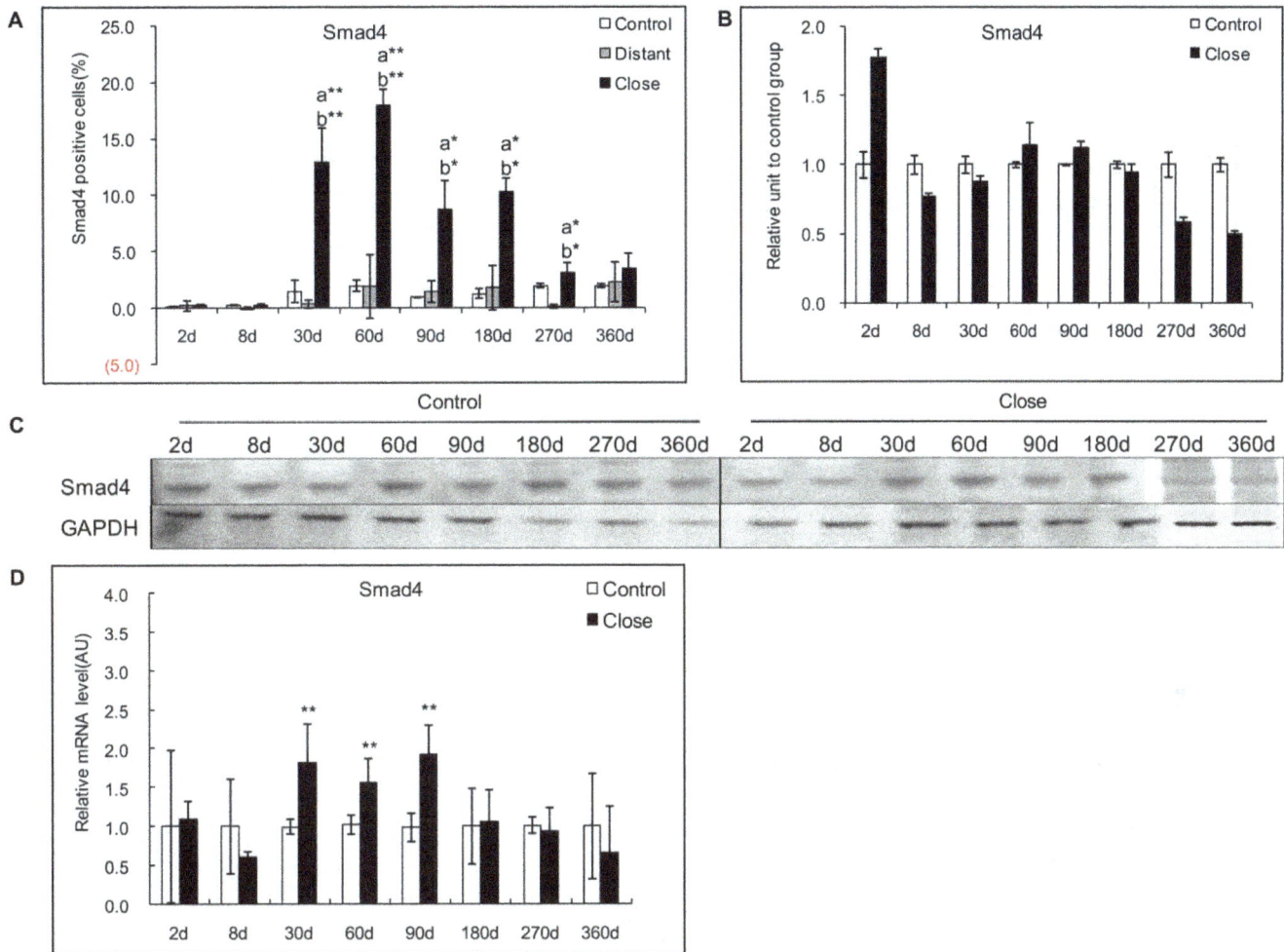

Figure 9. Course of Smad4 expression in the liver of mice during *E. multilocularis* infection in experimental mice. A: Course of Smad4 expression observed by immune-staining in the liver from *E. multilocularis* infected mice compared to control mice, calculated as the percent of positive cells to the total number of counted cells (see Materials and Methods section). B: Relative amount of Smad4 calculated from semi-quantitative analysis of the Western blot using densitometry. C: Representative example of the course of Smad4 protein measured by Western Blot in experimental mice. D: Course of Smad4 mRNA expression measured by real time RT-PCR in experimental mice. a: 'close' versus 'control'; b: 'close' versus 'distant'. *P<0.05; **P<0.01. 'Control', non-infected mice; 'Lesion': *E. multilocularis* metacestode and surrounding immune infiltrate; 'Close': liver parenchyma close to *E. multilocularis* lesion; 'Distant': liver parenchyma distant from *E. multilocularis* lesion.AU: arbitrary units; GAPDH: glyceraldehyde-3-phosphate dehydrogenase.

elevated levels of TGF-β1 present in *E. multilocularis*-infected liver, were functional to regulate the activities of immune cells as well as hepatocytes and cells involved in fibrosis. This was confirmed by the changes also observed in various Smad components of the TGF-β pathway, with usually a marked increase since the middle stage of the chronic phase of the disease in *E. multilocularis* infected mice, which suggested an activation of the Smad cascade and thus an activation of the signal transduction of TGF-β1. Expression of the receptors and of Smads and phosphorylation of Smad 2/3 in the liver of human patients with hepatic AE, with various types of gradient in the liver depending on the cascade component, confirmed the significant activation of the system at the middle/late stage of *E. multilocularis* infection.

Fibrosis is a hallmark of AE, leading to a complete disappearance of the liver parenchyma in the periparasitic area, and to fibrosis in portal spaces. Fibrosis protects the host against the parasitic growth, but at the same time it distorts the liver parenchyma, contributes to bile duct and vessel obstruction and

can lead to secondary biliary cirrhosis [5,7]. The irreversible acellular keloid scar-like fibrosis observed in AE is the ultimate result of cytotoxic and fibrogenetic events related to the immune response of the host which are taking place initially in the granulomatous area surrounding the young parasite larvae [13]. Previous observations in experimental models of AE have suggested that progression of fibrosis in AE involves an early deposition of type III collagen pro-peptide and type III collagen at the periphery of the granulomas, and a subsequent remodeling of fibrosis with bundles of type I collagen in the periparasitic central area [4]. Stellate cell–derived myofibroblasts have been observed in AE liver, both in humans [7] and in the experimental mouse model [4]. It was noted that in some regions of the liver where the parenchyma was totally replaced with dead parasitic lesions and fibrosis, HSC were the only cellular remnants present [7]. We confirmed that α-SMA, a specific cell marker for MFB, as well as type I and III collagens, were highly expressed in tissues surrounding AE lesions; the expression of collagen I increased

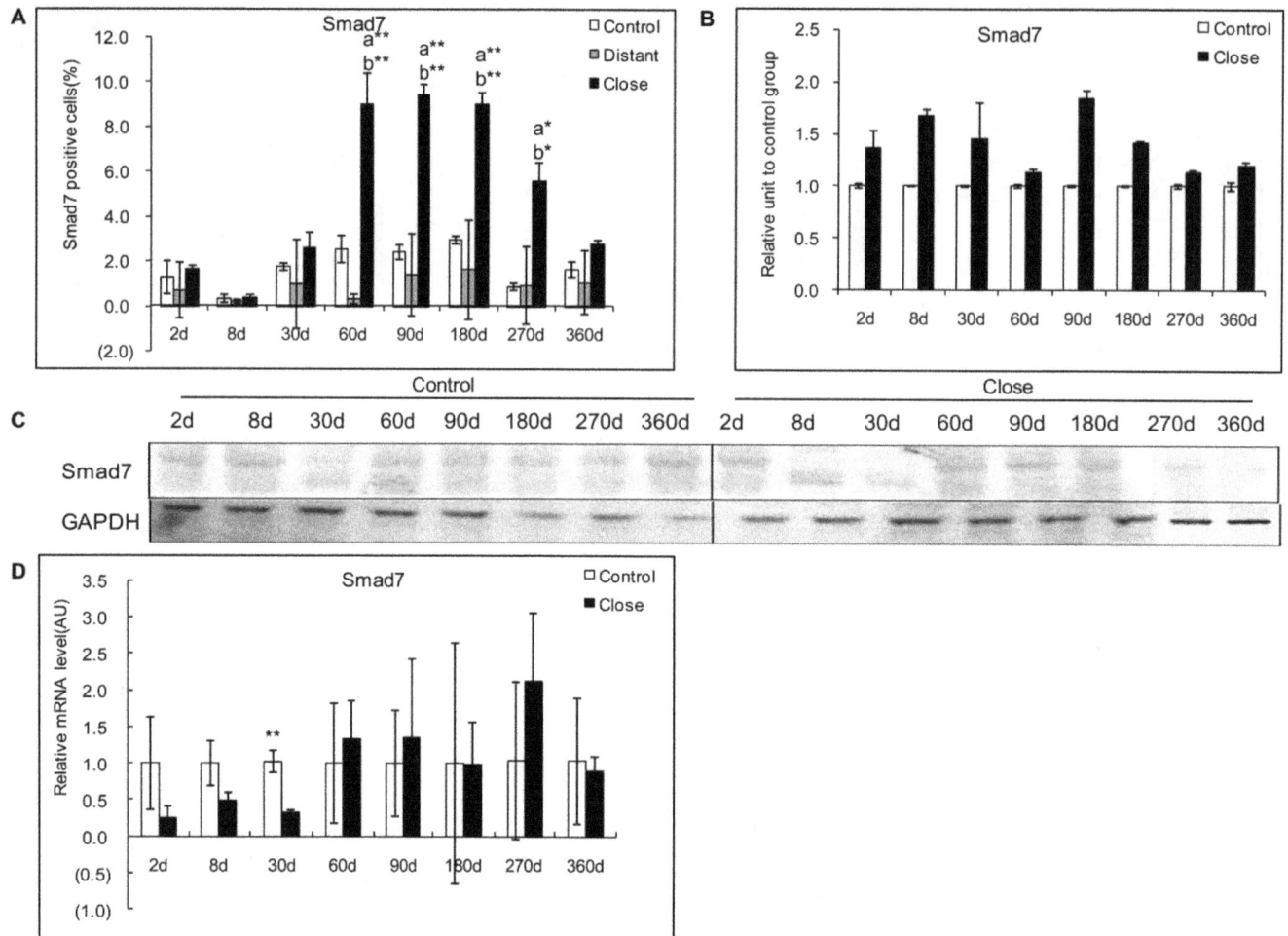

Figure 10. Course of Smad7 expression in the liver of mice during *E. multilocularis* infection in experimental mice. A: Course of Smad7 expression observed by immune-staining in the liver from *E. multilocularis* infected mice compared to control mice, calculated as the percent of positive cells to the total number of counted cells (see Materials and Methods section). B: Relative amount of Smad7 calculated from semi-quantitative analysis of the Western blot using densitometry. C: Representative example of the course of Smad7 protein measured by Western Blot in experimental mice. D: Course of Smad7 mRNA expression measured by real time RT-PCR in experimental mice. a: 'close' versus 'control'; b: 'close' versus 'distant'. *$P<0.05$; **$P<0.01$. 'Control', non-infected mice; 'Lesion': *E. multilocularis* metacestode and surrounding immune infiltrate; 'Close': liver parenchyma close to *E. multilocularis* lesion; 'Distant': liver parenchyma distant from *E. multilocularis* lesion. AU: arbitrary units; GAPDH: glyceraldehyde-3-phosphate dehydrogenase.

steadily through the course of the infection, whereas collagen III rapidly reached its maximum level of expression at day 8; this sequence of events, which is usual in fibrotic processes (collagen III being produced quickly by fibroblasts before collagen I is synthesized) was already noticed in the first studies on AE fibrosis in the experimental model; in humans, as well as in mice at later stages, location of collagen III in areas of recent larval development supported this sequence [4,7].

The positive correlation we found between their expression and expression of TGF-β1, both in the experimental model and in human livers, is an indirect argument for a significant role of this cytokine in AE fibrosis. The major peak of TGF-β1 at the middle stage of infection in experimental animals, and its expression in AE patients who are diagnosed at a similar stage, suggest that although lower levels may initiate immune tolerance as early as the early stage, the cytokine becomes prominent later, when both mainte-nance of the tolerance state and development of fibrosis are at stake (Fig. 11). Several cytokines are involved in fibrosis development [27,28]. The role of pro-inflammatory cytokines,

and especially tumor necrosis factor (TNF-α), in the protection of the host against *E. multilocularis* has been demonstrated, and it is likely that they act at least in part through the development of fibrosis [29]. In human livers with hepatic AE, the mRNAs of pro-inflammatory cytokines, interleukin (IL)-1β, IL-6, and TNF-α have been found in macrophages located at the periphery of granulo-mas, in those areas which were shown to be at the initiation of fibrogenesis [30]. IL-12, which inhibits the development of the parasitic vesicles after *E. multilocularis* infection, was also shown to induce a fast development of peri-vesicle fibrosis [31]. However, TGF-β is probably the most decisive cytokine and HSCs the most significant cells involved in liver fibrosis [32]; and the involvement of TGF-β and HSCs in the development of the fibrosis in other liver parasitic diseases, such as schistosomiasis, has been well documented [33,34]. During the development of chronic liver injury, including inflammation, fibrosis and regeneration, TGF-β1 plays a prominent role in stimulating liver fibrogenesis by MFBs derived from HSCs. TGF-β1 can be secreted by Kupffer cells, biliary cells, infiltrated inflammatory cells, and the HSC them-

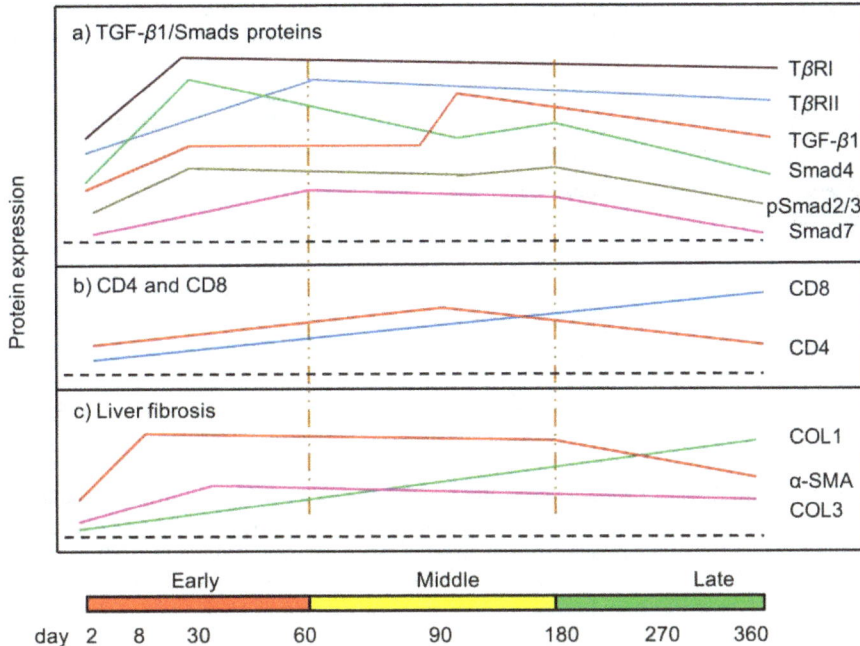

Figure 11. Course of the changes in the protein expression of TGF-β1/Smads (a), T cell subpopulation CDs (b) and liver fibrosis markers (c) during the process of *E. multilocularis*-induced liver injury in mice.

selves; it inhibits hepatocyte proliferation, induces hepatocyte apoptosis, and activates HSC to differentiate into MFBs and secrete ECM components, including collagens, acting via both paracrine and autocrine pathways; TGF-β1 also inhibits ECM degradation and enhances accumulation of ECM in the liver [35]. Our results highly suggest that TGF-β and its signaling pathway are in the position to play this major role regarding fibrosis in AE.

The Smad family of proteins mediates signaling from the TGF-β R to the nucleus. In the current study, there was an increased expression of TGF-β R, Smad3 mRNA, and especially of Smad4 which is a central mediator in TGF-β superfamily signaling [20]. A few discrepancies between RNA expression and the amount of protein regarding TGF-β R and Smads may be explain by post-transcriptional events, and deserve further studies, since such events could be caused by parasite components. On the other hand, information given by immunostaining and Western Blot analysis is different, albeit complementary, since the type and microenvironment of the producing cells may compensate

otherwise lower amounts of the protein. Our study showed that expression of Smad4 was higher in areas surrounding lesions than in distant liver in the patients with AE. Smad7, which is induced by TGF-β itself, is responsible for the fine-tuning of TGF-β signals [36]. It prevents the phosphorylation of Smad proteins, associates with ubiquitin ligases involved in TGF-β R-degradation, and acts as a transcriptional repressor inhibiting Smad-dependent promoter activation [37]. In physiological situations, its increase decreases the phosphorylation of Smad2/3, and thus decreases TGF-β functions. In chronic hepatic injury, the expression of Smad7 is paradoxically decreased [38]; as a result, TGF-β signal transduction cannot be effectively inhibited, and TGF-β functions are enhanced. An aberrant expression of Smad7 may thus disrupt the balanced activity of TGF-β under pathophysiological conditions. The low expression of Smad7 in the areas surrounding the lesions and its negative correlation with α-SMA and Collagen III highly suggest that in AE too the normal feed-back loop might not work properly, and that fibrosis might be permanently activated through

Table 4. Primers and cycling parameters of real time RT-PCR detection of TGF-β1 signaling pathway (mouse).

Gene	Genbank Accession	Primer Sequences	Annealing Temperature	Expected Size
TGF-β1	NM_011577	F:5'-GTGTGGAGCAACATGTGGAACTCTA-3' R:5'-TTGGTTCAGCCACTGCCGTA-3'	52.1°C	143 bp
TGF-β RI	NM_009370.2	F: 5'-TGCAATCAGGACCACTGCAATAA-3' R: 5'-GTGCAATGCAGACGAAGCAGA-3'	60.0°C	133 bp
TGF-β RII	NM_009371.2	F: 5'-AAATTCCCAGCTTCTGGCTCAAC-3' R: 5'-TGTGCTGTGAGACGGGCTTC-3'	60.0°C	100 bp
Smad2	NM_010754	F: 5'-AACCCGAATGTGCACCATAAGAA-3' R: 5'-GCGAGTCTTTGATGGGTTTACGA-3'	60.0°C	198 bp
Smad3	NM_016769	F: 5'-GTCAACAAGTGGTGGCGTGTG-3' R: 5'-GCAGCAAAGGCTTCTGGGATAA-3'	60.0°C	150 bp
Smad4	NM_008540	F: 5'-TGACGCCCTAACCATTTCCAG-3' R: 5'-CTGCTAAGAGCAAGGCAGCAAA-3'	60.0°C	136 bp
Smad7	NM_001042660	F: 5'-AGAGGCTGTGTTGCTGTGAATC-3' R: 5'-CCATTGGGTATCTGGAGTAAGGA-3'	60.0°C	126 bp
β-actin	NM_007393	F: 5'-AACTCCATCATGAAGTGTGA-3' R: 5'-ACTCCTGCTTGCTGATCCAC-3'	56.0°C	248 bp

Table 5. Primers and cycling parameters of real time RT-PCR detection of TGF-β1 signaling pathway (Human).

Gene	Genbank Accession	Primer Sequences	Annealing Temperature	Expected Size
TGF'-β1	A23751.1	F:5'-ACACCAACTATTGCTTCAG-3' R:5'-TGTCCAGGCTCCAAATG-3'	55.7°C	159 bp
TGF-β RI	NM_001130916	F: 5'-AATTCCTCGAGATAGGCCGT-3' R: 5'-TGCGGTTGTGGCAGATATAG-3'	60.0°C	244 bp
TGF-β RII	NM_003242.5	F: 5'-AACAACATCAACCACAACACAG-3' R: 5'-CCGTCTTCCGCTCCTCAG-3'	56.2°C	250 bp
Smad2	NM_005901.4	F: 5'-GTCTCTTGATGGTCGTCTC-3' R: 5'-GGCGGAAGTTCTGTTAGG-3'	53.3°C	249 bp
Smad3	NM_001145104.1	F: 5'-GTGCTCCATCTCCTACTAC-3' R: 5'-CCTCTTCCGATGTGTCTC-3'	56.5°C	183 bp
Smad4	BC002379.2	F: 5'-CAGGACAGCAGCAGAATG-3' R: 5'-CAATACTCAGGAGCAGGATG-3'	55.6°C	232 bp
Smad7	NM_001190823.1	F: 5'-TTTGTGTATTTATTTCTTTCTCTC-3' R: 5'-CACTCTCGTCTTCTCCTC-3'	54.5°C	194 bp
β-actin	NM_002046.3	F: 5'-GCACCGTCAAGGCTGAGAAC-3' R: 5'-TGGTGAAGACGCCAGTGGA-3'	50.8°C	138 bp

that mechanism. As TGF-β is likely to be crucial to maintain the immune tolerance state and T-reg generation/function essential to the parasite, *E. multilocularis* could be responsible for the paradoxical decrease of Smad7 in the periparasitic granuloma and nearby liver; this might be one of the mechanisms for the early induction of immune tolerance and for the progression from chronic hepatic injury to hepatic fibrosis during *E. multilocularis* infection. All results obtained in the mouse model however do not fully support an essential role for the inhibitory Smad7 feed-back loop: Smad7 was indeed high in the middle stage of *E. multilocularis* infection, and Smad7 expression negatively correlated globally with expression of collagen I and III in infected mice, but this elevation did not seem to markedly decrease pSmad2/3, and Smad4 expression; the light decrease of these components at day 90, could be an indication of its partial intervention; other mechanisms of regulation of the TGF-β pathway at that crucial stage of the disease, to maintain a high level of activity of the pathway are thus likely. In fact, TGF-β also induces other non-SMAD signaling pathways, which include activation of several MKKs (MAP kinase Kinase) and MEKs (MAPK/ERK Kinase) pathways (including JNK/SPAK, p38, and ERK1/2) through upstream mediators RhoA, Ras, TAK1 (TGF-βActivated Kinase), TAB1 (TAK1 Binding Protein); and the proteins XIAP (Xenopus Inhibitor of Apoptosis), HPK1 (Haematopoietic Progenitor Kinase-1) are also involved in this link [39]. Thus, TGF-β itself or its receptors, more than down-stream Smads, represent an attractive target for the development of therapeutics that simultaneously attack the pathogen and its micro-environment, the pleiotropic nature of TGF-β signaling, its role in tissue homeostasis and its dual role in pathogenesis present unique challenges that must be considered in pre-clinical and clinical drug development programs.

In preliminary *in vitro* studies (data not shown) we observed a secretion of TGF-β1 and an activation of the TGF-β pathway in rat hepatocyte cultures incubated with vesicle fluid of parasitic origin, in the absence of inflammatory cells, thus of immune cell-related cytokines. This is an intriguing finding which reinforces the hypothesis of a "cross-talk" between the parasitic larva and its host, already provided by a number of observations which suggested that the larval development of *E. multilocularis* is triggered by cell signaling originating from the intermediate host [40,41] and that *E. multilocularis* metacestode was thus able to "sense" host factors, which may result in an activation of the parasite metabolic pathway cascades [42]. Conversely, the parasite might also influence signaling mechanisms of host cells through the secretion of various molecules which might bind to host cell surface

receptors or to the temporary storage of host-derived molecules in the vesicle fluid. Such interactions could contribute to immuno-modulatory activities of *E. multilocularis*, to pathological consequences on the host's tissues, and/or be involved in mechanisms of organotropism [14]. In our previous study, a significant influence of *E. multilocularis* metacestode on the activation of MAPKs signalling pathways was found in the liver cells both in vivo in infected patients and in vitro in cultured rat hepatocytes [43]. A recent study has also provided evidence for the induction of apoptosis in host DC through *Echinococcus* E/S-products of early infectious stages of *E. multilocularis* [44]. These observations suggest that parasitic components, and not only factors from host origin, are actually acting on the host [44]. Further studies are, however, necessary to determine the parasite and/or host components actually involved in the activation of the TGF-β/Smad pathway.

Materials and Methods

Ethics Statement

The clinical investigation has been conducted according to the principles expressed in the Declaration of Helsinki. For research involving human participants, informed written consent has been obtained from the patients, as part of a research project approved by the Ethical Committee of First Affiliated Hospital of Xinjiang Medical University (20080812-5). The animal study was performed in strict accordance with the recommendations in the Guide for the Care and Use of Laboratory Animals. The protocol was approved by the Animal Care and Use Committee and the Ethical Committee of First Affiliated Hospital of Xinjiang Medical University (20081205-2). All surgery was performed under sodium pentobarbital anesthesia, and every effort was made to minimize suffering.

Experimental Design, Tissue Sampling and Histological Examination

Experimental animals. One hundred and twenty pathogen-free female BALB/c mice (8–10-week old) were housed in cages with a 12-h light/dark cycle and provided with rodent chow and water. BALB/c mice were infected by *E. multilocularis* and tissue samples were collected and detected as previously described [26,45]. For each autopsy time-point, ten experimentally infected mice were used in *E. multilocularis* group (n = 10) and compared with five control mice (n = 5), which received an intra-hepatic injection of 0.1 mL of saline in the anterior liver lobe using the same surgical procedure. Mice were killed at 2, 8, 30, 60, 90, 180, 270 and 360 days, respectively. Tissue samples from *E. multi-*

locularis lesions were taken and processed for histopathological examination and immunostaining. In addition, liver tissue samples were taken 1) close to the parasitic lesions, i.e. 1–2 mm from the macroscopic changes due to the metacestode/granuloma lesion, thus avoiding liver contamination with infiltrating immune cells and parasitic tissue, and 2) distant from the parasitic lesion, in another lobe of the liver, in *E. multilocularis* infected mice; in control mice, samples were taken in the injected lobe and in a non-injected lobe of the liver.

Patients. In humans, the diagnosis of *E. multilocularis* infection (AE) was based on positive serology with ELISA using crude *E. multilocularis* antigen, Antigen B, Em2 and Em18 (Xinjiang Bei Si Ming, Urumqi, China) and characteristic liver lesions observed on ultrasound- and CT scans. All diagnoses were confirmed by histological examination of the lesions [35]; tissue samples taken for diagnosis were also used for immunostaining. In addition, to measure proteins in the liver using Western Blot and mRNA using real time RT-PCR, paired liver specimens (0.5 cm3 each) were obtained at surgery by an experienced surgeon from 16 patients with AE at the First Affiliated Hospital of Xinjiang Medical University, Urumqi, China. From each patient, one specimen was taken close to the parasitic lesions (0.5 cm from the macroscopic changes due to the metacestode/granuloma lesion), and one was taken in the liver distant from the lesions (the non-diseased lobe of the liver whenever possible, or at least at 10 cm from the lesion), according to a previously described procedure [35].

Processing of tissue samples. Liver samples were separated into two parts and either deep-frozen in liquid nitrogen for RNA isolation or formalin-fixed for histopathological examination. For histological and immunohistochemical studies, the liver samples were fixed in 4% paraformaldehyde in neutral buffered formalin for a minimum of 24 h, embedded in paraffin, and cut into 4 μm serial sections. Paraffin-embedded liver tissue samples of experimental mice and AE patients were stained by Hematoxylin and Eosin (H&E) and Masson's trichrome for pathological observations.

Immunohistochemistry Analysis

Immunohistochemistry was performed on formalin-fixed, paraffin-embedded tissue. Briefly, 4 μm tissue sections were deparaffinized in xylene and rehydrated in gradual dilutions of ethanol. Endogenous peroxidase was blocked with 3% hydrogen peroxide. To increase staining, sections were pretreated by microwave heating for 15 min in antigen unmasking solution (pH 6.8, 0.1 M citrate buffer, Zhongshan Jinqiao Biology Corporation, Beijing). To block non-specific background, the sections were incubated with non-immune goat serum for 30 min. Sections were then incubated overnight at 4°C with the primary antibody diluted in pH 7.3 phosphate-buffered saline (PBS) (α-SMA 1:200, Collagen 1 (COL 1) 1:200, Collagen 3 (COL3) 1:200, CD4 1:100, CD8 1:100, TGF-β1 1:100, TGF-β receptor I (TGF-β RI) 1:200, TGF-β receptor II (TGF-β RII) 1:200, pSmad2/3 1:200, Smad4 1:200, and Smad7 1:100) (Santa Cruz Corporation, CA, USA). After 3 washes in PBS, the sections were subsequently incubated with horseradish peroxidase conjugated host-specific secondary antibodies and 3, 3′-diaminobenzidine was used as chromogen. Sections were counterstained with hematoxylin for 5 min, dehydrated, and covered with slips. For all samples, negative controls consisted of substitution of the isotype-matched primary antibody with PBS.

Western Blot Analysis

Western Blot analysis of cell lysates was performed by SDS-PAGE using NuPAGE (Invitrogen, California, USA) followed by transfer to nitrocellulose membrane (Invitrogen, California, USA). Ponceau S (Sigma, Missouri, USA) staining was used to ensure equal protein loading and electrophoretic transfer. Using the appropriate antibodies, TGF-β1, TGF-β RI, and RII, pSmad2/3, Smad4 and Smad7 (Cell Signaling Technology, Massachusetts, USA) and GAPDH (Santa Cruz Biotechnology, California, USA) were detected with WesternBreeze Kit (Invitrogen, California, USA). The expression levels of respective proteins (in "relative units") in the liver of control mice and *E. multilocularis* infected mice, as well as in the liver of AE patients, were quantified using Quantity One software (Bio-Rad, Hercules, USA).

Quantitative Real-time RT- PCR Analysis

After removing contaminated DNA from the isolated RNA using DNaseI (Fermentas, Vilnius, Lithuania), 1 μg of total RNA was reverse transcribed into cDNA in 20 mL reaction mixtures containing 200 U of Moloney murine leukemia virus reverse transcriptase (MMLV, Promega, Madison, USA); 100 ng per reaction of oligo (dT) primers; and 0.5 mM each of dNTPs, dATP, dCTP, dGTP, and dTTP. The reaction mixture was then incubated at 42°C for 1 hour and at 95°C for 5 min to deactivate the reverse transcriptase.

The real time RT-PCR was run in a thermocycler (iQ5 Bio-Rad, Hercules, CA, USA) with the SYBR Green PCR premix (TaKaRa, Dalian, China) following the manufacturer's instructions. Thermocycling was performed in a final volume of 20 μL containing 2 μL cDNA and 10 pM of each primer (Table 4 and 5). To normalize for gene expression, mRNA expression of the housekeeping gene GAPDH was measured. For every sample, both the housekeeping and the target genes were amplified in triplicate using the following cycle scheme: after initial denaturation of the samples at 95°C for 1 min, 40 cycles of 95°C for 5 s and 60°C (or other) for 30 s were performed. Fluorescence was measured in every cycle, and a melting curve was analyzed after the PCR by increasing the temperature from 55 to 95°C (0.5°C increments). A defined single peak was obtained for all amplicons, confirming the specificity of the amplification.

Expression of the Data and Statistical Analysis

Immunostaining of α-SMA, Collagen I, Collagen III, CD4 and CD8 was semi-quantified by calculating "expression scores" that consider both staining intensity and the percentage of cells stained at a specific range of intensities. A score of zero indicated the percentage of positive cells <5%, 1+ = 5–25%, 2+ = 25–50%, 3+ = 50–75%, 4+>75%. The staining intensity of each specimen was judged relative to the intensity of a control slide including an adjacent section stained with an irrelevant negative control antibody that was matched by species and isotype to the specimen. Staining of the section labeled with the negative reagent control was considered as background. A score of zero indicated no staining relative to background, 1+ = weak staining, 2+ = moderate staining, and 3+ = strong staining. According to standard pathology practice, staining intensity was reported at the highest level of intensity observed in all tissue elements, except the distinctive tissue element for which an expanded scoring scheme was reported. The "expression scores" were calculated by multiplying the percent of positive cells (0–4) and the staining intensity scores (0–3). For example: for a specimen with 30% of positive cells (3+), and a moderate staining intensity (2+), the "expression score" was 3×2 = 6. Three pathologists read the sections and established the scores, and they were blinded to each other results. Immunostaining of TGF-β1/Smads was quantified by calculating "positive cells". Cells with a positive immunostaining were counted in five random visual fields of 0.95 square mm each, at initial magnification: ×20, for each sample, and the result was expressed as the percent of positive cells to the total number of cells counted.

All the data were analyzed by SPSS 17.0. The results were presented as means ± SD. One-way ANOVA and Student's t-test were used to compare the differences between groups, and Spearman's rho was used to analyze the correlation coefficient. $P<0.05$ was considered to indicate statistical significance.

References

1. Vuitton DA, Zhou H, Bresson-Hadni S, Wang Q, Piarroux M, et al. (2003) Epidemiology of alveolar echinococcosis with particular reference to China and Europe. Parasitology 127 Suppl: S87–107.
2. Vuitton DA, Zhang SL, Yang Y, Godot V, Beurton I, et al. (2006) Survival strategy of Echinococcus multilocularis in the human host. Parasitol Int 55 Suppl: S51–55.
3. Grenard P, Bresson-Hadni S, El Alaoui S, Chevallier M, Vuitton DA, et al. (2001) Transglutaminase-mediated cross-linking is involved in the stabilization of extracellular matrix in human liver fibrosis. J Hepatol 35: 367–375.
4. Guerret S, Vuitton DA, Liance M, Pater C, Carbillet JP (1998) Echinococcus multilocularis: relationship between susceptibility/resistance and liver fibrogenesis in experimental mice. Parasitol Res 84: 657–667.
5. Ricard-Blum S, Bresson-Hadni S, Guerret S, Grenard P, Volle PJ, et al. (1996) Mechanism of collagen network stabilization in human irreversible granulomatous liver fibrosis. Gastroenterology 111: 172–182.
6. Ricard-Blum S, Bresson-Hadni S, Vuitton DA, Ville G, Grimaud JA (1992) Hydroxypyridinium collagen cross-links in human liver fibrosis: study of alveolar echinococcosis. Hepatology 15: 599–602.
7. Vuitton DA, Guerret-Stocker S, Carbillet JP, Mantion G, Miguet JP, et al. (1986) Collagen immunotyping of the hepatic fibrosis in human alveolar echinococcosis. Z Parasitenkd 72: 97–104.
8. Ouellette MJ, Dubois CM, Bergeron D, Roy R, Lambert RD (1997) TGF beta 2 in rabbit blastocoelic fluid regulates CD4 membrane expression: possible role in the success of gestation. Am J Reprod Immunol 37: 125–136.
9. Cufi S, Vazquez-Martin A, Oliveras-Ferraros C, Martin-Castillo B, Joven J, et al. (2010) Metformin against TGFbeta-induced epithelial-to-mesenchymal transition (EMT): from cancer stem cells to aging-associated fibrosis. Cell Cycle 9: 4461–4468.
10. Feng M, Wang Q, Zhang F, Lu L (2011) Ex vivo induced regulatory T cells regulate inflammatory response of Kupffer cells by TGF-beta and attenuate liver ischemia reperfusion injury. Int Immunopharmacol 12: 189–196.
11. Jetten AM, Shirley JE, Stoner G (1986) Regulation of proliferation and differentiation of respiratory tract epithelial cells by TGF beta. Exp Cell Res 167: 539–549.
12. Harraga S, Godot V, Bresson-Hadni S, Mantion G, Vuitton DA (2003) Profile of cytokine production within the periparasitic granuloma in human alveolar echinococcosis. Acta Trop 85: 231–236.
13. Vuitton DA (2003) The ambiguous role of immunity in echinococcosis: protection of the host or of the parasite? Acta Trop 85: 119–132.
14. Zhang S, Hue S, Sene D, Penfornis A, Bresson-Hadni S, et al. (2008) Expression of major histocompatibility complex class I chain-related molecule A, NKG2D, and transforming growth factor-beta in the liver of humans with alveolar echinococcosis: new actors in the tolerance to parasites? J Infect Dis 197: 1341–1349.
15. Wu XW, Peng XY, Zhang SJ, Niu JH, Sun H, et al. (2004) [Formation mechanisms of the fibrous capsule around hepatic and splenic hydatid cyst]. Zhongguo Ji Sheng Chong Xue Yu Ji Sheng Chong Bing Za Zhi 22: 1–4.
16. Mondragon-de-la-Pena C, Ramos-Solis S, Barbosa-Cisneros O, Rodriguez-Padilla C, Tavizon-Garcia P, et al. (2002) Echinococcus granulosus down regulates the hepatic expression of inflammatory cytokines IL-6 and TNF alpha in BALB/c mice. Parasite 9: 351–356.
17. Bartram U, Speer CP (2004) The role of transforming growth factor beta in lung development and disease. Chest 125: 754–765.
18. Higashiyama H, Yoshimoto D, Okamoto Y, Kikkawa H, Asano S, et al. (2007) Receptor-activated Smad localisation in bleomycin-induced pulmonary fibrosis. J Clin Pathol 60: 283–289.
19. Banas MC, Parks WT, Hudkins KL, Banas B, Holdren M, et al. (2007) Localization of TGF-beta signaling intermediates Smad2, 3, 4, and 7 in developing and mature human and mouse kidney. J Histochem Cytochem 55: 275–285.
20. Heldin CH, Miyazono K, ten Dijke P (1997) TGF-beta signalling from cell membrane to nucleus through SMAD proteins. Nature 390: 465–471.
21. Zhou L, McMahon C, Bhagat T, Alencar C, Yu Y, et al. (2010) Reduced SMAD7 leads to overactivation of TGF-beta signaling in MDS that can be reversed by a specific inhibitor of TGF-beta receptor I kinase. Cancer Res 71: 955–963.
22. Sobral LM, Montan PF, Zecchin KG, Martelli-Junior H, Vargas PA, et al. (2010) Smad7 blocks transforming growth factor-beta1-induced gingival fibroblast-myofibroblast transition via inhibitory regulation of Smad2 and connective tissue growth factor. J Periodontol 82: 642–651.
23. Kamiya Y, Miyazono K, Miyazawa K (2010) Smad7 inhibits transforming growth factor-beta family type i receptors through two distinct modes of interaction. J Biol Chem 285: 30804–30813.
24. Chen HY, Huang XR, Wang W, Li JH, Heuchel RL, et al. (2010) The protective role of Smad7 in diabetic kidney disease: mechanism and therapeutic potential. Diabetes 60: 590–601.
25. Singh P, Wig JD, Srinivasan R (2011) The Smad family and its role in pancreatic cancer. Indian J Cancer 48: 351–360.
26. Zhang C, Wang J, Lu G, Li J, Lu X, et al. (2012) Hepatocyte proliferation/growth arrest balance in the liver of mice during E. multilocularis infection: a coordinated 3-stage course. PLoS One 7: e30127.
27. Przybyszewska M, Miloszewska J, Rzonca S, Trembacz H, Pysniak K, et al. (2011) Soluble TNF-alpha receptor I encoded on plasmid vector and its application in experimental gene therapy of radiation-induced lung fibrosis. Arch Immunol Ther Exp (Warsz) 59: 315–326.
28. Maille E, Trinh NT, Prive A, Bilodeau C, Bissonnette E, et al. (2011) Regulation of normal and cystic fibrosis airway epithelial repair processes by TNF-alpha after injury. Am J Physiol Lung Cell Mol Physiol 301: L945–955.
29. Amiot F, Vuong P, Defontaines M, Pater C, Dautry F, et al. (1999) Secondary alveolar echinococcosis in lymphotoxin-alpha and tumour necrosis factor-alpha deficient mice: exacerbation of Echinococcus multilocularis larval growth is associated with cellular changes in the periparasitic granuloma. Parasite Immunol 21: 475–483.
30. Bresson-Hadni S, Petitjean O, Monnot-Jacquard B, Heyd B, Kantelip B, et al. (1994) Cellular localisations of interleukin-1 beta, interleukin-6 and tumor necrosis factor-alpha mRNA in a parasitic granulomatous disease of the liver, alveolar echinococcosis. Eur Cytokine Netw 5: 461–468.
31. Emery I, Liance M, Deriaud E, Vuitton DA, Houin R, et al. (1996) Characterization of T-cell immune responses of Echinococcus multilocularis-infected C57BL/6J mice. Parasite Immunol 18: 463–472.
32. Wallace K, Burt AD, Wright MC (2008) Liver fibrosis. Biochem J 411: 1–18.
33. Allen JT, Spiteri MA (2002) Growth factors in idiopathic pulmonary fibrosis: relative roles. Respir Res 3: 13.
34. Anthony B, Mathieson W, de Castro-Borges W, Allen J (2010) Schistosoma mansoni: egg-induced downregulation of hepatic stellate cell activation and fibrogenesis. Exp Parasitol 124: 409–420.
35. Acharya SS, Dimichele DM (2008) Rare inherited disorders of fibrinogen. Haemophilia 14: 1151–1158.
36. Itoh S, Taketomi A, Tanaka S, Harimoto N, Yamashita Y, et al. (2007) Role of growth factor receptor bound protein 7 in hepatocellular carcinoma. Mol Cancer Res 5: 667–673.
37. Schmierer B, Hill CS (2007) TGF beta-SMAD signal transduction: molecular specificity and functional flexibility. Nat Rev Mol Cell Biol 8: 970–982.
38. Del Pilar Alatorre-Carranza M, Miranda-Diaz A, Yanez-Sanchez I, Pizano-Martinez O, Hermosillo-Sandoval JM, et al. (2009) Liver fibrosis secondary to bile duct injury: correlation of Smad7 with TGF-beta and extracellular matrix proteins. BMC Gastroenterol 9: 81.
39. Moustakas A, Pardali K, Gaal A, Heldin CH (2002) Mechanisms of TGF-beta signaling in regulation of cell growth and differentiation. Immunol Lett 82: 85–91.
40. Spiliotis M, Konrad C, Gelmedin V, Tappe D, Bruckner S, et al. (2006) Characterisation of EmMPK1, an ERK-like MAP kinase from Echinococcus multilocularis which is activated in response to human epidermal growth factor. Int J Parasitol 36: 1097–1112.
41. Gelmedin V, Caballero-Gamiz R, Brehm K (2008) Characterization and inhibition of a p38-like mitogen-activated protein kinase (MAPK) from Echinococcus multilocularis: antiparasitic activities of p38 MAPK inhibitors. Biochem Pharmacol 76: 1068–1081.
42. Brehm K, Spiliotis M, Zavala-Gongora R, Konrad C, Frosch M (2006) The molecular mechanisms of larval cestode development: first steps into an unknown world. Parasitol Int 55 Suppl: S15–21.
43. Lin RY, Wang JH, Lu XM, Zhou XT, Mantion G, et al. (2009) Components of the mitogen-activated protein kinase cascade are activated in hepatic cells by Echinococcus multilocularis metacestode. World J Gastroenterol 15: 2116–2124.

Acknowledgments

We would like to thank Hui Liu, Tao Jiang and Chun Zhang for their excellent technical assistance.

Author Contributions

Conceived and designed the experiments: RL DV HW. Performed the experiments: JW CZ XW GL. Analyzed the data: RL JW DV. Contributed reagents/materials/analysis tools: OB GM XL. Wrote the paper: RL JW DV HW.

13

Human Amniotic Epithelial Cell Transplantation Induces Markers of Alternative Macrophage Activation and Reduces Established Hepatic Fibrosis

Ursula Manuelpillai[1], Dinushka Lourensz[2,5], Vijesh Vaghjiani[1], Jorge Tchongue[2,5], Derek Lacey[3], Jing-Yang Tee[1], Padma Murthi[4,6], James Chan[2], Alexander Hodge[2,5], William Sievert[2,5]*

1 Center for Reproduction and Development, Monash Institute of Medical Research, Monash University, Melbourne, Australia, 2 Center for Inflammatory Diseases, Monash University, Melbourne, Australia, 3 University of Melbourne, Arthritis and Inflammation Research Centre, Royal Melbourne Hospital, Melbourne, Australia, 4 Department of Obstetrics and Gynecology, University of Melbourne, Melbourne, Australia, 5 Gastroenterology and Hepatology Unit, Southern Health, Melbourne, Australia, 6 Pregnancy Research Center, Department of Perinatal Medicine, Royal Women's Hospital, Melbourne, Australia

Abstract

Chronic hepatic inflammation from multiple etiologies leads to a fibrogenic response that can progress to cirrhosis and liver failure. Transplantation of human amniotic epithelial cells (hAEC) from term delivered placenta has been shown to decrease mild to moderate hepatic fibrosis in a murine model. To model advanced human liver disease and assess the efficacy of hAEC therapy, we transplanted hAEC in mice with advanced hepatic fibrosis. Immunocompetent C57BL/6 mice were administered carbon tetrachloride (CCl_4) twice weekly resulting in bridging fibrosis by 12 weeks. hAEC (2×10^6) were infused via the tail vein at week 8 or weeks 8 and 10 (single and double dose, respectively). Human cells were detected in mouse liver four weeks after transplantation showing hAEC engraftment. CCl_4 treated mice receiving single or double hAEC doses showed a significant but similar decrease in liver fibrosis area associated with decreased activation of collagen-producing hepatic stellate cells and decreased hepatic protein levels of the pro-fibrogenic cytokine, transforming growth factor-beta1. CCl_4 administration caused hepatic T cell infiltration that decreased significantly following hAEC transplantation. Hepatic macrophages play a crucial role in both fibrogenesis and fibrosis resolution. Mice exposed to CCl_4 demonstrated increased numbers of hepatic macrophages compared to normal mice; the number of macrophages decreased significantly in CCl_4 treated mice given hAEC. These mice had significantly lower hepatic protein levels of the chemokine monocyte chemoattractant protein-1 than mice given CCl_4 alone. Alternatively activated M2 macrophages are associated with fibrosis resolution. CCl_4 treated mice given hAEC showed increased expression of genes associated with M2 macrophages including YM-1, IL-10 and CD206. We provide novel data showing that hAEC transplantation induces a wound healing M2 macrophage phenotype associated with reduction of established hepatic fibrosis that justifies further investigation of this potential cell-based therapy for advanced hepatic fibrosis.

Editor: Partha Mukhopadhyay, National Institutes of Health, United States of America

Funding: Australian National Health & Medical Research Council (www.nhmrc.gov.au) project grants #606473 to UM and WS and #509140 to PM and JC by program grant #436634 with support from the Victorian Government's Operational Infrastructure Support Program (http://www.business.vic.gov.au/BUSVIC/STANDARD/PC_60698.html). The funders had no role in study design, data collection and analysis, decision to publish, or preparation of the manuscript.

Competing Interests: The authors have declared that no competing interests exist.

* E-mail: william.sievert@monash.edu

Introduction

Chronic hepatic inflammation from diverse causes including alcohol, steatohepatitis, autoimmune disease and viral infection leads to a wound healing, pro-fibrogenic response. In some patients with ongoing liver injury, this response can progress to cirrhosis, portal hypertension and liver failure [1]. These outcomes are associated with a significant mortality rate for which liver transplantation is the only curative therapy [2,3]. However, low donor numbers, high procedural costs and the requirement for life-long immunosuppression limit the number of patients who undergo transplantation and consequently alternative therapies have been sought. Among these, the transplantation of hematopoietic and mesenchymal stem cells derived from adult bone marrow and placenta have shown beneficial effects in animal models of hepatic fibrosis [4,5,6,7] leading to

early phase clinical trials using autologous bone marrow derived cells [8,9,10,11]. Most of the clinical trials have been small, often with less than ten patients, and uncontrolled but have shown short-term clinical benefits [12]. Recently, we have shown that transplantation of placenta derived human amniotic epithelial cells (hAEC) into immunocompetent mice with carbon tetrachloride (CCl_4) induced liver fibrosis can constrain hepatic fibrogenesis [13]. This outcome may be related to several factors linked to hAEC transplantation including reduction in the expression of pro-inflammatory and pro-fibrogenic cytokines coupled with the induction of matrix metalloproteinases to promote a collagen-degrading environment [13].

During pregnancy, hAEC form a monolayer lining the inner of two membranes retaining the amniotic fluid surrounding the fetus. Unlike adult bone marrow derived stem cells, hAEC are highly abundant and easily harvested from term delivered amnion membranes typically yielding over 150×10^6 cells/membrane and thereby minimizing the need for expensive and time consuming cell expansion [14]. hAEC are derived from embryonic epiblast cells prior to gastrulation and possess some features of their founder pluripotent stem cells including the ability to differentiate into multiple lineages derived from the primary germ layers [14,15]. Importantly, like other fetal-derived placental cells that evade maternal immune recognition and secrete factors known to dampen maternal immune responses against the fetal semi-allograft, hAEC have also been shown to have low immunogenicity and the capacity to modulate innate and adaptive immune cell responses [14,16,17]. Collectively, these features make hAEC an attractive source of cells for potential therapeutic applications.

While we have shown ameliorative effects of hAEC transplantation on hepatic fibrosis, our study and others investigating stem cells were carried out predominantly in models of acute or short-term inflammation in which primarily mild fibrosis was evident [5,6,13]. Therefore, the effects of cellular therapy in models of chronic inflammation with well established fibrosis, which better reflect the clinical problem of advanced liver disease and cirrhosis, remain uncertain. Furthermore, there is no data on the efficacy of an additional cell dose or the generation of antibodies against the transplanted cells which may influence the timing and donor selection for subsequent treatments. Thus, using mice chronically injured with long-term CCl_4 treatment, we investigated the efficacy of a single versus double hAEC dose and the effect of transplanted hAEC on host T cells and anti-hAEC antibody generation. In order to gain an understanding of potential anti-fibrotic mechanisms, we studied the effects of hAEC transplantation on hepatic macrophages that play a pivotal role in mediating fibrogenesis and fibrosis resolution [18,19].

Materials and Methods

Ethics Statement

The study was approved by the Southern Health and Royal Women's Hospital Human Research Ethics Committees and Monash University and University of Melbourne Institutional Review Boards. Informed, written consent was obtained from healthy women with a normal singleton pregnancy prior to elective cesarean section at term (37–40 weeks gestation; n = 16). Six week old male C57BL/6 mice were purchased from Monash Animal Services, Melbourne, Australia. Experimentation on C57BL/6 mice was approved by the Animal Ethics Committee, Monash University (approval number MMCB 2008/17).

Isolation of hAEC

hAEC were isolated from amnion membranes and purity assessed as described previously [20]. Briefly, amnion membranes were cut into small pieces and digested twice in 0.05% trypsin:EDTA (Gibco, Grand Island, NY) for 40 min at 37°C. Following inactivation of trypsin with newborn calf serum, dispersed cells were washed in DMEM/F12 medium (Gibco) and erythrocytes lysed in hypotonic solution. Batches ≥99% positive for the epithelial markers cytokeratin-7 and 8/18 (Dako, Glostrup, Denmark) by flow cytometry and displaying a cobblestone epithelial morphology in culture [21], were transplanted into C57BL/6 mice (Figure S1).

hAEC-splenocyte Co-culture

hAEC have been shown to suppress T cell proliferation in hAEC-splenocyte co-culture assays [17,22]. To explore whether apoptosis played a role, hAEC were co-cultured with murine splenocytes stimulated with the mitogen Concanavalin A. The CD45+/CD3+/Annexin V+ cell population was determined by flow cytometry. Primary antibodies were linked to PE, Cy7 and FITC (BD Biosciences) and diluted 1:200, 1:50 and 1:20, respectively.

Murine Hepatic Stellate Cell (HSC) Isolation and Atreatment

HSC were isolated as described previously [23]. Briefly livers were perfused and digested with collagenase and pronase. HSC were isolated by Nycodenz density gradient centrifugation and purity was determined by vitamin A autofluorescence. To examine the effects of factors secreted by hAEC on transforming growth factor beta-1 (TGFβ-1) and collagen, murine HSC were grown in 24 well plates and stimulated with 25% hAEC conditioned media for 48 h. TGFβ-1 was measured by ELISA and collagen synthesis by the ^{3}H-proline incorporation assay. HSC were washed, incubated on ice with trichloroacetic acid and sodium hydroxide added. Equal volumes of lysate and hydrochloric acid were added to 10 parts scintillation fluid and the beta emission was measured.

Induction of Hepatic Fibrosis and hAEC Transplantation

Intraperitoneal injections of CCl_4 (Merck, Darmstadt, Germany; 1 µl/g body weight diluted 1:10 in olive oil) were administered to mice twice weekly for 12 weeks. hAEC (2×10^6) were injected via the tail vein at week 8 (single dose group) or at weeks 8 and 10 (double dose group) of CCl_4 treatment. The number of hAEC infused was based on previous experiments to identify the optimal dose [13]. Control groups consisted of mice given CCl_4 only and healthy, untreated mice. Each cohort consisted of n = 8 mice. The animals were culled at 12 weeks and blood and liver tissue collected.

Detection of Anti-hAEC Antibodies in Murine Serum

hAEC (2×10^6; n = 4) were injected into healthy C57BL/6 mice (n = 4) and blood collected two weeks later (single cell dose group). Cell injection was repeated immediately after the first blood collection and blood collected again after a further two weeks (double cell dose group). To determine if there were anti-hAEC antibodies, the murine serum was diluted 1:100 and mixed with suspensions of the same batches of hAEC that had been injected previously. The hAEC and serum were incubated for 30 min to enable anti-hAEC antibodies present in the murine serum to bind to the cells. Following three washes, the hAEC were incubated for 30 min with rabbit anti-mouse AlexaFluro-488 secondary antibody (1:100; Molecular Probes, Eugene, OR). Cells were washed thoroughly and analysed by flow cytometry. hAEC alone and cells incubated with serum from healthy, non-injected mice served as negative controls.

Immunohistochemistry

Mouse liver tissue was fixed in 10% neutral buffered formalin. Paraffin sections, 4 µm in thickness were dewaxed and rehydrated. hAEC present in the liver were identified by detecting human inner mitochondrial membrane (IMM; 1:100; Millipore, Billerica, MA) protein and human leukocyte antigen (HLA)-G (1:50; BD Biosciences, San Jose, CA) on serial sections following antigen retrieval in 0.01 M citrate buffer [13]. To examine if hAEC in the liver displayed features of mature hepatocytes, serial sections were stained for human albumin (1:5000; Abcam, Cambridge, UK) and hepatic nuclear factor 4 alpha (HNF4α; 1:150; Cell Signalling Technology, Danvers, MA) after antigen retrieval in citrate buffer. Hepatic macrophages were identified by staining with F4/80 (1:250; a gift from Dr Richard Kitching, Monash University); T cells with biotinylated CD3 (1:200; BD Biosciences), CD4 and CD8 (1:100 and 1:50, respectively; from Dr R Kitching) and activated HSC or myofibroblasts using α-smooth muscle actin (α-SMA; 1:5000; Sigma-Aldrich, St Louis, MO).

Briefly, endogenous peroxidase activity was quenched by adding 0.3–3% H_2O_2 (IMM, HLA-G, F4/80, albumin, CD4, CD8, HNF4α) or peroxidase block (Dako; α-SMA, CD3). Non-specific binding was minimized with CAS protein blocking solution (Invitrogen, Camarillo, CA). Primary antibodies were incubated at room temperature for 30 min (α-SMA) or overnight at 4°C. Primary antibodies were either omitted from negative controls (F4/80, albumin, HNF4α) or incubated with isotype matched IgG (α-SMA) or pre-immune serum (IMM, HLA-G, CD3, CD4, CD8). After several washes sections were incubated with biotinylated rabbit anti-mouse IgG2a (Invitrogen; 1:300; α-SMA, IMM, HLA-G, CD3), goat anti-rabbit IgG (Vector Laboratories, Burlingame, CA; 1:200; albumin, HNF4α) or rabbit anti-rat IgG (Dako; 1:150; F4/80, CD4, CD8). Antibody binding was detected using ABC kit reagents (Vector Laboratories) followed by DAB chromogen (Sigma-Aldrich). Slides were lightly counterstained with hematoxylin and mounted in DPX.

Picrosirius Red Staining and Computer-assisted Morphometry

To identify the extent of histological fibrosis, 4 μm thick deparaffinized liver sections were stained as previously described [13]. Briefly, sections were incubated in picrosirius red (Sigma-Aldrich; Direct Red 80, 0.1% wt/vol in saturated picric acid) for 90 min and washed with acetic acid and water (1:200). Fifteen non-overlapping fields were acquired, images digitized and fibrosis area measured by computer-assisted morphometry using Scion Image for Windows (vAlpha 4.0.3.2, Scion Corporation, Frederick, MD).

Enzyme-linked Immunosorbent Assays (ELISA)

The concentrations of TGFβ-1, fractalkine (CX3CL1) and monocyte chemoattractant protein-1 (MCP-1) in liver tissue were measured by ELISA. Snap frozen liver tissue (~150 mg) was homogenized in lysis buffer (50 mM Tris-HCl, 150 mM NaCl, 1 mM EDTA, 1% Triton X-100, 0.5% Tween-20, 0.1% SDS) containing a protease inhibitor cocktail (Roche, Mannheim, Germany). Lysates were sonicated and centrifuged at 14,000 g for 15 min at 4°C and supernatants collected. For TGFβ-1 measurement samples were activated with acetic acid/urea. ELISA plates were coated with antibodies against murine TGFβ-1 and CX3CL1 (R&D Systems, Minneapolis, MN) and murine MCP-1 (BD Pharmingen, San Diego, CA). Tissue lysates or media from murine HSC cultures were added and plates incubated for 2 h at room temperature. After several washes detection reagents were added and absorbencies read on a microplate reader (Magellan, Tecan, Austria). The concentrations were calculated from the standard curve generated by the plate reader software. The data was normalized against total protein concentrations that were measured using the BCA assay (Thermo Scientific, Rockford, IL).

Real Time Quantitative Polymerase Chain Reaction (RT-qPCR)

The expression of M1 and M2 associated macrophage genes and matrix metalloproteinase (MMP) genes was studied by RT-qPCR. Total RNA was isolated from snap frozen liver tissue using

the RNeasy mini kit (Qiagen, Hilden, Germany). RNA was converted to cDNA using the High-Capacity Reverse Transcription Kit (Applied Biosystems, Foster City, CA) and amplified using Power Sybr Green (Applied Biosystems, Warrington, UK) on a Rotor Gene 3000 light cycler (Qiagen, Sydney, Australia). The nucleotide sequences of primers used in the PCR are listed in Table 1. Samples were denatured at 95°C for 15 sec and annealed/extended at 60°C for 1 min for 40 cycles. Data was normalized to GAPDH and fold change calculated by the $^{\Delta\Delta}CT$ method using healthy mice as the calibrator.

Statistical Analysis

Data were analysed by one-way ANOVA with Tukey's post hoc test for multiple comparisons. Planned comparisons of numbers of hAEC engrafted in the liver following a single and double dose were analysed by Student's t test. Analyses were carried out using GraphPad Prism software (v5.0d for Mac OS X, San Diego, CA). $P<0.05$ was considered to be statistically significant. Data are shown as mean±SEM.

Results

Histological Liver Fibrosis Increases Over Time Following CCl_4 Administration

The extent of histological fibrosis was determined in picrosirius red-stained liver tissue sections. Twice weekly intraperitoneal administration of CCl_4 to wild type C57BL/6 mice over a period of 4–12 weeks resulted in a progressive increase in histological fibrosis. Minimal fibrosis was seen at 4 weeks while there was clear evidence of bridging fibrosis at 12 weeks (Figure S2A). Fibrosis area, determined by computer-assisted morphometry, increased by nearly 50% from 4 to 8 weeks of CCl_4 treatment (mean values of 2.07% and 3.01% at 4 and 8 weeks, respectively) and to 3.9 and 4.25% fibrosis area by weeks 10 and 12, respectively ($P<0.05$ vs 4 weeks; Figure S2B). Based on these findings, hAEC were transplanted at week 8 of CCl_4 administration to test the antifibrotic efficacy of a single dose. To test the effect of a second dose in advanced fibrosis, hAEC were injected into a separate group of mice at week 8 and again at week 10. CCl_4 administration continued until week 12, when both treated and control animals were culled.

hAEC Engraft in Mouse Liver and Decrease CCl_4-induced T Cell Infiltration

Intravenously infused hAEC were detected in liver tissue by immunohistochemistry for IMM protein and HLA-G. Intact, positively stained cells for both human markers were identified in serial tissue sections of animals given single and double hAEC doses (Figure 1A). hAEC were scattered throughout the hepatic acinus but were found predominantly in zone 1. These findings confirm that the infused hAEC had migrated, engrafted and remained in the injured liver for 2 to 4 weeks following cell transplantation. The number of IMM and HLA-G positive cells present in the liver increased with the second injection (mean ± SEM/high power microscopic field = 3.03±0.41 and 4.83±0.52 for single and double doses, respectively; $P<0.05$). Infused hAEC express several hepatocyte specific genes including albumin but lack HNF4α, a key transcription factor present in mature hepatocytes [24]. Engrafted hAEC (HLA-G+ cells) were albumin positive and some were HNF4α+ (Figure S3), suggesting that some of the engrafted hAEC had differentiated into mature hepatocyte-like cells in the liver.

Given the presence of hAEC in mouse liver, we next determined whether there was an effect on T cells that could

Table 1. Primers used to analyze expression of M1 and M2 macrophage genes and MMP.

Gene	Forward 5′→3′	Reverse 5′→3′
M1		
CCL17	CGAGAGTGCTGCCTGGATTACT	GGTCTGCACAGATGAGCTTGCC
CCL5	CCTGCTGCTTTGCCTACCTCTC	ACACACTTGGCGGTTCCTTCGA
IL-12b	CTCAGAAGCTAACCATCTCCTGG	CACAGGTGAGGTTCACTGTTTC
M2		
Cnrip-1	CGGCATCTATGACACAGAAGGTG	GGCAATGGTCTCGCTTGTGGTA
CD206	GTTCACCTGGAGTGATGGTTCTC	AGGACATGCCAGGGTCACCTTT
IL-10	CGGGAAGACAATAACTGCACCC	CGGTTAGCAGTATGTTGTCCAGC
YM-1	CCAGCATATGGGCATACCTT	AGACCTCAGTGGCTCCTTCA
Arg-1	CATTGGCTTGCGAGACGTAGAC	GCTGAAGGTCTCTTCCATCACC
Cadm-1	ACTTCTGCCAGCTCTACACGGA	CCCTTCAACTGCCGTGTCTTTC
CD36	GGACATTGAGATTCTTTCCTCTG	GCAAAGGCATTGGCTGGAAGAAC
MMP		
MMP-9	CTGGACAGCCAGACACTAAAG	CTCGCGGCAAGTCTTCAGAG
MMP-12	CATGAAGCGTGAGGATGTAGAC	TGGGCTAGTGTACCACCTTTG
Housekeeping		
GAPDH	TGTTCCTACCCCCAATGTGT	TGTGAGGGAGATGCTCAGTG

contribute to hepatic inflammation and to cell mediated rejection of the engrafted hAEC. We found an increase in hepatic CD3 positive T cells with CCl_4 treatment, consistent with reports of elevated T cell numbers in liver inflammation and fibrosis [25], (Figure 1B). Interestingly, subsequent to the single and double hAEC doses, the number of CD3 positive cells was reduced ($P<0.05$ and 0.01 for CCl_4 vs single and double doses, respectively). Dense cellular infiltration typically seen in cell-mediated graft rejection was not observed in the liver sections. Analysis of T cell sub-populations showed that the number of CD4+ cells remained unaltered whereas CD8+ cells were lower in hAEC treated mice ($P<0.05$ for CCl_4 vs single dose; Figure 1B and Figure S4). We explored if hAEC induced apoptosis contributed to the overall reduction in T cell numbers. However, the CD45+/CD3+/annexin V+ population remained unaltered when murine splenocytes were co-cultured with hAEC (data not shown).

Transplanted hAEC Elicit an Antibody Response

In separate experiments, we examined whether a humoral response with murine anti-hAEC antibodies was generated against the transplanted cells by analysing sera collected two weeks after healthy mice were given single and double hAEC doses. Similar levels of anti-hAEC antibodies were present in mice given single and double cell doses as shown by the mean fluorescence intensities of antibody bound hAEC analysed by flow cytometry (172.6 ± 51.1 and 226.8 ± 46 for single and double doses, respectively; $P=0.46$, Figure 1C), indicating that a second hAEC infusion did not lead to further increases in circulating anti-hAEC antibodies.

hAEC Transplantation Reduces Established Hepatic Fibrosis in CCl_4 Treated Mice

Given the evidence of a humoral immune response against hAEC, we then examined whether the cells would be effective in reducing established hepatic fibrosis. Computer-assisted

morphometry of picrosirius red-stained liver sections showed significantly less fibrosis area in CCl_4-treated mice given hAEC compared to mice given CCl_4 alone ($P<0.05$; Figure 2A). There was no further reduction in animals receiving a second hAEC dose. HSC are the principal collagen producing cell in the liver and when activated to a myofibroblast phenotype show increased expression of α-SMA. Mice given CCl_4 plus hAEC showed fewer activated HSC compared to those given CCl_4 alone ($P<0.01$; Figure 2B) with further reduction seen in mice receiving the double hAEC dose ($P<0.001$ compared to mice given CCl_4 only). TGFβ-1 drives HSC activation and is thought to be the most potent pro-fibrogenic cytokine in the liver [26]. We measured TGFβ-1 protein in liver tissue lysates and found that mice given CCl_4 plus hAEC had significantly less TGFβ-1 compared to mice given CCl_4 alone ($P<0.01$; Figure 2C). TGFβ-1 levels declined further in mice treated with a double hAEC dose ($P<0.001$ compared to mice given CCl_4 alone). We then explored if hAEC secreted factors acting directly on HSC could contribute to the reduction in hepatic fibrosis and TGFβ-1. Murine HSC were stimulated with media conditioned by hAEC. TGFβ-1 output and collagen synthesis declined significantly in the treated cultures ($P=0.016$ and 0.003, respectively; Figure 2D).

hAEC Transplantation Reduces Hepatic Macrophage Numbers and Induces an M2 Phenotype

Macrophages play a pivotal role in hepatic fibrogenesis as well as fibrosis resolution depending on their phenotype and local environment [27,28]. Previous studies have reported a large influx of bone marrow derived F4/80 positive monocytes in response to elevated levels of hepatic chemokines such as MCP-1 and fractalkine following injection of toxins such as CCl_4 [25,29,30]. Consistent with these studies, the number of F4/80 positive macrophages was elevated in CCl_4 treated animals compared to healthy mice ($P<0.001$; Figure 3A). However, the number of F4/80 positive cells was significantly lower in mice treated with hAEC

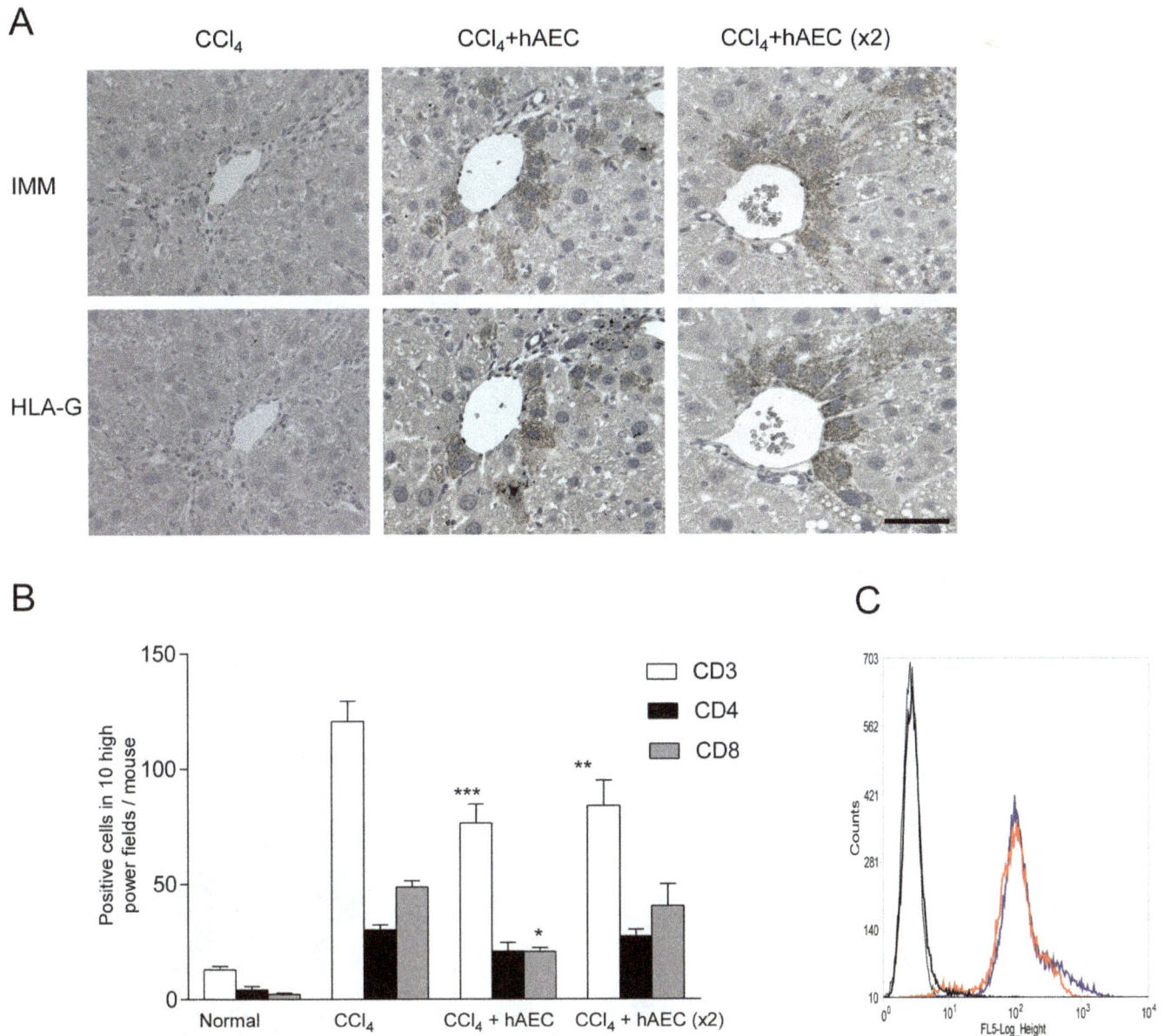

Figure 1. Engraftment of human amniotic epithelial cells (hAEC) in the liver and immune surveillance. A single or double hAEC dose was infused intravenously into C57BL/6 mice with established fibrosis induced by prolonged carbon tetrachloride (CCl₄) treatment. Engrafted hAEC were identified by immunohistochemistry for human inner mitochondrial membrane (IMM) protein and HLA-G on serial tissue sections (A). The numbers of CD3 and CD8 positive T cells in the liver were significantly lower in mice treated with hAEC (B). Serum from mice injected with hAEC contained anti-hAEC antibodies that bound to hAEC and were detected by flow cytometry. Red and blue lines on the representative flow plot shown correspond to single and double hAEC infusions, respectively. Controls (grey lines) consisted of hAEC alone or hAEC reacted with serum from non-injected mice (C). Scale bar $=50$ μm (IMM/HLA-G). *, ** and *** = $P<0.05$, 0.01 and 0.001, respectively.

($P<0.001$ and 0.05 for single and double doses, respectively). To explore potential mechanisms that could lead to a reduction in macrophage numbers, we measured MCP-1 protein in mouse liver tissue lysates and found less MCP-1 in mice treated with hAEC ($P<0.05$ vs. CCl₄ treated animals; Figure 3B). In contrast, hepatic fractalkine protein levels increased in mice treated with hAEC ($P<0.01$ and 0.001 for single and double hAEC doses, respectively).

The polarization of macrophages to a M2 alternatively activated phenotype is associated with hepatic wound healing [30]. We therefore examined the phenotype of the hepatic macrophage population by determining gene expression of known macrophage associated markers in whole liver extracts. We found that CCl₄-treated mice which had been infused with hAEC had increased mRNA expression of M2 associated markers YM-1 ($P<0.05$), CD206 and IL-10 ($P<0.01$; Figure 4A) compared with mice given CCl₄ alone. Cnrip-1 expression also increased in hAEC treated mice but did not reach significance while Arg-1 and Cadm-1 mRNA expression remained unaltered. We also examined the expression of classically activated M1 macrophages that have been linked to fibrosis progression [30]. We found no change in the expression of M1 associated markers CCL17 and CCL5 in hAEC treated mice compared with mice given CCl₄ alone (Figure 4B). We also examined the ratio of IL-12b mRNA, which

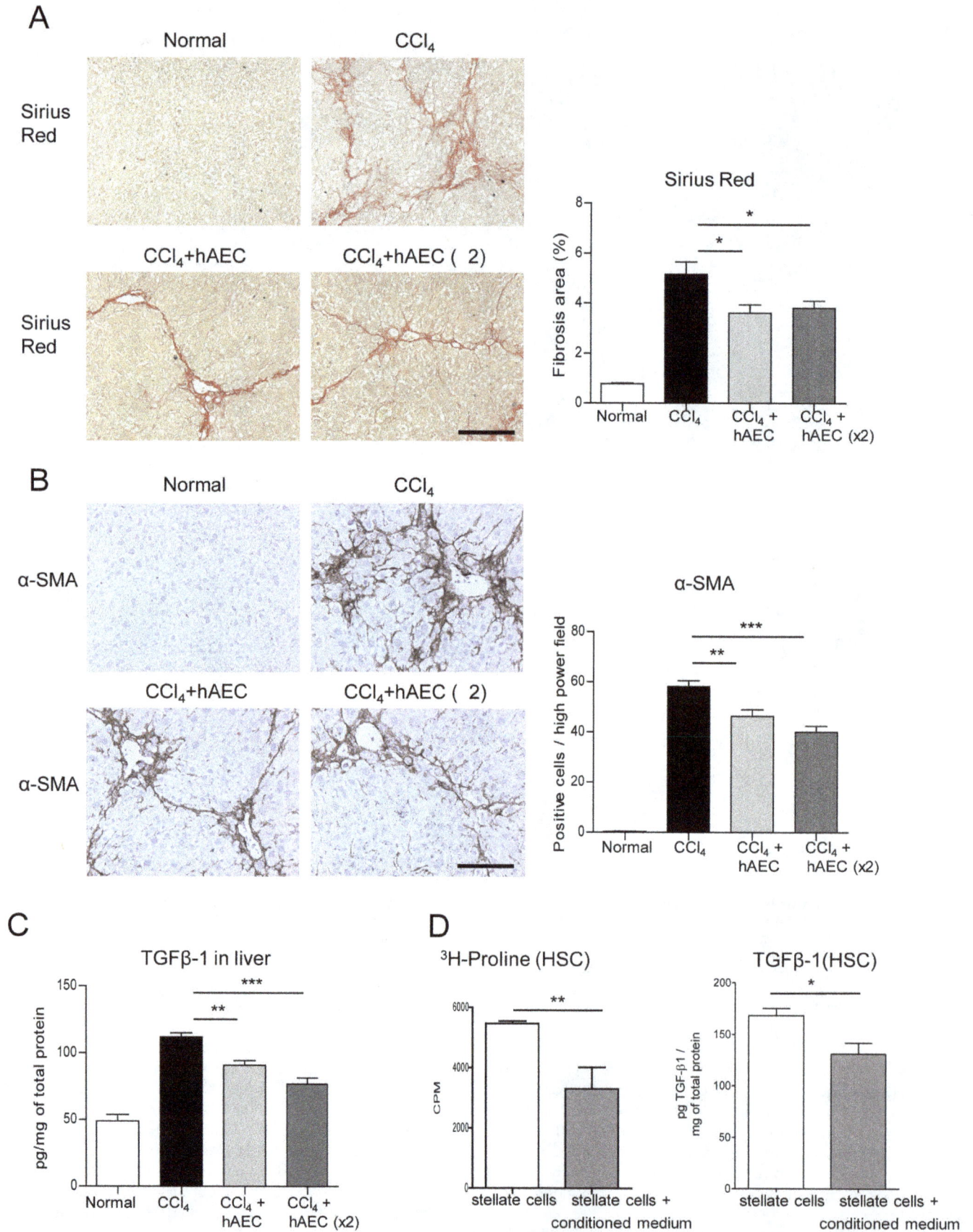

Figure 2. Human amniotic epithelial cell transplantation reduces established fibrosis. Sirius red staining of collagen and α-smooth muscle actin (α-SMA) immunohistochemistry of activated hepatic stellate cells (HSC) and quantitation are shown. C57BL/6 mice with established fibrosis

induced by prolonged carbon tetrachloride (CCl_4) administration were given a single or double hAEC dose. The hAEC-treated mice had significantly reduced fibrosis area (A) and numbers of activated HSC (B). The concentrations of the main pro-fibrogenic cytokine TGFβ-1 in the liver was measured by ELISA and found to be significantly lower in hAEC-treated mice (C). Murine HSC were treated with hAEC conditioned medium. TGFβ-1 and collagen synthesis declined significantly in HSC exposed to conditioned medium (D). Scale bars = 100 µm. *, ** and *** P<0.05, 0.01 and 0.001, respectively.

is expressed by M1 macrophages [31], to IL-10 mRNA to determine whether the macrophage phenotype was skewed towards M1 or M2. hAEC treated mice had increased IL-10 mRNA expression and a significant decrease in the IL-12b:IL-10 ratio consistent with skewing towards M2 macrophages (P<0.001 and <0.05 for single and double doses respectively; Figure 4C). Macrophages express MMP-9 and MMP-12, which are important regulators of fibrolysis [27,31]. MMP-9 expression

was elevated while MMP-12 decreased in hAEC treated mice (P<0.05; Figure 4C).

Discussion

In this study we have shown that intravenously delivered human AEC engraft in injured livers of immunocompetent mice and lead to significant changes in hepatic macrophage numbers and phenotype and significantly reduce the extent of established

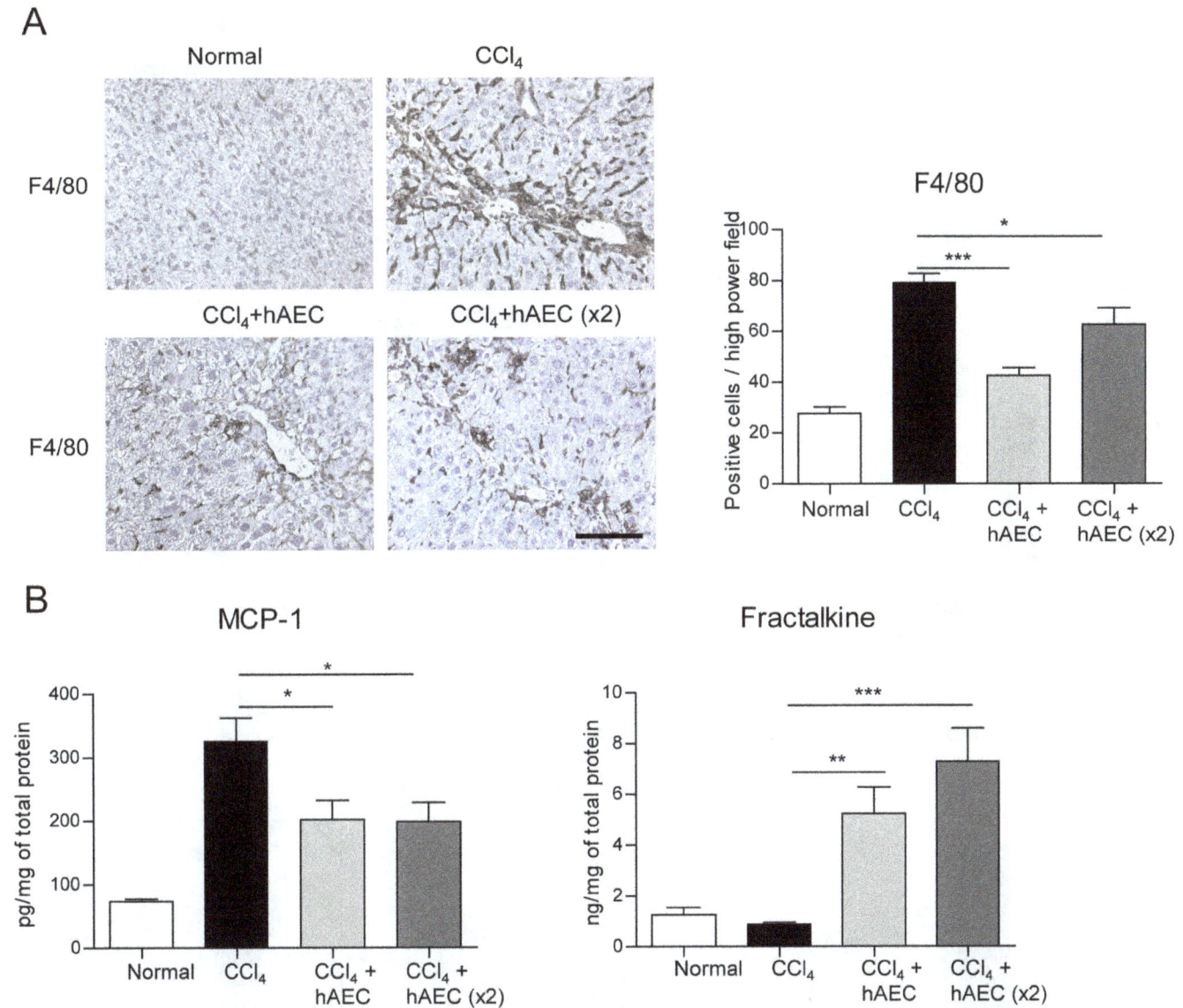

Figure 3. Human amniotic epithelial cell transplantation lowers hepatic macrophage number and alters monocyte recruitment factors. Hepatic macrophages were identified by F4/80 immunohistochemistry. C57BL/6 mice with established fibrosis treated with single or double hAEC doses had significantly lower number of F4/80 positive macrophages in the liver compared with animals given carbon tetrachloride (CCl_4) only (A). The concentrations of monocyte recruitment factors measured by ELISA showed that hAEC treatment led to a significant reduction in MCP-1 and increased levels of fractalkine in the liver compared to CCl_4 treated control animals (B). Scale bar = 100 µm. *, ** and *** P<0.05, 0.01 and 0.001, respectively.

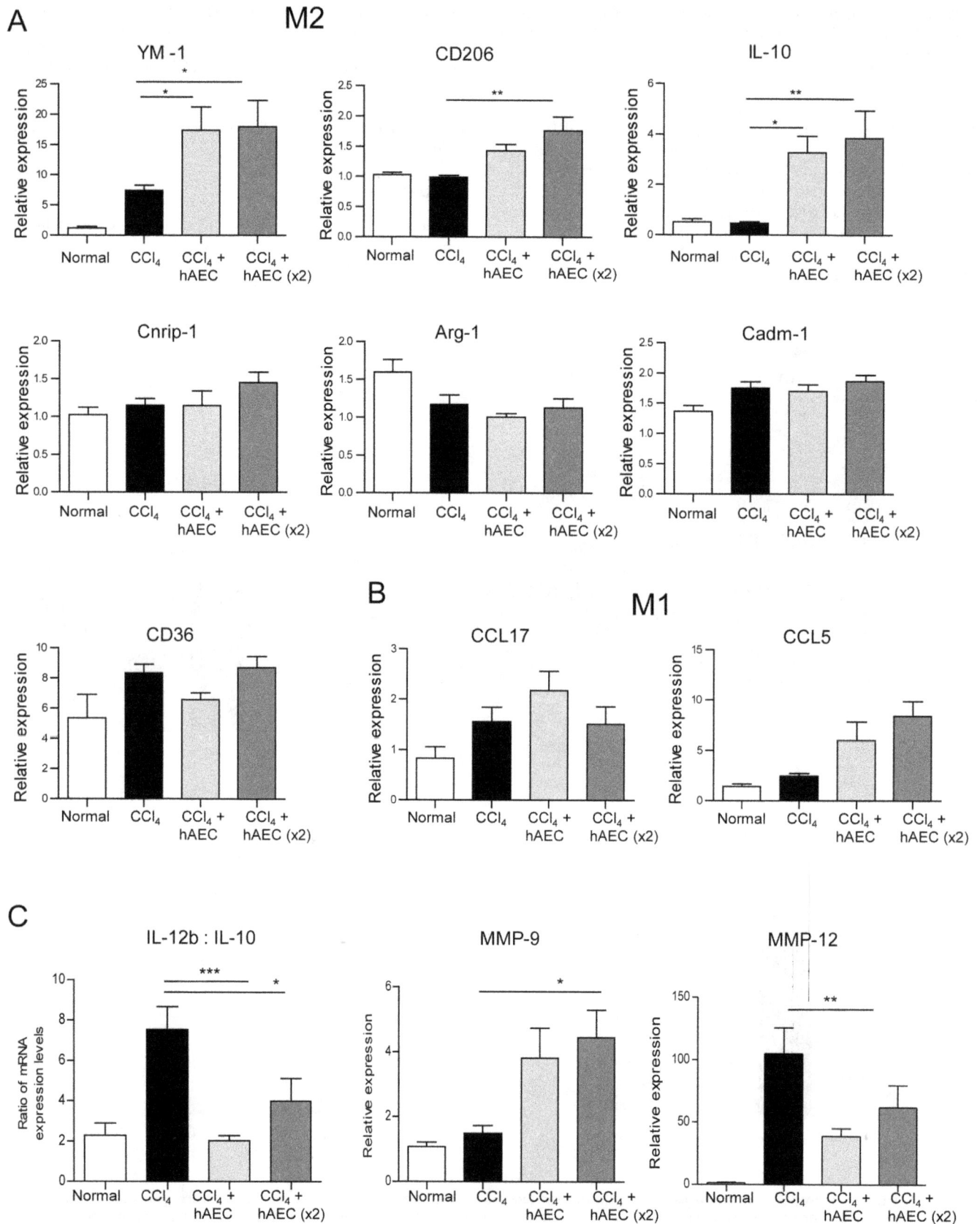

Figure 4. Human amniotic epithelial cell transplantation induces expression of genes associated with alternately activated (M2) macrophages. mRNA expression of classically (M1) and alternately activated M2 macrophage genes were analyzed by real time quantitative PCR and the fold change calculated by the $^{\Delta\Delta}$CT method. Expression of M2 associated YM-1, CD206 and IL-10 was significantly elevated in livers of mice

treated with hAEC compared to animals given carbon tetrachloride (CCl$_4$) alone (A). M1 associated genes CCL17 and CCL5 were expressed but levels did not alter with hAEC treatment (B). IL-12b:IL-10 ratio was skewed towards an M2 phenotype. MMP-9 increased and MMP-12 expression decreased with hAEC treatment (C). *, ** and *** P<0.05, 0.01 and 0.001, respectively.

fibrosis. hAEC engraftment was demonstrated by the presence of intact human IMM protein and HLA-G positive cells up to four weeks post transplantation. Similar outcomes showing grafted hAEC remaining several weeks after transplantation have also been reported in immunocompetent animals with brain, spinal cord and lung injury [32,33,34,35]. Low levels of HLA Class IA expression, lack of co-stimulatory molecules CD80/86 and secreted factors such as TGF-β and IL-6 from hAEC that can suppress T cell expansion may have limited the surveillance of the engrafted cells by host T cells [14,16,22,33]. However, anti-human antibodies were generated against the transplanted hAEC and it would be important to identify the antigens responsible, immunoglobulin sub-classes and the survival of hAEC following multiple infusions. Further, chemokines and adhesion molecules that regulate migration of intravenously infused hAEC to injury sites and subsequent engraftment remain uncertain.

The importance of our current findings in relation to human liver disease relates to the use of a model of established hepatic fibrosis and the evaluation of a second hAEC dose. We transplanted hAEC into mice only after advanced fibrosis was established and then continued CCl$_4$ administration following cell transplantation to simulate the clinical scenario of advanced liver disease due to persistent liver injury such as that from chronic viral hepatitis or continued excessive alcohol use. Despite continuing liver injury from CCl$_4$ exposure, hAEC transplantation resulted in a significant reduction in hepatic fibrosis area that was accompanied by a decrease in the number of α-SMA positive activated HSC. The decreased output of TGFβ-1, the principal profibrogenic and regulatory cytokine for HSC activation, in livers of mice that received hAEC treatment may have led to lower numbers of collagen-producing HSC. This is supported by our *in vitro* finding that hAEC conditioned medium reduced TGFβ-1 and collagen synthesis by murine hepatic stellate cells. Mice receiving two hAEC infusions showed a marginal increase in the number of engrafted cells and a small decrease in HSC activation and TGFβ-1 protein levels compared to mice receiving a single infusion. However in this model, two hAEC infusions did not decrease fibrosis area to a greater extent than a single infusion. This finding may relate to the timing of the second hAEC dose with less time for engraftment (two weeks compared to four weeks after a single injection). Additionally, the number of cells infused or the route of cell administration may have been a factor in this outcome. Overall, these findings extend our previous observations [13] by demonstrating that hAEC transplantation is effective in reducing advanced hepatic fibrosis and supports the concept that hAEC should be further investigated in regard to optimal cell numbers for multiple transplantations, alternative routes of delivery (intrahepatic or intrasplenic) to test for maximal cell engraftment and long term outcomes in this and other animal models of chronic hepatic fibrosis.

We also investigated the potential role of macrophages in hepatic fibrosis reduction in this model. Consistent with previous studies, we found that CCl$_4$-induced liver injury was associated with a significant increase in hepatic MCP-1, extensive infiltration of spindle-shaped F4/80 positive macrophages into the liver parenchyma and increased fibrosis compared to untreated controls [19,36]. MCP-1 signalling via its receptor CCR2 on monocytes has been shown to induce the

trafficking of these cells to sites of injury. Importantly, mice treated with hAEC had significantly lower levels of hepatic MCP-1 that correlated with reduced numbers of F4/80 positive macrophages and reduced fibrosis compared to mice receiving CCl$_4$ alone. The importance of reduced MCP-1/CCR2 expression on fibrosis has been demonstrated in recent studies showing that blocking MCP-1 by RNA oligonucleotides significantly decreases CCl$_4$-induced murine hepatic fibrosis [37], and that CCR2 knockout mice treated with CCl$_4$ had significantly reduced hepatic fibrosis [36]. In contrast, we found that hepatic fractalkine (CX3CL1) protein levels increased significantly in hAEC treated mice compared to CCl$_4$ alone. Increases in fractalkine have been shown to reduce HSC activation and fibrogenesis by inducing IL-10 and Arg-1 in hepatic macrophages [29]. Further, the interaction of fractalkine and its receptor, CX3CR1, leads to differentiation of macrophages having an anti-inflammatory phenotype (M2) and prolongs their survival leading to reduced fibrosis [38]. Our findings showing elevated IL-10 mRNA expression characteristic of alternately activated macrophages in livers of hAEC treated mice with increased levels of fractalkine lend support to this potential mechanism of fibrosis reduction.

The importance of macrophage plasticity in wound healing and hepatic tissue regeneration is increasingly recognised since alternatively activated M2 macrophages are thought to contribute to wound healing by secreting anti-inflammatory cytokines and collagen degrading enzymes [27,30,39]. Given the changes in F4/80 positive macrophage numbers and fibrosis with hAEC treatment, we explored whether the macrophage population displayed a phenotype consistent with wound healing and tissue remodelling. M2 macrophages express several distinct genes including YM-1, Cadm-1, CD206, CD36 and Cnrip-1. Analysis of hepatic mRNA expression showed that YM-1 mRNA, a chitinase family member, the anti-inflammatory cytokine IL-10 and the mannose receptor CD206 produced by alternatively activated macrophages, were significantly increased in CCl$_4$-treated mice following hAEC transplantation compared to control animals given CCl$_4$ alone. A decrease in the ratio of IL-12b to IL-10 expression further supports skewing towards a M2 phenotype. In addition, macrophages are an important source of matrix degrading enzymes. Liver from hAEC treated mice demonstrated significantly greater expression of MMP-9, which effectively degrades collagen, and significantly less MMP-12, which has been reported to inhibit the production of MMP-9 and increase hepatic fibrosis [40]. These are important new findings as there are few reports describing the effects of exogenous stem cells on macrophage phenotype. Mesenchymal stem cells have very recently been shown to regulate the switching of macrophages to a M2 phenotype in a murine model of myocardial infarction [41] and multipotent adult progenitor cells to induce a beneficial shift from M1 to M2 in a rat model of spinal cord injury [42]. Recently a therapeutic avenue using M2 macrophages has been suggested as CCl$_4$-treated mice infused with alternatively activated macrophages showed reduced hepatic fibrosis [39]. Therefore, it will be important to determine the influence of exogenous stem cells on hepatic macrophages in the setting of liver injury.

In summary, these findings suggest that hAEC induce changes to macrophage recruitment and promote a wound-healing phenotype that is associated with amelioration of hepatic fibrosis. Our results offer novel insights into potential mechanisms underlying the resolution of established hepatic fibrosis induced by exogenously delivered stem-like cells derived from the human placenta.

Supporting Information

Figure S1 Cytokeratin staining of human amniotic epithelial cells. Isolated hAEC show positive staining for cytokeratin (CK)-7 and CK8/18 by flow cytometry and immunocytochemistry. Scale bar = 100 μm.

Figure S2 The extent of hepatic fibrosis following long term carbon tetrachloride administration. Sirius red stained collagen in liver tissue sections obtained from immunocompetent C57BL/6 mice given twice weekly injections of CCl4 showed increased scarring with bridging fibrosis after 10–12 weeks (A). Quantitative computer assisted morphometry of Sirius red stained fibrosis area reflects the significant increase in collagen

deposition with prolonged CCl4 administration (B). Scale bar = 200 μm. * P<0.05.

Figure S3 Human amniotic epithelial cells in liver show features of hepatocytes. HLA-G positive hAEC stained for albumin. Some of these cells were also positive for HNF4α. (+VE = positive, -VE = negative; Scale bar = 50 μm).

Figure S4 T cell populations in liver of human amniotic epithelial cell treated mice. CD3, CD4 and CD8 populations in liver of hAEC treated and control groups of mice are shown. Scale bar = 50 μm.

Author Contributions

Conceived and designed the experiments: UM D. Lourensz JC AH WS. Performed the experiments: UM D. Lourensz JT D. Lacey VV J-YT JC AH. Analyzed the data: UM D. Lourensz VV D. Lacey JT PM JC AH WS. Contributed reagents/materials/analysis tools: D. Lacey PM. Wrote the paper: UM WS.

References

1. Friedman SL (2008) Mechanisms of hepatic fibrogenesis. Gastroenterology 134: 1655–1669.
2. Friedman LS (2010) Surgery in the patient with liver disease. Trans Am Clin Climatol Assoc 121: 192–204; discussion 205.
3. Hanje AJ, Patel T (2007) Preoperative evaluation of patients with liver disease. Nat Clin Pract Gastroenterol Hepatol 4: 266–276.
4. Gilchrist ES, Plevris JN (2010) Bone marrow-derived stem cells in liver repair: 10 years down the line. Liver Transpl 16: 118–129.
5. Tsai PC, Fu TW, Chen YM, Ko TL, Chen TH, et al. (2009) The therapeutic potential of human umbilical mesenchymal stem cells from Wharton's jelly in the treatment of rat liver fibrosis. Liver Transpl 15: 484–495.
6. Sakaida I, Terai S, Yamamoto N, Aoyama K, Ishikawa T, et al. (2004) Transplantation of bone marrow cells reduces CCl4-induced liver fibrosis in mice. Hepatology 40: 1304–1311.
7. Fang B, Shi M, Liao L, Yang S, Liu Y, et al. (2004) Systemic infusion of FLK1(+) mesenchymal stem cells ameliorate carbon tetrachloride-induced liver fibrosis in mice. Transplantation 78: 83–88.
8. Couto BG, Goldenberg RC, da Fonseca LM, Thomas J, Gutfilen B, et al. (2011) Bone marrow mononuclear cell therapy for patients with cirrhosis: a Phase 1 study. Liver Int 31: 391–400.
9. Kharaziha P, Hellstrom PM, Noorinayer B, Farzaneh F, Aghajani K, et al. (2009) Improvement of liver function in liver cirrhosis patients after autologous mesenchymal stem cell injection: a phase I-II clinical trial. Eur J Gastroenterol Hepatol 21: 1199–1205.
10. Pai M, Zacharoulis D, Milicevic MN, Helmy S, Jiao LR, et al. (2008) Autologous infusion of expanded mobilized adult bone marrow-derived CD34+ cells into patients with alcoholic liver cirrhosis. Am J Gastroenterol 103: 1952–1958.
11. Levicar N, Pai M, Habib NA, Tait P, Jiao LR, et al. (2008) Long-term clinical results of autologous infusion of mobilized adult bone marrow derived CD34+ cells in patients with chronic liver disease. Cell Prolif 41 Suppl 1: 115–125.
12. Stutchfield BM, Forbes SJ, Wigmore SJ (2010) Prospects for stem cell transplantation in the treatment of hepatic disease. Liver Transpl 16: 827–836.
13. Manuelpillai U, Tchongue J, Lourensz D, Vaghjiani V, Samuel CS, et al. (2010) Transplantation of human amnion epithelial cells reduces hepatic fibrosis in immunocompetent CCl-treated mice. Cell Transplant 19: 1157–1168.
14. Manuelpillai U, Moodley Y, Borlongan CV, Parolini O (2011) Amniotic membrane and amniotic cells: Potential therapeutic tools to combat tissue inflammation and fibrosis? Placenta 32 Suppl 4: S320–325.
15. Ilancheran S, Moodley Y, Manuelpillai U (2009) Human fetal membranes: a source of stem cells for tissue regeneration and repair? Placenta 30: 2–10.
16. Parolini O, Alviano F, Bagnara GP, Bilic G, Buhring HJ, et al. (2008) Concise review: isolation and characterization of cells from human term placenta: outcome of the first international Workshop on Placenta Derived Stem Cells. Stem Cells 26: 300–311.
17. Wolbank S, Peterbauer A, Fahrner M, Hennerbichler S, van Griensven M, et al. (2007) Dose-dependent immunomodulatory effect of human stem cells from amniotic membrane: a comparison with human mesenchymal stem cells from adipose tissue. Tissue Eng 13: 1173–1183.
18. Ramachandran P, Iredale JP (2009) Reversibility of liver fibrosis. Ann Hepatol 8: 283–291.
19. Karlmark KR, Wasmuth HE, Trautwein C, Tacke F (2008) Chemokine-directed immune cell infiltration in acute and chronic liver disease. Expert Rev Gastroenterol Hepatol 2: 233–242.
20. Miki T, Marongiu F, Dorko K, Ellis EC, Strom SC (2007) Isolation of amniotic epithelial stem cells. Curr Protoc Stem Cell Biol Chapter 1: Unit 1E 3.
21. Ilancheran S, Michalska A, Peh G, Wallace EM, Pera M, et al. (2007) Stem cells derived from human fetal membranes display multilineage differentiation potential. Biol Reprod 77: 577–588.
22. Pratama G, Vaghjiani V, Tee JY, Liu YH, Tan C, et al (2011) Changes in culture expanded human amniotic epithelial cells: implications for potential therapeutic applications. PLoS One 6:e26136.
23. Patella S PD, Tchongue J, de Kretser DM, Sievert W (2006) Follistatin attenuates early liver fibrosis: effects of hepatic stellate cell activation and hepatocyte apoptosis. American Journal of Physiology Gastrointestinal and Liver Physiology 290: G137–144.
24. Takashima S, Ise H, Zhao P, Akaike T, Nikaido T (2004) Human amniotic epithelial cells possess hepatocyte-like characteristics and functions. Cell Struct Funct 29: 73–84.
25. Wasmuth HE, Tacke F, Trautwein C (2010) Chemokines in liver inflammation and fibrosis. Semin Liver Dis 30: 215–225.
26. Kisseleva T, Brenner DA (2007) Role of hepatic stellate cells in fibrogenesis and the reversal of fibrosis. J Gastroenterol Hepatol 22 Suppl 1: S73–78.
27. Wynn TA, Barron L (2010) Macrophages: master regulators of inflammation and fibrosis. Semin Liver Dis 30: 245–257.
28. Kolios G, Valatas V, Kouroumalis E (2006) Role of Kupffer cells in the pathogenesis of liver disease. World J Gastroenterol 12: 7413–7420.
29. Aoyama T, Inokuchi S, Brenner DA, Seki E (2010) CX3CL1-CX3CR1 interaction prevents carbon tetrachloride-induced liver inflammation and fibrosis in mice. Hepatology 52: 1390–1400.
30. Heymann F, Trautwein C, Tacke F (2009) Monocytes and macrophages as cellular targets in liver fibrosis. Inflamm Allergy Drug Targets 8: 307–318.
31. Murray PJ, Wynn TA (2011) Protective and pathogenic functions of macrophage subsets. Nature reviews Immunology 11: 723–737.
32. Yang X, Song L, Wu N, Liu Z, Xue S, et al. (2010) An experimental study on intracerebroventricular transplantation of human amniotic epithelial cells in a rat model of Parkinson's disease. Neurol Res 32: 1054–1059.
33. Moodley Y, Ilancheran S, Samuel C, Vaghjiani V, Atienza D, et al. (2010) Human amnion epithelial cell transplantation abrogates lung fibrosis and augments repair. Am J Respir Crit Care Med 182: 643–651.
34. Cargnoni A, Gibelli L, Tosini A, Signoroni PB, Nassuato C, et al. (2009) Transplantation of allogeneic and xenogeneic placenta-derived cells reduces bleomycin-induced lung fibrosis. Cell Transplant 18: 405–422.
35. Liu T, Wu J, Huang Q, Hou Y, Jiang Z, et al. (2008) Human amniotic epithelial cells ameliorate behavioral dysfunction and reduce infarct size in the rat middle cerebral artery occlusion model. Shock 29: 603–611.
36. Seki E, de Minicis S, Inokuchi S, Taura K, Miyai K, et al. (2009) CCR2 promotes hepatic fibrosis in mice. Hepatology 50: 185–197.
37. Baeck C, Wehr A, Karlmark KR, Heymann F, Vucur M, et al. (2011) Pharmacological inhibition of the chemokine CCL2 (MCP-1) diminishes liver macrophage infiltration and steatohepatitis in chronic hepatic injury. Gut 61:416–26.
38. Karlmark KR, Zimmermann HW, Roderburg C, Gassler N, Wasmuth HE, et al. (2010) The fractalkine receptor CXCR1 protects against liver fibrosis by controlling differentiation and survival of infiltrating hepatic monocytes. Hepatology 52: 1769–1782.

39. Thomas JA, Pope C, Wojtacha D, Robson AJ, Gordon-Walker TT, et al. (2011) Macrophage therapy for murine liver fibrosis recruits host effector cells improving fibrosis, regeneration, and function. Hepatology 53: 2003–2015.

40. Madala SK, Pesce JT, Ramalingam TR, Wilson MS, Minnicozzi S, et al. (2010) Matrix metalloproteinase 12-deficiency augments extracellular matrix degrading metalloproteinases and attenuates IL-13-dependent fibrosis. Journal of Immunology 184: 3955–3963.

41. Dayan V, Yannarelli G, Billia F, Filomeno P, Wang XH, et al. (2011) Mesenchymal stromal cells mediate a switch to alternatively activated monocytes/macrophages after acute myocardial infarction. Basic Res Cardiol 106:1299–1310.

42. Busch SA, Hamilton JA, Horn KP, Cuascut FX, Cutrone R, et al. (2011) Multipotent adult progenitor cells prevent macrophage-mediated axonal dieback and promote regrowth after spinal cord injury. J Neurosci 31: 944–953.

14

MMP Mediated Degradation of Type VI Collagen is Highly Associated with Liver Fibrosis – Identification and Validation of a Novel Biochemical Marker Assay

Sanne Skovgård Veidal[1,2]*, Morten Asser Karsdal[1], Efstathios Vassiliadis[1,2], Arkadiusz Nawrocki[2], Martin Røssel Larsen[2], Quoc Hai Trieu Nguyen[1], Per Hägglund[4], Yunyun Luo[3], Qinlong Zheng[3], Ben Vainer[5], Diana Julie Leeming[1]

1 Nordic Bioscience A/S, Herlev, Denmark, 2 Faculty of Health Science, University of Southern Denmark, Odense, Denmark, 3 Nordic Bioscience Beijing, Beijing, China, 4 Department of Systems Biology, Technical University of Denmark, Kgs. Lyngby, Denmark, 5 Department of Pathology, Rigshospitalet, Copenhagen University Hospital, Copenhagen, Denmark

Abstract

Background and Aims: During fibrogenesis, in which excessive remodeling of the extracellular matrix occurs, both the quantity of type VI collagen and levels of matrix metalloproteinases, including MMP-2 and MMP-9, increase significantly. Proteolytic degradation of type VI collagen into small fragments, so-called neo-epitopes, may be specific biochemical marker of liver fibrosis. The aim of this study was to develop an ELISA detecting a fragment of type VI collagen generated by MMP-2 and MMP-9, and evaluate this assay in two preclinical models of liver fibrosis.

Methods: Mass spectrometric analysis of cleaved type VI collagen revealed a large number of protease-generated neo-epitopes. A fragment unique to type VI collagen generated by MMP-2 and MMP-9 was selected for ELISA development. The CO6-MMP assay was evaluated in two rat models of liver fibrosis: bile duct ligation (BDL) and carbon tetrachloride (CCl4)-treated rats.

Results: Intra- and inter-assay variation was 4.1% and 10.1% respectively. CO6-MMP levels were significantly elevated in CCl_4-treated rats compared to vehicle-treated rats at weeks 12 (mean 30.9 ng/mL vs. 12.8 ng/mL, p = 0.002); week 16 (mean 34.0 ng/mL vs. 13.7 ng/mL, p = 0.0018); and week 20 (mean 35.3 ng/mL vs. 13.3 ng/mL, p = 0.0033) with a tight correlation between hepatic collagen content and serum levels of CO6-MMP ($R^2 = 0.58$, p<0.0001) in CCl_4- treated rats. In BDL rats, serum levels of CO6-MMP were significantly elevated compared to the levels in sham-operated animals both at 2 weeks (mean 29.5 ng/mL vs. 14.2 ng/mL, p = 0.0001) and 4 weeks (mean 33.0 ng/mLvs. 11.8 ng/mL, p = 0.0003).

Conclusions: This novel ELISA is the first assay enabling assessment of MMP degraded type VI collagen, allowing quantification of type VI collagen degradation, which would be relevant for different pathologies. The marker was highly associated with liver fibrosis in two liver fibrosis animal models, suggesting type VI turnover to be a central player in fibrogenesis.

Editor: Donald Gullberg, University of Bergen, Norway

Funding: The authors gratefully acknowledge the funding from the Danish Research Foundation (den Danske Forskningsfond) supporting this work. The funders had no role in study design, data collection and analysis, decision to publish, or preparation of the manuscript.

Competing Interests: Sanne S. Veidal, Morten A. Karsdal, Quoc H.T. Nguyen, Efstathios Vassiliadis and Diana J. Leeming are employees of Nordic Bioscience. Morten A. Karsdal owns stocks and shares in Nordic Bioscience.

* E-mail: ssv@nordicbioscience.com

Introduction

Liver fibrosis due to viral or alcohol-induced injury is one of the leading causes of death worldwide [1]. To date no curative treatment for liver fibrosis is available and patients are dependent on the success of inactivation or removal of the injurious agent or in the case of end-stage cirrhosis, on liver transplantation. Assessment of liver fibrosis is important to estimate the prognosis for the progression to liver cirrhosis and to determine surveillance strategies. At present, liver biopsy is the most commonly used method for fibrosis assessment, but it is invasive, associated with patient discomfort and, in rare cases, with serious complications [2]. In addition, the accuracy of liver biopsy is limited due to sampling error and significant intra- and inter-observer variability in histological staging [3,4]. Therefore, research has focused on the evaluation of non-invasive methods for the assessment of liver fibrosis [5].

Fibrosis may be described as extensive scar formation, observed as increased deposition and abnormal distribution of extracellular matrix (ECM) components such as collagens and proteoglycans. ECM remodeling is a key process of tissue homoeostasis [6–8], and specific proteolytic activities are a prerequisite for a range of cellular functions and interactions during the process [9]. The specific proteolytic activities are precisely coordinated under physiological situations, with a specified sequence of events resulting in controlled tissue turnover. In pathological situations, including inflammations, fibrosis and cancer, the normal damage/repair balance is displaced [10], leading to excessive remodeling. As a consequence of this tissue turnover, there is a release of several protein degradation fragments specific for the combination of the involved proteases, the affected organ and the disease. The fragmentation results in exposure of new peptide ends (so-called neo-epitopes) to which specific antibodies can be developed. These neo-epitopes may be used for the design of molecular biochemical markers [11].

Endopeptidases such as metalloproteinases (MMPs) play a major part in the degradation of extracellular macromolecules such as collagens and during fibrogenesis the levels of MMPs increase [12,13]. With respect to excessive proteolytic activity in the fibrous tissue, the gelatinases MMP-2 and MMP-9 have been investigated and documented to be highly regulated [12,13]. Type VI collagen degradation yields several unique fragments, including the CO6-MMP fragment (YRGPEGPQGP). The combination of active and over-expressed MMPs and increased levels of type VI collagen poses the interesting hypothesis that a MMP-generated fragment of type VI collagen could be used as a biomarker of liver fibrosis.

Type VI collagen is a ubiquitous ECM protein. It is a heterotrimer composed of three different α-chains with short triple helical domains [14]. Following secretion into the ECM, type VI collagen tetramers aggregate into filaments and form an independent microfibrillar network in virtually all connective tissues, except for bone [15]. Type VI collagen has been identified within most tissues and it is generally accepted that it plays a role in the maintenance of tissue integrity since it participates in both cell-matrix and matrix-matrix interactions [16]. Type VI collagen interacta with many other ECM proteins, including fibronectin [17], type IV collagen [18], decorin, biglycan and type II collagen [19]. In close association with other collagen types, type VI collagen forms filaments and has therefore been described as a connecting protein [14,20]. It is mainly found in a pericellular localization around a number of cell types – in the liver, mainly around hepatic stellate cells and around hepatocytes in fetal liver [14,16]. In previous studies, total collagen type VI, a putative marker of mesenchymal activation, has been suggested to be an indicator of early architectural remodeling in liver fibrosis [21–24]. Serum levels of type VI collagen has been found to be elevated in patients with alcoholic cirrhosis [23,24]. During fibrogenesis, the total amount of type VI collagen is increased [14,24–26], and even though it represents only a minor fraction of the ECM collagens, the release to measurable products into the serum is significant, even in healthy individuals, indicating a considerable turnover [24,27].

Several animal models for liver fibrosis have been developed, most of them in small rodents [28], each with individual strengths and weaknesses. These different rodent models are complementary as they represent different pathways to fibrosis, as also seen in human disease. Bile duct ligation (BDL) in rats has been used as a model of chronic liver injury due to its resemblance to hepatocyte damage, hepatic stellate cell activation, and liver fibrosis observed in human cholestatic liver diseases [1,28]. Carbon tetrachloride (CCl4) is a hepatotoxin that causes acute liver injury and, when given repetitively at a low dose, induces liver fibrosis. It is a highly reproducible and robust model which is used to resemble alcoholic and non-alcoholic steatohepatitis with the consequent fibrosis and cirrhosis in humans [1,28].

We hypothesized that specific MMP-2 and MMP-9 mediated degradation of type VI collagen was measurable in serum during liver fibrogenesis. The aim of this work was to develop a novel competitive enzyme-linked immunosorbent assay (ELISA) for measuring MMP-2 and MMP-9 mediated turnover of type VI collagen and to measure the neo-epitopes in two complementary experimental models of liver fibrosis induced by BDL or CCl4.

Materials and Methods

Ethics Statement

The BDL experiments were approved by the Experimental Animal Committee of the Danish Ministry of Justice and were performed according to the European Standard for Good Clinical Practice (2008/561-1450).

The CCl4 study was approved by the Ethical Committee of Animal Experimentation of the University of Barcelona (B-NNP-233/09) and was performed according to the criteria of the Investigation and Ethics Committee of the Hospital Clinic Universitari (Barcelona, Spain).

Reagents

All reagents used for the experiments were standard high-quality chemicals from companies such as Merck (Whitehouse Station, NJ, USA) and Sigma Aldrich (St.Louis, MO, USA). The synthetic peptides used for monoclonal antibody production were purchased from the Chinese Peptide Company, Beijing, China.

In vitro cleavage

Purified type VI collagen from human placenta (cat. no. ab7538, Abcam, Cambridge, UK) was cleaved with pro-MMP-2 or pro-MMP-9 (cat. no. 444213; 444231; Calbiochem, Merck, Whitehouse Station, NJ, USA). Fifty μg MMP-2 or MMP-9 was activated with 20 μl 1 mM 4-aminophenylmercuric acetate (AMPA) in dimethyl sulfoxide and incubated at 37°C for 3 hours. Type VI collagen was delivered dissolved in 0.5 M acetic acid. To facilitate MMP cleavage, the protein was dialyzed for two days to remove the acetic acid. The liquid was filtered to remove proteins below 10 kDa (Microcon Ultracel YM-10, cat. no. 42407, Millipore, Billerica, MA, USA). Each MMP cleavage was performed separately by mixing 100 μg type VI collagen and 1 μg of either MMP-2 or MMP-9 in MMP buffer (100 mM Tris-HCl, 100 mM NaCl, 10 mM $CaCl_2$, 2 mM Zn acetate, pH 8.0). As control, 100 μg of collagen was mixed with MMP buffer alone. The solutions were incubated for 24 hours at 37°C. The cleavage reaction was stopped using 50 μM ethylenediaminetetraacetic acid (EDTA) to a final concentration of 1 μM. Cleavage was verified by visualization using the SilverXpress® Silver Staining Kit (cat. no. LC6100, Invitrogen, Carlsbad, Ca, USA) according to the manufacturer's instructions.

Pepsin cleavage was performed by mixing 100 μg type IV collagen and 1 μg of pepsin in pepsin buffer (0.2 M sodium acetate buffer, pH 4.0). The resultant enzyme/protein mixture was incubated at 37°C for 2 hours. At the designated time, 2 M Trizma Base was added to adjust pH to neutral to stop the reactions.

Peptide identification

Peptide fragments in the in vitro cleaved samples were identified using liquid chromatography (LC) coupled to electrospray ionization (ESI) tandem mass spectrometry (LC-MS/MS). LC-MS samples were ultra-filtrated to remove proteins above 10 kDa, the pH was adjusted to 2.0 using formic acid, and a 4 μl sample was analyzed by LC-MS/MS. LC was performed on a nanoACQUITY UPLC BEH C_{18} column (Waters, Milford, MA, USA) using a formic acid/acetonitril gradient. MS and MS/MS were performed on a Synapt High Definition Mass Spectrometry quadruple time of flight MS (QUAD-TOF; Waters, Milford, MA, USA), with an acquisition range of 350–1600 m/z in MS and 50–2000 m/z, in MS/MS. The software "ProteinLynx Global SERVER (PLGS)" (Waters, Milford, MA, USA) was used to analyze spectra and generate peak lists. To identify peptides, MS and MS/MS data was searched against a type VI collagen (FASTA) protein database using the Mascot 2.2 (Matrix Science, Boston, MA, USA) software with the ESI-QUAD-TOF settings and carbamidomethyl (C), oxidation of methionine (M), oxidation of lysine (K) and oxidation of proline (P) as variable modifications.

The six amino acids in the N- or C-terminal of the peptides identified by MS were regarded as a neo-epitope generated by the protease in question. All protease-generated sequences were analyzed for homology and distance to other cleavage sites and tested for homology using NPS@: network protein sequence analysis (Combet C, Blanchet C, Geourjon C, Deleage G. NPS@:network protein sequence analysis. Trends Biochem Sci 2000; 25: 147–50).

Peptide conjugation

The peptide conjugation was performed using the Maleidide Activated Immunogen Conjugation Kit (Sigma-Aldrich, MO, USA). Briefly, the cysteine-containing immunogenic neo-epitope (YRGPEGPQGP-GGC, 400 µl peptide at 5 mg/ml) with one free sulfhydryl (-SH) group was mixed in conjugation buffer with the maleimide-activated ovalbumin (OVA) (180 µl OVA at 10 mg/ml) as a carrier protein with an available maleimide group that could react with sulfhydryl-containing peptides and incubated for 2 hours at room temperature. Conjugated products were cleared of EDTA and sodium azide by desalting or dialysis for two days. For the biotin-conjugated peptides, the biotin-conjugated lysine was added in the solid-phase peptide synthesis procedure.

Monoclonal antibody development

4–6 weeks-old Balb/C mice were immunized subcutaneously with about 200 µl emulsified antigen and 50 µg of the neo-epitope CO6-MMP (YRGPEGPQGP-GGC-OVA). Consecutive immunizations were performed at 2-week intervals until stable sera titer levels were reached in Freund's incomplete adjuvant. Blood samples were collected from the 2nd immunization. At each blood sampling, the serum titer was determined and the mouse with highest antiserum titer was selected for fusion. After the 4th immunization, this mouse was rested for 1 month and then boosted intravenously with 50 µg CO6-MMP in 100 µl 0.9% sodium chloride solution three days before isolation of the spleen for cell fusion.

Fusion and antibody screening

The fusion procedure performed as described by Gefter et al [29]. Briefly, mouse spleen cells were fused with SP2/0 myeloma fusion partner cells. The hybridoma cells were cloned using a semi-solid medium method and transferred into 96-well microtiter plates for further growth and incubated in a CO_2-incubator. Standard limited dilution was used to promote monoclonal growth. Supernatants were screened using an indirect ELISA with streptavidin-coated microtitre plates and YRGPEGPQGP-K-Biotin as a capture peptide.

Characterization of clones

Native reactivity and peptide binding of the monoclonal antibodies was evaluated by displacement of native samples (human/rat/mouse serum, plasma and urine) in a preliminary ELISA using 10 ng/mL biotinylated peptide coater on a streptavidin-coated microtitre plate and the supernatant from the growing monoclonal hybridoma. Specificities of the clones to a free peptide (YRGPEGPQGP), a non-sense peptide, and an

elongated peptide (GYRGPEGPQG) were tested. Isotyping of the monoclonal antibodies was performed using the Clonotyping System-HRP kit, cat. no. 5300-05 (Southern Biotech, Birmingham, AL, USA). The selected clones were purified using protein G columns according to manufacturer's instructions (GE Healthcare Life Science, Little Chalfont, Buckinghamshire, UK). Selected monoclonal antibodies were labeled with horseradish peroxidase (HRP) using the Lightning link HRP labeling kit according to the instructions of the manufacturer (Innovabioscience, Babraham, Cambridge, UK).

CO6-MMP ELISA methodology

In preliminary experiments, we optimized the reagents, their concentrations and the incubation periods by performing several checkerboard analyses. The CO6-MMP ELISA was developed as follows: A 96-well streptavidin plate was coated with biotinylated synthetic peptide YRGPEGPQGP-K-Biotin dissolved in assay buffer (25 mM Tris, 1% BSA, 0.1% Tween-20, pH 7.4) and incubated 30 minutes at 20°C. Twenty µl of peptide calibrator or sample were added to appropriate wells, followed by 100 µL of conjugated monoclonal antibody and incubated 1 hour at 20°C. Finally, 100 µL tetramethylbenzinidine (TMB) (Kem-En-Tec cat. no. 438OH) was added and the plate was incubated 15 minutes at 20°C in the dark. All the above incubation steps included shaking at 300 rpm. After each incubation step the plate was washed five times in washing buffer (20 mM Tris, 50 mM NaCl, pH 7.2). The TMB reaction was stopped by adding 100 µl stopping solution (1% HCL) and measured spectrophotometrically at 450 nm with 650 nm as the reference. A standard curve was performed by serial dilution of the CO6-MMP peptide and plotted using a 4-parametric mathematical fit model. Standard concentrations were 0, 0.39, 7.8, 15.6, 31.3, 62.5, 125 250 ng/mL.

Technical evaluation

From 2-fold dilutions of pooled serum and plasma samples, lincarity was calculated as a percentage of recovery of the 100% sample. The lower detection limit (LDL) was calculated from 21 determinations of the lowest standard (the zero standard) and calculated as the mean +3x standard deviation. The inter- and intra-assay variation was determined by 10 independent runs of 5 QC samples, with each run consisting of two replicas of double determinations of the samples. Finally, for each assay, a master calibrator prepared from synthetic peptides accurately quantified by amino acid analysis was used for calibration purposes.

The analyte stability was determined for six serum samples (three rat and three human) for 10 freeze and thaw cycles.

ELISA characterization

The developed CO6-MMP ELISA was evaluated using 20 µl of the cleavage-samples: type VI collagen, type VI collagen cleaved with MMP-2, type VI collagen cleaved with MMP-9 described under "In vitro cleavage". The negative control was in vitro cleaved type VI collagen with fibroblast activation protein (FAP). Cross-reactivity was tested using intact or in vitro cleaved type I or IV collagen using 20 µL peptide solution of 1000 ng/mL for each test in the assay. Neo-epitope specificity was tested using cleaved (by either MMP-2 or MMP-9) and non-cleaved type VI collagen and by an elongated CO6-MMP amino acid sequence (GYRGPEGPQG).

Bile duct ligation

A total of 40 female Sprague-Dawley rats aged 6 months were housed at the animal research facilities at Nordic Bioscience,

Denmark. The rats were kept in standard type III-H cages at 18–22°C with bedding and nest material (Altromin 1324; Altromin, Lage, Germany) and water *ad libitum*. Rats were kept under conditions of a 12-hour light: dark cycle. Experiments began after 1 week of acclimatization. Bile duct ligation (BDL) was performed in anaesthetized rats by ligation of the bile duct in two places and dissection between the ligations in an open-surgery procedure. In sham-operated rats, the abdomen was closed without BDL. BDL- or sham-operated rats were sacrificed after 2 or 4 weeks.

CCl₄ inhalation

The study included 52 3-months old male Wistar rats treated with CCl_4 and 28 Wistar control rats (Charles-River, Saint Aubin les Elseuf, France). Complete details of the study are described elsewhere (Segovia-Silvestre T et al.). Liver damage was induced as previously described [30], and in short included administration by inhalation of CCl_4 twice weekly. Phenobarbital (0.3 g/l) was added to the drinking water. Animals were stratified into groups receiving 8, 12, 16 or 20 weeks of CCl_4 (n = 13 for CCl_4; n = 7 control for each group). Control rats received Phenobarbital only. Four animals from the CCl_4 groups died during the study. After the stated weeks of CCl4 administration the rats were weighed, anesthetized with pentobarbital (50 mg/kg) and terminated by decapitation.

Blood and tissue sampling

Blood samples were taken under light CO_2/O_2 anesthesia at baseline and at termination from the retro-orbital sinus of rats which had fasted for at least 14 hours. The collected blood was left for 30 min at room temperature to clot, followed by centrifugation at 3000 *g* for 10 min. All clot-free liquid was transferred to new tubes and centrifuged again at 3000 *g* for 10 min. The serum was then transferred to clean tubes and stored at −80°C.

Livers were carefully dissected, weighed, fixed in 4% formaldehyde for a minimum of 24 hours, cut into appropriate slices and embedded in paraffin. Liver sections (4–5 µm thick) were stained with 0.1% Sirius Red F3B (Sigma-Aldrich, St. Louis, MO) in saturated picric acid (Sigma-Aldrich).

Histology image analysis

Relative fibrosis area (expressed as a percentage of total liver area) was assessed by analyzing 36 fields of Sirius Red-stained liver sections per animal. Each field was acquired at 10× magnification [E600 microscope (Nikon) and RT-Slider SPOT digital camera (Diagnostic Instruments, Inc., Sterling Heights, Michigan, US)]. Results were analyzed using a computerized Bioquant Life Science morphometry system. To evaluate the relative fibrosis area, the measured collagen area was divided by the net field area and then multiplied by 100. Subtraction of vascular luminal area from the total field area yielded the final calculation of the net fibrosis area. From each animal analyzed, the amount of fibrosis as a percentage was measured and the average value presented [31].

Immunohistochemistry

Liver sections (4 µm) were de-paraffinised, hydrated and further peroxidase activity was blocked with the addition of 0.4% hydrogen peroxide. Sections were then incubated with a polyclonal antibody against type VI collagen (1:100; Abcam, Cambridge, UK). Sections were then rinsed and the antibody binding was depicted using the Super Sensitive Polymer-HRP IHC Detection System combined with AEC substrate, according to the supplier's instructions (Biogenex, Taby, Sweden). Sections were counterstained with Mayer's haematoxylin. Digital photographs were taken using an Olympus B×60 microscope with ×40 magnification and an Olympus 5050-zoom digital camera (Olympus, Tokyo, Japan).

Results

In vitro cleavage and selection of peptides

High molecular bands of type VI collagen were seen by silver staining in the *in vitro* control sample not exposed to proteases. These bands were abolished in the MMP-2 and MMP-9 cleaved samples, indicating that type VI collagen was degraded by these proteases (data not shown). Fragments of type VI collagen cleaved by MMP-2 or MMP-9 were identified with a statistically significant Mascot score ($p < 0.05$). All protease-generated neo-epitopes were tested for homology. Among 184 MMP-2 or MMP-9 generated neo-epitopes five sequences were selected for immunizations since blasting showed that these sequences were unique to type VI collagen, and conserved throughout species:

1. 573'.YRGPEGPQGPPG'584; CO6A1 generated by MMP-2 or MMP-9
2. 1164'GIGIGNADIT.'1173; CO6A3 generated by MMP-2
3. 1164'.GIGIGNADIT'1173; CO6A3 generated by MMP-2
4. 2279'GPKGGIGNRG.'2288; CO6A3 generated by MMP-9
5. 2176'.LGPMGVPGRD'2185; CO6A3 generated by MMP-9

The sequence 573'.YRGPEGPQGPPG'584 (CO6-MMP) in the alpha 1 chain of type VI collagen generated by MMP-2 and MMP-9 was selected consequent to the best technical performance as the antibodies were able to distinguish between cleaved and uncleaved type VI collagen. In addition, this sequence is 100% homologous to human, rat and mouse (Figure 1).

Clone characterization

The antibody with the best native reactivity, affinity and stability in the assay was chosen from the antibody-producing clones generated after the fusion between spleen cells and myeloma cells. The clone selected was determined to be the IgG1 subtype.

The clone was reactive to human serum and plasma (Figure 2A), rat serum and plasma (Figure 2B) and mouse serum (Figure 2B).

Technical evaluation

The typical standard curve is presented in Figure 2A and 2B, showing a 4-parametric fit for the assay. The lower limit of detection (LDL) for the assay was 0.30 ng/mL. Dilution recovery was within 100±20% (Table 1). The inter- and intra-assay variation was a mean 4.0 and 10.1% respectively (Table 2). The analyte stability was acceptable for 2–10x freeze/thaw cycles within 100+/−20% (Table 3).

Antibody bindingsite

CO6A1 MOUSE   YRGPEGPQGP
CO6A1 RAT   YRGPEGPQGP
CO6A1 HUMAN   YRGPEGPQGP

Figure 1. Alignment. Alignment of part of type VI collagen alpha 1 sequence for mouse, rat and human.

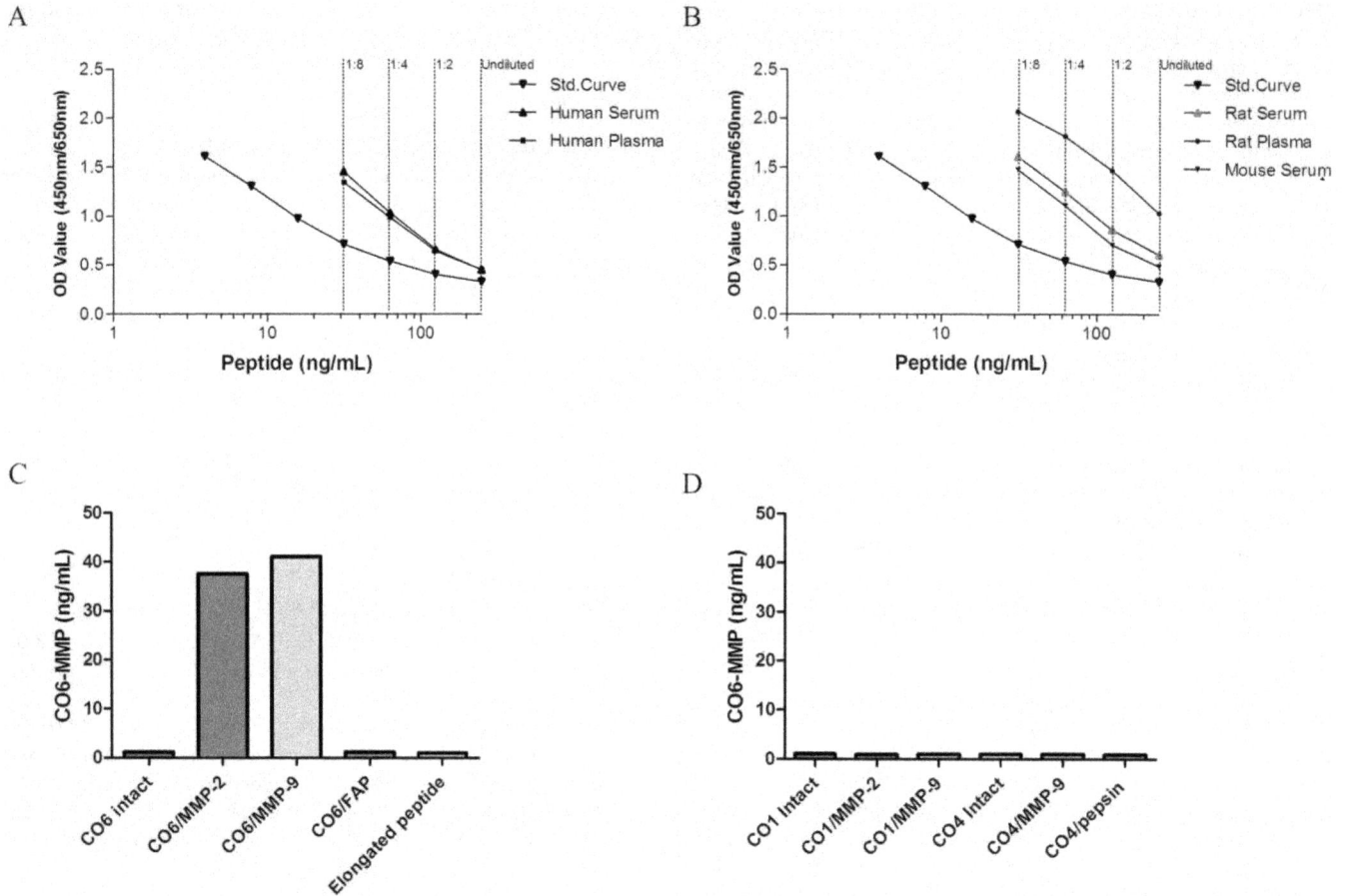

Figure 2. Assay characteristics. (A+B) ELISA run showing typical standard curves and native reactivity against (A) Human serum, plasma, (B) Rodent: Rat serum and plasma; mouse serum, plasma and urine. Native material was run undiluted, 1:2, 1:4, and 1:8 as indicated (—).The signal is seen as the optical density at 450 nm, subtracting the background at 650 nm, as a function of peptide concentration; (C+D) Characterization of the CO6-MMP assay with regards to reactivity against (C) intact type VI collagen (CO6 intact), type VI collagen cleaved by MMP-2 (CO6/MMP-2), type VI collagen cleaved by MMP-9 (CO6/MMP-9), type VI collagen cleaved by fibroblast activation protein (FAP) (CO6/FAP), elongated peptide with extension of one amino acid at the neo-epitope site; (D) Intact type I collagen (CO1), type I collagen cleaved by MMP-2 (CO1/MMP-2), type I collagen cleaved by MMP-9 (CO1/MMP-9), intact type IV collagen (CO4), type IV collagen cleaved by MMP-2 (CO4/MMP-2), type IV collagen cleaved by MMP-9 (CO4/MMP-9), type IV collagen cleaved by pepsin (CO4/pepsin).

ELISA characterization

To characterize the analytes detected in the assay, different collagens were cleaved with different proteases. Both MMP-2 and MMP-9 were able to generate the CO6-MMP fragment from

Table 1. Percentage dilution recovery for the CO6-MMP assay.

CO6-MMP ng/mL	HS1 44.7	HS2 36.5	RS1 9.92	RS2 14.11
Undil	100%	100%	100%	100%
Dilution 1:2	91%	87%	113%	109%
Dilution 1:4	98%	90%	110%	105%
Dilution 1:8	98%	86%	102%	96%
Dilution 1:16	93%	92%	93%	101
Mean	95%	89%	104%	103%

HS = human serum; RS = rat serum.

Table 2. Inter- and intra-assay variation for the CO6-MMP assays using human serum quality control samples.

CO6-MMP Sample	Amount (ng/mL)	Intra-assay variability %	Inter-assay variability %
HS1	7.6	4.5	10.1
HS2	11.7	4.8	13.3
HS3	10.5	2.9	8.7
HS4	13.1	4.3	9.4
HS5	13.8	3.7	9.2
HS6	13.3	4.2	10.5
HS7	17.8	3.8	9.8
HS8	21.3	4.3	9.9
Mean	13.6	4.1	10.1

The variation was calculated as the mean variation between 10 individual determinations of each sample.

Table 3. Analyte stability in three rat- and three human serum samples in 10 freeze/thaw cycles.

Analyte stability	Percent recovery compared to 1 ×freeze/thaw	
Freeze/thaw cycles	Human CO6-MMP	Rat CO6-MMP
2x	95.2	93.6
3x	86.1	96.0
4x	102.7	92.9
5x	105.7	103.6
6x	90.1	96.7
7x	98.1	99.2
8x	92.4	95.1
9x	91.4	99.7
10x	85.2	104.6

All data are shown as percent recovery compared to day 0 or 1 freeze/thaw cycle.

collagen type VI (Figure 2C). In contrast, the fragment was not found in either intact or FAP-cleaved type VI collagen. Finally, no cross-reactivity was seen between CO6-MMP and intact or cleaved type I or IV collagens, which have high homology with the immunization sequence of type VI collagen (Figure 2D). No reactivity was seen against the elongated synthetic peptide, as expected proving neo-epitope reactivity (Figure 2C).

Evaluations performed in the BDL study

During the 4 weeks, 3 of 40 rats, 2 BDL and 1 Sham, were put down due to excessive weight loss.

Levels of CO6-MMP were significantly elevated in BDL rats compared to sham levels at both the two-(mean BDL 29.5 ng/mL, mean sham: 14.2 ng/mL, p = 0.0001) and four week (mean BDL: 33.0 ng/ml, mean sham: 11.8 ng/mL, p = 0.0003) termination point (Figure 3).

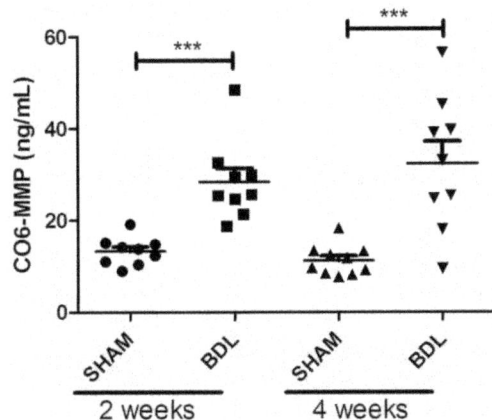

Figure 3. CO6-MMP serum levels in BDL-rats. BDL rat liver fibrosis model. Serum CO6-MMP was assessed in BDL and sham operated rats at termination. Termination time points were 2 and 4 weeks after surgery. Levels of CO6-MMP were significantly elevated in BDL rats compared to sham levels at both the two-(mean BDL 29.5 ng/mL, mean sham: 14.2 ng/mL, p = 0.0001) and four week mean BDL: 33.0 ng/ml, (mean sham: 11.8 ng/mL, p = 0.0003) termination point.

By immunohistochemistry, collagen type VI deposition was found exclusively in the venous wall of healthy rats (Figure 4B). In contrast, in BDL rats in which marked ductal proliferation was seen around the portal tract with the formation of multiple neo-bile ducts, more extensive type VI collagen was found (Figure 4B).

Evaluations performed in the CCL4 study

In the CCL4 rat model, levels of CO6-MMP were significantly elevated at all time points compared to baseline levels, except at week 8 (week 12: mean CCl4 30.9 ng/mL, mean control 12.8 ng/mL, p = 0.0015; week 16: mean CCl4 34.0 ng/mL, mean control 13.7 ng/mL, p = 0.0018, week 20: mean CCl4 35.3 ng/mL, mean control 13.3 ng/mL, p = 0.0033) (Figure 5A). When CCl4- treated rats were classified by the total amount of collagen in the liver evaluated by histology (Sirius Red) (Figure 5B), it clearly seen that the marker was elevated in the lowest quartile of total collagen (quartile 1), as well as in quartiles 2–4 compared to control animals (mean Q1: 18.1 ng/mL, p>0.03; mean Q2: 22.0 ng/mL, p<0.05; mean Q3: 36.7 ng/mL, p<0.0001; mean Q4: 46.1 ng/mL, p = 0.0018; mean across all controls 13.4 ng/mL). The correlation between CO6-MMP and total collagen was highly significant in CCl4-treated rats (p<0.0001, $R^2 = 0.58$) (Figure 5C), however this was not seen in control rats (p = ns, $R^2 = 0.04$) (Figure 5D).

By immunohistochemistry, collagen type VI deposition was found exclusively in the venous wall of control rats (Figure 4D). In contrast, in CCl4-treated rats type VI collagen was located along the fibrotic bands (figure 4D).

Discussion

This is, to our knowledge, the first study to present the development of an assay specific for a fragment of type VI collagen generated by MMPs. Our main findings were: 1) A technically robust assay was developed with monoclonal antibodies highly specific for the CO6-MMP fragment. The assay had acceptable inter-, and intra-assay variation, dilution recovery and a low limit of detection; 2) CO6-MMP levels were assessed in two different animal models of liver fibrosis: CCl4 and BDL. In both models we found significant increased levels in liver fibrotic rats compared to controls. In addition CO6-MMP levels were significantly correlated to collagen deposition in the CCl4 model of liver fibrosis.

ECM remodeling is an essential part of tissue homeostasis. Extensive ECM remodeling is associated with a range of pathologies [7,8,20,26,32,33] in which fibrosis is of particular relevance. Biochemical markers consisting of protein fragments from pathologic tissue remodeling may be useful for diagnostic and prognostic purposes [34]. Such an approach focusing on neo-epitopes have primarily been useful for the arthritis and bone field [35], and for liver fibrosis in monitoring degradation of collagen type III [36,37].

The gelatinases MMP-2 and MMP-9 have been investigated and documented to be highly regulated in fibrous tissue [12,13]. Cleavage of type VI collagen with these two proteases generated several fragments. Among these CO6-MMP was chosen due to it being unique and conversed among species. Several assays already exist for measuring total type VI collagen in different pathologies, using polyclonal antibodies (antibodies-online GmbH) or monoclonal antibodies (Uscn Life Science). Circulating levels of total type VI collagen patients with alcoholic liver disease have been investigated by Stickel *et al* [24], who found an significant elevation in alcoholic patients compared to controls. In addition they concluded that total collagen type VI already waselevated in early fibrotic states and therefore seem to be an important indicator of

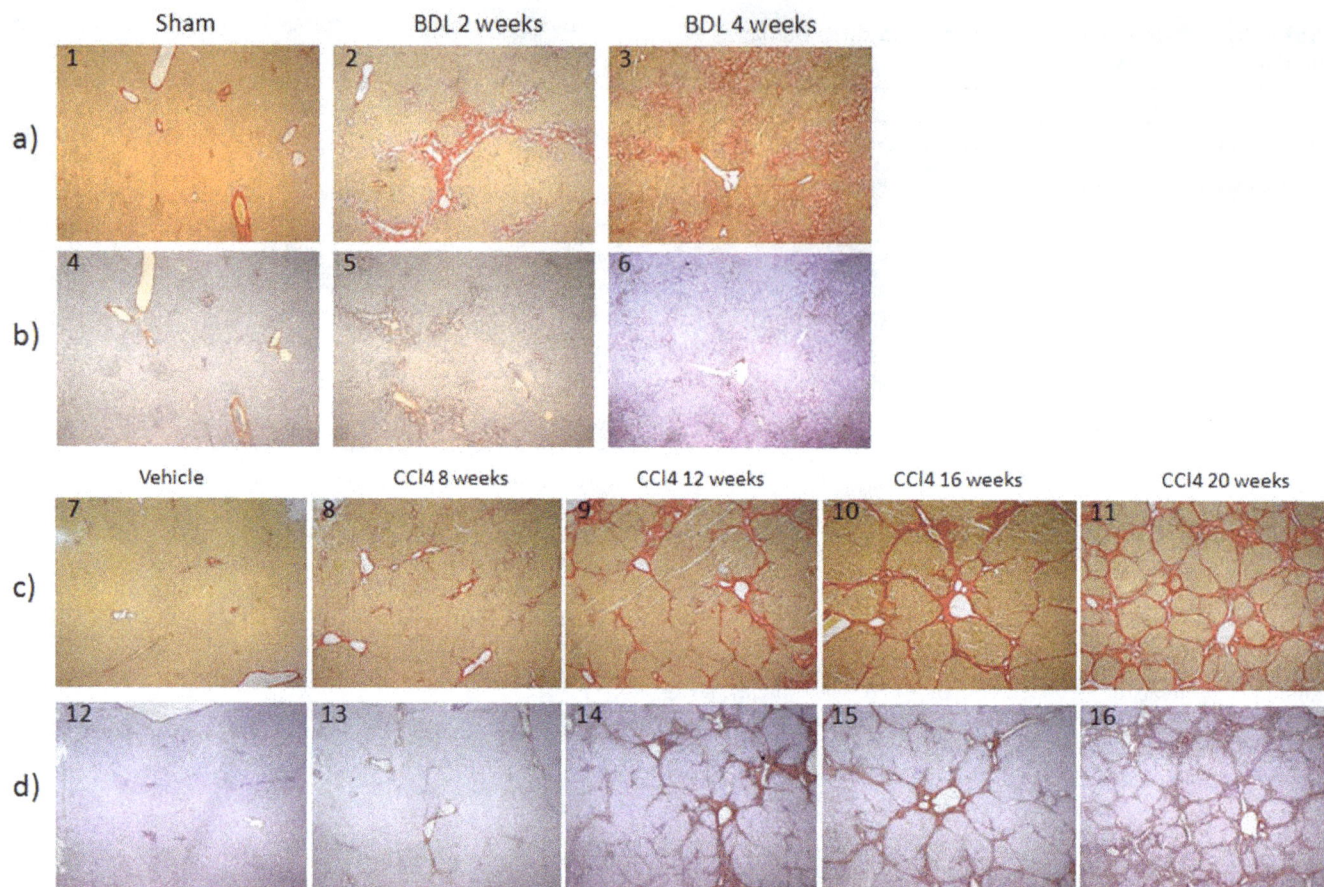

Figure 4. Type VI collagen in the liver. (A) Sirius Red photomicrographs showing the hepatic structure in rats 4 weeks after a sham operation (1), 2 weeks after BDL (2) and 4 weeks after BDL (3) (B) Immunohistochemical analysis of type VI collagen. Type VI collagen is localized around fibrotic structures. (C) Sirius Red photomicrographs showing the hepatic structure in rats 20 weeks after vehicle treatment (7), 8 weeks of CCl4 treatment (8), 12 weeks of CCl4 treatment (9), 16 weeks of CCl4 treatment (10) and 20 weeks of CCl4 treatment (11). (D) Immunohistochemical analysis of type VI collagen. Type VI collagen is localized around the fibrotic bands. Original magnification ×40.

early fibrotic transformation [24]. These data are consistent with our data indicating CO6-MMP is an early marker for fibrosis and they are in alignment with the fact that collagen type VI may be a good candidate biomarker. The CO6-MMP assay provides additional information on protease mediated tissue destruction in face of the total collagen markers. Such a careful deconstruction of the information entailed in the precise analyte may prove important to understand the processes that are leading to increased tissue formation as well as tissue degradation, and therefore eventually resolution of diseases. This may be assisted by the measurement of protein degradation and protein formation, in face of a crude measure of total protein [11,36,38]. The competitive ELISA was technically stable with a acceptable dilution recovery, as well as inter- and intra-variation for all matrices tested. The highest sensitivity for the assay was observed in the range of 4–125 ng/mL. Characterization of the selected monoclonal antibody revealed strong reactivity towards human, mouse and rat serum as well as the CO6-MMP peptide, strongly suggesting that the antibody recognizes this amino acid sequence for type VI collagen in native samples in complicated matrices. Characterizations using the final ELISA format showed that the recognized peptide fragment was generated by MMP-2 and MMP-9. Furthermore, it was seen that the antibody was specific against the neo-epitope generated in type VI collagen, as no response was detected when type I or type IV collagen was cleaved

by MMP-2 and -9. In addition the antibody did not recognise the elongated peptide, indicating neo-epitope specificity. The analyte stability was very good for both human- and rat serum CO6-MMP all recoveries within 100+/−20%.

It is well-appreciated that the BDL and the CCl4 models describe two different fibrotic processes in which increased ECM remodelling and excessive collagen deposition are key characteristics. The CO6-MMP was significantly related to liver fibrosis in CCL4 treated rats treated for 12–20 weeks. Furthermore, when rats were classified into quartiles according to the extent of fibrosis defined as the amount of collagen in the liver, we observed that the marker was elevated in all quartiles. The marker also correlated highly significantly to total collagen in the livers of CCL4-treated rats; however this was not the case in control rats, strongly indicating liver specific pathological relevance of the neo-epitope.

In the BDL model of liver fibrosis, serum CO6-MMP was elevated 2 and 4 weeks after BDL surgery compared to baseline and sham levels. These data are in agreement with the previous studies highlighting that type VI is generated during fibrogenesis by the activated hepatic stellate cells in the liver [2,37] and that MMP levels become elevated and unbalanced during fibrosis [1]. These data suggest that liver fibrosis is a high turnover disease, not may nor exclusively be described as an accumulation disease with increased collagen formation. Additionally, our data are in alignment investigating the collagen turnover profile in fibrotic

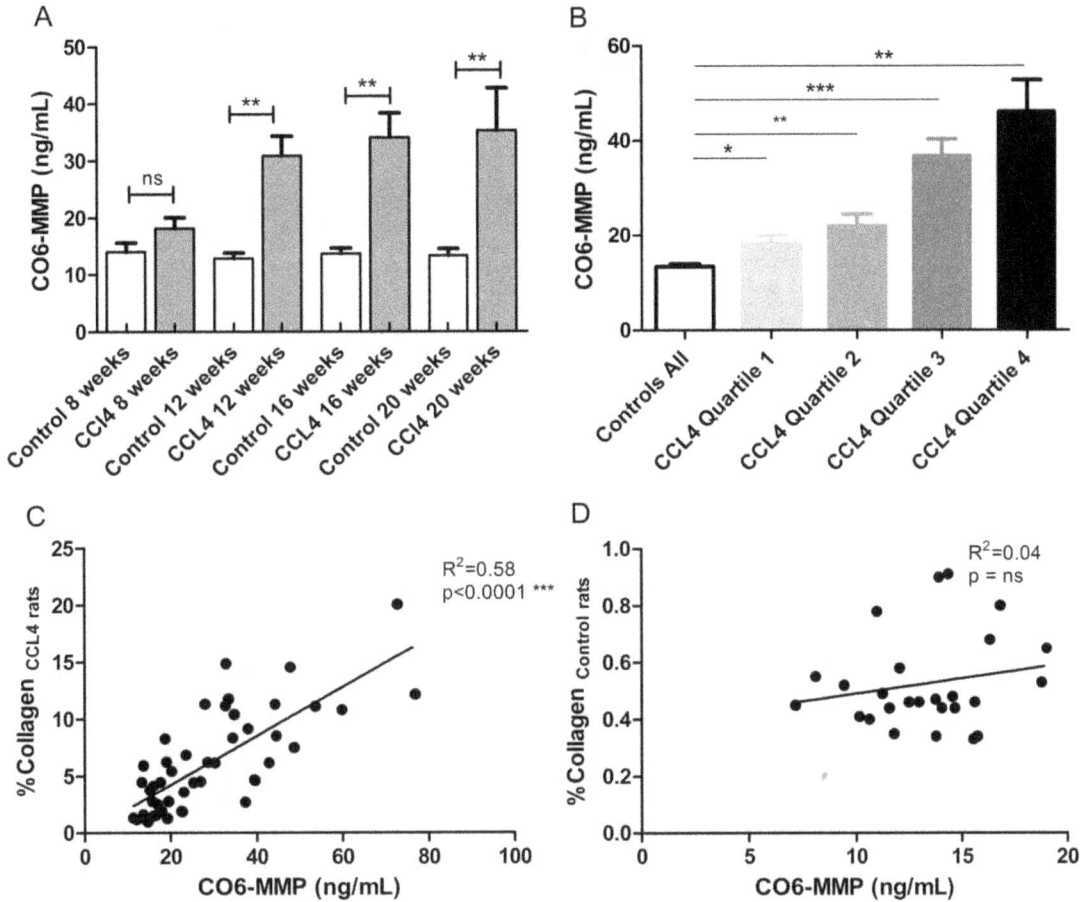

Figure 5. CO6-MMP serum levels in CCl4-treated rats. CCl4 rat liver fibrosis model: (A) Serum CO6-MMP was assessed in control rats at termination (controls) as well as in CCl4-treated rats at termination (CCl4) at weeks 8, 12, 16, 20. Results shown are mean ± standard error of the mean (SEM); (B) Serum CO6-MMP in all controls pooled and CCl4 rat stratified in quartiles according to total collagen in the liver; (C) Correlations between CO6-MMP and Sirius red in (C) CCl4 rats and in (D) control rats; Asterisks indicate statistical significance as indicated by bars. (** = $p<0.05$; *** = $p<0.001$, ns = non-significant difference).

rats, which demonstrated that a MMP-9 generated fragment of collagen type III (CO3-610) was elevated in the BDL rat model [37]. These combined data, past and present, indicate that liver fibroses may be a high collagen turnover disease with both increased collagen formation [23,38] and collagen degradation. This further emphasis the need of measuring the individual processes, enabling discovery of pathways leading to a resolution of the disease – by lowering tissue formation and increasing tissue degradation transiently. Such an investigation may not be obtained by exclusively measuring the total protein levels.

The systemic level of a biochemical marker is the result of the activity level and number/area of affected tissues. As such, levels of the CO6-MMP analyte are a systemic measurement of several local events. Type VI collagen has been identified within most tissues in different quantities [16]. In addition chronic liver diseases are associated with co-morbidities like osteoporosis, protein and calorie malnutrition [39], which may cause increased CO6-MMP levels originating from secondary tissues. The increased CO6-MMP levels in the presented two animal models may primarily derive from fibrosis in the liver but there may be confounded by effects from other tissues e.g. bone loss or muscular dystrophy, albeit bone only contain minute quantities of type IV collagen [39]. The exact contribution to the systemic pool of CO6-MMP from different

tissues, healthy and disease affected remains to be more carefully investigated.

This study carries some limitations. One major limitation of this study is that it is carried out in homogeneous, inbred laboratory rats with a synchronous induction of liver disease, which that bear little resemblance to the highly complicated presentation of clinical description of liver fibrosis. Further investigations in clinical settings are needed to provide more information on the usefulness of CO6-MMP.

In conclusion, we have developed an assay using a specific monoclonal antibody for the detection of CO6-MMP, a collagen type VI fragment generated by MMP-2 and -9. It was demonstrated that this marker was elevated in two pre-clinical models of fibrosis, the BDL and the CCl4 rat model, indicating that there is a high potential for the use of neo-epitope biomarkers in ECM-related diseases.

Author Contributions

Conceived and designed the experiments: SSV MAK DJL. Performed the experiments: SSV EV AN QHTN YL. Analyzed the data: SSV MAK EV AN BY DJL. Contributed reagents/materials/analysis tools: MRL PH QZ BV. Wrote the paper: SSV MAK BV DJL.

References

1. Friedman SL (2003) Liver fibrosis – from bench to bedside. J Hepatol 38 Suppl 1: S38–S53.
2. Gressner OA, Weiskirchen R, Gressner AM (2007) Biomarkers of liver fibrosis: clinical translation of molecular pathogenesis or based on liver-dependent malfunction tests. Clin Chim Acta 381: 107–113.
3. Bedossa P, Dargere D, Paradis V (2003) Sampling variability of liver fibrosis in chronic hepatitis C. Hepatology 38: 1449–1457.
4. Maharaj B, Maharaj RJ, Leary WP, Cooppan RM, Naran AD, et al. (1986) Sampling variability and its influence on the diagnostic yield of percutaneous needle biopsy of the liver. Lancet 1: 523–525.
5. Veidal SS, Bay-Jensen AC, Tougas G, Karsdal MA, Vainer B (2010) Serum markers of liver fibrosis: combining the BIPED classification and the neo-epitope approach in the development of new biomarkers. Dis Markers 28: 15–28.
6. Kumar V, Abbas AK, Fausto N (2005) Tissue renewal and repair: regeneration, healing, and fibrosis. Pathologic basis of disease. Philadelphia, Pennsylvania, USA: Elsevier Saunders. pp 87–118.
7. Schuppan D (1990) Structure of the extracellular matrix in normal and fibrotic liver: collagens and glycoproteins. Semin Liver Dis 10: 1–10.
8. Schuppan D, Ruehl M, Somasundaram R, Hahn EG (2001) Matrix as a modulator of hepatic fibrogenesis. Semin Liver Dis 21: 351–372.
9. Lochter A, Bissell MJ (1999) An odyssey from breast to bone: multi-step control of mammary metastases and osteolysis by matrix metalloproteinases. APMIS 107: 128–136.
10. Karsdal MA, Madsen SH, Christiansen C, Henriksen K, Fosang AJ, et al. (2008) Cartilage degradation is fully reversible in the presence of aggrecanase but not matrix metalloproteinase activity. Arthritis Res Ther 10: R63.
11. Karsdal MA, Henriksen K, Leeming DJ, Mitchell P, Duffin K, et al. (2009) Biochemical markers and the FDA Critical Path: how biomarkers may contribute to the understanding of pathophysiology and provide unique and necessary tools for drug development. Biomarkers 14: 181–202.
12. Hemmann S, Graf J, Roderfeld M, Roeb E (2007) Expression of MMPs and TIMPs in liver fibrosis - a systematic review with special emphasis on anti-fibrotic strategies. J Hepatol 46: 955–975.
13. Kirimlioglu H, Kirimlioglu V, Yilmaz S (2008) Expression of matrix metalloproteinases 2 and 9 in donor liver, cirrhotic liver, and acute rejection after human liver transplantation. Transplant Proc 40: 3574–3577.
14. Gelse K, Poschl E, Aigner T (2003) Collagens–structure, function, and biosynthesis. Adv Drug Deliv Rev 55: 1531–1546.
15. von der MH, Aumailley M, Wick G, Fleischmajer R, Timpl R (1984) Immunochemistry, genuine size and tissue localization of collagen VI. Eur J Biochem 142: 493–502.
16. Ricard-Blum S, Dublet B, van der Rest M (2000) Unconventional Collagens Oxford University Press, United States. pp 4–20.
17. Chang J, Nakajima H, Poole CA (1997) Structural colocalisation of type VI collagen and fibronectin in agarose cultured chondrocytes and isolated chondrons extracted from adult canine cartilage. J Anat 190: 523–532.
18. Kuo HJ, Maslen CL, Keene DR, Glanville RW (1997) Type VI collagen anchors endothelial basement membranes by interacting with type IV collagen. J Biol Chem 272: 26522–26529.
19. Bidanset DJ, Guidry C, Rosenberg LC, Choi HU, Timpl R, et al. (1992) Binding of the proteoglycan decorin to collagen type VI. J Biol Chem 267: 5250–5256.
20. Martinez-Hernandez A, Amenta PS (1993) The hepatic extracellular matrix. I. Components and distribution in normal liver. Virchows Arch A Pathol Anat Histopathol 423: 1–11.
21. Gerling B, Becker M, Staab D, Schuppan D (1997) Prediction of liver fibrosis according to serum collagen VI level in children with cystic fibrosis. N Engl J Med 336: 1611–1612.
22. Ji X, Li S, Kong X, Xu G, Chen J, et al. (1997) Clinical significance of serum 7S collagen and type VI collagen levels for the diagnosis of hepatic fibrosis. Chin Med J (Engl) 110: 198–201.
23. Shahin M, Schuppan D, Waldherr R, Risteli J, Risteli L, et al. (1992) Serum procollagen peptides and collagen type VI for the assessment of activity and degree of hepatic fibrosis in schistosomiasis and alcoholic liver disease. Hepatology 15: 637–644.
24. Stickel F, Urbaschek R, Schuppan D, Poeschl G, Oesterling C (2001) Serum collagen type VI and XIV and hyaluronic acid as early indicators for altered connective tissue turnover in alcoholic liver disease. Dig Dis Sci 46: 2025–2032.
25. Gressner AM, Weiskirchen R (2006) Modern pathogenetic concepts of liver fibrosis suggest stellate cells and TGF-beta as major players and therapeutic targets. J Cell Mol Med 10: 76–99.
26. Martinez-Hernandez A, Amenta PS (1993) The hepatic extracellular matrix. II. Ontogenesis, regeneration and cirrhosis. Virchows Arch A Pathol Anat Histopathol 423: 77–84.
27. Schuppan D, Ruhlmann T, Hahn EG (1985) Radioimmunoassay for human type VI collagen and its application to tissue and body fluids. Anal Biochem 149: 238–247.
28. Weiler-Normann C, Herkel J, Lohse AW (2007) Mouse models of liver fibrosis. Z Gastroenterol 45: 43–50.
29. Gefter ML, Margulies DH, Scharff MD (1977) A simple method for polyethylene glycol-promoted hybridization of mouse myeloma cells. Somatic Cell Genet 3: 231–236.
30. Clariá J, Jimenez W (1999) Renal dysfunction and ascites in carbon tetrachloride-induced cirrhosis in rats. The Liver and the Kidney. Blackwell Science, Boston. pp 379–396.
31. Munoz-Luque J, Ros J, Fernandez-Varo G, Tugues S, Morales-Ruiz M, et al. (2008) Regression of fibrosis after chronic stimulation of cannabinoid CB2 receptor in cirrhotic rats. J Pharmacol Exp Ther 324: 475–483.
32. Botney MD, Kaiser LR, Cooper JD, Mecham RP, Parghi D, et al. (1992) Extracellular matrix protein gene expression in atherosclerotic hypertensive pulmonary arteries. Am J Pathol 140: 357–364.
33. Sondergaard BC, Wulf H, Henriksen K, Schaller S, Oestergaard S, et al. (2006) Calcitonin directly attenuates collagen type II degradation by inhibition of matrix metalloproteinase expression and activity in articular chondrocytes. Osteoarthritis Cartilage 14: 759–768.
34. Bagger YZ, Tanko LB, Alexandersen P, Karsdal MA, Olson M, et al. (2005) Oral salmon calcitonin induced suppression of urinary collagen type II degradation in postmenopausal women: a new potential treatment of osteoarthritis. Bone 37: 425–430.
35. Schaller S, Henriksen K, Hoegh-Andersen P, Sondergaard BC, Sumer EU, et al. (2005) In vitro, ex vivo, and in vivo methodological approaches for studying therapeutic targets of osteoporosis and degenerative joint diseases: how biomarkers can assist? Assay Drug Dev Technol 3: 553–580.
36. Barascuk N, Veidal SS, Larsen L, Larsen DV, Larsen MR, et al. (2010) A novel assay for extracellular matrix remodeling associated with liver fibrosis: An enzyme-linked immunosorbent assay (ELISA) for a MMP-9 proteolytically revealed neo-epitope of type III collagen. Clin Biochem 43: 899–904.
37. Veidal SS, Vassiliadis E, Barascuk N, Zhang C, Segovia-Silvestre T, et al. (2010) Matrix metalloproteinase-9-mediated type III collagen degradation as a novel serological biochemical marker for liver fibrogenesis. Liver Int 30: 1293–1304.
38. Veidal SS, Vassiliadis E, Bay-Jensen AC, Tougas G, Vainer B, et al. (2010) Procollagen type I N-terminal propeptide (PINP) is a marker for fibrogenesis in bile duct ligation-induced fibrosis in rats. Fibrogenesis Tissue Repair 3: 5.
39. Mehta G, Rothstein KD (2009) Health maintenance issues in cirrhosis. Med Clin North Am 93: 901–9ix.

15

Suppression of CB1 Cannabinoid Receptor by Lentivirus Mediated Small Interfering RNA Ameliorates Hepatic Fibrosis in Rats

Si-Wen Chen[1]*, Ben-Yan Wu[1], Shi-Ping Xu[1], Ke-Xing Fan[2], Li Yan[1], Yuan Gong[1], Jun-Bao Wen[1], Dao-Hong Wu[1]

1 Department of Gastroenterology, NanLou Clinic, General Hospital of PLA, Beijing, China, 2 International Joint Cancer Institute, The Second Military Medical University, Shanghai, China

Abstract

It is recognized that endogenous cannabinoids, which signal through CB1 receptors in hepatic stellate cells (HSCs), exert a profibrotic effect on chronic liver diseases. In this study, we suppressed CB1 expression by lentivirus mediated small interfering RNA (CB1-RNAi-LV) and investigated its effect on hepatic fibrosis in vitro and in vivo. Our results demonstrated that CB1-RNAi-LV significantly inhibited CB1 expression, and suppressed proliferation and extracellular matrix production in HSCs. Furthermore, CB1-RNAi-LV ameliorated dimethylnitrosamine induced hepatic fibrosis markedly, which was associated with the decreased expression of mesenchymal cell markers smooth muscle α-actin, vimentin and snail, and the increased expression of epithelial cell marker E-cadherin. The mechanism lies on the blockage of Smad signaling transduction induced by transforming growth factor β1 and its receptor TGF-β RII. Our study firstly provides the evidence that CB1-RNAi-LV might ameliorate hepatic fibrosis through the reversal of epithelial-to-mesenchymal transition (EMT), while the CB1 antagonists AM251 had no effect on epithelial-mesenchymal transitions of HSCs. This suggests that CB1 is implicated in hepatic fibrosis and selective suppression of CB1 by small interfering RNA may present a powerful tool for hepatic fibrosis treatment.

Editor: Partha Mukhopadhyay, National Institutes of Health, United States of America

Funding: This work was supported by Grant from National Natural Science Foundation of China (No. 30900668), http://www.nsfc.gov.cn/Portal0/default152.htm. The funders had no role in study design, data collection and analysis, decision to publish, or preparation of the manuscript.

Competing Interests: The authors have declared that no competing interests exist.

* E-mail: chensiwenfj@yahoo.com.cn

Introduction

Hepatic fibrosis is a reversible wound-healing response characterized by an imbalance between excessive synthesis of extracellular matrix (ECM) and altered matrix degradation. The fibrogenic process is consecutive to proliferation and accumulation of myofibroblastic cells deriving from activated hepatic stellate cells (HSCs) and hepatic myofibroblasts (MFs). Both cell types express smooth muscle α-actin (α-SMA) and synthesize fibrogenic cytokines (transforming growth factor β1, TGF-β1), chemokines, fibrosis components (fibronectin, procollagen type I, and so on) and inhibitors of matrix degradation [1].

Endogenous cannabinoids are a family of molecules derived from arachidonic acid that signal through CB1 and CB2 receptors. Several studies have showed that chronic liver disease, including hepatic fibrosis, liver cirrhosis, alcoholic fatty liver and nonalcoholic fatty liver, all associated with the upregulation of endocannabinoids and their receptor, CB1 [2–10]. Increased activity of the hepatic CB1 also play a prominent role in both liver regeneration and liver carcinoma [11]. Major endogenous ligands of cannabinoids are anandamide, 2-arachidonylglycerol (2-AG), noladin ether and virodhamine [12]. It is recognized that endocannabinoids exert a profibrotic effect that is possibly mediated by CB1 receptors. This is compatible with the finding of increased CB1 expression in HSCs and hepatic MFs in the cirrhotic human liver

and in the fibrotic livers of mice [13]. Genetic or pharmacological ablation of CB1 receptors protected mice against liver injury; this was reflected by the reduced expression of α-SMA and TGF-β1 [13]. The profibrotic effects of CB1 activation could provide a rationale for the use of CB1 antagonists in the medical management of advanced liver cirrhosis. And CB1 have increasingly emerged as crucial targets during liver diseases [13].

In this study, we inhibited the CB1 expression by RNA interference to block its intracellular signaling transduction and investigated its effect on the biological characteristics of HSCs in vitro, and aimed to examine the therapeutic effect of CB1 small interference RNA (siRNA) on chronic liver disease and consider their implications regarding disease mechanism and the development of new therapeutic modalities. Furthermore, we compared the effect of CB1 siRNA with CB1 antagonists on biological characteristics of HSCs in vitro, and present CB1 siRNA as a powerful tool for hepatic fibrosis treatment.

Materials and Methods

Lentivirus vectors for CB1 RNAi

Four different CB1-specific target sequences were chosen using the CB1 reference sequence (Gene Bank Accession No NM_012784). Double-stranded DNA were synthesized according to the structure of a pGCSIL-GFP viral vector

(Genechemgene, Shanghai, China) and then inserted into a linearized vector. The positive clones were identified as lentiviral vectors named KD1, KD2, KD3 and KD4. Among the four vectors, KD4 (target sequence: 5'-GGAGACACAACAAA-CATTA-3') induced the highest levels of downregulation. So KD4 vector and viral packaging system were cotransfected into 293 cells to replicate competent lentivirus. The lentivirus containing the rat CB1 shRNA (short hairpin RNA) expressing cassette was used as a positive control for lentivirus production and denoted as CB1-RNAi-LV in the next experiments. The pGCSIL/U6 mock vector was also packaged and used as a negative control, denoted as NC-LV, which has no significant homology to rat gene sequences. For Annexin V/PI detection, we modified the lentivirus with deleting the GFP tag. The titers averaged 1×10^8 TU/mL.

Cell culture and transfection

Primary HSCs were isolated from SD rats (about 400 g body weight) by in situ perfusion, followed by centrifugation on a discontinuous gradient of metrizamide, as described previously [14]. The isolated HSCs were identified by their intrinsic vitamin A autofluorescence and by staining for desmin. Their purity was >95%. Cells were seeded in Dulbecco's modified medium containing 10% fetal bovine serum. Activated HSCs were obtained by subcultivation of HSCs at day 7 and then the cells were plated on new culture dishes for screening the efficacy of CB1 shRNA.

To examine the effect of CB1-RNAi-LV on activation and ECM production of HSCs, primary HSCs were transduced with lentiviral vectors CB1-RNAi-LV or NC-LV after expansion. For transduction, cells were seeded at 2000 cells/cm^2 in a T-75 cm^2 flask. The following day virus particles were added at a multiplicity of infection (m.o.i.) of 40 for 36 hours. Then cells were washed and cultured continually. 60 hours later, freshmedium with CB1 antagonists AM251 (1 µM, Santa Cruz, Santa Cruz, USA) was added to the cultured cells. The following day fresh medium with the endogenous cannabinoid ligands 2-AG (1 µM, Tocris Bioscience, Bristol, UK) was added to the cultured cells. 24 hours later, cells were collected for reverse transcription-polymerase chain reaction (RT-PCR) and western blot analysis.

To explore the effect of CB1-RNAi-LV on proliferation and the expression of PDGF receptor β subunit (PDGFR-β) of HSCs, primary HSCs treated with 20 ng/ml platelet-derived growth factor-BB (PDGF-BB; Sigma, St Louis, USA) for 48 h were transduced with lentiviral vectors CB1-RNAi-LV or NC-LV for another 48 h. Cells were then collected and total RNA was isolated with Trizol reagent (Invitrogen, Carlsbad, USA).

RT-PCR assay

cDNA was amplified from RNA with the use of the RT–PCR (Reverse transcriptional-PCR) kit (Takara, Otsu, Japan). Primers were designed according to Pubmed Genbank and synthesized by Shanghai Sangon Biological Engineering and Technology and Service Co. Ltd (China) (Table 1). Briefly, PCR was performed at 95°C with initial denaturation for 15 secs, followed by 45 cycles of amplification at 95°C (5 secs) and 60°C (30 secs). Finally, the samples were extended at 72°C for 10 min. For each gene, crossing point (Cp) values were determined and normalized by subtraction of the Cp value for GAPDH (generating a ΔCp value). Relative change was determined by subtraction of the ΔCp value for the control sample from the ΔCp value for the treated sample (ΔΔCp value). Fold change was subsequently calculated using the formula $2^{-\Delta\Delta Cp}$, which was denoted as the relative mRNA expression of each gene. Aliquots of the synthesized PCR products

Table 1. PCR primer sequences for RT-PCR detection.

GAPDH	114 bp	Forward	5'-TTCAACGGCACAGTCAAGG-3'
		Reverse	5'-CTCAGCACCAGCATCACC-3'
Cnr1	142 bp	Forward	5'-GACCTACCTGATGTTCTGGATTG-3'
		Reverse	5'-GTGGATGATGATGCTCTTCTGG-3'
α-SMA	191 bp	Forward	5'-CACCATCGGGAATGAACG-3'
		Reverse	5'-TGTCAGCAATGCCTGGGTA-3
PDGFRβ	233 bp	Forward	5'-GCCATCCTGAGGTCCCAA-3'
		Reverse	5'-TCGCAGGAGATGGTGGAAG-3'
TGFβ1	301 bp	Forward	5'-GCAACAACGCAATCTATGAC-3'
		Reverse	5'-TTCCTCTGCCTTATGTCCC-3'
TGFβR II	193 bp	Forward	5'-TCACCTACCACGGCTTCAC-3'
		Reverse	5'-ACGCCCGTCACTTGGATA-3'
Fibronectin	312 bp	Forward	5'-TCAGCTGTACCATTGCAAATC-3
		Reverse	5'-TGGTGTCCTGATCATTGCAT-3'
Procollagen Type I	142 bp	Forward	5'-CCTCCCAGCGGTGGTTAT-3'
		Reverse	5'-GGCTCTTGAGGGTAGTGTCC-3'
E-cadherin	196 bp	Forward	5'-GTCAAACGGCATCTAAAGC-3'
		Reverse	5'-TCAGACCCTGGTGAAAGC-3'
Snail	216 bp	Forward	5'-TCCTTGCTCCACAAACACCA-3'
		Reverse	5'-TGCCTTCCATCAGCCATCT-3'
Vimentin	132 bp	Forward	5'-TCCCTGAACCTGAGAGAAAC-3'
		Reverse	5'-ATCGTGGTGCTGAGAAGTC-3'

were separated by electrophoresis on a 1.5% agarose gel and analyzed by Gel-Pro 3.1 software.

Proliferation assay

After lentivirus transfected and/or PDGF-BB stimulation, primary HSCs cultured in 96 wells plate were stimulated with 10 µl/well 5-bromodeoxyuridine (BrdU, Roche, Mannheim, Germany) for 24 h, followed by being fixed with 200 µl/well FixDenat solution for 30 minutes. Cells were then incubated with 5–10% BSA for 30 minutes. Subsequently, 100 µl/well anti-BrdU-POD solutions were added to the cells. The immune complexes are detected by the subsequent substrate reaction. The reaction product is quantified by measuring the absorbance at the 450 nm wavelength using a scanning multiwell spectrophotometer (ELISA reader). The developed color and thereby the absorbance values directly correlate to the amount of DNA synthesis hereby to the number of proliferating cells in the respective microcultures. Results were expressed as mean±SD of cells that had incorporated BrdU (percentage of BrdU-positive cells).

Apoptosis assay

Apoptosis assay was performed according to the protocol of the Annexin V/PI Apoptosis Assay Kit (Jingmei, Shanghai, China). In brief, primary HSCs stimulated by AM251 and/or 2-AG and/or transfected by lentivirus mentioned above were harvested and washed in ice-cold phosphate-buffered saline. The cells were then resuspended in 250 µl binding buffer to a final concentration of 1×10^6 cells per ml, and 100 µl of the cell suspension was aliquot into each test tube. Five µl of Annexin/FITC and 10 µl PI (20 µg/ml) were added. FACS Aria Flow Cytometer System (BD, San Jose, USA) was used to analyze cell apoptosis.

Western blot analysis

After lentivirus transfection and/or AM251 treatment, whole cells were homogenized in lysis buffer. Phosphatase inhibitor (Sigma, St Louis, USA) was added to prevent protein dephosphorylation. A Bio-Rad Rapid Coomassie kit (Bio-Rad, Hercules, CA) was used to determine the total protein concentration. Sixty micrograms of protein were run on a 10% SDS-poly-acrylamide gel and transferred to a polyvinylidene difluoride membrane. Immunoblotting was performed with primary antibodies against CB1 (Alomone labs, CA, USA), αSMA (Boster, Wuhan, China), TGF-β1 (CST, Beverly, USA), transforming growth factor β receptor II (TGF-β RII, CST, Beverly, USA), fibronectin (Santa Cruz, Santa Cruz, USA), procollagen Type I (Santa Cruz, Santa Cruz, USA), E-cadherin (Santa Cruz, Santa Cruz, USA), snail (CST, Beverly, USA), vimentin (CST, Beverly, USA) and GAPDH (Santa Cruz, Santa Cruz, USA), followed by incubation with horseradish peroxidase-conjugated anti-mouse- or anti-rabbit IgG (Santa Cruz, Santa Cruz, CA, USA) as secondary antibodies. The blot was developed with a chemiluminescence system (ECL; Amersham, Piscataway, NJ) according to the manufacturer's protocol. The optical densities of the bands were measured with a Model GS-700 Imaging Densitometer (Bio-Rad, Hercules, CA).

Animal model of hepatic fibrosis

All animals (male SD rats) weighing about 160 g were housed in cages with stainless steel wire tops and with 12-h light-dark cycles under standard animal laboratory conditions in the SPF-grade animal room of the experimental animal center of General Hospital of PLA in China. The rats had free access to standard rat chow and water. This study was carried out in strict accordance with the recommendations in the Guide for the Care and Use of Laboratory Animals of the National Institutes of Health. The protocol was approved by the Local Ethical Committee of General Hospital of PLA (Permit Number: 2012-87).

To induce the hepatic fibrosis animal model, 48 male SD rats were randomly divided into the normal group (n = 12) and the DMN (dimethylnitrosamine, Tianjin Chemical Reagent Research Institute, Tianjin, China)-treatment group (n = 36). All the animals in the DMN-treatment group received DMN dissolved in saline at a dose of 10 ml DMN/kg by a peritoneal injection for three consecutive days each week for 3 weeks, and were randomly assigned to the following three groups (12 in each): CB1-RNAi-LV treatment group (1×10^8 TU CB1-RNAi-LV dissolved in Ringer's solution was injected through the tail vein on the day before DMN injection), Ringer's solution group and NC-LV treatment group (1×10^8 TU NC-LV dissolved in Ringer's solution was injected through the tail vein on the day before DMN injection) as the negative control group.

At the end of 3 weeks, the rats were killed and serum samples were collected for biochemical tests. The right lobes of livers were taken and soaked with 10% neutral formaldehyde for histology.

Evaluation of hepatic fibrosis

To evaluate the pathogenesis of hepatic fibrosis semiquantita-tively, Masson's trichrome staining was used. The stage of fibrosis was graded as follows: stage 0, normal connective tissue (no fibrosis); stage 1, fibrous portal expansion; stage 2, periportal fibrosis with short septa extending into lobules or rare porto-portal septa (intact architecture); stage 3, fibrous septa reaching adjacent portal tracts and terminal hepatic venule (architecture distortion, but no obvious cirrhosis); stage 4, diffuse nodular formation (cirrhosis).

Immunohistochemistry examination for liver sections

The paraffin sections were deparaffinized using xylene and alcohol and hydrated to water, then treated with primary antibodies including α-SMA polyclone antibody, CB1 polyclone antibody and E-cadherin monoclone antibody, followed by

biotinylated second antibody and then streptavidin peroxidase. The integrated optical intensity of α-SMA, CB1 and E-cadherin was semiquantified using Image-Pro Plus software.

Statistical analysis

Results were presented as means of three independent experiments ($\pm$SD). In the semiquantitive analysis of histological staging, nonparametric tests (Wilcoxon test) were used and other statistical analyses performed with an unpaired Student's t-test. Differences were considered as significant or highly significant at $p<0.05$ or $p<0.01$, respectively.

Results

RNA interference knockdown the expression of CB1 in HSCs

In this study, we constructed four pairs of shRNA expressing lentivirus vectors named KD1, KD2, KD3 and KD4 to knockdown CB1 mRNA expression in the activated HSCs. RT–PCR detection showed that KD4 had the highest gene-silencing efficacy among all the four pairs of lentivirus vectors (Figure 1A). KD4 deduced CB1 mRNA expression by about 75% at 24 h, and protein expression by about 80% at 48 h, respectively (Figure 1B). So in the subsequent experiments, we selected KD4 (also named CB1-RNAi-LV in the ensuing paragraphs) to knock down CB1 expression and investigate its effect on hepatic fibrosis in vitro and in vivo.

CB1-RNAi-LV inhibits the activation and ECM production of HSCs

To investigate the effect of CB1-RNAi-LV on the activation and ECM production of HSCs, we detected mRNA and protein expression of α-SMA, TGF-β1, TGF-β RII, fibronectin and procollagen type I by RT-PCR and western blot. The results showed that the expressions of all the five molecules in HSCs increased significantly by 2-AG stimulation or by 2-AG stimula-tion and NC-LV transfection, and the expressions of all in HSCs with 2-AG stimulation decreased significantly when stimulated by AM-251, the CB1 antagonist (Figure 2). In HSCs stimulated by 2-AG and transfected with CB1-RNAi-LV, mRNA and protein expression of the five molecules also decreased markedly, compared with that in HSCs stimulated by 2-AG and transfected with NC-LV (Figure 2). Furthermore, mRNA and protein expression of α-SMA, TGF-β1, TGF-β RII and fibronectin in HSCs with 2-AG stimulation and CB1-RNAi-LV transfection declined significantly, when compared with that in HSCs stimulated by 2-AG and treated with AM251. We deduced that CB1 could promote the activation and ECM production of HSCs, which could be blocked by CB1 siRNA and CB1 antagonist, and the inhibition effect of CB1 siRNA on HSCs activation was more significant than the CB1 antagonist.

CB1-RNAi-LV suppresses HSC proliferation induced by PDGF-BB

PDGF is recognized as the most potent mitogen for HSCs, which impedes HSCs proliferation via its receptor β subunit (PDGFR-β). To investigate the effect of CB1-RNAi-LV on HSCs proliferation pretreated with PDGF-BB, BrdU incorporation was used. Results showed that PDGF-BB significantly promoted HSCs proliferation, which was constrained by CB1-RNAi-LV (Figure 3A). Furthermore, RT-PCR detection showed that PDGFR-β mRNA expression in HSCs increased markedly by PDGF-BB pretreatment, and decreased markedly by CB1-RNAi-

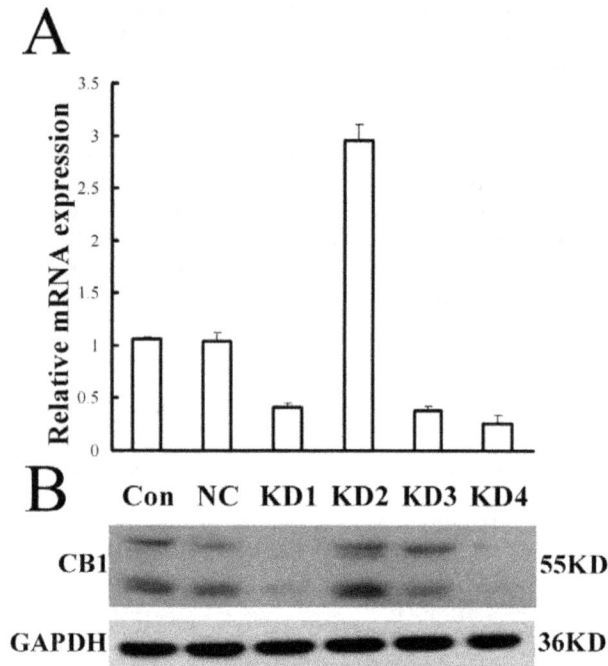

Figure 1. Effect of shRNA expressing lentivirus against CB1 on CB1 expression in primary hepatic stellate cells. (A) The statistical results of CB1 mRNA expression in primary hepatic stellate cells (HSCs) transfected with 4 pairs of shRNA expressing lentivirus named KD1, KD2, KD3 and KD4 by RT-PCR detection. The pGCSIL/U6 mock vector named Con was used as a negative control. KD4 displayed the highest gene-silencing efficacy among all the 4 pairs of lentivirus. Relative expression levels of mRNA were normalized against those of GAPDH mRNA. **(B)** The CB1 protein expression in HSCs transfected with 4 pairs of shRNA expressing lentivirus and the negative control lentivirus, respectively. The results demonstrated that KD4 deduced CB1 mRNA expression by about 75%, and protein expression by about 80%, which had the highest gene-silencing efficacy among all the four pairs of lentivirus vectors.

LV transfection (Figure 3B). It was deduced that CB1 siRNA could suppress PDGFR-β mRNA expression, and inhibit HSCs proliferation induced by PDGF.

CB1-RNAi-LV does not affect HSCs apoptosis induced by 2-AG

It is recognized that hepatic fibrosis is reversible by apoptosis of hepatic MFs [1]. In this study, results showed that the percentage of apoptotic HSCs increased markedly by 2-AG stimulation ($14.3 \pm 3.8\%$ vs $7.4 \pm 2.1\%$, $p < 0.01$), and no significant differences of the percentage of apoptotic HSCs were shown between HSCs with 2-AG stimulation and HSCs with 2-AG stimulation and NC-LV transfection ($14.3 \pm 3.8\%$ vs $12.9 \pm 4.3\%$, $p > 0.05$). Furthermore, there were also no significant differences of the percentage of apoptotic HSCs between HSCs with 2-AG stimulation and NC-LV transfection and HSCs with 2-AG stimulation and CB1-RNAi-LV transfection ($12.9 \pm 4.3\%$ vs $14.1 \pm 5.3\%$, $p > 0.05$), and between HSCs with 2-AG stimulation and HSCs with 2-AG stimulation and AM251 treatment ($14.3 \pm 3.8\%$ vs $13.6 \pm 4.7\%$, $p > 0.05$). These data revealed that 2-AG could increase the apoptosis of culture-activated HSCs, but neither CB1 shRNA nor CB1 antagonist AM251 could affect the HSCs apoptosis induced by 2-AG, indicating that 2-AG-induced HSCs apoptosis was independent of its receptor CB1.

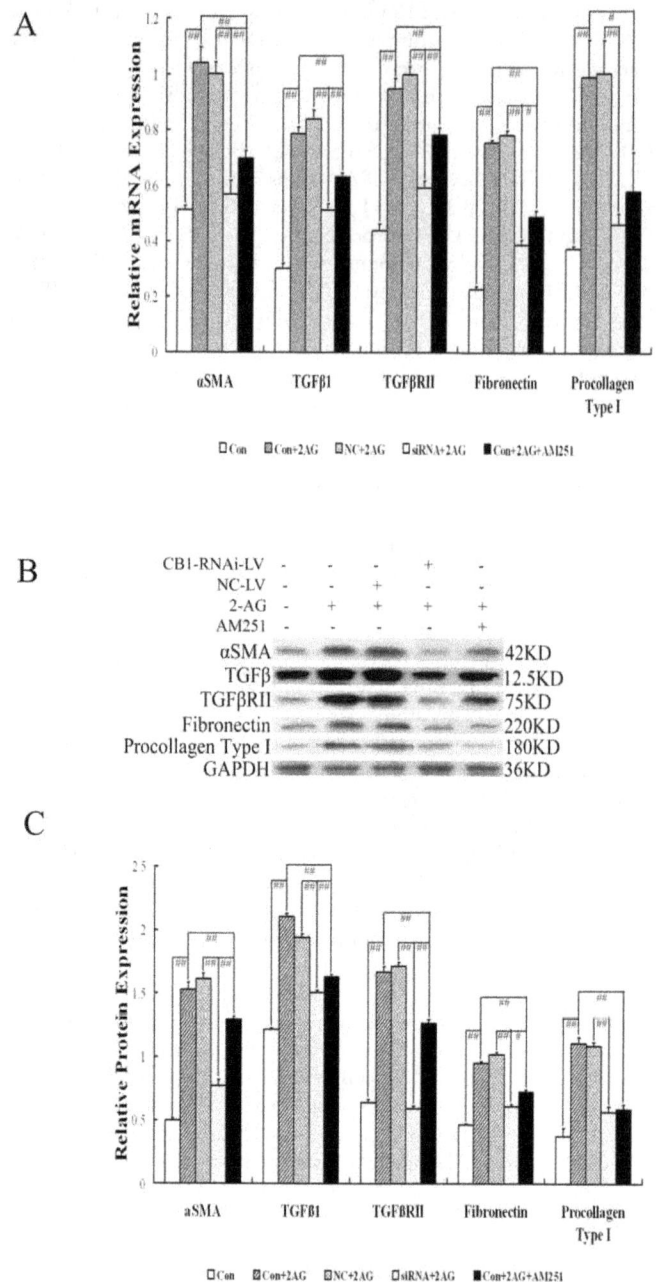

Figure 2. Effect of CB1-RNAi-LV on activation and ECM production of primary hepatic stellate cells. (A) The statistical results of α-SMA, TGF-β1, TGF-β RII, fibronectin and procollagen type I mRNA expression in HSCs (named Con), HSCs with 2-AG (named Con+2AG), HSCs with NC-LV and 2-AG (named NC+2AG), HSCs with CB1-RNAi-LV and 2-AG (named siRNA+2AG), HSCs with 2-AG and AM251 (named Con+2AG+AM251) by RT-PCR analysis. Relative expression levels of mRNA were normalized against those of GAPDH mRNA. **(B)** shows representative graphs of α-SMA, TGF-β1, TGF-β RII, fibronectin and procollagen type I protein expression by Western blot analysis and **(C)** shows the statistical results. Results demonstrated that the mRNA and protein expressions of α-SMA, TGF-β1, TGF-β RII, fibronectin and procollagen type I in HSCs were all increased significantly after 2-AG stimulation, which were all decreased significantly when stimulated with AM251 or transfected with CB1-RNAi-LV. Furthermore, the mRNA expression of α-SMA, TGF-β1, TGF-β RII and fibronectin in HSCs stimulated by 2-AG and AM251 was higher significantly than that in HSCs stimulated by 2-AG and transfected with CB1-RNAi-LV. "#" $p < 0.05$, "# #" $p < 0.01$.

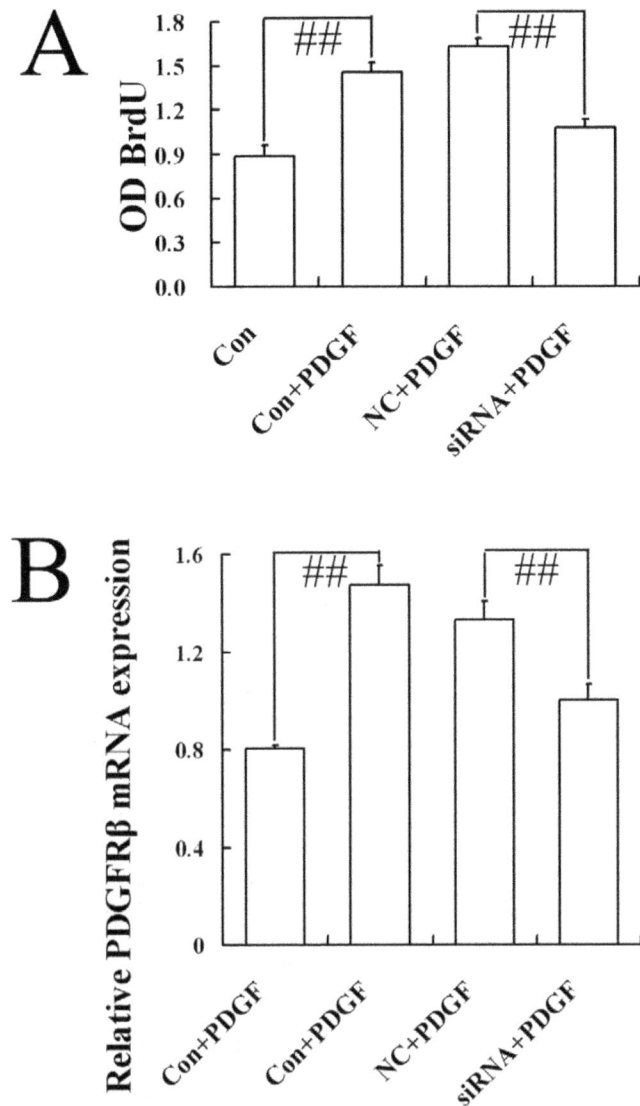

Figure 3. Effect of CB1-RNAi-LV on the proliferation of primary hepatic stellate cells. (A) The statistical results of the optical density (OD) value of BrdU incorporative cells in HSCs (named Con), HSCs with PDGF (named Con+PDGF), HSCs with NC-LV and PDGF (named NC+PDGF), HSCs with CB1-RNAi-LV and PDGF (named siRNA+PDGF) by ELISA method. "# #" $p<0.01$. Results showed that the proliferation of HSCs stimulated by PDGF-BB elevated significantly than HSCs alone. NC-LV transfection did not affect the proliferation of HSCs stimulated by PDGF-BB. Furthermore, the proliferation of HSCs stimulated with PDGF-BB and transfected with CB1-RNAi-LV decreased markedly than that of HSCs stimulated with PDGF-BB and transfected with NC-LV. **(B)** The statistical results of PDGFR-β mRNA expression in HSCs (named Con), HSCs with PDGF (named Con+PDGF), HSCs with NC-LV and PDGF (named NC+PDGF), HSCs with CB1-RNAi-LV and PDGF (named siRNA+PDGF) by RT-PCR analysis. Relative expression levels of mRNA were normalized against those of GAPDH mRNA. "# #" $p<0.01$. Results showed that PDGFR-β mRNA expression increased markedly by PDGF-BB pretreatment or by PDGF-BB pretreatment plus NC-LV transfection, while PDGFR-β mRNA expression in HSCs pretreated with PDGF-BB and transfected with CB1-RNAi-LV decreased markedly than that in HSCs pretreated with PDGF-BB and transfected with NC-LV.

CB1-RNAi-LV induce Mesenchymal-Epithelial Transition in HSCs

Several lines of evidence support an important role of Epithelial-to-Mesenchymal Transition (EMT) and Mesenchymal-to-Epithelial Transition (MET) in the pathogenesis of hepatic fibrosis [15,16]. RT-PCR and western blot analysis indicated that the levels of E-cadherin, the epithelial phenotype gene, were down-regulated significantly in the HSCs stimulated by 2-AG, compared with the HSCs alone (Figure 4), and were up-regulated significantly in the HSCs transfected by CB1-RNAi-LV, compared with the HSCs transfected by NC-LV (Figure 4). These data indicated that the CB1 siRNA could promote the epithelial phenotype expression in activated HSCs. On the other hand, the expression of vimentin and snail in HSCs, which indicated mesenchymal phenotype and mesenchymal defining function, was significantly up-regulated by 2-AG stimulation, which could be down-regulated by CB1-RNAi-LV transfection (Figure 4). These data demonstrated that deactivation of activated HSCs could be achieved by inducing the MET process ascribed to down-regulation of CB1, revealing an important role of CB1 for HSCs in restoring biological characteristics of activated state.

CB1-RNAi-LV relieves liver injury in DMN rats

To further investigate the effect of CB1-RNAi-LV on liver injury, the DMN rats model was used. Serum levels of alanine aminotransferase (ALT) and aspartate aminotransferase (AST) elevated significantly in DMN rats as compared with the normal rats (Figure 5). However, CB1-RNAi-LV treatment markedly reduced the serum levels of ALT and AST as compared with NC-LV treatment (Figure 5), illustrating that CB1 siRNA could relieve liver injury induced by DMN.

CB1-RNAi-LV knocked down CB1 expression in DMN rats

We have confirmed that CB1-RNAi-LV could suppress CB1 expression in primary isolated HSCs, so we transfected DMN rats with CB1-RNAi-LV to identify the efficacy of CB1-RNAi-LV on CB1 expression in vivo. Immunohistochemical examination showed almost no CB1 expression in normal liver, which increased markedly in DMN rats. However, CB1-RNAi-LV transfection markedly decreased the expression of CB1 in DMN rats, revealing that CB1 siRNA could also knock down CB1 expression in vivo (Figure 6).

CB1-RNAi-LV inhibits HSC activation and ameliorates hepatic fibrosis in DMN rats

Immunohistochemical examination revealed that CB1 and α-SMA protein expressions increased significantly in the DMN rats, which were suppressed by CB1-RNAi-LV treatment (Figure 6). Masson's trichrome staining of liver sections in the DMN rats and the NC-LV treatment rats showed periportal fibrosis with short septa extending into lobules or porto-portal septa, and severe cholestasis and bile duct hyperplasia were also observed, the semiquantitative analysis of the fibrosis stage pathologically showed that hepatic fibrosis was significantly ameliorated in the CB1-RNAi-LV treatment rats as compared with the NC-LV treatment rats (Figure 6A and Table 2). These results clearly indicated that CB1 shRNA could ameliorate hepatic fibrosis induced by DMN.

CB1-RNAi-LV induces Mesenchymal-Epithelial Transition in livers of DMN rats

To further investigate whether CB1-RNAi-LV could induce the MET process in hepatic fibrosis animal model, we treated hepatic against those of GAPDH mRNA. "# #" $p < 0.01$. (**B**) shows representative graphs of E-cadherin, Snail and Vimentin protein expression by Western blot analysis and (**C**) shows the statistical results. These data indicated that the mRNA and protein expressions of E-cadherin in HSCs were down-regulated significantly by 2-AG stimulation, while the levels of Snail and Vimentin were up-regulated significantly by 2-AG stimulation. On the other hand, the expression level of E-cadherin in HSCs with CB1-RNAi-LV transfection and 2-AG stimulation were increased markedly than that in HSCs with NC-LV transfection and 2-AG stimulation, while the expression levels of Vimentin and Snail in HSCs with CB1-RNAi-LV transfection and 2-AG stimulation were decreased markedly than that in HSCs with NC-LV transfection and 2-AG stimulation. The results also revealed that the expression levels of E-cadherin, Snail and Vimentin in HSCs stimulated by 2-AG were not affected by AM251 treatment.

fibrosis rats induced by DMN with CB1-RNAi-LV or its negative control, NC-LV. Immunochemical examination showed that DMN treatment declined E-cadherin expression significantly compared with normal rats, while E-cadherin expression elevated significantly by CB1-RNAi-LV transfection, compared with NC-LV transfected rats (Figure 6). These results demonstrated that EMT played important roles in the progression of hepatic fibrosis, which can be reversed by CB1 siRNA.

Discussion

Many studies have demonstrated the up-regulation of the expression of CB1 in hepatic MFs and vascular endothelial cells, as well as increased concentration of endocannabinoids in liver in the course of chronic progressive liver diseases [8,9,13,17]. Teixeira-Clerc et al [9] have provided evidence for the involvement of CB1 in regulation of hepatic fibrosis and the profibrogenic effect of CB1 signaling. Moreover, the effect of CB1 inactivation was demonstrated in three experimental models of liver injury induced by CCl4, thioacetamide or biliary cholestasis. The favorable anti-

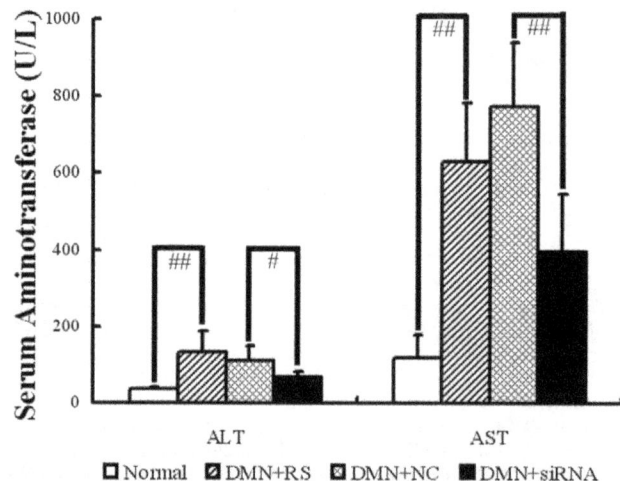

Figure 5. Effect of CB1-RNAi-LV on serum aminotransferase in DMN induced hepatic fibrosis. The statistical results of serum alanine aminotransferase (ALT) and aspartate aminotransferase (AST) levels in normal rats, rats with DMN treatment and Ringer's solution (RS) injected, rats with DMN treatment and NC-LV injected, rats with DMN treatment and CB1-RNAi-LV injected. "#" $p < 0.05$ and "# #" $p < 0.01$. The data demonstrated that serum ALT and AST elevated significantly in DMN rats as compared with the normal rats. However, CB1-RNAi-LV treatment markedly reduced the serum ALT and AST as compared with NC-LV treatment rats.

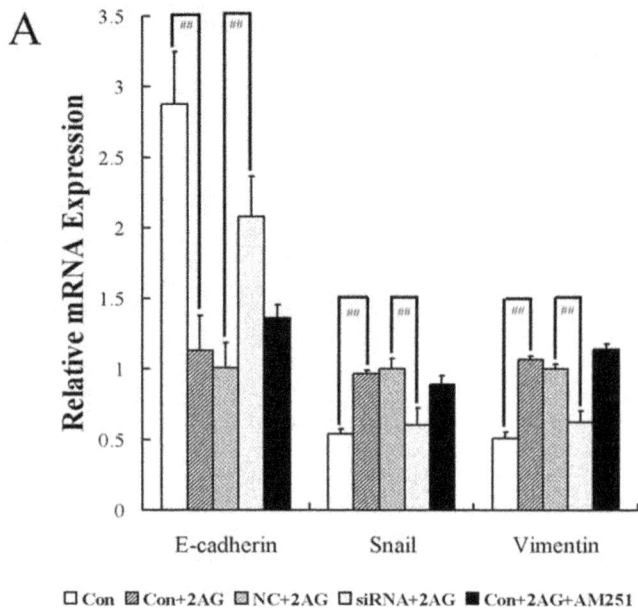

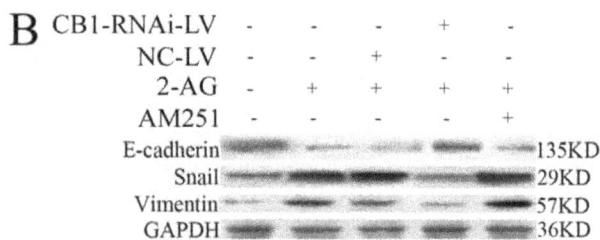

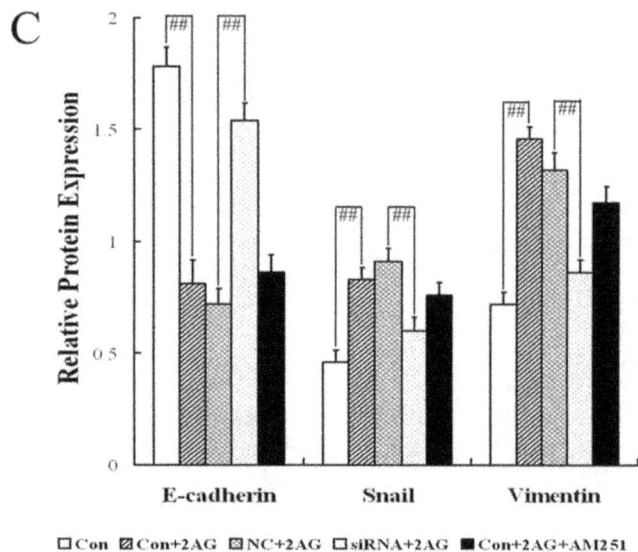

Figure 4. Effect of CB1-RNAi-LV on Mesenchymal-Epithelial Transitions of primary hepatic stellate cells. (**A**) The statistical results of E-cadherin, Snail and Vimentin mRNA expression in HSCs (named Con), HSCs with 2-AG (named Con+2AG), HSCs with NC-LV and 2-AG (named NC+2AG), HSCs with CB1-RNAi-LV and 2-AG (named siRNA+2AG), HSCs with 2-AG and AM251 (named Con+2AG+AM251) by RT-PCR analysis. Relative expression levels of mRNA were normalized

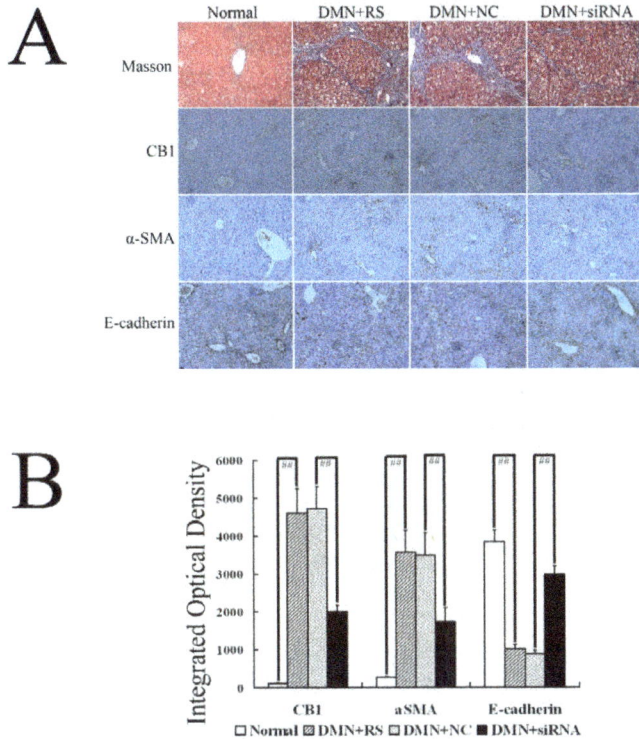

Figure 6. Effect of CB1-RNAi-LV on hepatic fibrosis and epithelial- mesenchymal transitions in livers of DMN rats. (A) The first line showed the representative graph of Masson's trichrome staining (magnification of 20×) in normal rats (Normal), rats with DMN treatment and Ringer's solution injected (DMN+RS), rats with DMN treatment and NC-LV injected (DMN+NC-LV), rats with DMN treatment and CB1-RNAi-LV injected (DMN+RNAi-LV). The second, the third and the fourth line showed the representative graph of CB1, α-SMA and E-cadherin immunohistochemical examination (magnification of 20×) in normal rats (Normal), rats with DMN treatment and Ringer's solution injected (DMN+RS), rats with DMN treatment and NC-LV injected (DMN+NC-LV), rats with DMN treatment and CB1-RNAi-LV injected (DMN+RNAi-LV). **(B)** Shows statistical results of CB1, α-SMA and E-cadherin immunohistochemical staining. Masson's trichrome staining of liver sections in the DMN rats and the NC-LV treatment rats showed periportal fibrosis with short septa extending into lobules or porto-portal septa, and severe cholestasis and bile duct hyperplasia were also observed, whereas hepatic fibrosis was significantly ameliorated in the CB1-RNAi-LV treatment rats as compared with the NC-LV treatment rats. Immunohistochemical examination revealed that CB1 and α-SMA protein expressions increased significantly in the DMN rats, which were suppressed by CB1-RNAi-LV treatment. Immunochemical examination also showed that DMN treatment declined E-cadherin expression significantly compared with normal rats, while E-cadherin expression elevated significantly in DMN rats transfected with CB1-RNAi-LV, compared with that in DMN rats transfected with NC-LV. "# #" $p < 0.01$.

Table 2. Effect of CB1 shRNA on hepatic fibrosis of DMN rats.

Group/Stage	0–1	1–2	2–3	3–4	U
Normal	12	0	0	0	/
DMN+RS	0	0	10	0	4.3875**
DMN+NC-LV	0	0	6	2	/
DMN+RNAi-LV	0	8	0	0	3.4668##

To score the stage of fibrosis, three fields of microscope in the liver section of each rat were scored, and the average score was the stage of fibrosis.
**$p < 0.01$ compared with the normal rats.
##$p < 0.01$ compared with the DMN+NC-LV rats.

fibrogenic results were obtained either by pharmacological inactivation with rimonabant, a selective antagonist of CB1 receptor, or via genetic inactivation in homozygous CB1-deficient mice, and decreased progression of fibrosis was accompanied by reduced hepatic TGF-β1 expression, and inhibited proliferation and increased apoptosis of MFs. In the present study, RNA interference technique was used firstly to knockdown the CB1 expression, and lentivirus based shRNA expressing vector named CB1-RNAi-LV was applied firstly in hepatic fibrosis animal model.

Several lines of evidence indicate that TGF-β1 from autocrine or paracrine sources plays a role in activating HSCs and increasing

the synthesis of ECM proteins and cellular receptors for various matrix proteins [18,19]. In response to TGF-β1, type II TGF-β1 receptors autophosphorylated and transmitted the signal by which regulatory Smad molecules (Smad3/2) are phosphorylated and form an active complex with co-Smad (Smad4) [20]. The fibrogenic effect of TGF-β in liver can be inhibited by neutralizing antibodies against TGF-β or soluble TGF-β-RII [21,22]. In the present study, reduced expressions of TGF-β1, its receptor TGF-β RII and snail, the important intracellular transcription factor closely related to the intracellular signaling transduction pathway of TGF-β1, were induced by CB1-RNAi-LV in cultured HSCs, furthermore, the antifibrogenic effect of CB1-RNAi-LV was also confirmed in vitro and in vivo, demonstrating that the restorative effect of CB1-RNAi-LV on hepatic fibrosis might be partially attributed to the decreased expression of TGF-β1 and its receptor, and the blockage of its intracellular signaling transduction pathway subsequently.

Epithelial cells are adherent cells that closely attach to each other, forming coherent layers in which cells exhibit apico-basal polarity. Mesenchymal cells, in contrast, are non-polarized cells, capable of moving as individual cells because they lack intercellular connections. EMT describes the process by which cells gradually lose their epithelial signatures while acquiring the characteristics of mesenchymal cells. MET refers to the reverse process. Organ fibrosis is a potential outcome of EMT, which is associated with inflammation, when inflammation persists, EMT generates fibroblastic cells that accumulate and cause progressive fibrosis [23].

A series of recent studies strongly suggested that EMT is an important contributor to the progression of hepatic fibrosis [16,24–26]. The adhesion junction protein E-cadherin is critical for the disappearance of cell-cell junctions and apical-basal polarity of epithelia. As one of intermediate filament proteins, vimentin will accumulate dramatically in the cytoplasm during EMT. The expression of E-cadherin can be repressed by transcriptional factors including snail [27,28]. HSCs are the most accepted myofibroblast progenitors in the liver [19]. Recently, several studies pointed out that HSCs in the quiescent state contain epithelial characteristics, and the activation of HSCs might be considered as an EMT phenomenon [25,29,30].

The paracrine activity of HSCs may also affect the cell phenotype of hepatocytes, the main epithelial cells in liver, which may be another mechanism of EMT in liver. Jeong WI, et al [31] reported chronic alcohol feeding could promote CB1 expression in hepatocytes in vivo, which could be replicated in vitro by co-culturing control hepatocytes with HSCs isolated from ethanol-fed mice, implicating HSCs-derived mediators in the regulation of hepatic CB1. HSCs are a rich source of retinoic acid (RA). Mukhopadhyay B et al [10] confirmed that the HSCs-derived 2-

AG also promoted CB1 expression in hepatocytes, which was mediated indirectly via RA, because it was absent in hepatocytes from mice lacking retinaldehyde dehydrogenase1, the enzyme catalyzing the generation of RA from retinaldehyde.

Since EMT is dynamic and bidirectional, we deduce that fibrogenic cells such as activated HSCs can undergo MET and revert back to an epithelial phenotype, which results in the reverse of hepatic fibrosis. Actually, bone morphogenic protein-7, a negative regulator of EMT, has been proven as an effective agent to control liver fibrosis [32].

In our present study, we have confirmed that expression of vimentin, snail and α-SMA was increased during HSCs activation, accompanying the down-regulation of E-cadherin. Significant different expression of both epithelial and mesenchymal cell markers strongly suggests that HSCs activation is closely related to the EMT process. More importantly, our study has clearly demonstrated that decreased expression of CB1 gene could increase the expression of epithelial markers in favor of down-regulating mesenchymal markers expression and suppressing the known fibroblast functions. In addition, we also demonstrated that CB1 siRNA deactivates the MFs through inducing the MET process of activated HSCs and robustly inhibited their proliferation. All of these results provided direct evidence for the potential role of EMT in activation of HSCs and suggested that CB1 siRNA could block and reverse liver fibrosis partly through the inhibition of the EMT state of activated HSCs.

It was reported that TGF-β1 was important triggers to EMT in fibrotic liver [18]. During EMT, TGF-β1 inhibits E-cadherin expression by up-regulating transcriptional repressors such as Snail, Zeb, and Twist [27,28]. This process is receptor-dependent. Considering the downregulation of TGF-β1 and its receptor TGF-β RII, and inhibition of EMT in HSCs transfected by CB1-RNAi-LV, we deduced that the decrease expression of CB1 could promote MET in HSCs via suppressing the expression of TGF-β1 and its intracellular signal transduction subsequently.

E-cadherin is an epithelial marker. Il Je Cho et al [33] reported that overexpression of E-cadherin could reduce the expression of TGF-β and block the intracellular Smad signaling pathway mediated by TGF-β in HSCs. We provide the hypothesis that a negative feedback exists in Smad signaling pathway mediated by TGF-β and the E-cadherin expression: TGF-β promotes EMT of HSCs via Smad signaling pathway and results in decreased expression of E-cadherin subsequently, but overexpression of E-cadherin also inhibit Smad signaling pathway and decrease the expression of TGF-β.

As one major endocannabinoids ligands, 2-AG is the likely fibrogenic mediator because its hepatic level is preferentially increased in the CCl4 treated mice [3,4]. Previous study reported that 2-AG induce apoptosis in activated HSCs in vitro, which means that 2-AG has antifibrotic activity in vitro [34,35]. In the present study, we also found that extrinsic supplement of 2-AG could incresse HSCs apoptosis, but 2-AG-induced HSCs apoptosis was independent of its receptor CB1, which was in accordance with the previous study [34,35]. It means that the ameliorate effect on hepatic fibrosis by CB1 shRNA can not explained by the increase of HSCs apoptosis.

AM251, the CB1 antagonists, was added to the activated HSCs to inactivate CB1 receptor in the present study. Results showed decreased expression of α-SMA, TGF-β1, TGF-β RII, fibronectin and procollagen Type I, and reduced ECM production after AM-251 treatment in HSCs, indicating the antifibrotic effect of AM251 on hepatic fibrosis in vitro, which was agreed with the previous study reported by Yang YY et al [36], in which AM-251 treatment could inhibit hepatic TGF-β1 expression and reduce hepatic collagen deposition in cirrhotic livers induced by common bile-duct ligation. Interestingly, our study also revealed that the antifibrotic effect of CB1 siRNA on hepatic fibrosis was superior to AM251. These data indicated that gene therapy based on siRNA had superiority over chemical therapy based on receptor antagonists.

In summary, the present study first provides strong evidence for the striking suppression effect of CB1 siRNA on hepatic fibrosis, which is associated with inhibition of activation and proliferation of HSCs. This study also confirmed firstly that the suppression effect of CB1 siRNA on hepatic fibrosis was superior to CB1 antagonist. Furthermore, reversal of EMT of HSCs secondary to CB1 knocking down is also defined firstly in this study. These results suggest that CB1 siRNA might emerge as a therapeutic agent to control liver fibrosis. In this study, we also present the MET of HSCs in the fibrotic liver as a new therapeutic strategy for chronic liver diseases.

Author Contributions

Conceived and designed the experiments: SWC BYW SPX. Performed the experiments: SWC BYW SPX LY YG JBW DHW. Analyzed the data: SPX LY YG. Contributed reagents/materials/analysis tools: SWC KXF DHW. Wrote the paper: SWC SPX KXF DHW.

References

1. Fallowfield JA (2011) Therapeutic targets in liver fibrosis. Am J Physiol Gastrointest Liver Physiol 300:G709–715.

2. Reichenbach V, Ros J, Fernández-Varo G, Casals G, Melgar-Lesmes P, et al. (2012) Prevention of Fibrosis Progression in CCl4-Treated Rats: Role of the Hepatic Endocannabinoid and Apelin Systems. J Pharmacol Exp Ther 340:629–637.

3. Mallat A, Teixeira-Clerc F, Deveaux V, Manin S, Lotersztajn S (2011) The endocannabinoid system as a key mediator during liver diseases: new insights and therapeutic openings. Br J Pharmacol 163:1432–1440.

4. Huang L, Quinn MA, Frampton GA, Golden LE, DeMorrow S (2011) Recent advances in the understanding of the role of the endocannabinoid system in liver diseases. Dig Liver Dis 43:188–193.

5. Yang YY, Lee KC, Huang YT, Lee FY, Chau GY, et al. (2009) Inhibition of hepatic tumour necrosis factor-alpha attenuates the anandamide-induced vasoconstrictive response in cirrhotic rat livers. Liver Int 29:678–685.

6. Domenicali M, Caraceni P, Giannone F, Pertosa AM, Principe A, et al. (2009) Cannabinoid type 1 receptor antagonism delays ascites formation in rats with cirrhosis. Gastroenterology 137:341–349.

7. Magen I, Avraham Y, Berry E, Mechoulam R (2008) Endocannabinoids in liver disease and hepatic encephalopathy. Curr Pharm Des 14:2362–2369.

8. Di Marzo V (2009) The endocannabinoid system: its general strategy of action, tools for its pharmacological manipulation and potential therapeutic exploitation. Pharmacol Res 60:77–84.

9. Teixeira-Clerc F, Belot MP, Manin S, Deveaux V, Cadoudal T, et al. (2010) Beneficial paracrine effects of cannabinoid receptor 2 on liver injury and regeneration. Hepatology 52:1046–1059.

10. Mukhopadhyay B, Liu J, Osei-Hyiaman D, Godlewski G, Mukhopadhyay P, et al. (2010) Transcriptional regulation of cannabinoid receptor-1 expression in the liver by retinoic acid acting via retinoic acid receptor-gamma. J Biol Chem 285:19002–19011.

11. Mukhopadhyay B, Cinar R, Yin S, Liu J, Tam J, et al. (2011) Hyperactivation of anandamide synthesis and regulation of cell-cycle progression via cannabinoid type 1 (CB1) receptors in the regenerating liver. Proc Natl Acad Sci U S A 108:6323–6328.

12. Kano M, Ohno-Shosaku T, Hashimotodani Y, Uchigashima M, Watanabe M (2009) Endocannabinoid-mediated control of synaptic transmission. Physiol Rev 89:309–380.

13. Wasmuth HE, Trautwein C (2007) CB1 cannabinoid receptor antagonism: a new strategy for the treatment of liver fibrosis. Hepatology 45:543–544.

14. Racine-Samson L, Rockey DC, Bissell DM (1997) The role of alpha1beta1 integrin in wound contraction. A quantitative analysis of liver myofibroblasts in vivo and in primary culture. J Biol Chem 272:30911–30917.

15. Kaimori A, Potter J, Kaimori JY, Wang C, Mezey E, et al. (2007) Transforming growth factor-beta1 induces an epithelial-to-mesenchymal transition state in mouse hepatocytes in vitro. J Biol Chem 282:22089–22101.

16. Choi SS, Diehl AM (2009) Epithelial-to-mesenchymal transitions in the liver. Hepatology 50:2007–2013.

17. Tam J, Liu J, Mukhopadhyay B, Cinar R, Godlewski G, et al. (2011) Endocannabinoids in liver disease. Hepatology 53:346–355.

18. Bi WR, Yang CQ, Shi Q (2012) Transforming Growth Factor-β1 Induced Epithelial-Mesenchymal Transition in Hepatic Fibrosis. Hepatogastroenterology 59(118). [Epub ahead of print]

19. Friedman SL (2008) Mechanisms of hepatic fibrogenesis. Gastroenterology 134:1655–1669.

20. Derynck R, Zhang YE (2003) Smad-dependent and Smad-independent pathways in TGF-beta family signalling. Nature 425:577–584.

21. Qi Z, Atsuchi N, Ooshima A, Takeshita A, Ueno H (1999) Blockade of type beta transforming growth factor signaling prevents liver fibrosis and dysfunction in the rat. Proc Natl Acad Sci U S A 96:2345–2349.

22. George J, Roulot D, Koteliansky VE, Bissell DM (1999) In vivo inhibition of rat stellate cell activation by soluble transforming growth factor beta type II receptor: A potential new therapy for hepatic fibrosis. Proc Natl Acad Sci U S A 96:12719–12724.

23. Kalluri R, Weinberg RA (2009) The basics of epithelial-mesenchymal transition. J Clin Invest 119:1420–1428.

24. Yue HY, Yin C, Hou JL, Zeng X, Chen YX, et al. (2010) Hepatocyte nuclear factor 4alpha attenuates hepatic fibrosis in rats. Gut 59:236–246.

25. Ikegami T, Zhang Y, Matsuzaki Y (2007) Liver fibrosis: possible involvement of EMT. Cells Tissues Organs 185:213–221.

26. Robertson H, Kirby JA, Yip WW, Jones DE, Burt AD (2007) Biliary epithelial-mesenchymal transition in posttransplantation recurrence of primary biliary cirrhosis. Hepatology 45:977–981.

27. Fabris L, Strazzabosco M (2011) Epithelial-mesenchymal interactions in biliary diseases. Semin Liver Dis 31:11–32.

28. Peinado H, Olmeda D, Cano A (2007) Snail, Zeb and bHLH factors in tumour progression: an alliance against the epithelial phenotype. Nat Rev Cancer 7:415–428.

29. Povero D, Busletta C, Novo E, di Bonzo LV, Cannito S, et al. (2010) Liver fibrosis: a dynamic and potentially reversible process. Histol Histopathol 25:1075–1091.

30. Gressner OA, Weiskirchen R, Gressner AM (2007) Evolving concepts of liver fibrogenesis provide new diagnostic and therapeutic options. Comp Hepatol 6:7.

31. Jeong WI, Osei-Hyiaman D, Park O, Liu J, Batkai S, et al. (2008) Paracrine activation of hepatic CB1 receptors by stellate cell-derived endocannabinoids mediates alcoholic fatty liver. Cell Metab 7:227–235.

32. Zeisberg M, Yang C, Martino M, Duncan MB, Rieder F, et al. (2007) Fibroblasts derive from hepatocytes in liver fibrosis via epithelial to mesenchymal transition. J Biol Chem 282:23337–23347.

33. Cho IJ, Kim YW, Han CY, Kim EH, Anderson RA, et al. (2010) E-Cadherin Antagonizes Transforming Growth Factor β1 Gene Induction in Hepatic Stellate Cells by Inhibiting RhoA-Dependent Smad3 Phosphorylation. Hepatology 52:2053–2064.

34. Siegmund SV, Qian T, de Minicis S, Harvey-White J, Kunos G, et al. (2007) The endocannabinoid 2-arachidonoyl glycerol induces death of hepatic stellate cells via mitochondrial reactive oxygen species. FASEB J 21:2798–2806.

35. Lim MP, Devi LA, Rozenfeld R (2011) Cannabidiol causes activated hepatic stellate cell death through a mechanism of endoplasmic reticulum stress-induced apoptosis. Cell Death Dis 2:e170.

36. Yang YY, Lin HC, Huang YT, Lee TY, Hou MC, et al. (2007) Effect of chronic CB1 cannabinoid receptor antagonism on livers of rats with biliary cirrhosis. Clin Sci (Lond) 112:533–542.

16

Hydrogen Sulfide Attenuates Carbon Tetrachloride-Induced Hepatotoxicity, Liver Cirrhosis and Portal Hypertension in Rats

Gang Tan[1], Shangha Pan[1], Jie Li[3], Xuesong Dong[1], Kai Kang[2], Mingyan Zhao[2], Xian Jiang[1], Jagat R. Kanwar[4], Haiquan Qiao[1], Hongchi Jiang[1]*, Xueying Sun[1,5]*

1 Department of General Surgery, The Hepatosplenic Surgery Center, The First Affiliated Hospital of Harbin Medical University, Harbin, China, 2 Department of ICU, The First Affiliated Hospital of Harbin Medical University, Harbin, China, 3 Department of Hepatobiliary Surgery, Affiliated Qianfoshan Hospital of Shandong University, Jinan, China, 4 Laboratory of Immunology and Molecular Biomedical Research, Centre for Biotechnology and Interdisciplinary Biosciences, Institute for Technology and Research Innovation, Deakin University, Geelong, Victoria, Australia, 5 Department of Molecular Medicine and Pathology, Faculty of Medical and Health Sciences, The University of Auckland, Auckland, New Zealand

Abstract

Background: Hydrogen sulfide (H_2S) displays vasodilative, anti-oxidative, anti-inflammatory and cytoprotective activities. Impaired production of H_2S contributes to the increased intrahepatic resistance in cirrhotic livers. The study aimed to investigate the roles of H_2S in carbon tetrachloride (CCl_4)-induced hepatotoxicity, cirrhosis and portal hypertension.

Methods and Findings: Sodium hydrosulfide (NaHS), a donor of H_2S, and DL-propargylglycine (PAG), an irreversible inhibitor of cystathionine γ-lyase (CSE), were applied to the rats to investigate the effects of H_2S on CCl_4-induced acute hepatotoxicity, cirrhosis and portal hypertension by measuring serum levels of H_2S, hepatic H_2S producing activity and CSE expression, liver function, activity of cytochrome P450 (CYP) 2E1, oxidative and inflammatory parameters, liver fibrosis and portal pressure. CCl_4 significantly reduced serum levels of H_2S, hepatic H_2S production and CSE expression. NaHS attenuated CCl_4-induced acute hepatotoxicity by supplementing exogenous H_2S, which displayed anti-oxidative activities and inhibited the CYP2E1 activity. NaHS protected liver function, attenuated liver fibrosis, inhibited inflammation, and reduced the portal pressure, evidenced by the alterations of serum alanine aminotransferase (ALT), aspartate aminotransferase (AST), hyaluronic acid (HA), albumin, tumor necrosis factor (TNF)-α, interleukin (IL)-1β, IL-6 and soluble intercellular adhesion molecule (ICAM)-1, liver histology, hepatic hydroxyproline content and α-smooth muscle actin (SMA) expression. PAG showed opposing effects to NaHS on most of the above parameters.

Conclusions: Exogenous H_2S attenuates CCl_4-induced hepatotoxicity, liver cirrhosis and portal hypertension by its multiple functions including anti-oxidation, anti-inflammation, cytoprotection and anti-fibrosis, indicating that targeting H_2S may present a promising approach, particularly for its prophylactic effects, against liver cirrhosis and portal hypertension.

Editor: Antonio Bertoletti, Singapore Institute for Clinical Sciences, Singapore

Funding: Grants from the National Natural Scientific Foundation of China (30872987 and 30973474)(www.nsfc.gov.cn), and Heilongjiang Provincial Scientific and Technology Bureau, China (QC06C075)(http://www.hljkjt.gov.cn). The funders had no role in study design, data collection and analysis, decision to publish, or preparation of the manuscript.

Competing Interests: The authors have declared that no competing interests exist.

* E-mail: k.sun@auckland.ac.nz (XS); jianghc@vip.163.com (HJ)

Introduction

Hydrogen sulfide (H_2S) has displayed many physiological and pathological activities [1]. Administration of H_2S limited myocardial infarct size caused by ischemia reperfusion injury (IRI) [2,3], suppressed development of gastric ulcer [4], alleviated hypoxic pulmonary hypertension [5], attenuated neuronal injury [6], and prevented the development of hypertension [7]. An H_2S-releasing molecule, GYY4137, protected endotoxic shock by decreasing the production of proinflammatory cytokines including tumor necrosis factor-α (TNF-α) and interleukin-6 (IL-6) [8]. The multiple actions of H_2S mainly involve inhibiting oxidative stress [9], production of lipid peroxidation and inflammatory factors [4], and activating ATP sensitive potassium (K_{ATP}) channels [10].

H_2S has also shown regulatory effects on hepatic physiology and pathology [11]. H_2S is endogenously produced in mammalian tissues by cystathionine γ-lyase (CSE) and cystathionine β-synthase (CBS) [1], but CBS accounts for only 3% of H_2S production in livers [12]. CSE-derived H_2S contributes to hepatic arterial buffer response, mediates vasorelaxation of the hepatic artery via activation of K_{ATP} channels [13], and modulates biliary bicarbonate excretion [14]. H_2S has exhibited anti-inflammatory and cytoprotective activities against hepatic IRI [15], and protected acetaminophen-induced hepatotoxicity in mice [16]. Diallyl trisulfide, an H_2S-releasing chemical, protected from carbon tetrachloride (CCl_4)-induced liver injury [17,18].

The reduction of H_2S production and CSE expression is related to the development of increased intrahepatic resistance and portal hypertension in a rat model of liver cirrhosis induced by CCl_4 [19], and H_2S counteracts the impaired vasodilation and hepatic stellate cell contraction, which contribute to the dynamic component of portal hypertension [20]. These two studies have focused on the regulatory effects of H_2S in already established portal hypertension mainly by its vasodilative activities via activating K_{ATP} channels. As mentioned in one report [20], liver fibrosis represents the main causative factor in portal hypertension in cirrhosis, but the role of H_2S in the development of cirrhosis remains unclear. CCl_4 has been widely used to induce liver injury and cirrhosis in animal models, as it is rapidly metabolized into the trichloromethyl radical by cytochrome P450 (CYP) 2E1, and the reactive intermediate attacks membrane lipids, resulting in the formation of lipid peroxide molecules and necrosis of hepatocytes [21]. Given that H_2S displays anti-oxidative, anti-inflammatory and cytoprotective activities, an anti-fibrotic effect against pulmonary fibrosis [22], and a regulatory effect on hypoxic pulmonary hypertension [23] and portal hypertension [19,20], we hypothesized that H_2S might have a protective effect against CCl_4-induced acute hepatotoxicity, and the resulting liver cirrhosis and portal hypertension.

Methods

Ethics Statement

All the procedures and care administered to the animals have been approved by the institutional ethic committee, under a permit of animal use (SYXK20020009) in the First Affiliated Hospital of Harbin Medical University, compliance with the Experimental Animal Regulations by the National Science and Technology Commission, China.

Animals

Male Wistar rats (weighing 210-230 g) were supplied by the Animal Research Center at the First Affiliated Hospital of Harbin Medical University, Harbin, China. They were housed in the animal facility with a 12-h-light/-dark cycle and the temperature was maintained at 22-23°C.

Acute hepatotoxicity experiment

The rats received phenobarbital sodium (0.35 g/L) in drinking water for 3 days, followed by a single i.p. injection of CCl_4 (Nanjing Chem. Ltd., Nanjing, China) diluted in equal volume of paraffin oil at a dose of 3 ml/kg body weight. Then the rats were randomly assigned to 3 groups (each group had 6 rats): control, NaHS and PAG, receiving an i.p. injection of 1 ml of physiological saline, NaHS (Sigma-Aldrich) solution (14 μmol/kg body weight), or PAG (Sigma-Aldrich) solution (50 mg/kg body weight), respectively. The injection was repeated every 6 h. The rats were killed 48 h after CCl_4 administration. Six untreated rats served as healthy controls. Blood was collected via cardiac puncture, and serum was prepared by centrifugation at 2000 × g for 10 min, and stored at -80°C. Livers were divided into two parts, one fixed in 10% buffered formalin, the other stored at -80°C.

Induction of liver cirrhosis

Liver cirrhosis was induced by CCl_4 as described previously [20,21]. Briefly, rats received phenobarbital sodium (0.35 g/L) in drinking water for 3 days, followed by i.p. injections of 1 ml/kg body weight of CCl_4 diluted in an equal volume of paraffin oil twice a week for 12 weeks.

Prevention experiment

Thirty-six rats receiving i.p. injections of CCl_4 as above were randomly assigned into 3 groups (each had 12 rats): saline, NaHS and PAG, receiving i.p. injections of 1 ml of saline, NaHS solution (10 μmol/kg body weight) and PAG solution (30 mg/kg body weight), respectively, every two days for 12 weeks, starting on the same day of CCl_4 administration. 300 μl of blood samples were collected by tail tipping at indicated time points. At completion of the experiments, the rats were weighed, and the portal pressure measured as below, and 300 μl of blood sample was collected from the portal vein. The spleen was weighed as % of bodyweight and used as a parameter for portal hypertension. Blood was collected via cardiac puncture, and then the liver and spleen were collected. Serum and liver samples were prepared and stored as above.

Measurement of portal pressure

The methodology has been described previously [24]. Briefly, under anesthesia by an i.p. injection of sodium pentobarbital (50 mg/kg body weight), rats underwent laparotomy, and a PE-tube (23G, 0.6×30 mm) was inserted over the ileocolic vein and advanced toward the confluence of the portal and splenic veins. This cannula was used to monitor portal pressure for 5 min by a Medlab-Ug4Cs bio-signal processing system (Nanjing Medease Science and Technology co., Ltd, Nanjing, China).

Treatment experiment

Rats with liver cirrhosis induced by 12-week administration of CCl_4 as above were randomly assigned to 3 groups (each had 6 rats): saline, NaHS and PAG, receiving daily injection of 1 ml of saline, NaHS solution (10 μmol/kg) and PAG solution (30 mg/kg), respectively, for 5 days. At completion of the experiments, the portal pressure measured, and then serum and liver samples were prepared.

Measuring H_2S production in livers and H_2S concentration in sera

The methods have been described previously [15,25]. All samples were assayed in triplicate and H2S was calculated against a calibration curve of NaHS (0.122–250 μmol/L). The H2S producing activity was expressed as μmole of H2S formed/g tissues.

RT-PCR analysis

The analysis of CES mRNA by RT-PCR has been described previously [15]. A pair of primers 5'- GAC CTC AAT AGT CGG CTT CGT TTC -3' and 5'- CAG TTC TGC GTA TGC TCC GTA ATG -3' to generate a 618 bp product of CSE mRNA. A 497 bp PCR product was amplified from glyceraldehyde 3-phosphate dehydrogenase (GAPDH) cDNA as an internal control, with a pair of primers: 5'-GAAGGTGAAGGTCGGAGT-3' and 3'-TGAAACCATAGCACCTTCC-5'. PCR products underwent a 2% agarose gel electrophoresis, and the density of each band was evaluated using the gel image analyzer (UV ChemiDOC, USA). The relative density of mRNA levels was calculated as the following formula: band density/ GAPDH band density.

Measurement of serum parameters

The serum levels of alanine aminotransferase (ALT), aspartate aminotransferase (AST), hyaluronic acid (HA) and albumin were measured with an auto-biochemical analyzer (Toshiba, Japan). The serum levels of TNF-α, IL-6, interleukin-1β (IL-1β) and soluble intercellular adhesion molecule-1 (ICAM-1) were measured with ELISA kits (BPB Biomedicals, Inc., USA).

Measurement of CYP2E1 activity in livers

The CYP2E1 activity was assayed using p-nitrophenol (Sigma-Aldrich) as a substrate as described previously [26].

Measurement of hepatic malondialdehyde (MDA) and glutathione (GSH)

Liver tissue was homogenized in a buffer containing 9 volumes of 0.15 mol/L KCl-1.0 mmol/L EDTA to obtain 1:10 (w/v) homogenates. Homogenates were then centrifuged at 10,000 g (4°C) for 30 min to collect the supernatant for determining the concentrations of MDA, GSH and total protein. MDA was evaluated by the thiobarbituric acid reactive substances (TBARS) method [27]. The final concentration of MDA was expressed as μmol/g protein. GSH were measured using commercially available kits (Jiancheng Institute of Biotechnology, Nanjing, China) and expressed as nmol/mg protein. Protein concentration of liver homogenate was determined by the Bradford method, using bovine serum albumin as a standard [28].

Measurement of hepatic hydroxyproline

Hepatic hydroxyproline was measured as described previously [29].

Histological analysis

Formalin-fixed liver specimens were embedded in paraffin, sectioned, stained with hematoxylin and eosin (HE) or Masson, and examined under light microscopy. Quantifying liver fibrosis was performed by measuring blue pixels of the images taken from Masson-stained sections. Ten photographs (200 × magnification) were randomly taken from each liver at fixed exposure time and conditions. The pictures were saved as JPEG (Joint photographic experts group). The histogram function in Adobe Photoshop CS4 was used to count the blue pixels, and the numbers of red pixels were recorded for each picture.

Western Blot analysis

The methodology has been described previously [15]. The Abs against CSE or α-smooth muscle actin (α-SMA) (Santa Cruz Biotechnology, Inc. Santa Cruz, CA) were used. The levels of proteins were normalized with respect to band density of β-actin, as an internal control.

Statistics

Results were expressed as mean values ± standard deviation (SD). A one-way analysis of variance (ANOVA) followed by the post-hoc Dunnett's test was used for evaluating statistical significance (SPSS 17.0). A value of $P<0.05$ was considered significant.

Results

H$_2$S protects livers from CCl$_4$-induced acute toxicity

Administration of NaHS significantly attenuated, while PAG further raised, the elevated serum levels of ALT and AST by CCl$_4$ (Table 1). The impaired liver function by CCl$_4$ and the protective effects of H2S were supported by the histological alterations (Figure S1). The liver sections from healthy control rats showed normal histology (Figure S1A). CCl$_4$-treated livers had focal midzonal necrosis and ballooning degeneration (Figure S1B). NaHS attenuated the necrosis and vacuolization (Figure S1C), while PAG further aggravated the hepatotoxicity and caused more inflammatory cells infiltration (Figure S1D). NaHS also significantly reduced the activity of CYP2E1, the major enzyme to metabolize CCl$_4$, in livers from CCl$_4$-treated rats, compared with saline, while either CCl$_4$ or PAG had no effects on its activity (Table 1). CCl$_4$-treated rats had a significant higher level of hepatic MDA (a marker of lipid peroxidation) and a significantly lower level of hepatic GSH, compared to healthy controls. NaHS significantly attenuated the increase of hepatic MDA, and restored hepatic GSH, but PAG only had slight effects on hepatic MDA and GSH, in CCl$_4$-treated rats, compared with saline (Table 1).

Serum levels of H$_2$S, production of H$_2$S and CSE expression in the acute experiment

The serum levels of H$_2$S in CCl$_4$ + saline-treated rats were significantly lower than that in healthy controls ($P<0.05$) (Fig. 1A), supported by that CCl$_4$ significantly ($P <0.05$) reduced hepatic H$_2$S producing activity (Fig. 1B). Hepatic expressions of CSE mRNA (Fig. 1C and D) and protein (Fig. 1E and F) were significantly (Both $P<0.05$) lower in CCl$_4$-treated rats than that in healthy controls. NaHS significantly ($P<0.001$) increased the levels of H$_2$S (Fig. 1A), but had no effect on hepatic H$_2$S producing activity (Fig. 1B) and the expression of CSE mRNA (Fig. 1C and D) and protein (Fig. 1E and F), in CCl$_4$-treated rats, compared saline. However, PAG significantly (Both $P<0.05$) reduced the levels of H$_2$S (Fig. 1A) and H$_2$S producing activity (Fig. 1B), but had no effect on the expression of CSE mRNA (Fig. 1C and D) and protein (Fig. 1E and F), in CCl$_4$-treated rats, compared with saline.

H$_2$S production in cirrhotic rats induced by CCl$_4$

Among the rats in the prevention experiment, one from the CCl$_4$ + saline group and two from the CCl$_4$ + PAG group died

Table 1. Serum ALT and AST, and hepatic CYP2E1, MDA and GSH in hepatotoxicity experiment*.

	Healthy control	CCl$_4$		
		saline	NaHS	PAG
	(n = 6)	(n = 6)	(n = 6)	(n = 6)
Serum ALT (IU/L)	36.2±7.5	245.8±36.5[a]	149.6±25.7[a,b]	268.7±46.9[a,b]
Serum AST (IU/L)	78.9±11.4	657.0±96.1[a]	427.6±102.3[a,b]	835.2±133.5[a,b]
Liver CYP2E1(μmol/g protein)	2.8±0.2	2.7±0.4	1.4±0.3[a,b]	3.1±1.0
Liver MDA (μmol/g protein)	1.6±0.3	5.9±1.2[a]	3.8±0.7[a,b]	6.3±1.5[a]
Liver GSH (μmol/g protein)	11.5±2.4	5.7±1.8[a]	10.7±3.0[a,b]	4.6±1.1[a]

*The blood and liver samples were collected from the rats 48 h after CCl$_4$ administration. Data are expressed as means ± SD, and statistical analysis was performed by one-way ANOVA analysis followed by the post-hoc Dunnett's test.
[a]Significant difference ($P<0.05$) from healthy controls.
[b]Significant difference ($P<0.05$) from saline -treated rats.

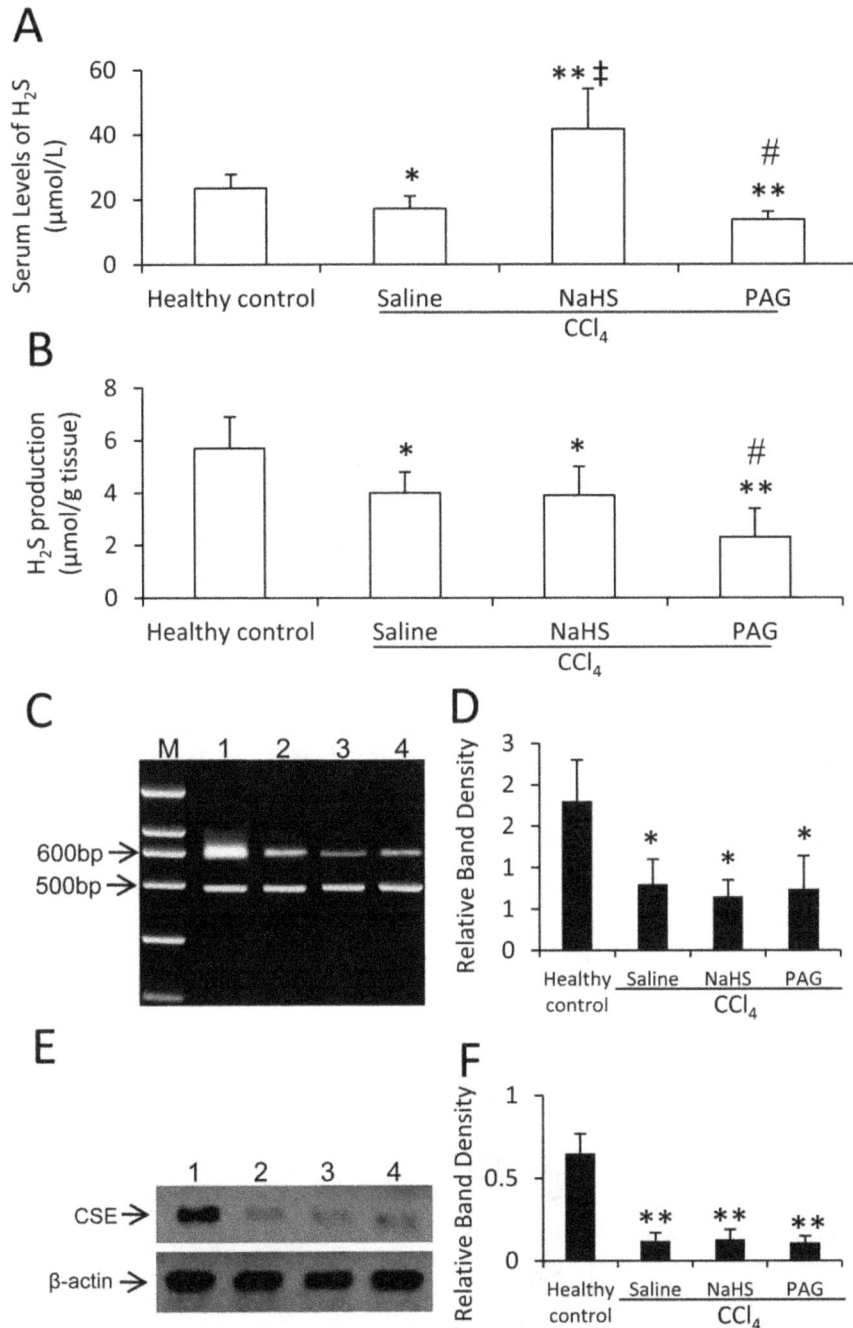

Figure 1. Serum levels of H₂S, H₂S production and CSE expression in CCl₄-induced acute hepatotoxicity. Healthy rats, or CCl₄-treated rats receiving administrations of saline, NaHS or PAG, were killed 48 h after CCl₄ administration, blood and liver samples were collected. The levels of H₂S in sera (A) and H₂S producing activity in livers (B) were measured. (C-F) The expression of CSE mRNA (C, D) and protein (E, F) was detected in liver tissues from healthy rats (lane 1), or CCl₄-treaed rats receiving administration of saline (lane 2), NaHS (lane 3) or PAG (lane 4), by RT-PCR (C, D) or Western blot analysis (E, F), respectively. M, DNA marker. (D) The density of each band from (C) was measured and compared to that of the internal control, GAPDH. (F) The density of each band from (E) was measured and compared to that of the internal control, β-actin. Results are expressed as mean ± SD (n = 6). Compared to the healthy controls, a significant difference is denoted by "*", and a highly significant difference by "**" (P<0.001). Compared to rats treated with CCl₄ + saline, a significant increase is denoted by "‡", and a significant reduction is denoted by "#".

before completion of the experiment, and were excluded from the study. Blood samples were collected at indicated time points to measure the serum levels of H₂S in rats. The healthy rats had a stable serum level of H₂S, while the H₂S levels in CCl₄-induced cirrhotic rats receiving injection of saline declined at week 4 after CCl₄ administration, and continued dropping as the H₂S levels

were even lower at week 8 and 12 than that at week 4 (Fig. 2A). However, NaHS significantly (P<0.05) elevated the serum level of H₂S at week 4 after CCl₄ administration in CCl₄-induced cirrhotic rats, compared with saline, and serum H₂S was maintained at a higher level at week 8 and 12 (Fig. 2A). Administration of PAG resulted in significantly (All P<0.05) lower serum levels of H₂S in

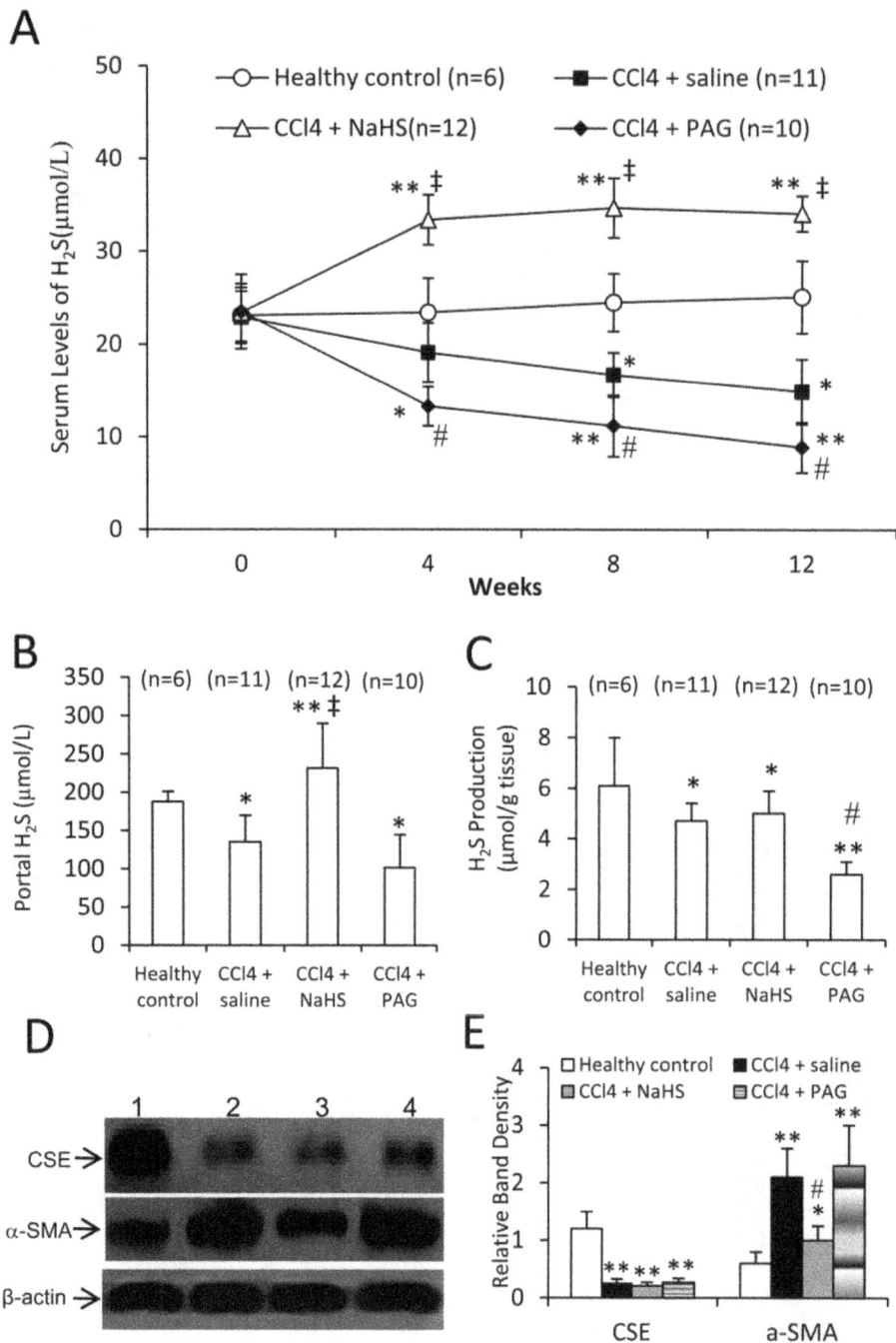

Figure 2. Serum H₂S levels, H₂S production, and expression of CSE and α-SMA in the prevention experiment. The rats were treated with CCl_4 + saline, CCl_4 + NaHS or CCl_4 + PAG for 12 weeks. Untreated rats served as healthy controls. (A) Blood samples were collected at indicated time points, and the serum levels of H_2S were measured. The statistical comparison between two groups was done at the respective time point. (B-E) The rats were killed at the completion of experiment. Blood samples were collected from portal vein, and livers harvested. The levels of H_2S in sera from the portal vein (B), and H_2S producing activity in livers (C) were measured. (D) The expression of CSE and α-SMA was detected in livers from healthy controls (lane 1), or rats treated saline+CCl_4 (lane 2), NaHS+CCl_4 (lane 3) or PAG+CCl_4 (lane 4) by Western blot analysis. (E) The density of each band was measured and compared to that of the internal control, β-actin. Results are expressed as mean ± SD. n, number of samples. Compared to the healthy controls, a significant difference is denoted by "*", a highly significant difference by "**" (P<0.001). Compared to saline + CCl_4-treated rats, a significant increase is denoted by "‡", and a significant reduction is denoted by "#".

CCl_4-induced cirrhotic rats, than saline, at all the three time points (Fig. 2A). The portal serum levels of H_2S at the completion of experiment was significantly (P<0.05) lower in CCl_4-induced cirrhotic rats receiving injection of saline than the healthy controls (Fig. 2B). However, NaHS significantly (P<0.05) elevated, but

PAG did not significantly (P>0.05) decrease, the portal serum levels of H_2S, in CCl_4-induced cirrhotic rats, compared with saline (Fig. 2B). We further examined the H_2S producing activity (Fig. 2 C) in livers from CCl_4-induced cirrhotic rat receiving injections of saline, NaHS or PAG, and the similar results were obtained as

Table 2. Serum biochemicals and inflammatory factors in cirrhotic rats*.

	Healthy control	CCl$_4$ + saline	CCl$_4$ + NaHS	CCl$_4$ + PAG
	(n = 6)	(n = 11)	(n = 12)	(n = 10)
ALT (IU/L)	34.4±8.9	198.8±26.7[a]	137.6±20.3[a,b]	208.5±36.4[a]
AST(IU/L)	80.3±12.5	466.7±46.4[a]	317.5±78.2[a,b]	515.0±97.6[a,b]
HA (µg/L)	113.5±20.1	482.6±51.4[a]	296.3±32.1[a,b]	549.0±47.3[a,b]
Albumin (g/L)	472.5±43.8	314±51.6[a]	443.7±80.5[a,b]	294.3±32.8[a]
TNF-α (ng/L)	43.9±6.8	143.5±21.4[a]	109.3±22.6[a,b]	176.3±28.5[a,b]
IL-1β(ng/L)	20.3±5.0	75.4±10.2[a]	50.6±9.8[a,b]	80.2±17.4[a]
IL-6 (ng/L)	87.0±15.9	297.1±55.4[a]	216.4±42.1[a,b]	320.6±51.4[a]
ICAM-1(ng/L)	69.2±8.7	180.8±19.7[a]	153.6±22.8[a,b]	207.2±31.3[a,b]

*Data are expressed as means ± SD, and statistical analysis was performed by one-way ANOVA analysis followed by the post-hoc Dunnett's test.
[a]Significant difference (P<0.05) from healthy controls.
[b]Significant difference (P<0.05) from CCl$_4$+saline-treated rats.

shown in the acute hepatotoxicity experiment (Fig. 1B), supported by the results of hepatic CES expression (Fig. 2D and E), where CCl$_4$ significantly downregulated, while NaHS or PAG had no effect on, the expression of CES.

H$_2$S attenuates the impaired liver function and elevated inflammatory factors in cirrhotic rats

Cirrhotic rats induced by 12-week administration of CCl$_4$ had significantly higher levels of ALT, AST, HA and lower level of albumin, than healthy controls (Table 2). However, simultaneous administration of NaHS resulted in significantly lower levels of ALT, AST and HA, and higher level of albumin, while PAG led to significantly higher levels of AST and HA, slight increase of ALT level and slight reduction of albumin level, in CCl$_4$-induced cirrhotic rats, compared with saline (Table 2).

Cirrhotic rats had significantly higher levels of proinflammatory cytokines including TNF-α, IL-1β and IL-6, and soluble ICAM-1 (Table 2), which have been shown to play important roles in development of cirrhosis. However, simultaneous administration of NaHS resulted in significantly lower levels of all the four parameters in CCl$_4$-induced cirrhotic rats than saline, while PAG led to significantly higher levels of TNF-α and soluble ICAM, and slight increase of IL-1β and IL-6, in CCl$_4$-induced cirrhotic rats, compared with saline (Table 2).

H$_2$S attenuates CCl$_4$-induced liver cirrhosis and portal hypertension

The Masson-stained liver sections from healthy controls had almost no collagen fibers of blue color (Fig. 3A), but those from CCl$_4$-induced cirrhotic rats injected with saline had abundant and widespread fibers of blue color (Fig. 3B). However, the liver sections from CCl$_4$-induced cirrhotic rats injected with NaHS had fewer fibers (Fig. 3C), while those from PAG-injected cirrhotic rats (Fig. 3D) had even more fibers, compared with those from saline-injected cirrhotic rats. The numbers of blue pixels in Masson-stained liver sections were measured to quantify collagen fibers. CCl$_4$ highly significantly (P<0.001) increased the number of blue pixels in liver sections (Fig. 3E). However, administration of NaHS resulted in a significant (P<0.05) lower number of blue pixels, but PAG, a significant (P<0.05) higher number of blue pixels, in CCl$_4$-induced cirrhotic rats, compared with saline (Fig. 3E). We further measured hydroxyproline, a marker of fibrosis, and found that CCl$_4$-treated rats had significantly (P<0.001) higher hepatic

hydroxyproline content than the healthy controls. However, administration of NaHS significantly (P<0.05) reduced, but PAG did not significantly (P>0.05) increase, the hepatic hydroxyproline contents in CCl$_4$-induced cirrhotic rats, compared with saline (Fig. 3F). Next, we detected hepatic expression of α-SMA, another marker of liver fibrosis, and found that the CCl$_4$-treated rats had significantly higher hepatic expression of α-SMA, compared to the healthy controls. However, administration of NaHS significantly (P<0.05) downregulated, but PAG did not significantly (P>0.05) increase, hepatic expression of α-SMA in CCl$_4$-induced cirrhotic rats, compared with saline (Fig. 2D and E).

The spleen weight and portal pressure were used as parameters for portal hypertension. The spleen weight of CCl$_4$-treated rats was highly significantly (P<0.001) higher than that of healthy controls (Fig. 3G). However, administration of neither NaHS nor PAG resulted in significant difference in spleen weight of CCl$_4$-induced cirrhotic rats, compared with saline (Fig. 3G). CCl$_4$-induced cirrhotic rats had a significantly (P<0.001) higher portal pressure than the healthy controls (Fig. 3H). However, administration of NaHS resulted in a significant (P<0.05) lower level of portal pressure, while PAG, a significant (P<0.05) higher level of portal pressure, in CCl$_4$-induced cirrhotic rats, than saline (Fig. 3H).

The therapeutic effect of H$_2$S on liver cirrhosis and portal hypertension

Given that H$_2$S displayed a preventive effect against CCl$_4$-induced liver cirrhosis and portal hypertension, we next investigated whether H$_2$S could have a similar therapeutic effect in already established liver cirrhosis. Liver cirrhosis was induced in rats by 12-week administration of CCl$_4$ as above, and then saline, NaHS or PAG was administered to the cirrhotic rats, respectively, for 5 days. Administration of NaHS significantly (Both P<0.05) elevated the levels of H$_2$S in sera from the peripheral blood (Fig. 4A) and portal vein (Fig. 4B), but again had no effect on H$_2$S production activity in livers (Fig. 4C). PAG significantly (P <0.05) reduced the levels of H$_2$S in sera from the systemic circulation (Fig. 4A), marginally significantly (P = 0.07) reduced the levels of H$_2$S in the portal vein (Fig. 4B), and significantly (P <0.05) reduced the H$_2$S production in livers (Fig. 4C). NaHS or PAG had no significantly influence on the histological alterations of livers (Data not shown), and the hepatic hydroxyproline in NaHS or PAG-treated rats were not significant different from the saline-

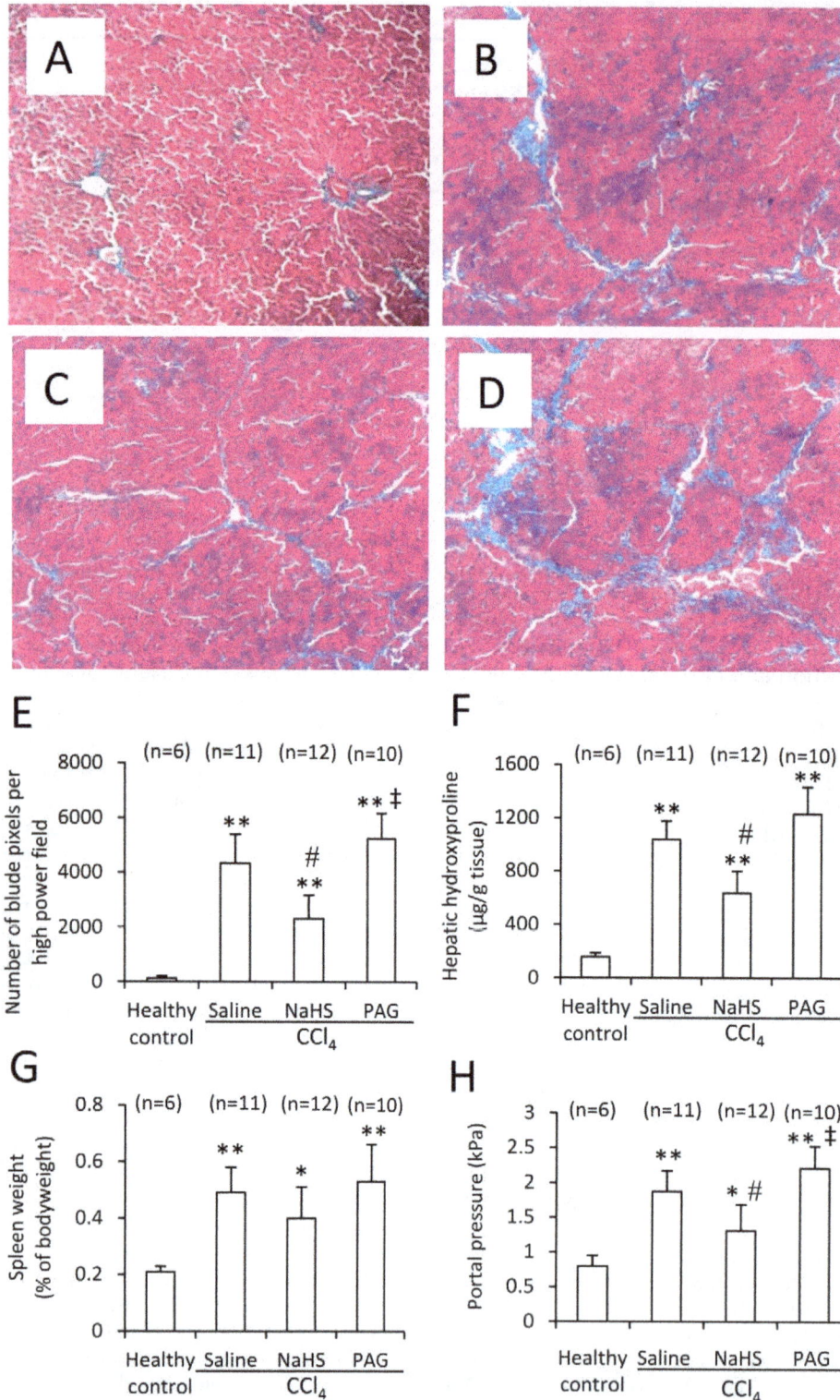

Figure 3. Histology of liver cirrhosis, hepatic hydroxyproline, spleen weight and portal pressure in the prevention experiment.
Representative illustrations (200 × magnification) of Masson-stained liver sections were taken from healthy controls (A), or rats treated with CCl$_4$ + saline (B), CCl$_4$ + NaHS (C) or CCl$_4$ + PAG (D), for 12 weeks. (E) The numbers of blue pixels of each image of the above Masson-stained liver sections were counted, and the average number of blue pixels for each liver was calculated. (F) The level of hydroxyproline in livers taken from the above rats was measured. (G) Each spleen was weighed as % of bodyweight. (H) The portal pressure of each was measured. Data were expressed mean ± SD. n, number of samples. Compared to the healthy controls, a significant difference is denoted by "*", and a highly significant difference, by "**" (P<0.001). Compared to saline + CCl$_4$-treated rats, a significant increase is denoted by "‡", and a significant reduction is denoted by "#".

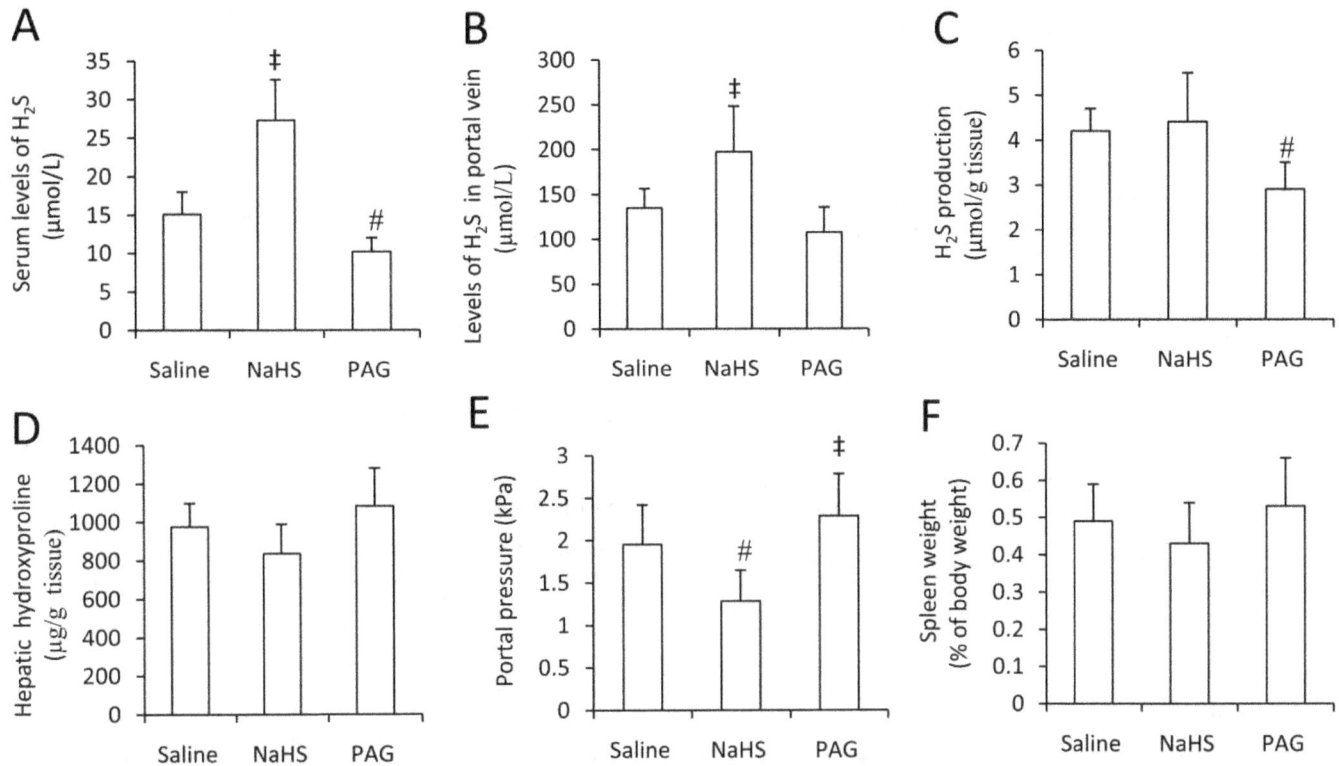

Figure 4. H₂S levels and production, hepatic hydroxyproline, portal pressure and spleen weight in the treatment experiment. Liver cirrhosis was induced in rats as in Figure 3, and then the rats were assigned to three groups (Each group had 6 rats), and received daily injection of saline, NaHS or PAG, respectively, for 5 days, and then killed. (A) Blood samples were collected and the serum levels of H_2S were measured. (B) Blood samples were collected from portal vein to measure the levels of H_2S in portal vein (B). The hepatic H_2S producing activity (C) and hydroxyproline contents (D) were measured. The portal pressure was measured (E), and each spleen was weighed as % of bodyweight (F). Results are expressed as mean ± SD. A significant increase from saline-treated rats is denoted by "‡", and a significant reduction by "#".

injected rats (Fig. 4D). However, administration of NaHS significantly ($P<0.05$) reduced the portal pressure, while PAG significantly ($P<0.05$) elevated the portal pressure, compared with saline (Fig. 4E), but their effects on spleen weight were not significant, compared with saline (Fig. 4F).

Discussion

CCl_4 has been widely used as a chemical model to induce hepatotoxicity, liver cirrhosis and portal hypertension, since it is metabolized into trichloromethyl radical, leading to increased lipid peroxidation, depletion of GSH, impaired hepatic anti-oxidant activity and necrosis of hepatocytes [21,30]. The present study has demonstrated that CCl_4 downregulated the expression of CSE, the major enzyme accounting for 97% of H_2S production in livers [1,12,19], resulting in decreased hepatic H_2S producing activity. Administration of NaHS, a donor of H_2S, attenuated CCl_4-induced acute hepatotoxicity, evidenced by the reduction of serum levels of AST and ALT, and attenuation of histopathological alterations, in accordance with the previous reports on its cytoprotective effects against myocardial IRI [2], endotoxin-induced cardiac injury [31], hepatic IRI [15], acetaminophen-induced hepatotoxicity [16], or gastric mucosa damage caused by stress [4], nonsteroidal anti-inflammatory drugs [32] or oxidative stress [33]. The protective effects of H_2S may rely on its anti-oxidative activity by reducing the production of lipid peroxides, as NaHS inhibited the activity of CYP2E1, one of the major enzymes metabolizing CCl_4 [21]. The vasodilative activity of H_2S may also contribute this protective

activity, as H_2S-induced vasorelaxation [34] can improve micro-circulation of livers, which help livers to get rid of excessive lipid peroxides. In addition, though not investigated herein, the anti-apoptotic activity of H_2S as demonstrated against hepatic IRI [15], may also contribute to this action.

The effects of CCl_4 on H_2S production were shown to be accumulative as the serum levels of H_2S declined in a time-dependent course. NaHS had no effect on either hepatic CSE expression or H_2S producing activity, and led to a relatively higher but stable level of H_2S in sera, implying that the body has the ability to adjust endogenous production of H_2S or get rid of excessive H_2S, which has been recognized as a "toxic gas" in environmental pollution [35]. In both the acute and prevention experiments, PAG, an irreversible inhibitor of CSE, significantly suppressed the H_2S producing activity and reduced the H_2S levels, thus showing opposite effects to NaHS on liver function, lipid peroxides, and liver fibrosis, but had no impact on CSE expression, in accordance with previous reports [3,15].

The present study has for the first time demonstrated the anti-fibrotic activity of H_2S against liver cirrhosis, evidenced by reduced number of collagenous fibers in livers, and hepatic hydroxyproline content and expression of α-SMA. Besides the direct mechanism on fibrogenesis, the protective effect of H_2S on hepatic injury also contributes to its anti-fibrotic activity. In addition, NaHS inhibited the production of inflammatory factors including TNF-α, IL-1β, IL-6, soluble ICAM-1. The anti-inflammatory effect, particular inhibition of IL-6 production by H_2S, can contribute to its anti-fibrotic activity, as IL-6 is upregulated in cirrhotic livers and contributes to the fibrogenic process in an autocrine/paracrine manner [36].

The regulation of sinusoidal resistance depends on the contraction of hepatic stellate cells (HSCs) around sinusoidal endothelial cells [19]. It has been demonstrated that H_2S is an autocrine mediator involved in regulating HSCs contraction and maintaining portal venous pressure by targeting KATP channels [19]. H_2S can counteract the impaired vasodilation and HSC contraction, thus reducing portal hypertension, cirrhotic livers [20]. The results presented herein further support the effects of H_2S on portal hypertension as administration of NaHS showed prophylactic and therapeutic effects in reducing portal hypertension. The protective effects of H_2S on liver cirrhosis may also attributes to this effect in the prevention experiment, as liver fibrosis represents the main causative factor in portal hypertension [20]. However, H_2S did not show significant therapeutic effects on liver cirrhosis in the treatment experiment, based on the histological alterations and hepatic hydroxyproline contents in cirrhotic rats, indicating H_2S may not have the ability to reverse the process of liver fibrosis.

In conclusion, the present study has for the first time systemically investigated the potential protective role of H_2S on CCl_4-induced acute hepatotoxicity, the prophylactic effect of H_2S on long-term CCl_4-induced cirrhosis and portal hypertension, and the therapeutic effect of H_2S on portal hypertension, by its multiple functions including anti-oxidation, anti-inflammation, cytoprotection and anti-fibrosis. The results indicate that targeting H_2S may present a potent approach, particularly for its prophylactic effects, against liver cirrhosis and portal hypertension. Preclinical trials by applying some promising H_2S-relesaing chemicals have already been launched though at their infancy. For instance, diallyl trisulfide, a stable H_2S donor and organic polysulfide compound [37], has been shown to protect from carbon tetrachloride (CCl_4)-induced liver injury [17,18]. However, cautions must be taken as H_2S has been recognized as a "toxic gas" [35], and more preclinical trials are required before H_2S-releasing agents reach the clinics for use in preventing liver cirrhosis and portal hypertension.

Author Contributions

Conceived and designed the experiments: GT XS JL HJ. Performed the experiments: GT SP XD KK MZ HQ XJ. Analyzed the data: JL HQ HJ XS. Contributed reagents/materials/analysis tools: JL JK XS. Wrote the paper: XS GT SP JK HJ.

References

1. Łowicka E, Betowski J (2007) Hydrogen sulfide (H2S) - the third gas of interest for pharmacologists. Pharmacol Rep 59: 4–24.
2. Elrod JW, Calvert JW, Morrison J, Doeller JE, Kraus DW, et al. (2007) Hydrogen sulfide attenuates myocardial ischemia-reperfusion injury by preservation of mitochondrial function. Proc Natl Acad Sci U S A 104: 15560–15565.
3. Gao Y, Yao X, Zhang Y, Li W, Kang K, et al. (2011) The protective role of hydrogen sulfide in cardiac ischemia reperfusion-induced injury in diabetic rats. Int J Cardiol;doi:10.1016/j.ijcard.2010.07.012.
4. Lou LX, Geng B, Du JB, Tang CS (2008) Hydrogen sulphide-induced hypothermia attenuates stress-related ulceration in rats. Clin Exp Pharmacol Physiol 35: 223–228.
5. Chunyu Z, Junbao D, Dingfang B, Hui Y, Xiuying T, et al. (2003) The regulatory effect of hydrogen sulfide on hypoxic pulmonary hypertension in rats. Biochem Biophys Res Commun 302: 810–816.
6. Zhang LM, Jiang CX, Liu DW (2009) Hydrogen sulfide attenuates neuronal injury induced by vascular dementia via inhibiting apoptosis in rats. Neurochem Res 34: 1984–1992.
7. Zhong G, Chen F, Cheng Y, Tang C, Du J (2003) The role of hydrogen sulfide generation in the pathogenesis of hypertension in rats induced by inhibition of nitric oxide synthase. J Hypertens 21: 1879–1885.
8. Li L, Salto-Tellez M, Tan CH, Whiteman M, Moore PK (2009) GYY4137, a novel hydrogen sulfide-releasing molecule, protects against endotoxic shock in the rat. Free Radic Biol Med 47: 103–113.
9. Kimura Y, Goto Y, Kimura H (2010) Hydrogen sulfide increases glutathione production and suppresses oxidative stress in mitochondria. Antioxid Redox Signal 12: 1–13.
10. Zhong GZ, Li YB, Liu XL, Guo LS, Chen ML, et al. (2010) Hydrogen sulfide opens the KATP channel on rat atrial and ventricular myocytes. Cardiology 115: 120–126.
11. Fiorucci S, Distrutti E, Cirino G, Wallace JL (2006) The emerging roles of hydrogen sulfide in the gastrointestinal tract and liver. Gastroenterology 131: 259–271.
12. Kabil O, Vitvitsky V, Xie P, Banerjee R (2011) The Quantitative Significance of the Transsulfuration Enzymes for H2S Production in Murine Tissues. Antioxid Redox Signal 15: 363–372.
13. Siebert N, Cantré D, Eipel C, Vollmar B (2008) H2S contributes to the hepatic arterial buffer response and mediates vasorelaxation of the hepatic artery via activation of K(ATP) channels. Am J Physiol Gastrointest Liver Physiol 295: G1266–1273.
14. Fujii K, Sakuragawa T, Kashiba M, Sugiura Y, Kondo M, et al. (2005) Hydrogen sulfide as an endogenous modulator of biliary bicarbonate excretion in the rat liver. Antioxid Redox Signal 7: 788–794.
15. Kang K, Zhao M, Jiang H, Tan G, Pan S, et al. (2009) Role of hydrogen sulfide in hepatic ischemia reperfusion-induced injury in rats. Liver Transpl 15: 1306–1314.
16. Morsy MA, Ibrahim SA, Abdelwahab SA, Zedan MZ, Elbitar HI (2010) Curative effects of hydrogen sulfide against acetaminophen-induced hepatotoxicity in mice. Life Sci 87: 692–698.
17. Hosono-Fukao T, Hosono T, Seki T, Ariga T (2009) Diallyl trisulfide protects rats from carbon tetrachloride-induced liver injury. J Nutr 139: 2252–2256.
18. Fukao T, Hosono T, Misawa S, Seki T, Ariga T (2004) Chemoprotective effect of diallyl trisulfide from garlic against carbon tetrachloride-induced acute liver injury of rats. Biofactors 21: 171–174.
19. Fiorucci S, Antonelli E, Mencarelli A, Orlandi S, Renga B, et al. (2005) The third gas: H2S regulates perfusion pressure in both the isolated and perfused normal rat liver and in cirrhosis. Hepatology 42: 539–548.
20. Distrutti E, Mencarelli A, Santucci L, Renga B, Orlandi S, et al. (2008) The methionine connection: homocysteine and hydrogen sulfide exert opposite effects on hepatic microcirculation in rats. Hepatology 47: 659–667.
21. Weber LW, Boll M, Stampfl A (2003) Hepatotoxicity and mechanism of action of haloalkanes: carbon tetrachloride as a toxicological model. Crit Rev Toxicol 33: 105–136.
22. Fang L, Li H, Tang C, Geng B, Qi Y, et al. (2009) Hydrogen sulfide attenuates the pathogenesis of pulmonary fibrosis induced by bleomycin in rats. Can J Physiol Pharmacol 87: 531–538.
23. Qingyou Z, Junbao D, Weijin Z, Hui Y, Chaoshu T, et al. (2004) Impact of hydrogen sulfide on carbon monoxide/heme oxygenase pathway in the pathogenesis of hypoxic pulmonary hypertension. Biochem Biophys Res Commun 317: 30–37.
24. Steib CJ, Hennenberg M, Beitinger F, Hartmann AC, Bystron M, et al. (2010) Amiloride reduces portal hypertension in rat liver cirrhosis. Gut 59: 827–836.
25. Bhatia M, Wong FL, Fu D, Lau HY, Moochhala SM, et al. (2005) Role of hydrogen sulfide in acute pancreatitis and associated lung injury. FASEB J 19: 623–625.
26. Chang TK, Crespi CL, Waxman DJ (1998) Spectrophotometric analysis of human CYP2E1-catalyzed p-nitrophenol hydroxylation. Methods Mol Biol 107: 147–152.
27. Ohkawa H, Ohishi N, Yagi K (1979) Assay for lipid peroxides in animal tissues by thiobarbituric acid reaction. Anal Biochem 95: 351–358.
28. Bradford MM (1976) A rapid and sensitive method for the quantification of microgram quantities of protein utilizing the principle of protein–dye binding. Anal Biochem 72: 248–254.
29. Stegemann H, Stalder K (1967) Determination of hydroxyproline. Clin Chim Acta 18: 267–273.
30. Yuan L, Kaplowitz N (2009) Glutathione in liver diseases and hepatotoxicity. Mol Aspects Med 30: 29–41.
31. Sivarajah A, McDonald MC, Thiemermann C (2006) The production of hydrogen sulfide limits myocardial ischemia and reperfusion injury and contributes to the cardioprotective effects of preconditioning with endotoxin, but not ischemia in the rat. Shock 26: 154–161.

32. Fiorucci S, Santucci L, Distrutti E (2007) NSAIDs, coxibs, CINOD and H(2)S-releasing NSAIDs: What lies beyond the horizon. Dig Liver Dis 39: 1043–1051.

33. Yonezawa D, Sekiguchi F, Miyamoto M, Taniguchi E, Honjo M, et al. (2007) A protective role of hydrogen sulfide against oxidative stress in rat gastric mucosal epithelium. Toxicology 241: 11–18.

34. Zhao WM, Wang R (2002) H2S-induced vasorelaxation and underlying cellular and molecular mechanisms. Am J Physiol Heart Circ Physiol 283: H474–H480.

35. Guidotti TL (1996) Hydrogen sulphide. Occup Med (Lond) 46: 367–371.

36. Dranoff JA, Wells RG (2010) Portal fibroblasts: underappreciated mediators of biliary fibrosis. Hepatology 51: 1438–1444.

37. Predmore BL, Grinsfelder DB, Aragon JP, Elston M, Calvert JW, et al. (2010) The stable hydrogen sulphide donor, diallyl trisulfide, protects against acute myocardial infarction in mice. J Am Coll Cardiol 55: A116.

17

Dietary Supplementation of Blueberry Juice Enhances Hepatic Expression of Metallothionein and Attenuates Liver Fibrosis in Rats

Yuping Wang[1], Mingliang Cheng[2]*, Baofang Zhang[2], Fei Nie[3], Hongmei Jiang[1]

1 Department of Clinical Microbiology and Immunology, Affiliated Hospital of Guiyang Medical College, Guiyang, Guizhou Province, China, **2** Department of Infectious Diseases, Affiliated Hospital of Guiyang Medical College, Guiyang, Guizhou Province, China, **3** Guizhou Academy of Sciences, Guiyang, Guizhou Province, China

Abstract

Aim: To investigate the effect of blueberry juice intake on rat liver fibrosis and its influence on hepatic antioxidant defense.

Methods: Rabbiteye blueberry was used to prepare fresh juice to feed rats by daily gastric gavage. Dan-shao-hua-xian capsule (DSHX) was used as a positive control for liver fibrosis protection. Liver fibrosis was induced in male Sprague-Dawley rats by subcutaneous injection of CCl_4 and feeding a high-lipid/low-protein diet for 8 weeks. Hepatic fibrosis was evaluated by Masson staining. The expression of α-smooth muscle actin (α-SMA) and collagen III (Col III) were determined by immunohistochemical techniques. The activities of superoxide dismutase (SOD) and malondialdehyde (MDA) in liver homogenates were determined. Metallothionein (MT) expression was detected by real-time RT-PCR and immunohistochemical techniques.

Results: Blueberry juice consumption significantly attenuates CCl_4-induced rat hepatic fibrosis, which was associated with elevated expression of metallothionein (MT), increased SOD activity, reduced oxidative stress, and decreased levels of α-SMA and Col III in the liver.

Conclusion: Our study suggests that dietary supplementation of blueberry juice can augment antioxidative capability of the liver presumably via stimulating MT expression and SOD activity, which in turn promotes HSC inactivation and thus decreases extracellular matrix collagen accumulation in the liver, and thereby alleviating hepatic fibrosis.

Editor: Partha Mukhopadhyay, National Institutes of Health, United States of America

Funding: This study was supported by a grant from the Department of Science and Technology of Guizhou Province for Traditional Chinese Medicine Modernization (Grant No. ZY[2012]3017), a grant from the Foundation of the Governor of Guizhou Province ([2012] 44), and a grant from the National Foundation for Educational Teams of China ([2009]12). The funders had no role in study design, data collection and analysis, decision to publish, or preparation of the manuscript.

Competing Interests: The authors have declared that no competing interests exist.

* E-mail: chengml@21cn.com

Introduction

Hepatic fibrosis is a repair response to chronic liver injury [1]. It is a progressive pathological process and a common pathological change in chronic liver diseases. Oxidative stress is an important pathogenic factor for many liver diseases, which can cause hepatocyte damage through lipid peroxidation and protein alkylation [2–5]. Superoxide dismutase (SOD) and catalase are important antioxidant enzymes that function as endogenous free radical scavengers. Recently, metallothionein (MT) was identified as a more efficient scavenger for reactive oxygen species (ROS) [6]. There are two major isoforms of MT, Mt-1 and Mt-2, which are ubiquitously distributed in almost all tissues [7]. Interestingly, MT was shown to be able to enhance SOD activity in vitro [8]. Cardiac overexpression of MT has been shown to effectively attenuate diabetic cardiomyopathy via suppression of reactive oxygen species (ROS) production and oxidative stress [9]. Currently, there are no effective drugs available to prevent or treat liver fibrosis, and some natural substances with antioxidant properties are under investigation for developing new therapeutic reagents.

Blueberries are perennial flowering plants belonging to *Vaccinium spp.* of the family *Ericaceae*. In recent years, Human Nutrition Research Center of the United States has carried out a series of studies, demonstrating that blueberry contains a high level of anthocyanins and appears to have the highest antioxidant capacity among fruits and vegetables [10,11]. Blueberry and probiotics were shown to have protective effects on acute liver injury induced by d-galactosamine and lipopolysaccharide [12]. Proanthocyanidin isolated from blueberry leaves was able to inhibit hepatitis-c virus (HCV) replication [13]. Furthermore, proanthocyanidin derived from the leaves of *Vaccinium virgatum* suppresses platelet-derived growth factor-induced proliferation of the human hepatic stellate cell line LI90 [14]. Increasing blueberry consumption seems to be a practical and effective strategy to reduce oxidative stress and thus protect tissue injury [15].

Table 1. Major active ingredients of the blueberry juice.

Ingredients	Anthocyanin(mg/kg)	SOD (U/kg)
	3507.6±56.12	$3.7 \times 10^4 \pm 101.23$

The aim of this research work was to examine the effect of blueberry juice on CCl_4-induced rat liver fibrosis and its effects on hepatic levels of the endogenous antioxidant components.

Materials and Methods

Reagents and animal treatments

"Rabbiteye Blueberry" was produced by Guizhou Academy of Sciences in the Blueberry Production Field at Ma-Jiang, Guizhou, China. The blueberry was stored at $-20°C$ until experimental use.

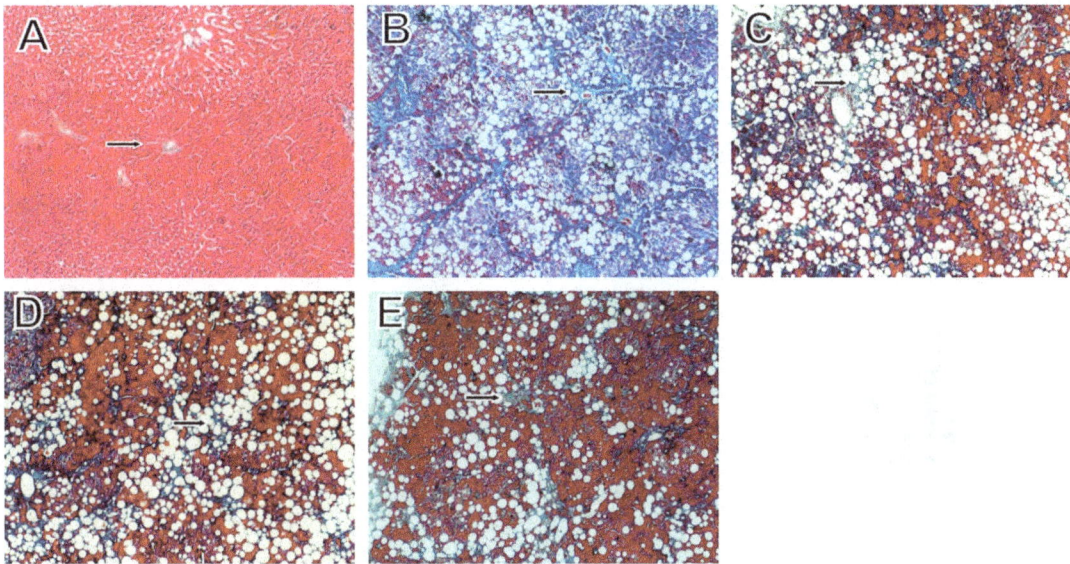

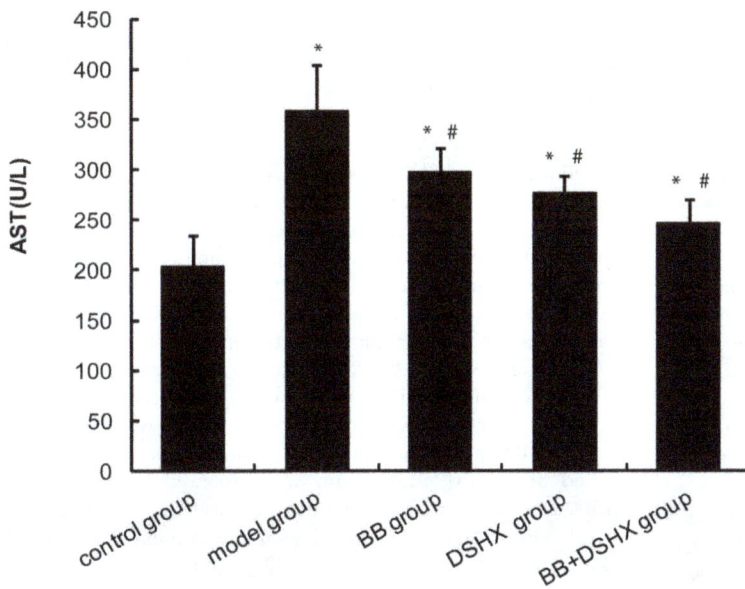

Figure 1. Effect of blueberry juice on CCl₄-induced liver fibrosis and liver damage. Liver fibrosis was induced in rats by subcutaneous injection of CCl_4 and subsequently feeding a high-lipid/low-protein diet for 8 weeks with or without daily blueberry juice gavage. After 8 weeks, the degree of hepatic fibrosis was evaluated by Masson staining. *The upper panel images* show the representative liver histology changes in the livers of the normal control group (**A**), CCl_4-induced hepatic fibrosis group (the model group, **B**), blueberry juice prevention group (BB group, **C**), Dan-shao-hua-xian capsule prevention group (DSHX group, **D**), and blueberry juice+DSHX prevention group (BB+DSHX group, **E**), Original magnification 100×, arrows indicate collagen fibers. *The lower panel* illustrates serum aspartate aminotransferase (AST) levels in the five groups of rats as indicated. *p<0.05 *vs.* the control group, #p<0.05 *vs.* the model group.

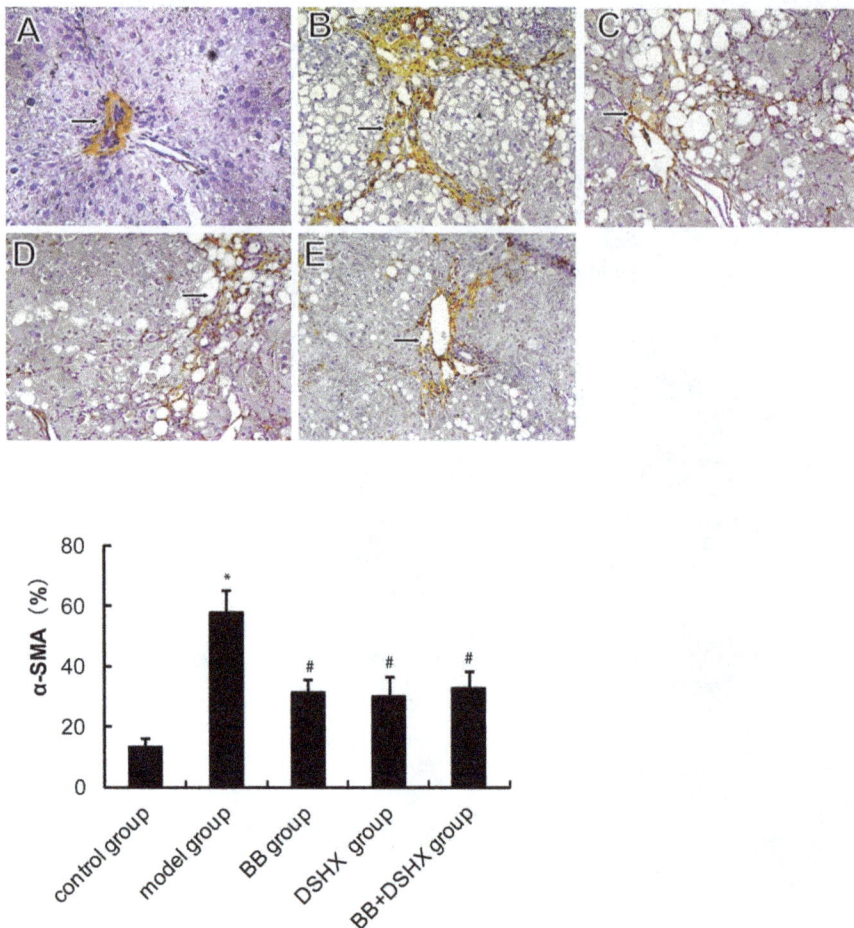

Figure 2. Effect of blueberry juice on α-SMA protein expression in rat livers. The same groups of rats were treated as described in Figure 1. *The upper panel images* show the representative liver α-SMA IHC staining in the normal control group (**A**), CCl$_4$-induced hepatic fibrosis group (the model group, **B**), blueberry juice prevention group (BB group, **C**), Dan-shao-hua-xian capsule prevention group (DSHX group, **D**), and blueberry juice+DSHX prevention group (BB +DSHXgroup, **E**). Original magnification 400×, arrows indicate positive cytoplasmic staining. *The lower panel* shows the quantification data of α-SMA IHC staining. *p<0.05 *vs.* the control group, #p<0.05 *vs.* the model group.

Fresh blueberry juice was prepared by homogenization of the frozen fruit right before the start of experiments (1 ml of blueberry juice contained about 2 g of dried blueberry). The major active ingredients of the blueberry juice was analyzed by HPLC-DAD and NBT methods and shown in Table 1. Dan-shao-hua-xian capsule (DSHX) capsules composed of five Chinese herbal medicines-Tetrandrine, Radix Salviae Miltiorrhizae, Radix Paeoniae Rubra, Astragalus Membranaceus and Ginkgleaf was purchased from Guiyang Pharmaceutical Company (Guizhou, China, lot number 20081011). We previously reported that DSHX is effective in preventing hepatic fibrosis [16], and it was therefore served as positive control for liver fibrosis protection.

Forty-five male Sprague–Dawley rats (200±20 g) were obtained from the Experimental Animal Center of Guiyang Medical College, Guiyang, China (Approval number SCXK (Guizhou) 2002-0001). Rats were randomly divided into five groups with nine rats in each group: control group, CCl$_4$-induced hepatic fibrosis group (model group), blueberry juice prevention group (BB group), Dan-shao-hua-xian capsule prevention group (DSHX group), and blueberry juice+DSHX prevention group (BB+DSHX group). Except in the control group, liver fibrosis was induced in by a complex method [17]. Rats in model group, BB group, DSHX group, and BB+DSHX group received subcutaneous injections of 40% CCl$_4$ solution (mixture of pure CCl$_4$ and peanut oil) at a dose of 3 ml/kg twice a week for 8 weeks (the first dose was 4 ml/kg). Rats were fed a high-lipid/low-protein diet (79.5% corn farina, 20% fat, and 0.5% cholesterol) each day. Rats in control group were fed a normal diet. At the same time, blueberry juice (15 g/kg, once a day, by gastric gavage), DSHX (1.0 g/kg, once a day, by gastric gavage), and blueberry juice+DSHX (15 g/kg, and 1.0 g/kg, once a day, by gastric gavage) were given to the rats in the corresponding groups. After 8 weeks, rats were killed to collect blood and livers. The same part of each liver was removed and fixed in 10% neutral formalin; the remaining portion of liver was stored at −80°C. Rat serum was prepared by centrifugation (1500 rpm for 15 min at room temperature) and stored at −80°C.

All animal studies complied with the Animal Care and Use Guidelines of Guiyang Medical College (Guiyang, China).

Histopathology and the measurement of serum AST levels

After fixation in 10% formalin for 24 h, liver samples were embedded in paraffin. Samples were then cut into 5-μm pieces and mounted on slides. They were then stained with hematoxylin and eosin (H&E) for histopathological examination, and with fibrosis-specific Masson stain for evaluation of the degree of liver fibrosis.

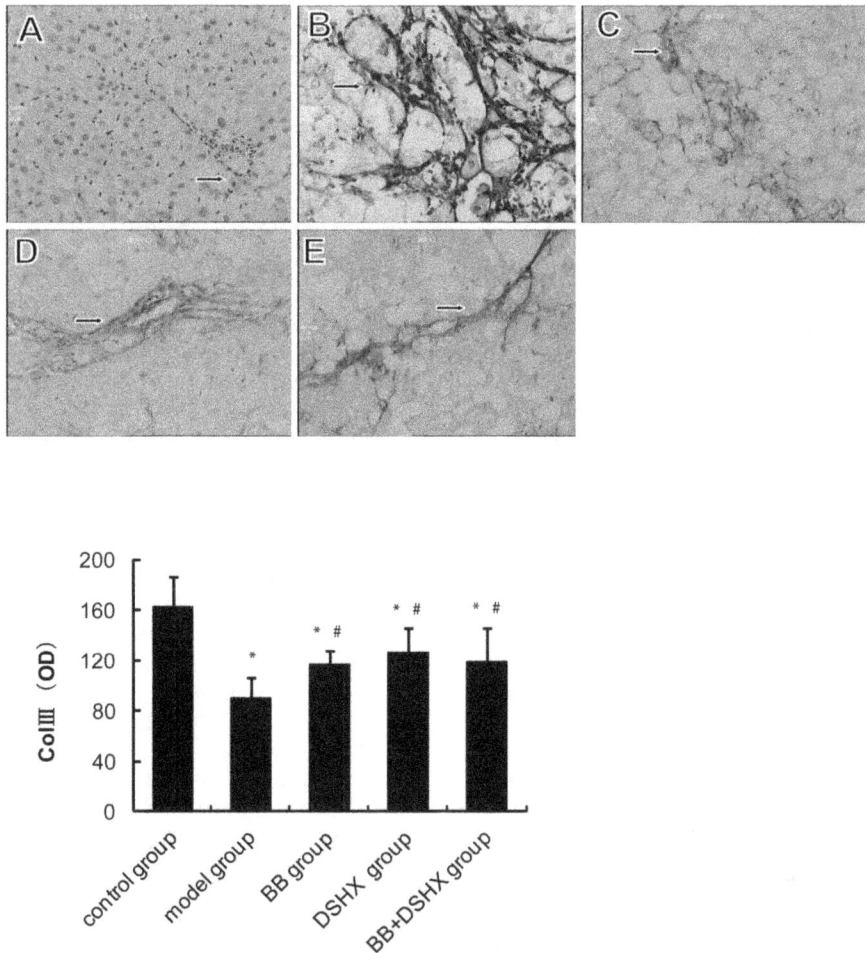

Figure 3. Effect of blueberry juice on Col III protein expression in rat livers. *The upper panel images* show the representative liver Col III IHC staining in the normal control group (**A**), CCl$_4$-induced hepatic fibrosis group (the model group, **B**), blueberry juice prevention group (BB group, **C**), Dan-shao-hua-xian capsule prevention group (DSHX group, **D**), and blueberry juice+DSHX prevention group (BB+DSHX group, **E**). Original magnification 400×, arrows indicate positive cytoplasmic staining. *The lower panel* shows the quantification data of Col III IHC staining by using the Biomias2000 image analysis system, which measures the transparence of the slides that is reversely related to the positivity of Col III IHC staining. *p<0.05 *vs.* the control group, #p<0.05 *vs.* the model group.

Histologic evaluation was performed twice by two pathologists blinded to the protocol on five low-power fields per slide. Modified Ishak scoring system was used with minor changes in order to define the degree of fibrosis [18].

Concentrations of serum AST were measured by an automatic biochemical analytic instrument (Siemens Advia 1650, Bensheim, Germany).

Immunohistochemical analysis

After de-paraffinization, rehydration, and antigen unmasking by heat treatment, liver sections were incubated in 3% H$_2$O$_2$ for 10 min. They were then incubated with anti-α-SMA (SC-32251, Santa Cruz Biotechnology, Santa Cruz, CA, USA), anti-Col III (SC-80564, Santa Cruz Biotechnology) and anti-MT (sc-11377, Santa Cruz Biotechnology) antibody (1:100) overnight at 4°C. Samples were then processed using an EnVision kit (lot number 10N1775A, Dako, Denmark) according to the manufacturer's protocols. Phosphate-buffered saline (PBS) was used as negative control. The cells with brown staining in the cytoplasm/nucleus were considered to be positive. Five high power microscopic fields (400× magnification) were randomly chosen per slide, and the

number of positive cells per field was counted (α-SMA and MT immunopositivity). For Col III staining, 5 high power fields were chosen randomly in each section and the images were analyzed by the Biomias2000 Image Analytic Instrument to quantify the transparency of the immunopositive areas in the section (data expressed as optical density (OD) that is in inverse proportion to the intensity of immunostaining signals).

Real-time reverse transcriptase-polymerase chain reaction (RT-PCR) analysis

Total RNA was extracted from liver tissues with Trizol reagent (lot number 13827390, Invitrogen, Carlsbad, CA, USA) according to the manufacturer's instructions. The RNA samples were used for reverse transcription with Moloney murine leukemia virus (MMuLV) reverse transcriptase and oligo (dT) primers (lot number 00033699, Fermentas, MBI, Burlington, ON, Canada). The SYBR Green DNA PCR kit (lot number 0804104, Applied Biosystems, Foster City, CA, USA) was used for real-time RT-PCR analysis. PCR primers were supplied by Dr. Jie Liu (The University of Kansas Medical Center, USA). The sequences of the primers are as follows. MT-I upstream 5'-TGTGCCTGAAGT-

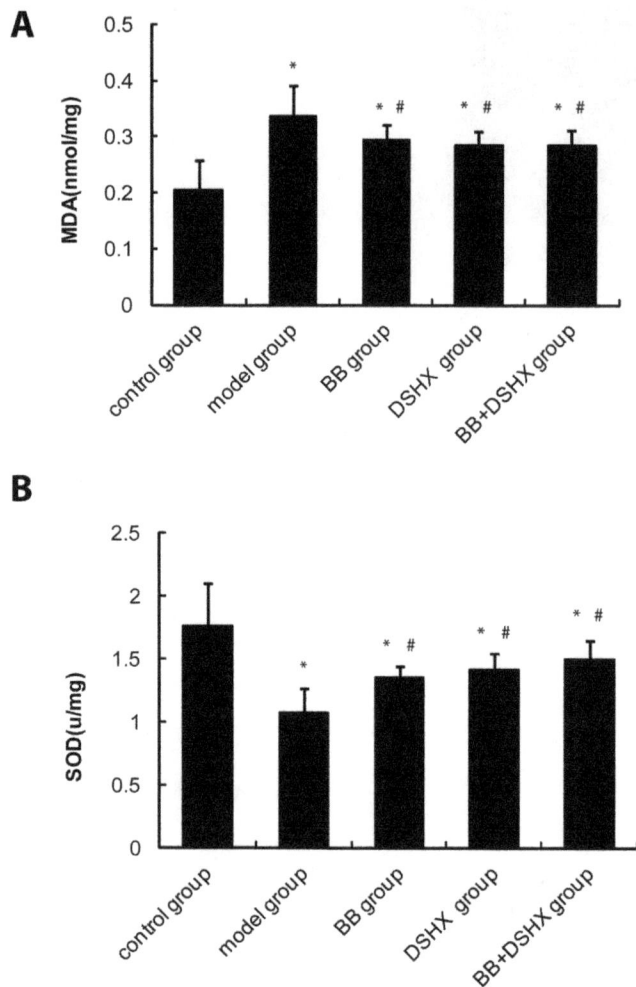

Figure 4. Effect of blueberry juice on hepatic SOD and MDA levels. Liver homogenates were prepared using the frozen liver tissues from rats in the indicated groups. SOD (**A**) and MDA (**B**) levels in the homogenates were measured. *p<0.05 *vs.* the control group, #p<0.05 *vs.* the model group.

GACGAACAG-3′,downstream 5′-TTCACATGCTCGGTA-GAAAACG-3′; Beta-actin upstream 5′-TCCTCCTGAGCG-CAAGTACTCT-3′,downstream 5′-GCTCAGTAACAGTCCG-CCTAGAA-3′.

The cycle time (C_t) values of the genes of interest were normalized with β-actin from the same sample. Relative differences between groups were calculated and expressed as relative increases, with the control set to 100%.

Measurement of levels of SOD and MDA in liver homogenates

Liver homogenates were prepared using the frozen liver tissues. SOD content was determined by the xanthine oxidase method and MDA content was tested by the thiobarbituric acid method according to the manufacturer's instructions (lot numbers 20090615, 20090616, respectively; Jiancheng Biologic Company, Nanjing, China).

Statistical analysis

Data analysis was carried out using SPSS 11.5 software (Chicago, IL, USA). Quantitative data were expressed as mean±SD and subjected to one-way analysis of variance, followed by Tukey's Post Test for multiple comparisons. Ordinal data were analyzed by Radit analysis. $P<0.05$ was considered statistically significant.

Results

Blueberry juice consumption attenuates CCl₄-induced rat hepatic fibrosis and liver injury

We established a rat hepatic fibrosis model with chronic CCl₄ injection and the degree of liver fibrosis was assessed by H&E and Masson staining (Figure 1). In control group, hepatocytes had a normal radial array surrounding the central veins, and no regenerating collagen fibers were present. In the fibrosis model group, the lobular structure of hepatocytes was destroyed, and the hepatic plates were disordered with diffuse, fatty degeneration. Collagen fibers expanded into the hepatic parenchyma, which formed fibrous septa surrounding and separating the normal lobules. Pseudolobules were observed in a few samples, and infiltration of numerous inflammatory cells was present in the portal area and fibrous septa. These histopathological changes indicate significant liver fibrotic changes in rats chronically treated with CCl₄. The hepatic fibrosis was significantly alleviated in BB group, DSHX group, and BB+DSHX group, as evidenced by much thinner fibrous septa these groups (Figure 1) with decreased hepatocyte fatty degeneration, bridging fibrosis, and less inflammatory cell infiltration [19]. We also measured serum AST concentrations to determine the degree of liver injury in the rats. Consistent with our histological data, rats fed blueberry juice had significantly lower levels of serum AST compared to the fibrosis model control group (Figure 1).

Blueberry juice consumption reduces α-SMA and Col III expression in the liver

We next examined the effect of blueberry on hepatic α-SMA and Col III expression, two markers for liver fibrosis and hepatic stellate cells (HSCs) activation. Immunohistochemical staining showed that, in control group, α-SMA -positive staining was restricted to the vascular walls in the portal areas and the central veins, while a significantly stronger immune staining was noted in the periportal sinusoid and around the bile ductules in the model group (Figure 2). The expression of α-SMA were significantly decreased in BB group, DSHX group and BB+DSHX group compared with model group ($P<0.05$, Figure 2).

A very low level of Col III expression was observed in the normal control group, which was mainly distributed in the periportal areas (Figure 3). In the fibrosis model group, abundant Col III positive fibers were detected in periportal areas and hepatic sinusoids, which expanded into the liver parenchyma to form fibrous septa that surrounded hepatocytes and formed pseudolobules (Figure 3). In the BB group, DSHX group and BB+DSHX group, the expression of Col III was significantly ameliorated compared with the model group ($P<0.05$, Figure 3).

Effect of blueberry juice on SOD and MDA levels in the rat liver

Next we wanted to examine whether blueberry juice affected hepatic reactive oxidative species (ROS), which are known to play an important role in CCl₄-induced liver damage and fibrosis formation. We measured the haptic tissue levels of malondialdehyde (MDA), a marker of oxidative stress. As shown in Figure 4A, blueberry juice consumption significantly reduced MDA levels in the liver compared to those in rats of the fibrosis group that

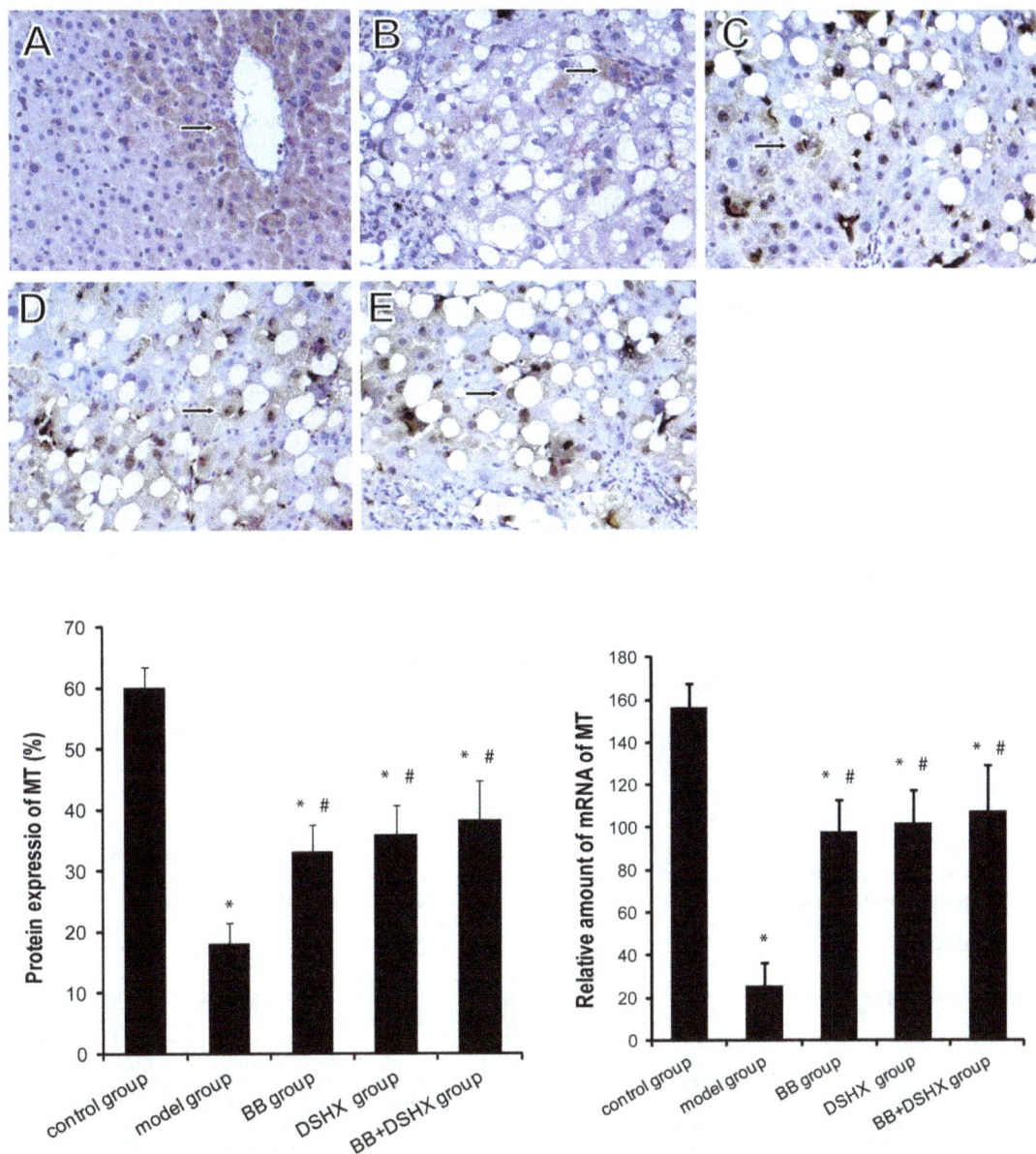

Figure 5. Effect of blueberry juice on MT expression in the rat livers. *The upper panel images* show the representative IHC staining of MT protein in the livers of normal control group (**A**), CCl$_4$-induced hepatic fibrosis group (the model group, **B**), blueberry juice prevention group (BB group, **C**), Dan-shao-hua-xian capsule prevention group (DSHX group, **D**), and blueberry juice+DSHX prevention group (BB+DSHX group, **E**). Original magnification 400×, arrows indicate positive cytoplasmic/nuclear staining. *The lower left panel* shows the quantification data of MT protein expression based on the MT IHC staining. *The lower right panel* shows the mRNA levels of MT in the livers assessed by RT-PCR. *p<0.05 *vs.* the control group, #p<0.05 *vs.* the model group.

received a control diet. Conversely, the levels of superoxide dismutases (SODs) were significantly increased in the livers of rats receiving blueberry juice feeding compared to rats in the fibrosis group that received a control diet (Figure 4B). These data suggest that the fibrosis protective effect of blueberry juice might be due to its enhancement of SOD activity and thereby decreasing oxidative stress in the liver.

Blueberry juice upregulates metallothionein (MT) expression in the liver

Metallothionein (MT) is another ROS scavenger with a more efficient antioxidant activity [20,21],and MT was recently shown

to be able to enhance SOD activity in vitro [8]. We performed immunohistochemistry satining and real-time RT-PCR analyses and found that hepatic MT protein and mRNA expression was significantly lower in rats with CCl$_4$-induced liver fibrosis; blueberry consumption markedly increased MT expression in the liver (Figure 5).

Discussion

Our previous work showed that blueberry can increase expression of *Nrf2* and HO-1 in primary hepatic stellate cells [22], and when given orally for 21 days, blueberry can increase the level of mRNA expression of *Nrf2*, Nqo1, and HO-1 in rat liver, and had protective effects against acute and chronic hepatic injury in rats [19,23]. In the present study, we demonstrated that blueberry juice consumption by rats attenuates CCl_4-induced hepatic fibrosis. We also showed that blueberry juice can stimulate hepatic expression of metallothionein (MT), increase SOD activity, and reduce oxidative stress in the liver, suggesting that the protection of liver fibrosis by blueberry juice might be through its enhancement of the antioxidative capability of the liver.

Chronic hepatic injury by carbon tetrachloride (CCl_4) is a well-established animal model of liver fibrosis. Reactive oxygen species and oxidative stress have been shown to play an important role in the etiopathogenesis of the hepatic fibrotic changes [24–26], and antioxidant treatment in vivo seems to be effective in preventing or reducing chronic liver damage and fibrosis [27]. Oxidative stress aggravates liver fibrosis via HSC activation, and lipid peroxidation stimulates transcription of the collagen gene. The expression of α-SMA is a characteristic feature of activated HSCs and this is considered as a marker for hepatic fibrosis [28]. Upon liver injury, HSCs become activated and differentiate into myofibroblast-like cells, which proliferate and contribute to collagen deposition in the extracelluar matrix (ECM) [29]. Collagen accounts for about 50% of the total protein in fibrous liver) [30]. Here we showed that blueberry significantly reduces type III collagen content and decrease α-SMA expression in the liver, indicating an inhibitory effect on HSC activation. We also found that blueberry juice can increase SOD activity and decrease oxidative stress in the liver. These data suggest that the fibrosis protective effect of blueberry juice might be due to its antioxidative effect in the liver.

Furthermore, we provided evidence showing that blueberry juice also has a remarkable stimulatory effect on metallothioneins (MTs) expression in the liver. Metallothioneins (MTs) are a family of low molecular mass (6–7 kDa), cysteine-rich, inducible, intracellular proteins that bind heavy metals with high affinity [31]. MT is considered one of the most important intracellular free

radical scavengers that plays an important role in defense of stress reactions and tissue injury [32,33]. It has been shown that mice which have developed a reversible liver fibrosis upon removal of CCl_4, had a high level of hepatic MT, but mice which developed an irreversible fibrosis, had low expression of MT [34]. Therefore, hepatic MT expression levels are inversely related to the severity of chronic liver damage [35]. Induction of MT synthesis protects animals from hepatotoxicity induced by various toxins including CCl_4; it also promotes repair and regeneration of injured liver [36]. In this study, we showed that blueberry juice significantly increased MT expression in the liver, which is associated with decreased liver fibrosis, suggesting a potentially important role of MT in blueberry juice-medicated protection against fibrosis.

In summary, our study demonstrated that the liver fibrosis protective effect of blueberry juice was associated with elevated hepatic expression of metallothionein (MT), increased SOD activity, reduced oxidative stress, and decreased levels of α-SMA and Col III in the liver. We therefore propose that dietary supplementation of blueberry juice can augment antioxidative capability of the liver presumably via stimulating MT expression and SOD activity, which in turn promotes HSC inactivation and thereby decreases extracellular matrix collagen accumulation in the liver.

Acknowledgments

The authors would like to thank Dr. Jie Liu for his help in the experimental research by providing the primers for MT real-time RT-PCR and his technical support.

Author Contributions

Conceived and designed the experiments: MC. Performed the experiments: YW BZ. Analyzed the data: MC YW BZ FN HJ. Contributed reagents/materials/analysis tools: MC. Wrote the paper: YW MC.

References

1. Ming LC, Chang QY (2008) Hepatic fibrosis. Beijing: Beijing People's Medical Publishing House. pp. 3–4.
2. Cederbaum AI, Lu Y, Wu D (2009) Role of oxidative stress in alcohol-induced liver injury. Arch Toxicol 83: 519–548.
3. Lai MM (2002) Hepatitis C virus proteins: direct link to hepatic oxidative stress, steatosis, carcinogenesis and more. Gastroenterology 122:568–571.
4. Weber LW, Boll M, Stampfl A (2003) Hepatotoxicity and mechanism of action of haloalkanes: carbon tetrachloride as a toxicological model. Crit Rev Toxicol 33:105–136.
5. Parola M, Robino G (2001) Oxidative stress-related molecules and liver fibrosis. J Hepatol 35:297–306.
6. Sato M, Kondoh M (2002) Recent studies on metallothionein: protection against toxicity of heavy metals and oxygen free radicals. J Exp Med 196: 9–22.
7. Kang YJ (2006) Metallothionein redox cycle and function. Exp Biol Med (Maywood) 231:1459–1467.
8. Koh M, Kim H.(2001) The effects of metallothionein on the activety of enzymes involved in removal of reactive oxygen species. Bull Korean Chem Soc 22:362–366.
9. Cai L, Wang YH, Zhou GH, Chen T, Song Y (2006) Attenuation by metallothionein of early cardiac cell death via suppression of mitochondrial oxidative stress results in a prevention of diabetic cardiomyopathy. J Am Coll Cardiol 48:1688–1697.
10. Wu X, Beecher GR, Holden JM, Haytowitz DB, Gebhardt SE, et al. (2004) Lipophilic and hydrophilic antioxidant capacities of common foods in the United States. J Agric Food Chem 52:4026–4037.
11. Prior RL, Cao G, Prior RL, Cao G (2000) Analysis of botanicals and dietary supplements For antioxidant capacity: a review. J AOAC Int 83: 950–956.
12. Osman N, Adawi D, Ahrné S, Jeppsson B, Molin G (2007) Endotoxin- and d-galactosamine-induced liver injury improved by the administration of Lactobacillus, Bifidobacterium and blueberry. Dig Liver Dis 39: 849–856.
13. Takeshita M, Ishida Y, Akamatsu E, Ohmori Y, Sudoh M, et al. (2009) Proanthocyanidin from blueberry leaves suppresses expression of subgenomic hepatitis C virus RNA J Biol Chem 284: 21165–21176.
14. Takami Y, Uto H, Takeshita M, Kai H, Akamatsu E, et al. (2010) Proanthocyanidin derived from the leaves of Vaccinium virgatum suppresses

15. platelet-derived growth factor-induced proliferation of the human hepatic stellate cell line LI90. Hepatol Res 40:337–345.
15. Wolfe KL, Kang X, He X, Dong M, Zhang Q, et al. (2008) Cellular Antioxidant Activity of Common Fruits. J Agric Food Chem 56: 8418–8426.
16. Geng XX, Yang Q, Xie RJ, Luo XH, Li CX, et al. (2004) Effects of Dan-Shao-Hua-Xian on the expression of collagen type I and III in rats with hepatic fibrosis. Hepatobiliary Pancreat Dis 3:558–563.
17. Yang Q, Xie RJ, Geng XX, Luo XH, Han B, et al. (2005) Effect of Danshao Huaxian capsule on expression of matrix metalloproteinase-1 and tissue inhibitor of metalloproteinase-1 in fibrotic liver of rats.World J Gastroenterol 11:4953–4956.
18. Ishak K, Baptista A, Bianchi L, Callea F, De Groote J, et al. (1995) Histological grading and staging of chronic hepatitis. J Hepatol 22: 696–699
19. Wang YP, Cheng ML, Zhang BF, Mu M, Wu J (2010) Effects of blueberry on hepatic fibrosis and Nrf2 transcription factor in rats. World J Gastroenterol 16:2657–2663.
20. Cai L, Klein JB, Kang YJ (2000) Metallothionein inhibits peroxynitrite-induced DNA and lipoprotein damage. J BiolChem 275: 38957–38960.
21. Eum WS, Chung IS, Li MZ, Kang JH, Kim DW, et al. (2004) HIV-1 Tat-mediated protein transduction of Cu,Zn-superoxide dismutase into pancreatic β cells in vitro and in vivo. Free Radic Biol Med 37:339–349.
22. Wang YP, Cheng ML, Wu YY, Zhang BF, Wu J (2010) Effects of Blueberry on hepatic stellate cell proliferation,activation and its mechanism. Zhong Hua Yi Xue Za Zhi 9: 2504–2508.
23. Wang YP, Cheng ML, Zhang BF, Mu M, Zhou MY, et al. (2010) Effect of blueberry on hepatic and immunological functions in mice. Hepatobiliary Pancreat Dis Int 9: 164–168.
24. Tahan G, Tarcin O, Tahan V, Eren F, Gedik N, et al. (2007) The effects of N-acetylcysteine on bile duct ligation-induced liver fibrosis in rats. Dig Dis Sci 52: 3348–3354.
25. Tahan V, Ozaras R, Canbakan B, Uzun H, Aydin S, et al. (2004) Melatonin reduces dimethylnitrosamine-induced liver fibrosis in rats. J Pineal Res 37: 78–84.
26. Poli G (2000) Pathogenesis of liver fibrosis: role of oxidative stress. Mol Aspects Med 21:49–98.

27. Parola M, Robino G (2001) Oxidative stress-related molecules and liver fibrosis. J Hepatol 35:297–306.

28. Campbell JS, Hughes SD, Gilbertson DG, Palmer TE, Holdren MS, et al. (2005) Plateletderived growth factor C induces liver fibrosis, steatosis, and Hepatocellular carcinoma. Proc Natl Acad Sci USA 102:3389–3394.

29. Friedman SL (2000) Molecular regulation of hepatic fibrosis, an integrated cellular response to tissue injury. J Biol Chem 275:2247–22550.

30. Wang YD, Jia LW, Li CM (2000) Hepatic content of collagens and laminin in rat model of experimental liver fibrosis. World J Gastroenterol 6 (Suppl 3):73.

31. Coyle P, Philcox JC, Carey LC, Rofe AM (2002) Metallothionein: the multipurpose protein. Cell Mol Life Sci 59:627–647.

32. Chiaverini N, De Ley M (2010) Protective effect of metallothionein on oxidative stress-induced DNA damage. Free Radic Res 44:605–613.

33. Nachman-Clewner M, Giblin FJ, Dorey CK, Blanks RH, Dang L, et al. (2008) Selective Degeneration of Central Photoreceptors after Hyperbaric Oxygen in Normal and Metallothionein-Knockout Mice. Invest Ophthalmol Vis Sci 49:3207–3215.

34. Jiang Y, Kang YJ (2004) Metallothionein gene therapy for chemical-induced liver fibrosis in mice. Mol Ther 10:1130–1139.

35. Carrera G, Paternain JL, Carrere N, Folch J, Courtade-Saïdi M, et al. (2003) Hepatic metallothionein in patients with chronic hepatitis C: relationship with severity of liver disease and response to treatment. Am J Gastroenterol 98:1142–1149.

36. Cherian MG, Kang YJ (2006) Metallothionein and liver cell regeneration. Exp Biol Med (Maywood) 231: 138–144.

18

Targeted Recombinant Fusion Proteins of IFNγ and Mimetic IFNγ with PDGFβR Bicyclic Peptide Inhibits Liver Fibrogenesis *In Vivo*

Ruchi Bansal[1,2]*, **Jai Prakash**[1,2], **Marieke De Ruiter**[2], **Klaas Poelstra**[2]

1 Department of Controlled Drug Delivery (Targeted Therapeutics), MIRA Institute for Biomedical Technology and Technical Medicine, University of Twente, Enschede, The Netherlands, **2** Department of Pharmacokinetics, Toxicology and Targeting, University of Groningen, Groningen, The Netherlands

Abstract

Hepatic stellate cells (HSCs), following transdifferentiation to myofibroblasts plays a key role in liver fibrosis. Therefore, attempts to attenuate this myofibroblastic phenotype would be a promising therapeutic approach. Interferon gamma (IFNγ) is a potent anti-fibrotic cytokine, but its pleiotropic receptor expression leading to severe adverse effects has limited its clinical application. Since, activated HSC express high-level of platelet derived growth factor beta receptor (PDGFβR), we investigated the potential of PDGFβR-specific targeting of IFNγ and its signaling peptide that lacks IFNγR binding site (mimetic IFNγ or mimIFNγ) in liver fibrosis. We prepared DNA constructs expressing IFNγ, mimIFNγ or BiPPB (PDGFβR-specific bicyclic peptide)-IFNγ, BiPPB-mimIFNγ fusion proteins. Both chimeric proteins alongwith IFNγ and mimIFNγ were produced in *E.coli*. The expressed proteins were purified and analyzed for PDGFβR-specific binding and *in vitro* effects. Subsequently, these recombinant proteins were investigated for the liver uptake (pSTAT1α signaling pathway), for anti-fibrotic effects and adverse effects (platelet counts) in CCl_4-induced liver fibrogenesis in mice. The purified HSC-targeted IFNγ and mimIFNγ fusion proteins showed PDGFβR-specific binding and significantly reduced TGFβ-induced collagen-I expression in human HSC (LX2 cells), while mouse IFNγ and mimIFNγ did not show any effect. Conversely, mouse IFNγ and BiPPB-IFNγ induced activation and dose-dependent nitric oxide release in mouse macrophages (express IFNγR while lack PDGFβR), which was not observed with mimIFNγ and BiPPB-mimIFNγ, due to the lack of IFNγR binding sites. *In vivo*, targeted BiPPB-IFNγ and BiPPB-mimIFNγ significantly activated intrahepatic IFNγ-signaling pathway compared to IFNγ and mimIFNγ suggesting increased liver accumulation. Furthermore, the targeted fusion proteins ameliorated liver fibrogenesis in mice by significantly reducing collagen and α-SMA expression and potentiating collagen degradation. IFNγ also induced reduction in fibrogenesis but showed significant decrease in platelet counts, which was restored with targeted proteins. These results suggest that these rationally designed proteins can be further developed as novel anti-fibrotic therapeutics.

Editor: Rafael Aldabe, Centro de Investigacion en Medicina Aplicada (CIMA), Spain

Funding: Work was supported by VICI grant-in-aid from Netherlands Organization for Scientific Research (NWO; http://www.nwo.nl/) and the Technical foundation (STW; http://www.stw.nl/). The funders had no role in study design, data collection and analysis, decision to publish, or preparation of the manuscript.

Competing Interests: KP is scientific advisor and shareholder of BiOrion Technologies B.V., a company dedicated to the commercialization of drug carriers, including the carrier presented here.

* E-mail: R.Bansal@utwente.nl

Introduction

IFNγ is a pleiotropic homodimeric Th1 cytokine mainly produced by activated inflammatory cells and has been documented to be highly effective in viral, immunological and malignant diseases [1,2]. IFNγ (Interferon gamma-1b) has also been explored in clinical trials in patients suffering from liver fibrosis, renal fibrosis or idiopathic pulmonary fibrosis [3–6]. However, despite its promising effects *in vivo*, all clinical trials failed due to a lack of efficacy and unfavorable adverse effects [4,7,8]. The clinical application of this potent cytokine is nowadays limited to only a very few diseases. Many attempts have been made to prolong the half-life of IFNγ by PEGylation or by increasing its activity through slow release by incorporation in nanoparticles, elastomers, microspheres or liposomes [9–11]. These approaches have shown to be beneficial, but adverse effects due to the longer exposure of IFNγ to non-target tissues can still be detrimental. Therefore, targeted approaches leading to an increased therapeu-

tic efficacy without eliciting adverse effects would be ideal to treat slowly progressing chronic diseases [12].

Liver fibrosis, induced by viral infections (e.g hepatitis B and C), alcohol abuse, metabolic syndrome or genetic disorders, is characterized by an excessive accumulation of matrix proteins in the liver [13,14]. Worldwide millions of people, suffering from one of these disorders, are at risk of developing liver fibrosis. Currently, there are no effective and clinically approved anti-fibrotic therapy available and the treatment is mainly based on the removal of the underlying cause of the disease [15,16]. Liver transplantation is the only option for the patients suffering from advanced liver fibrosis or end stage liver cirrhosis.

Hepatic stellate cells (HSC) are the key pathogenic cells involved in the progression of liver fibrosis. These cells gets activated following release of growth factors from damaged hepatocytes, kupffer cells and infiltrating inflammatory cells. These activated HSC are then transformed into proliferative and contractile myofibroblast-like cells that produce large amounts of extracellular matrix (ECM) proteins leading to impairment of the structure and function of liver [17,18]. Among the potent anti-fibrotic therapeutic cytokines, Interferon gamma (IFNγ) is shown to be highly efficacious *in vitro* and *in vivo* in liver fibrosis models [19], but it failed in clinical trials due to reduced efficacy and unwanted systemic effects [8].

Others and we have shown that activated HSC abundantly express the platelet derived growth factor receptor (PDGFβR) during liver fibrosis, while its expression is relatively weak on other cells and normal tissues [20–22]. Recently, we have shown that using PDGFβR-specific delivery of IFNγ to activated HSC; acute and advanced liver fibrosis *in vivo* could be significantly inhibited with minimal adverse effects [20,23]. The results of these chimerical constructs of IFNγ and PDGFβR binding moieties were remarkably potent and encouraged us to pursue this strategy and prepare a targeted fusion proteins that are inexpensive and can be feasibly applied in clinical trials.

To that end, we have now produced the recombinant proteins containing a bicyclic PDGFβR-recognizing peptide (BiPPB) fused to IFNγ to synthesize BiPPB-IFNγ or to the signaling moiety of IFNγ (mimetic IFNγ or mimIFNγ) lacking extracellular IFNγR binding site [24,25] to generate BiPPB-mimIFNγ in *E.coli*. IFNγ and mimetic IFNγ were also expressed in parallel as control proteins. These proteins were analyzed *in vitro* in human HSC cells and *in vivo* in acute liver fibrogenesis mouse model. Encouragingly, we found that the targeted fusion proteins (BiPPB-IFNγ and BiPPB-mimIFNγ) specifically bound to PDGFβR-expressing human HSC and induced significant reduction in major ECM production *in vitro* (collagen). *In vivo*, in the CCl4 mouse model, targeted proteins significantly stimulated the IFNγ-mediated pSTAT1α-signaling pathway, inhibited collagen accumulation, HSC activation and induced fibrolysis. Apart from therapeutic effects, BiPPB-mimIFNγ and to a lesser extent BiPPB-IFNγ did not affect circulating platelets counts as observed by untargeted IFNγ.

Materials and Methods

Plasmids, Bacterial Strains and Cell Culture

pET42a and pET39b protein expression vectors were purchased from Novagen (Madison, WI, USA). All the restriction enzymes were procured from New England Biolabs (Beverly, MA).

Escherichia coli strain JM109 was used for plasmid propagation and cloning. Strain BL21 (DE3) (Novagen) was used as a host for the production of recombinant proteins. Human hepatic stellate cells, LX2 were kindly provided by Prof. Scott Friedman (Mount Sinai Hospital, New York). LX2 cell line is a well-established human HSC cell line [26]. LX2 cells were cultured in DMEM-Glutamax (Invitrogen, Carlsbad, CA) supplemented with 10% FBS and antibiotics (50 U/ml penicillin and 50 ng/ml streptomycin). Mouse spleen cells, freshly isolated from healthy C57BL/6 mice, were grown in DMEM cell culture medium.

Plasmid Construction

(a) Preparation of pET42a-IFNγ and pET42a-mimIFNγ. Splenocytes (freshly isolated from the spleen of healthy C57BL/6 mice) were seeded in the presence of 20 μg/ml phytohemagglutinin (PHA) for 24 h. RNA was isolated from spleen cells was used for PCR amplification of mouse IFNγ and mimetic IFNγ using gene specific primers (primer 1, primer 2 for IFNγ and primer 3, primer 4 for mimIFNγ as listed in **Table 1**). The PCR product was purified and digested with Eco RI. The digested gene was inserted into Psh A1/Eco RI digested pET42a vector to produce pET42a-IFNγ or pET42a-mim IFNγ (**Figure S1 and S2**).

(b) Preparation of pET39b-BiPPB-IFNγ and pET39b-BiPPB-mimIFNγ. For synthesis of pET39b-BiPPB-IFNγ and pET39b-BiPPB-mimIFNγ, pET39b-BiPPB was prepared by PCR extension of annealed primers (primer 5, primer 6 and primer 7, primer 8 listed in **Table 1**). The resulting products (2 fragments) were then digested with Bam HI and Not I, purified and ligated to Sca I/Not I digested pET39b vector (**Figure S3**). Thereafter, PCR amplified IFNγ and mimIFNγ (primer 9, primer 10 for IFNγ and primer 11, primer 12 for mimIFNγ listed in **Table 1**) were digested with Not I/Xho I and inserted into Not I/Xho I digested and purified pET39b vector. The resulted recombinant vectors were termed as pET39b-BiPPB-IFNγ and pET39b-BiPPB-mimIFNγ that encodes for BiPPB and IFNγ or mimIFNγ plus a three amino-acid linker (AAA) between them (**Figure S4 and S5**).

All the DNA constructs were confirmed by DNA sequencing. pET42a-IFNγ and pET42a-mimIFNγ expressed proteins of 45.2 and 34.5 KDa respectively including GST tag, His tag, S tag and IFNγ or mimIFNγ. pET39b-BiPPB-IFNγ and pET39b-BiPPB-mimIFNγ

Table 1. Primers used for plasmids construction.

Primers	Sequence	Restriction sites
Primer 1	TGCCACGGCCACAGTCATTGAAAGC	–
Primer 2	GCGAATTCTCAGCAGCGACTCCTTTTC	Eco RI
Primer 3	GCCAAGTTTGAGGTCAACAACCCACAG	–
Primer 4	GCGAATTCTCAGCGACTCCTTTTCCG	Eco RI
Primer 5	TGTTCTAGAAACCTCATCGATTGTAAG	–
Primer 6	GCGGATCCCTTACAATCGATGAGGTT	Bam HI
Primer 7	GCGGATCCGGAGGTTGTTCACGTAATCTAATAG	Bam HI
Primer 8	TAGCGGCCGCTGAACAATCTATTAGATTA	Not I
Primer 9	GGGCGGCCGCATGTCATGGTACAGTCATTGAA	Not I
Primer 10	GCCTCGAGTTAGCAGCGACTCCTTTTCCG	Xho I
Primer 11	AAGCGGCCGCAGCCAAGTTTGAGGTCAACAAC	Not I
Primer 12	GCCTCGAGTTATCGACTCCTTTTCCGCTTCCTG	Xho I

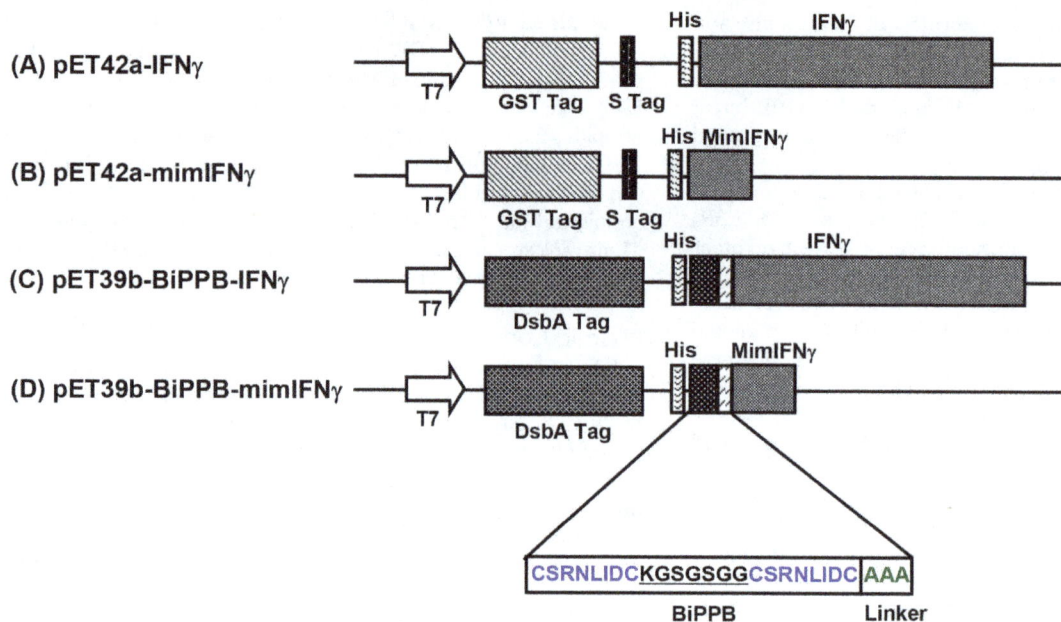

Figure 1. Schematic representation of the prokaryotic vectors used for the expression of the recombinant proteins. IFNγ (**A**) and mimetic IFNγ (**B**) were cloned in-frame upstream of His-tag in pET42a (+) vector to achieve cytoplasmic protein expression. The fusion proteins BiPPB-IFNγ (**C**) and BiPPB-mimIFNγ (**D**) were expressed in pET39b (+) vector for periplasmic expression of fusion proteins to ensure proper folding and disulfide bonds formation. For the synthesis of fusion proteins, BiPPB was fused to the N-terminal of IFNγ or mimetic IFNγ sequence through a flexible 3 amino acid linker (AAA) maintaining the open reading frame.

expressed 42.8 and 32.2 KDa fusion proteins respectively including Dsb tag, His tag, BiPPB, linker and IFNγ or mimIFNγ.

Expression and Purification of Recombinant Proteins

DNA constructs were transformed into CaCl₂ competent BL21 (DE3) and then induced with 1 mM IPTG at 37°C for 4 h.

For purification of IFNγ and mimIFNγ, the cell pellets were washed and suspended in binding buffer (500 mM NaCl, 20 mM sodium phosphate buffer, 20 mM Imidazole pH7.4), followed by enzymatic lysis (0.2 mg/ml lysozyme, 20 μg/ml DNase, 10 mM PMSF) for 30 min at 4°C and sonication for 10 min (10–15 short bursts). The cell debris was removed by centrifugation at 12,000 g

for 30 min at 4°C. The supernatant was extensively dialyzed against binding buffer.

For purification of periplasmic proteins BiPPB-IFNγ and BiPPB-mimIFNγ, the cell pellets were suspended in 0.03 mol/l Tris.HCl, 20% sucrose, 0.001 mol/l EDTA, pH8.0. The cells were incubated on ice for 5–10 min followed by centrifugation at 8000 g for 20 min at 4°C. The pellet was then resuspended in ice-cold 5 mM MgSO₄ and stirred for 10 min on ice bath. The cell debris was removed by centrifugation at 8000 g for 20 min at 4°C. The supernatant was extensively dialyzed against binding buffer.

The supernatants were then applied to Ni-charged chelating-Sepharose HisTrap High performance column (Pharmacia Biotech, Uppsala, Sweden). After being washed with binding

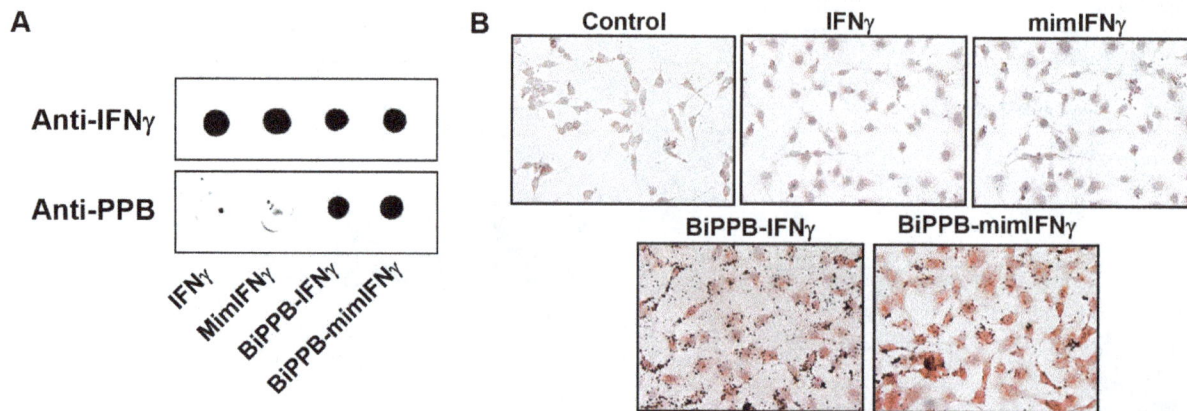

Figure 2. Dot-blot and *in vitro* binding of recombinant proteins in human HSC. (A) Dot-blot analysis of purified recombinant proteins IFNγ, mimetic IFNγ, BiPPB-IFNγ and BiPPB-mimIFNγ using anti-IFNγ and anti-PPB antibody. **(B)** Representative pictures showing binding of BiPPB-IFNγ and BiPPB-mimIFNγ to human HSC (LX2). Mouse IFNγ and mimIFNγ did not show any binding (similar to control) to human LX2 cells due to species differences and lack of IFNγR or PDGFβR binding sites respectively.

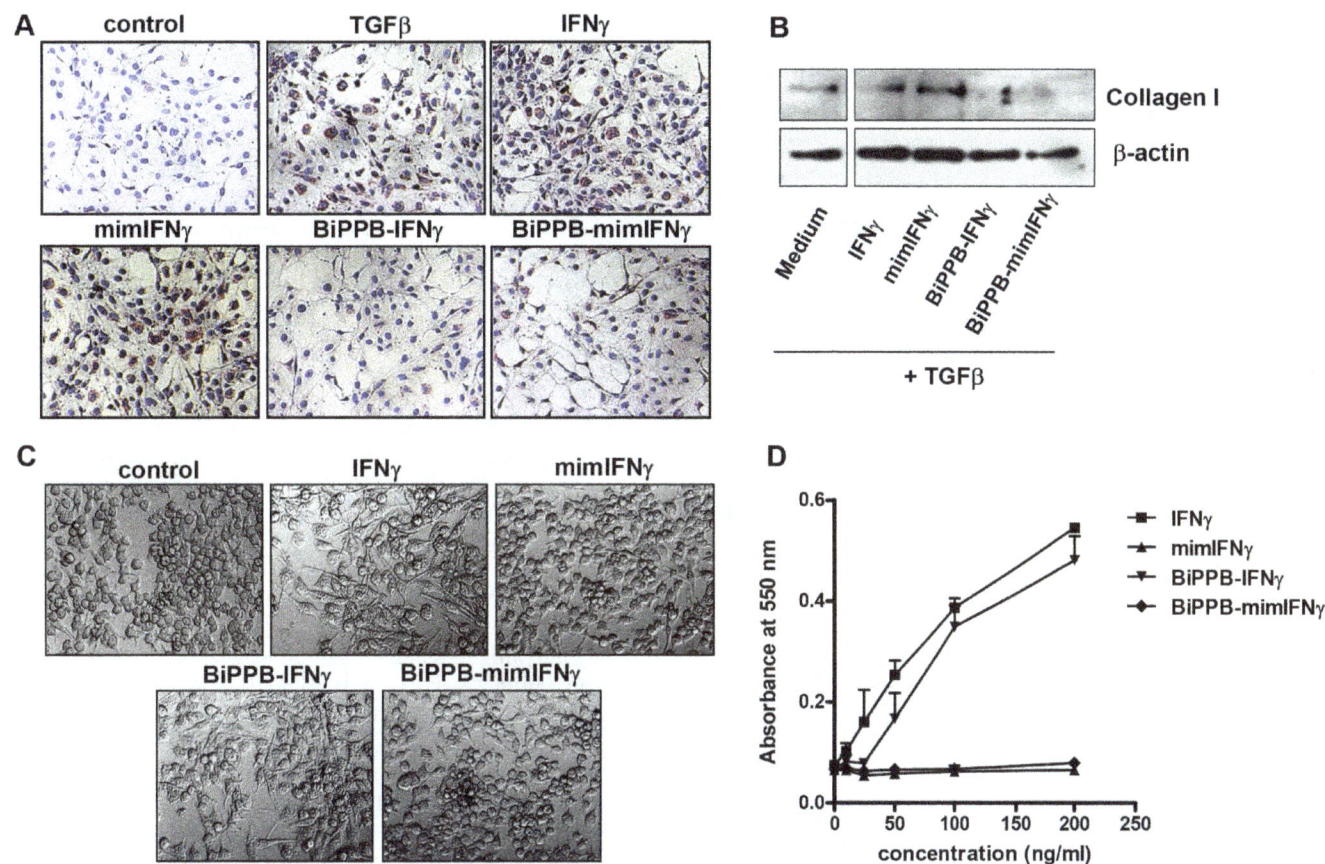

Figure 3. *In vitro* **effects of the recombinant proteins in human HSC and mouse macrophages.** Representative pictures (**A**) and western blot analysis (**B**) of collagen-I stained LX2 cells, incubated with TGFβ (5 ng/ml) in combination with different recombinant proteins (1 µg/ml). In human LX2 cells, only BiPPB-modified proteins attenuated collagen expression, whereas unmodified mouse IFNγ and mimIFNγ did not cause any reduction due to species restriction and lack of receptor binding sites respectively. (**C**) Representative microscopic photographs depicting the activation of mouse RAW macrophages after 24 h of incubation with mouse IFNγ and BiPPB-IFNγ (1 µg/ml) along with 100 ng/ml LPS. (**D**) Dose-dependent release of nitrogen oxide (NOx) in mouse RAW macrophages after incubation with unmodified IFNγ and BiPPB modified IFNγ fusion protein. MimIFNγ and BiPPB-mimIFNγ did not induce any NOx release due to absence of IFNγR binding site and/or lack of PDGFβR on RAW macrophages.

buffer, the protein was eluted with the elution buffer containing 500 mM imidazole and then dialysed against PBS buffer overnight.

Dot Blot Immunoassay

Purified proteins were applied on dehydrated PVDF membrane (Roche, Mannheim, Germany) in dot-blot apparatus (Bio-Rad, Hercules, CA, USA). The wells were then incubated with 200 µl blocking solution (1% BSA in TBS) for 1 h. After washing in TBST (0.05% tween 20 in TBS), the membrane was incubated for 1 h with either anti-IFNγ antibody (1:2000; Abcam, Cambridge, UK) or anti-PPB antibody (1:1000, custom-made, Harlan) followed by 1 h incubation with horseradish peroxidase-labeled secondary antibody. The membrane was washed again with TBST subsequent with incubation in substrate solution (0.06% diamino-benzidine (DAB), 0.08% hydrogen peroxide in TBS) for color development. The membranes were finally rinsed in distilled water and air-dried.

In vitro Binding of Recombinant Proteins in Human HSC (LX2 Cells)

Cells (30,000 cells/well) were seeded in 24-well culture plates (Becton Dickinson, Heidelberg, Germany) and grown overnight at

37°C/5%CO₂. Then, cells were incubated with IFNγ, mimIFNγ, BiPPB-IFNγ or BiPPB-mimIFNγ (1 µg/ml) for 2 h. Thereafter, cells were fixed and stained using anti-PPB antibody.

In vitro Effects of Recombinant Proteins in Human HSC

Cells were plated in 24 well (30,000 cells/well) and 12 well (75,000 cells/well) culture plates, grown overnight and were starved with 0.5% containing medium for 24 h. Starved cells were then incubated with medium alone, recombinant IFNγ, mimIFNγ, BiPPB-IFNγ or BiPPB-mimIFNγ (equivalent to 1 µg/ml) plus 5 ng/ml of human recombinant TGFβ1 (Roche) for 48 h. Subsequently, cells (24 well plates) were fixed and stained for collagen I (1:100, Southern Biotech, Birmingham, AL). In addition, cells (12 well plates) were lysed with 5x SDS-PAGE sample buffer constituted with β-mercaptoethanol (Stratagene, La Jolla, CA) to perform western blot analysis for collagen I (1:250; Southern Biotech) and β-actin (house-keeping gene) as per standard protocols.

Nitric Oxide (NO) Release Bioassay in Mouse RAW Macrophages

The biological activity of recombinant proteins were assessed by measuring the accumulation of nitrite NO2, a stable nitric oxide

pSTAT1α

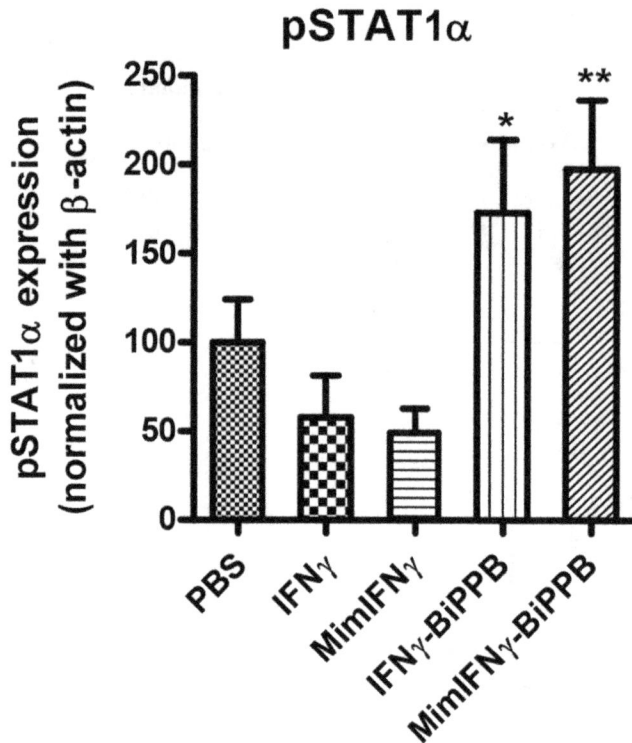

Figure 4. *In vivo* activation of IFNγ pSTAT1α signaling pathway by recombinant proteins. Western blot analysis of pSTAT1α after 24 h post intravenous administration of IFNγ (n = 6), MimIFNγ (n = 5), BiPPB-IFNγ (n = 6), BiPPB-mimIFNγ (n = 6) or PBS alone (n = 6). The graph shows significant increase in activation of pSTAT1α with HSC-targeted fusion proteins (BiPPB-IFNγ, BiPPB-mimIFNγ). Bars represent mean ± SEM of 5–6 mice per group. *P<0.05 and **P<0.01 versus PBS treated CCl4 mice. The groups were normalized to CCl4 group (treated with PBS).

(NO) metabolite produced by RAW macrophages as described previously [27]. Briefly, cells (1×10^5 cells/200 µl/well) were seeded in 96-well plates and grown overnight at 37°C/5%CO2. Then cells were incubated with either medium alone or recombinant proteins at different concentrations (10, 25, 50, 100 and 200 ng/ml) together with 100 ng/ml lipopolysaccharides (LPS from E. coli 055:B5, Sigma). After 24 h, the secreted nitrite was measured using Griess reagent (1% sulfanilamide; 0.1% naphthylethylendia-mine dihydrochloride; 3% H3PO4). The absorbance was determined at 550 nm using an ELISA plate reader.

Animal Experiments: Ethics Statement

All the animal experiments were performed in strict accordance with the guidelines and regulations for the Care and Use of Laboratory Animals, University of Groningen, The Netherlands. The protocols were approved by the Institutional Animal Ethics Committee of the University of Groningen, The Netherlands (Permit Number 5429A). Male 6- to 8-week old C57BL/6 mice were purchased from Harlan (Zeist, Netherlands) and kept at 12 h light/12 h dark cycles with ad libitum normal diet.

CCl4-induced Acute Liver Fibrogenesis Model in Mice

Acute liver injury was induced in male C57BL/6 mice by a single intra-peritoneal injection of carbon tetrachloride (CCl4; 1 ml/kg prepared in olive oil) at day 1. At day 2 and day 3, mice received intravenous injections of IFNγ (n = 6), mimIFNγ (n = 5),

BiPPB-IFNγ (n = 6), BiPPB-mimIFNγ (n = 6) (equivalent to 5 µg IFNγ/mouse/day) or PBS alone. At day 4, all mice were sacrificed under deep anesthesia by cervical dislocation; blood and livers were collected for subsequent measurements.

In vivo IFNγ (pSTAT1α) Signaling Pathway

The IFNγ signaling pathway was analyzed in the acute liver fibrogenesis model in mice after 24 h of administration with IFNγ (n = 6), mimIFNγ (n = 5), BiPPB-IFNγ (n = 6), BiPPB-mimIFNγ (n = 6) (equivalent to 5 µg IFNγ/mouse/day) or PBS alone. Liver tissues samples were homogenized in cold RIPA buffer (50 mM Tris-HCl, 150 mM NaCl, 0.1% SDS, 0.1% Igepal in 0.5% sodium deoxycholate, 1 tablet of protease inhibitor cocktail and 1 tablet of phosphatase inhibitor in 10 ml) on ice using a tissue homogenizer and the lysates were centrifuged at 12,000 rpm for 1 h at 4°C. 20 µg of protein was used for western blot analysis performed as per standard protocols using anti-pSTAT1α antibody (1:1000; cell signaling, Beverly, MA) or anti-β-actin antibody (1:5000; Sigma).

Immunohistochemistry and Immunofluorescence

The cells were fixed with acetone:methanol (1:1), dried and stored until immunostaining. Livers were harvested and transferred to Tissue-Tek OCT embedding medium, and snap frozen in isopentane chilled in a dry ice. Cryosections (4 µm) were cut using a Leica CM 3050 cryostat (Leica Microsystems, Nussloch, Germany). The sections were allowed to adhere to Superfrost microscopic glass slides (Menzel-Gläser, Braunschweig, Germany), air-dried and fixed with acetone for 10 min. Cells or tissue sections were rehydrated with PBS and incubated with the collagen I antibody (1:100; Southern Biotech), α-SMA antibody (1:600, Sigma) or PPB (1:100; custom-made, Harlan) for 1 h. Thereafter, cells or sections were washed thrice with PBS and incubated with horseradish peroxidase (HRP)-conjugated secondary antibody for 30 min. Cells or sections were washed again and further incubated with HRP-conjugated tertiary antibody for 30 min. Thereafter, peroxidase activity was developed with 3-amino-9-ethyl carbazole (Sigma, St. Louis,MO) for 20 min and nuclei were counterstained with hematoxylin (Fluka Chemie, Buchs, Switzerland). Cells or sections were then mounted with Kaiser's gelatin (Darmstadt, Germany), visualized and photographed using a light microscope (Olympus UK Ltd., Essex, UK).

Quantitative Real-time PCR

Total RNA from liver tissues was isolated using RNeasy mini kit (Qiagen, Hilden, Germany) according to manufacturer's instructions. RNA concentrations were quantitated by a Nanodrop UV spectrophotometer (NanoDrop Technologies, Wilmington, DE). Total RNA (1.6 µg) was reverse transcribed in a volume of 50 µl using cDNA synthesis kit (Promega, Madison, WI). All primers were purchased from Sigma-Genosys (Haverhill, UK). Following primers were used, MMP13 forward: CCAGAACTTCCCAAC-CATGT; MMP13 reverse: GTCTTCCCCGTGTTCTCAAA; TIMP1 forward: ATCAGTGCCTGCAGCTTCTT; TIMP1 reverse: TGACGGCTCTGGTAGTCCTC; GAPDH forward: ACAGTCCATGCCATCACTGC; GAPDH reverse: GATC-CACGACGGACACATTG. The reactions were performed with 20 ng cDNA using SYBR green PCR master mix (Applied Biosystems, Foster City, CA) according to manufacturer's instructions and were analyzed by ABI7900HT sequence detection system (Applied Biosystems). Finally, the threshold cycles (Ct) were calculated and relative gene expression was normalized with GAPDH (for mouse) as housekeeping gene.

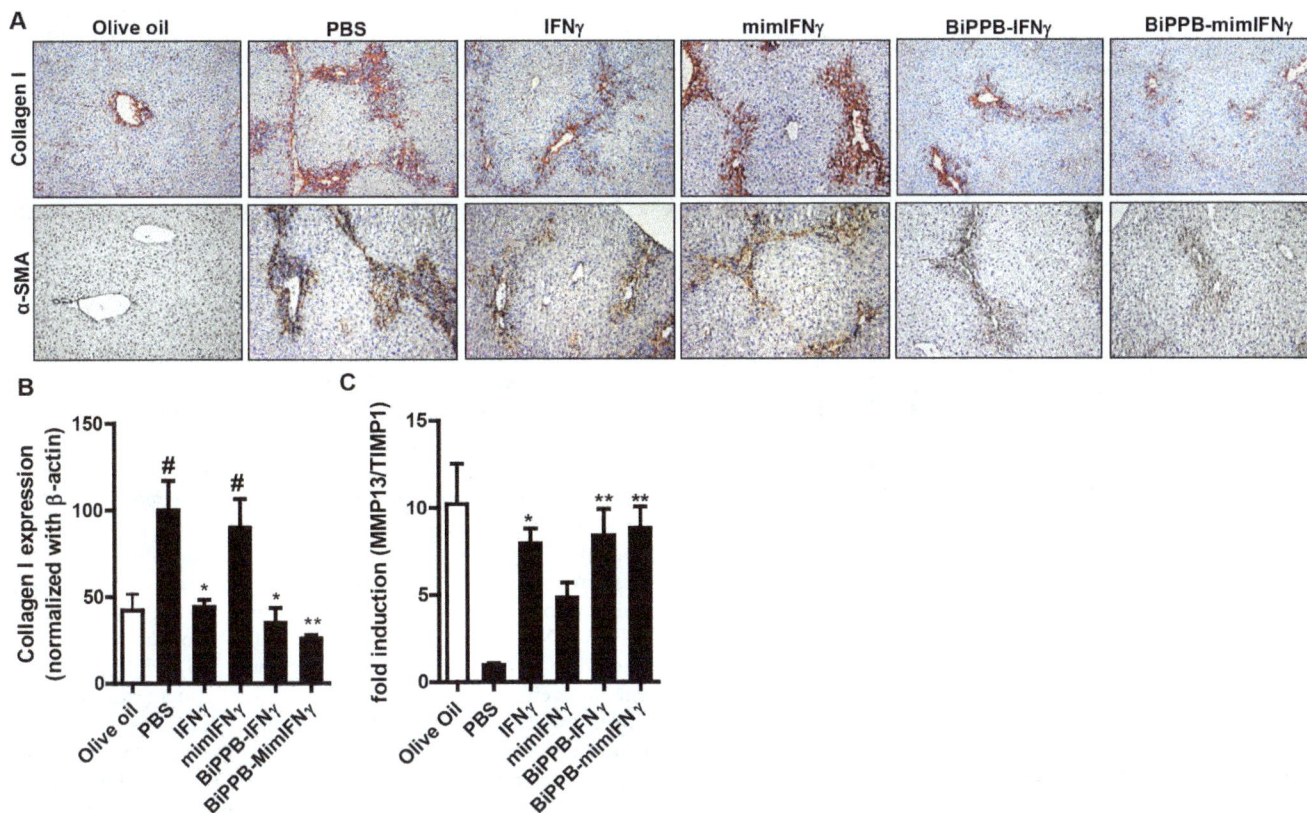

Figure 5. Effects of recombinant proteins on fibrotic parameters in vivo. (A) Representative pictures of collagen I and α-SMA stained liver sections from olive oil treated mice (normal) or CCl₄-treated mice (acute model) that were treated with IFNγ (n = 6), MimIFNγ (n = 5), BiPPB-IFNγ (n = 6), BiPPB-mimIFNγ (n = 6) or PBS alone (n = 6). Scale bars, 200 μm. **(B)** Whole-liver lysates from treated animals were subjected to western blot analysis using anti-collagen I antibody. Graph represents collagen I expression (normalized with β-actin) depicted as mean ± SEM from n = 5–6 mice per group. #P<0.05 denotes significance versus PBS treated olive oil mice and *P<0.05, **P<0.01 denotes significance versus PBS treated-CCl₄ mice. For quantitative analysis, the groups were normalized to vehicle group (PBS treated-CCl₄ mice). **(C)** Effect of recombinant proteins on intrahepatic fibrinolysis as determined by the ratio of MMP13 and TIMP-1 transcripts. The groups were normalized to vehicle group (PBS treated-CCl₄ mice). Bars represent mean ± SEM of 5–6 mice per group. *P<0.05, **P<0.01 denotes significance versus PBS treated-CCl₄ mice.

Statistical Analyses

Data are presented as mean ± standard error mean (SEM). Multiple comparisons between different groups were performed by one-way ANOVA with Bonferroni post-test using GraphPad Prism version 5.02 (GraphPad Prism Software, Inc., La Jolla, CA, USA).

Results

Construction and Expression of Recombinant Proteins

We synthesized four recombinant proteins: IFNγ, mimetic IFNγ (mimIFNγ), BiPPB-IFNγ and BiPPB-mimetic IFNγ (BiPPB-mimIFNγ) (**Figure 1**). IFNγ and mimetic IFNγ were expressed using pET42a derived bacterial expression vector to achieve cytoplasmic expression of the proteins (**Figure 1A, 1B and Figure S1, S2**). While, BiPPB-IFNγ and BiPPB-mimIFNγ fusion proteins were expressed using pET39b (+) expression vector (**Figure 1C, 1D and Figure S4, S5**) to yield periplasmic expression, required for their proper folding. DNA constructs were extensively analysed for the presence of inserts using specific restriction enzyme digestions and by automated DNA sequencing. Thereafter, constructs were transformed into *E. coli* strain BL21 (DE3) and protein expression was induced by 1 mM IPTG. Proteins of interest with the expected molecular weight were found in total cell pellets. Soluble proteins were purified from the

supernatant of lysed bacterial pellets through Ni-NTA affinity columns. Purified proteins were further dialysed against PBS and concentrated by ultrafiltration. The presence of IFNγ moieties or/ and PPB peptides in the prepared fusion proteins was confirmed in dot blots using anti-IFNγ and anti-PPB antibodies (**Figure 2A**).

In vitro Binding of Recombinant Proteins in Human HSC

The binding of IFNγ to its receptor is strictly species-specific, whereas PDGFβR binding is not. In order to demonstrate PDGFβR-specific binding of BiPPB containing fusion proteins, we used human LX2 hepatic stellate cells that are known to express PDGFβR. The results confirmed the species specificity of IFNγ; mouse IFNγ and mimetic IFNγ (lacking extracellular IFNγR binding site) did not show any binding to human HSC (**Figure 2B**). However, BiPPB-fused mouse IFNγ or mimetic IFNγ proteins showed high binding to human cells (**Figure 2B**).

In vitro Effects of Recombinant Proteins in Human HSC and Mouse Macrophages

Following the binding studies, we investigated the anti-fibrotic effects of the recombinant proteins in human HSC after their activation with TGFβ. In corroboration with the binding studies in human LX2 cells, TGFβ-induced collagen expression was strongly inhibited by treatment with the PDGFR-specific BiPPB-IFNγ and

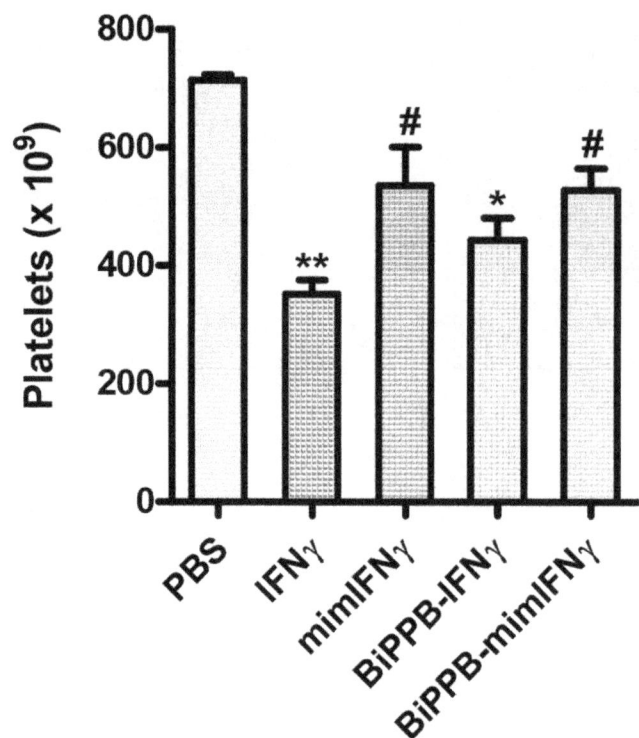

Figure 6. Effects of recombinant proteins on IFNγ-related adverse effect in the acute CCl₄ model. Graph represents platelet counts measured in CCl₄-treated mice receiving PBS (n = 6) or the different recombinant proteins IFNγ (n = 6), MimIFNγ (n = 5), BiPPB-IFNγ (n = 6), BiPPB-mimIFNγ (n = 6). Bars represent mean ± SEM of 5–6 mice per group. The results showed a significant reduction in platelet counts following two intravenous administration of IFNγ, which was significantly improved following treatment with BiPPB-mimIFNγ and to a lesser extent with BiPPB-IFNγ. MimIFNγ did not show significant change in platelets counts due to lack of binding to IFNγR or PDGFβR. *P<0.05, **P<0.01 denotes significance versus PBS treated CCl₄ mice. #P<0.05 denotes the significance versus IFNγ-treated CCl₄ mice.

-mimIFNγ fusion proteins (**Figure 3A, 3B**) as analyzed by immunostaining and western blot analysis. While both mouse IFNγ and mimIFNγ did not induce any effect in human cells due to species differences and the absence of a receptor-binding site respectively. On the other hand, mouse IFNγ and BiPPB-IFNγ strongly potentiated LPS-induced activation and dose-dependent release of nitric oxide in mouse RAW macrophages due to presence of mouse IFNγR (**Figure 3C, 3D**). However, mimIFNγ lacking the IFNγR binding site and mimIFNγ-BiPPB directed to PDGFβR did not induce any effect due to lack of PDGFβR expression on macrophages (**Figure 3C, 3D**).

In vivo Liver Uptake of BiPPB-modified Fusion Proteins in Acute CCl₄-induced Liver Fibrosis in Mice

Others and we have earlier demonstrated that PDGFβR is highly upregulated on activated HSC during acute and advanced liver fibrosis [20,21]. Our group has extensively studied the bio-distribution of proteins modified with PDGFβR-recognizing cyclic peptides (PPB), using radiolabeled and imaging studies, and showed high distribution of PPB-modified proteins to PDGFβR-expressing hepatic stellate cells in fibrotic livers [23]. In the present study, we assessed the intracellular activation of the pSTAT1α signaling pathway after 24 h of IFNγ, mimIFNγ, BiPPB-IFNγ and BiPPB-mimIFNγ administration in CCl₄-induced liver fibrosis in

mice. We found a significant increase in pSTAT1α activation after 24 h of treatment with BiPPB-IFNγ (p<0.05) and BiPPB-mimIFNγ (p<0.01) compared to PBS, IFNγ and mimIFNγ treatments indicating enhanced liver uptake of the fusion proteins due to high PDGFβR expression on activated HSC in the fibrotic livers (**Figure 4 and Figure S6**).

In vivo Effects of BiPPB-modified Fusion Proteins in Acute CCl₄-induced Liver Fibrosis Model in Mice

A single CCl₄ administration induced acute liver injury in mice, characterized by an increased intrahepatic expression of HSC activation marker (α-smooth muscle actin) and an increased deposition of extracellular matrix molecule (collagen I) as shown in **Figure 5A–5C**. IFNγ, mimIFNγ, BiPPB-IFNγ and BiPPB-mimIFNγ proteins were examined for their anti-fibrotic effects in this experimental model in mice. After two intravenous injections, a strong reduction in collagen I expression was observed with IFNγ (≈45% reduction, p<0.05), HSC-targeted BiPPB-IFNγ (≈50% reduction, p<0.05) and BiPPB-mimIFNγ (≈60% reduction, p<0.01) as analyzed by immunostaining and quantitative western blot analysis (**Figure 5A, 5B and Figure S7**). Furthermore, α-SMA expression was attenuated by HSC-targeted BiPPB-IFNγ administration and more strongly by BiPPB-mimIFNγ treatment as shown in **Figure 5A,** while IFNγ had only little effect and mimIFNγ did not induce any reduction in α-SMA expression levels (**Figure 5A**). Apart from collagen expression and deposition, the balance between collagen degrading matrix metalloproteinases-13 (MMP-13) and their major endogenous inhibitor, tissue inhibitor of metalloproteinases-1 (TIMP-1), is an important determinant of progression or reversal of fibrosis [28,29]. A significant increase in MMP13/TIMP1 transcript ratio was observed after treatment with IFNγ (p<0.05), BiPPB-IFNγ (p<0.01) and BiPPB-mimIFNγ (p<0.01) suggesting activation of fibrolysis and induction of reversal of fibrosis (**Figure 5C**). Of note, no effect was observed with mimetic IFNγ alone due to lack of an IFNγR binding site while the inhibitory effects of HSC-targeted BiPPB-modified fusion proteins on collagen deposition were higher compared to non-targeted IFNγ (**Figure 5**).

The main hurdles in IFNγ-based therapies are the adverse effects that led to the failure of clinical trials. IFN-mediated reduction in blood platelets is clinically relevant and a well-known side effect [30]. Indeed, we observed a significant reduction in the platelet counts following two intravenous treatments with IFNγ (p<0.001), which was significantly improved following treatment with BiPPB-mimIFNγ and to a lesser extent with BiPPB-IFNγ (**Figure 6**). MimIFNγ did not induce a significant change in platelets counts due to lack of binding to IFNγR or PDGFβR.

Discussion

Hepatocellular damage, hepatic inflammatory cell infiltration and extensive tissue remodeling ultimately culminate into the development of progressive fibrosis and cirrhosis [31]. During liver fibrosis, the interplay between growth factors and cytokines produced by the damaged hepatocytes; inflammatory cells and non-parenchymal cells activate quiescent hepatic stellate cells (HSC). These activated HSC in turn proliferate and accumulate in the injured liver producing large amounts of extracellular matrix proteins [32]. Therefore, therapeutic approaches to silence these activated HSC would be appropriate to inhibit or reverse liver fibrosis [12].

Fibrosis is an heterogeneous process e.g. CCl₄ intoxication results in hepatocyte damage, necrosis, inflammation, and fibrosis, leading to portal fibrosis or cirrhosis. While bile duct ligation (BDL) stimulates the proliferation of biliary epithelial cells and oval cells, resulting in proliferating bile ductules accompanied by portal inflammation leading to biliary cirrhosis (PBC). As documented in fibrotic animal models (BDL or CCL₄ etc.) and diseased human livers, PDGFβR is expressed abundantly on activated HSC or portal fibroblasts (collectively referred as myofibroblasts-like cells) [21,22]. The expression was found to be very weak in normal healthy tissues or cells (pericytes or smooth muscle cells) relative to expression levels in the fibrotic livers, which motivated us to examine the potential of using PDGFβR for a targeted delivery of anti-fibrotic or apoptotic drugs to the fibrotic livers [12]. In the present study, we have directed IFNγ or mimetic IFNγ (signaling moiety of IFNγ lacking extracellular IFNγR binding site while retaining activities of IFNγ) [33] to PDGFβR-expressing activated HSC using bicyclic PDGFβR peptides to inhibit liver fibrosis with reduced adverse effects.

IFNγ or mimetic IFNγ modified with bicyclic PDGFβR-recognizing peptide were generated via recombinant technology in E.coli. Unmodified IFNγ or mimetic IFNγ were also produced in parallel to serve as respective controls. BiPPB-IFNγ and BiPPB-mimIFNγ were produced from a periplasmic vector (pET39b), since this vector contains the DsbA tag that exports the expressed proteins to the periplasmic space (space between plasma membrane and outer membrane). DsbA, periplasmic enzyme catalyzes the sequential formation of disulfide bonds therefore favors proper folding of the fusion proteins containing bicyclic peptide (cyclized via bisulfide bonds) at the N-terminus of IFNγ and mimetic IFNγ. Unmodified IFNγ and mimetic IFNγ were produced using pET42a vector as cytoplasmic proteins. These proteins were expressed, purified and analyzed using immune dot-blots where the presence of IFNγ, mimIFNγ, BiPPB-IFNγ and BiPPB-mimIFNγ was confirmed using anti-IFNγ and anti-PPB antibodies.

The BiPPB-modified proteins were investigated for PDGFβR-specific binding in human HSC. BiPPB-IFNγ and BiPPB-mimIFNγ showed specific binding to PDGFβR-expressing human LX2 cells whereas unmodified mouse derived IFNγ and mimIFNγ did not show binding to these human cells due to species restrictive interaction of mouse IFNγ to mouse IFNγR, while PDGFβR interaction is not species-specific. BiPPB-IFNγ and BiPPB-mimIFNγ also induced a strong reduction in TGFβ-induced collagen I expression in human LX2 cells while IFNγ and mimIFNγ did not affect the collagen expression in these cells corroborating with the binding studies. We did not observe any difference in α-SMA expression in vitro after 48 hrs of treatment (data not shown) while significant reduction is observed in collagen expression (**Figure 3A, 3B**), since IFNγ has shown to have direct effect on collagen expression by directly acting on C/EBPbeta signaling pathway [34] while longer treatments might lead to inhibitory effects on α-SMA expression. These studies clearly demonstrate that directing IFNγ or mimetic IFNγ to the accessory PDGFβR can transform mouse (whose activity is restricted to mouse cells) and mim-IFNγ (unable to enter any cell), into highly active proteins in human LX2 cells. On the other hand, we studied effect of these recombinant proteins in mouse macrophages expressing IFNγR and lacking PDGFβR. Results showed that IFNγ or BiPPB-modified IFNγ containing IFNγR binding site activated mouse RAW cells and induced NO release while both mimIFNγ (lacking IFNγR binding site) or BiPPB-modified mimIFNγ (containing PDGFβR binding site and lacking IFNγR binding site) did not show any effect in macrophages. These results indicate that targeted mimIFNγ will not influence cell types (especially macrophages which are known to be highly influenced

by IFNγ) other than PDGFβR-expressing cells and therefore will not induce adverse effects in other normal cells or tissues.

In the past years, our group has extensively demonstrated the higher liver accumulation and HSC-specific distribution of PPB-modified proteins [35]. Here we examined the intra-hepatic activation of IFNγ signaling pathway in vivo in treated livers to assess the increased accumulation of our targeted proteins in fibrotic livers. IFNγ internalization results in the activation of the JAK–STAT pathway and subsequent phosphorylation of signal transducers and activators of transcription (STAT1) that binds to unique gamma-activated sequence (GAS) regulating IFNγ-responsive genes [36]. Both BiPPB-modified IFNγ and mimIFNγ induced a significant increase in intrahepatic pSTAT1α signalling compared to unmodified IFNγ and mimiFNγ implicating increased liver accumulation of targeted proteins.

Thereafter, we studied the anti-fibrotic effects of recombinant proteins in the CCl₄-induced liver fibrogenesis model in mice. This model is associated with HSC activation, enhanced PDGFR expression and ECM deposition, the key parameters of fibrogenesis. Two subsequent intravenous injections of IFNγ, BiPPB-IFNγ or BiPPB-mimIFNγ led to the highly significant reduction in collagen I expression (major extracellular matrix protein) and α-SMA (HSC activation marker) expression. Additionally, IFNγ, BiPPB-IFNγ and BiPPB-mimIFNγ enhanced the MMP13/TIMP1 transcripts ratio implying activation of fibrolysis. In this study, we observed anti-fibrotic effects with IFNγ in comparison with our previously reported studies [20,23], is attributed to the increased dose (5 μg) used here, as compared to 2.5 μg dose used earlier. MimIFNγ that cannot be internalized due to lack of receptor binding sites did not show any effect on these fibrotic PPB-modified proteins can block the PDGFβR in vitro [35,37] and this might also account for the observed antifibrotic effects. However, previous studies with PPB-peptides coupled to albumin have shown that this effect does not occur in vivo at the doses used [20,23]. To further reinforce this hypothesis, we used synthetic BiPPB as a control but did not observed any effect on the fibrotic parameters (data not shown).

Liver fibrosis or cirrhosis is a slowly progressing disease that develops over many years, therefore patients are treated for longer periods to cure or reverse the disease. Therefore, therapies with improved therapeutic efficacy and preferably without provoking off-target systemic effects would be highly favourable. In clinical trials with IFNγ, patients suffered from mild to severe adverse effects; therefore we investigated one of the well-known IFN-mediated adverse effects, significant reduction in circulating blood platelets (mainly produced by bone marrow) can lead to fatal disorders and also found to be associated with the serotonin levels associated to depression [30]. We found that only two intravenous injections of IFNγ led to a highly significant reduction in platelet counts (p<0.001) in comparison to PBS-treated mice. Furthermore, BiPPB-IFNγ that can still interact with IFNγR receptor showed a slight reduction in platelet counts (p<0.05), but mimIFNγ (without receptor binding sites) and BiPPB-mimIFNγ (only specific to PDGFβR) did not induce a reduction in platelet counts. Further studies in long-term fibrotic models are important to examine the adverse effects of targeted constructs due to the long-term administration. Since platelets are produced by bone marrow, it is also important to study the effect of these constructs on the bone marrow as these effects may influence other crucial biological processes.

In conclusion, the results in this paper clearly demonstrate that HSC-targeted mimIFNγ is capable of accumulating in PDGFβR-expressing fibrotic livers and exerting an inhibitory effect on fibrotic parameters, which makes this recombinant protein a highly attractive candidate to explore for the treatment of liver fibrosis. The recombinant synthesis of this chimeric compound will facilitate further translational research with this compound.

Supporting Information

Figure S1   Schematic representation depicting cloning strategy for preparation of pET42a-IFNγ. PCR amplified and EcoRI digested mouse IFNγ gene fragment was cloned in pET42a (+) prokaryotic vector at Psh A1/Eco RI site.

Figure S2   Schematic representation depicting cloning strategy for preparation of pET42a-mimIFNγ. PCR amplified and EcoRI digested mouse mimetic IFNγ gene fragment was cloned in pET42a (+) prokaryotic vector at Psh A1/Eco RI site.

Figure S3   Schematic representation depicting cloning strategy for preparation of pET39b-BiPPB. BiPPB was prepared by annealing and PCR extension of 2 sets of primers (refer to methods), which were linked together via Bam HI site and cloned in Sca I/Not I digested pET39b (+) prokaryotic vector.

Figure S4   Schematic representation depicting cloning strategy for preparation of pET39b-BiPPB-IFNγ. PCR amplified IFNγ prepared for fusion with BiPPB was digested with Not I/Xho I was cloned in pET39b vector at Not I/Xho I site. The resultant recombinant vector termed as pET39b-BiPPB-IFNγ encodes for BiPPB and IFNγ plus a three amino-acid linker (AAA) between them.

References

1. Bonnem EM, Oldham RK (1987) Gamma-interferon: physiology and speculation on its role in medicine. JBiolResponse Mod 6: 275–301.
2. Borden EC, Sen GC, Uze G, Silverman RH, Ransohoff RM, et al. (2007) Interferons at age 50: past, current and future impact on biomedicine. NatRevDrug Discov 6: 975–990.
3. Bouros D, Antoniou KM, Tzouvelekis A, Siafakas NM (2006) Interferon-gamma 1b for the treatment of idiopathic pulmonary fibrosis. ExpertOpinBiolTher 6: 1051–1060.
4. King TE, Jr., Albera C, Bradford WZ, Costabel U, Hormel P, et al. (2009) Effect of interferon gamma-1b on survival in patients with idiopathic pulmonary fibrosis (INSPIRE): a multicentre, randomised, placebo-controlled trial. Lancet 374: 222–228.
5. Knight B, Lim R, Yeoh GC, Olynyk JK (2007) Interferon-gamma exacerbates liver damage, the hepatic progenitor cell response and fibrosis in a mouse model of chronic liver injury. JHepatol 47: 826–833.
6. Oldroyd SD, Thomas GL, Gabbiani G, El Nahas AM (1999) Interferon-gamma inhibits experimental renal fibrosis. Kidney Int 56: 2116–2127.
7. Miller CH, Maher SG, Young HA (2009) Clinical Use of Interferon-gamma. AnnNYAcadSci 1182: 69–79.
8. Pockros PJ, Jeffers L, Afdhal N, Goodman ZD, Nelson D, et al. (2007) Final results of a double-blind, placebo-controlled trial of the antifibrotic efficacy of interferon-gamma1b in chronic hepatitis C patients with advanced fibrosis or cirrhosis. Hepatology 45: 569–578.
9. Bansal R, Post E, Proost JH, de Jager-Krikken A, Poelstra K, et al. (2011) PEGylation improves pharmacokinetic profile, liver uptake and efficacy of Interferon gamma in liver fibrosis. Journal of controlled release: official journal of the Controlled Release Society 154: 233–240.
10. Cleland JL, Jones AJ (1996) Stable formulations of recombinant human growth hormone and interferon-gamma for microencapsulation in biodegradable microspheres. PharmRes 13: 1464–1475.
11. Gu F, Younes HM, El-Kadi AO, Neufeld RJ, Amsden BG (2005) Sustained interferon-gamma delivery from a photocrosslinked biodegradable elastomer. JControl Release 102: 607–617.
12. Poelstra K, Schuppan D (2011) Targeted therapy of liver fibrosis/cirrhosis and its complications. Journal of hepatology 55: 726–728.
13. Friedman SL (2008) Hepatic fibrosis – overview. Toxicology 254: 120–129.
14. Guo J, Friedman SL (2007) Hepatic fibrogenesis. SeminLiver Dis 27: 413–426.

Figure S5   Schematic representation depicting cloning strategy for preparation of pET39b-BiPPB-mimIFNγ. PCR amplified mimIFNγ prepared for fusion with BiPPB was digested with Not I/Xho I was cloned in pET39b vector at Not I/Xho I site. The resultant recombinant vector termed as pET39b-BiPPB-mimIFNγ encodes for BiPPB and mimIFNγ plus a three amino-acid linker (AAA) between them.

Figure S6   *In vivo* activation of IFNγ pSTAT1α signaling pathway by recombinant proteins. Representative western blot images of pSTAT1α (upper panel) and β-actin (house-keeping protein, lower panel) after 24 h post intravenous administration of IFNγ (n = 6), MimIFNγ (n = 5), BiPPB-IFNγ (n = 6), BiPPB-mimIFNγ (n = 6) or PBS alone (n = 6). Figure shows the significant increase in activation of pSTAT1α with HSC-targeted fusion proteins (BiPPB-IFNγ, BiPPB-mimIFNγ).

Figure S7   Effects of recombinant proteins on fibrotic parameters in vivo. Representative western blot images of collagen I (upper panel) and β-actin (house-keeping protein, lower panel) from CCl$_4$-treated mice (acute model) that were treated with IFNγ (n = 6), MimIFNγ (n = 5), BiPPB-IFNγ (n = 6), BiPPB-mimIFNγ (n = 6) or PBS alone (n = 6). Figure shows the significant reduction in collagen expression after treatment with HSC-targeted fusion proteins (BiPPB-IFNγ, BiPPB-mimIFNγ).

Author Contributions

Conceived and designed the experiments: RB JP KP. Performed the experiments: RB MDR. Analyzed the data: RB JP. Wrote the paper: RB JP KP.

15. Gressner OA, Weiskirchen R, Gressner AM (2007) Evolving concepts of liver fibrogenesis provide new diagnostic and therapeutic options. Comp Hepatol 6: 7.
16. Popov Y, Schuppan D (2009) Targeting liver fibrosis: strategies for development and validation of antifibrotic therapies. Hepatology 50: 1294–1306.
17. Friedman SL (2004) Stellate cells: a moving target in hepatic fibrogenesis. Hepatology 40: 1041–1043.
18. Friedman SL (2008) Hepatic stellate cells: protean, multifunctional, and enigmatic cells of the liver. Physiol Rev 88: 125–172.
19. Baroni GS, D'Ambrosio L, Curto P, Casini A, Mancini R, et al. (1996) Interferon gamma decreases hepatic stellate cell activation and extracellular matrix deposition in rat liver fibrosis. Hepatology 23: 1189–1199.
20. Bansal R, Prakash J, Post E, Beljaars L, Schuppan D, et al. (2011) Novel engineered targeted interferon-gamma blocks hepatic fibrogenesis in mice. Hepatology 54: 586–596.
21. Borkham-Kamphorst E, Kovalenko E, van Roeyen CR, Gassler N, Bomble M, et al. (2008) Platelet-derived growth factor isoform expression in carbon tetrachloride-induced chronic liver injury. Lab Invest 88: 1090–1100.
22. Wong L, Yamasaki G, Johnson RJ, Friedman SL (1994) Induction of beta-platelet-derived growth factor receptor in rat hepatic lipocytes during cellular activation in vivo and in culture. JClinInvest 94: 1563–1569.
23. Bansal R, Prakash J, Ruijter M, Beljaars L, Poelstra K (2011) Peptide-modified albumin carrier explored as a novel strategy for a cell-specific delivery of interferon gamma to treat liver fibrosis. Molecular pharmaceutics 8: 1899–1909.
24. Johnson HM, Ahmed CM (2006) Gamma interferon signaling: insights to development of interferon mimetics. Cell MolBiol 52: 71–76.
25. Subramaniam PS, Flowers LO, Haider SM, Johnson HM (2004) Signal transduction mechanism of a peptide mimetic of interferon-gamma. Biochemistry 43: 5445–5454.
26. Xu L, Hui AY, Albanis E, Arthur MJ, O'Byrne SM, et al. (2005) Human hepatic stellate cell lines, LX-1 and LX-2: new tools for analysis of hepatic fibrosis. Gut 54: 142–151.
27. Kim YM, Son K (1996) A nitric oxide production bioassay for interferon-gamma. JImmunolMethods 198: 203–209.
28. Arthur MJ (2000) Fibrogenesis II. Metalloproteinases and their inhibitors in liver fibrosis. AmJPhysiol GastrointestLiver Physiol 279: G245–G249.
29. Benyon RC, Arthur MJ (2001) Extracellular matrix degradation and the role of hepatic stellate cells. SeminLiver Dis 21: 373–384.

30. Schafer A, Scheurlen M, Seufert J, Keicher C, Weissbrich B, et al. (2010) Platelet serotonin (5-HT) levels in interferon-treated patients with hepatitis C and its possible association with interferon-induced depression. JHepatol 52: 10–15.

31. Bataller R, Brenner DA (2005) Liver fibrosis. JClinInvest 115: 209–218.

32. Schuppan D, Afdhal NH (2008) Liver cirrhosis. Lancet 371: 838–851.

33. Ahmed CM, Burkhart MA, Mujtaba MG, Subramaniam PS, Johnson HM (2003) The role of IFNgamma nuclear localization sequence in intracellular function. JCell Sci 116: 3089–3098.

34. Ghosh AK, Bhattacharyya S, Mori Y, Varga J (2006) Inhibition of collagen gene expression by interferon-gamma: novel role of the CCAAT/enhancer binding protein beta (C/EBPbeta). J Cell Physiol 207: 251–260.

35. Beljaars L, Weert B, Geerts A, Meijer DK, Poelstra K (2003) The preferential homing of a platelet derived growth factor receptor-recognizing macromolecule to fibroblast-like cells in fibrotic tissue. BiochemPharmacol 66: 1307–1317.

36. Farrar MA, Schreiber RD (1993) The molecular cell biology of interferon-gamma and its receptor. AnnuRevImmunol 11: 571–611.

37. Beljaars L, Molema G, Schuppan D, Geerts A, De Bleser PJ, et al. (2000) Successful targeting to rat hepatic stellate cells using albumin modified with cyclic peptides that recognize the collagen type VI receptor. The Journal of biological chemistry 275: 12743–12751.

19

Predictive Value of Liver Enzymes and Inflammatory Biomarkers for the Severity of Liver Fibrosis Stage in HIV/HCV Co-Infected Patients

Charlotte Charpentier[1]*, **Karen Champenois**[2], **Anne Gervais**[3], **Roland Landman**[3], **Véronique Joly**[3], **Sylvie Le Gac**[3], **Lucile Larrouy**[1], **Florence Damond**[1], **Françoise Brun-Vézinet**[1], **Diane Descamps**[1], **Yazdan Yazdanpanah**[3]

1 Laboratoire de Virologie, Assistance Publique-Hôpitaux de Paris (AP-HP), Groupe Hospitalier Bichat-Claude Bernard, HUPNVS, Université Paris Diderot, Paris 7, PRES Sorbonne Paris Cité, EA4409, Paris, France, 2 Inserm ATIP-Avenir: "Modélisation, Aide à la Décision, et Coût-Efficacité en Maladies Infectieuses", Lille, France, 3 Service des Maladies Infectieuses et Tropicales, AP-HP, Groupe Hospitalier Bichat-Claude Bernard, HUPNVS, Université Paris Diderot, Paris 7, PRES Sorbonne Paris Cité, EA4409, Paris, France

Abstract

Objective: The aim of our study was to assess a possible association between plasma inflammatory biomarkers (CRP, IL-6, soluble CD14) and the extent of fibrosis or cirrhosis using a FibroScan® in HIV/HCV co-infected patients.

Methods: This cross-sectional study assessed 60 HIV/HCV co-infected patients who had paired plasma samples and FibroScan® values available. All included patients were controlled for HIV infection (HIV-1 RNA <50 copies/mL) and had detectable HCV RNA levels. Levels of three biomarkers were measured in all samples using commercial ELISA kits. Multivariate logistic regression models identified factors associated with the METAVIR stages of fibrosis (F0–F2 *vs.* F3–F4).

Results: In univariate logistic regression analyses, in addition to sCD14 (odds ratio [OR] = 3.23, 95% confidence interval [95%CI] = 1.30–7.97, $P = 0.01$), aspartate aminotransferase (AST), alanine aminotransferase, platelet counts, and CD4 cell counts were associated with the stage of liver fibrosis and, thus, were introduced into the model. However, only AST (OR = 1.06, 95%CI = 1.02–1.10, $P = 0.0009$) was independently associated with F3–F4 stage liver fibrosis.

Conclusions: In our study of HIV/HCV co-infected patients, sCD14 plasma level, a biomarker of monocyte activation, was not independently associated with the F3–F4 stage of liver fibrosis. We hypothesize that the higher levels of inflammation markers observed in HIV/HCV co-infected patients, compared to HCV mono-infected patients, prevent this association being observed within this population.

Editor: Cristian Apetrei, University of Pittsburgh Center for Vaccine Research, United States of America

Funding: This study was supported by French National Agency for Research on AIDS and viral hepatitis (Agence Nationale de Recherches sur le SIDA et les hépatites virales [ANRS]) and from the European Community's Seventh Framework Programme (FP7/2007–2013) under the project "Collaborative HIV and Anti-HIV Drug Resistance Network (CHAIN)" (grant no. 223131). The funders had no role in study design, data collection and analysis, decision to publish, or preparation of the manuscript.

Competing Interests: The authors have declared that no competing interests exist.

* E-mail: charlotte.charpentier@bch.aphp.fr

Introduction

Microbial translocation has been described as associated with chronic inflammation in both HIV-infected and hepatitis (HBV or HCV)-infected patients [1–4]. The mechanism of microbial translocation is positively correlated with the level of the bacterial product, lipopolysaccharide, and is indirectly reflected by the presence of soluble CD14 (sCD14), a plasma biomarker of monocyte/macrophage activation.

In HIV-infected patients, several studies reported that high sCD14 plasma levels predict disease progression and are positively correlated with all-cause mortality [2,3]. Higher levels of the inflammatory biomarkers, C-reactive protein (CRP) and interleukine-6 (IL-6), have been also previously associated with an increased risk of mortality or opportunistic diseases in large randomized clinical trials [5,6]. Similarly, the role of sCD14 has been reported in patients infected with HBV or HCV, as well as an association between high sCD14 plasma levels and cirrhosis; thus, the presence of sCD14 can predict progression to end-stage liver disease [4]. However, there are scarce data on the role and predictive value in the development of liver fibrosis of inflammatory biomarkers as high-sensitivity CRP (hsCRP) and IL-6, or of a monocyte/macrophage activation marker, such as sCD14.

The aim of our study was to assess the possible associations between plasma inflammatory biomarkers and the extent of liver fibrosis or cirrhosis in HIV/HCV co-infected patients.

Table 1. Characteristics of HIV/HCV co-infected patients ($n = 60$).

Characteristics	$n = 60$
Men n (%)	45 (75)
Age (years)	50 (46–53)
HCV RNA ($\log_{10}$ IU/mL)	6.46 (6.06–6.70)
HCV genotype 1 n (%)	36 (60)
AST (U/L)	48 (37–65)
ALT (U/L)	57 (42–83)
GGT (IU/L)	78 (44–133)
Creatinine (μM/L)	77 (64–88)
Platelet count (/μL)	174 (129–217)
CD4 cell count (/mm^3)	562 (291–771)
Nadir CD4 (/mm^3)	177 (70–255)
Duration since diagnosis of HIV infection (years)	19 (11–23)
CD4/CD8 ratio	0.69 (0.41–0.98)

Continuous variables were expressed as medians and interquartile ranges (IQR), and categorical variables were expressed as numbers and percentages.
ALT: alanine aminotransferase; AST: aspartate aminotransferase; GGT: gamma glutamyl transpeptidase.

Patients and Methods

This cross-sectional study included co-infected HIV/HCV patients from the Infectious Diseases Unit of Bichat Hospital (Paris, France). All enrolled patients were receiving an antiretroviral-based therapy and were virologically suppressed for HIV replication (HIV-1 RNA <50 copies/mL), they had detectable HCV RNA levels, and paired plasma samples and FibroScan® values were available. Plasma samples were obtained between 2009 and 2011, and stored at −80°C in Bichat Hospital virology lab.

This study's protocol was approved by an institutional ethics review board (Saint-Germain en Laye, France), and all patients provided their written informed consent.

Levels of three biomarkers were measured in all samples. hsCRP (human C-reactive protein [CRP] Quantikine ELISA Kit, R&D Systems, MN, USA), hsIL-6 (human IL-6 Quantikine High Sensitivity ELISA Kit, R&D Systems), and sCD14 (human sCD14 Quantikine ELISA Kit, R&D Systems) were measured using commercial ELISA assays. Lower levels of detection were 0.010 ng/mL, 0.039 pg/mL, and 0.125 μg/mL for hsCRP, IL-6, and sCD14, respectively.

Sociodemographic characteristics and clinical, virological, and biological data from patients were assessed using descriptive

statistical methods. We assessed the correlation between inflammatory biomarkers and FibroScan® values as continuous variables using Spearman's rank test. We also used a logistic regression model, as a dichotomous variable, to determine if there was an association between the level of inflammatory biomarkers and METAVIR stage of liver fibrosis (F0–F2 vs. F3–F4). Then we adjusted the model for those factors found, in univariate analyses, to be associated with METAVIR fibrosis stage (F0–F2 vs. F3–F4). We applied a forward-selection procedure for those variables with a univariate P-value of ≤0.20, and we retained a significance threshold of $P = 0.05$ to determine which factors were independently associated with the stage of liver fibrosis. Analyses were conducted with SAS software, version 9.2 (SAS Institute, Cary, NC).

Results

The characteristics of the 60 included patients are shown in Table 1. Their median age was 50 years (interquartile range [IQR] = 46–53) and 75% were men. Among all patients, 28 (47%) were receiving a protease inhibitor-based regimen, 15 (25%) a non nucleoside reverse transcriptase inhibitor-based regimen, and 17 (28%) a different antiretroviral-based regimen. Most patients ($n = 36$, 60%) were infected with HCV genotype 1, three (5%) with HCV genotype 2, six (10%) with HCV genotype 3, and fifteen (25%) with HCV genotype 4. Seventeen patients (28%) displayed METAVIR F3- or F4-stage liver fibrosis (FibroScan® value ≥10.5 kPa). The median time since diagnosis of HIV infection was 19 years (IQR = 11–23). The median CD4 cell count at the time of the study and nadir CD4 cell count were 562/mm^3 (IQR = 291–771) and 177/mm^3 (IQR = 70–255), respectively.

In the 60 patients, median sCD14, hsCRP, and IL-6 levels were 2.79 μg/mL (IQR = 2.39–3.46), 0.67 μg/L (IQR = 0.19–2.07), and 1.73 pg/mL (IQR = 0.47–4.91), respectively. The FibroScan® values correlated with sCD14 plasma levels (r = 0.40, P = 0.002), but not with IL-6 (r = 0.16, P = 0.23) or hsCRP-plasma levels (r = 0.14, P = 0.25) (Figure 1). In the logistic regression, which included only inflammatory markers, sCD14 was associated with the F3–F4 stage of liver fibrosis (odds ratio [OR] = 3.35, 95% confidence interval [95%CI] = 1.31–8.53, P = 0.01).

In the univariate logistic regression analyses, in addition to sCD14 and ALT, aspartate aminotransferase (AST) (P = 0.0009), platelet counts (P = 0.0055), and CD4 cell counts (P = 0.05) were associated with the stage of liver fibrosis and so were introduced into the model (Table 2). However, only AST (OR = 1.06, 95%CI = 1.02–1.10, P = 0.0009) was independently associated with the F3–F4 stage of liver fibrosis (Table 2).

Similar results were obtained in a multivariate regression model, which evaluated the association between inflammatory biomarkers and FibroScan® values, adjusted on other variables (data not shown).

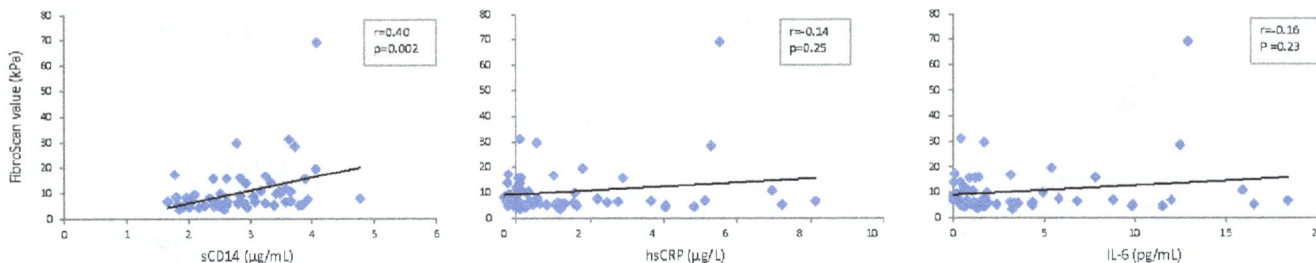

Figure 1. Correlation between FibroScan® values and inflammatory biomarkers (Spearman rank's test).

Table 2. Factors associated with the METAVIR liver fibrosis stage.

	F0–F1 n=43	F3–F4 n=17	OR	[95% CI]	P-value	aOR	[95% CI]	P-value
AST (U/L)	42 [34–56]	71 [56–107]	1.06	[1.02–1.10]	0.0009	1.06	[1.02–1.10]	0.0009
ALT (U/L)	52 [36–67]	97 [59–135]	1.03	[1.01–1.05]	0.0017	–		
Platelet count (/μL)	183 [155–231]	129 [76–194]	1.00	[1.00–0.01]	0.0055	–		
sCD14 (μg/mL)	2.57 [2.15–3.07]	3.33 [2.82–3.66]	3.23	[1.30–7.97]	0.01	–		
CD4 cell count (/mm³)	630 [453–788]	455 [248–567]	1.00	[0.99–1.00]	0.05	–		
Sex, men, n (%)	30 (70)	15 (88)	3.25	[0.64–16.30]	0.15	–		

Continuous variables were expressed as median and interquartile range (IQR).
ALT: alanine aminotransferase; aOR: adjusted odds ratio; AST: aspartate aminotransferase; OR [CI95%]: odds ratio and 95% confidence interval.

Discussion

In this study, based on 60 HIV/HCV co-infected patients, we found high levels of inflammatory biomarkers. However, sCD14 plasma level, the biomarker of monocyte activation, was not found to be independently associated with F3–F4 stage liver fibrosis.

A main limitation of our study was its limited sample size, which meant there was lack of statistical power; however, we assumed that the risk of selection bias was negligible. Furthermore, few studies have reported on the role of inflammatory biomarkers in HIV/HCV co-infection and, as yet, no large studies have been conducted.

In our study, the median sCD14 plasma level was 2.79 μg/mL (IQR = 2.39–3.46), which is a similar level to that observed in the study of Marchetti et al.: they assessed inflammatory biomarkers in HIV/HCV co-infected patients and found that median sCD14 plasma levels ranged from 2.79 to 3.09 μg/mL and was linked to the severity of the liver disease [3]. In a study by Sandler et al., which assessed the inflammatory biomarkers in hepatitis (HBV and HCV) mono-infected patients, the median sCD14 plasma levels were lower in patients with severe fibrosis (at 2.06 μg/mL) and in patients without fibrosis (at 1.74 μg/mL) [2]. Although we should be cautious when comparing these studies, sCD14 plasma levels seem to be lower in hepatitis mono-infected patients than in HIV/HCV co-infected patients [2,3]. These differences in plasma levels might be result from the accelerated mechanism of fibrogenesis observed in HIV/HCV co-infection, which includes patients who are receiving a suppressive antiretroviral therapy [7,8].

We found similar results to those of Marchetti et al. regarding the ability of inflammatory markers to predict the degree of liver inflammation and its progression to cirrhosis in HIV/HCV co-infected patients: these authors reported that a greater extent of fibrosis was not associated with higher sCD14 plasma levels [3]. This, however, contradicts Sandler et al.'s results, where sCD14 plasma levels were associated with cirrhosis and predicted progression to end-stage liver disease [4].

The difference between these studies is probably not related to differences in statistical power as (i) a similar number of patients were assessed in these studies; and (ii) sCD14 was associated with the stage of fibrosis, in univariate analyses, in both studies [4]. However, this difference may be because our study and Marchetti et al.'s study included HIV/HCV co-infected patients whereas Sandler et al.'s study focused on HBV/HCV mono-infected

patients [3,4]. HIV/HCV co-infected patients had higher levels of inflammatory biomarkers and sCD14 values because of the HIV co-infection, regardless of which stage of fibrosis. Thus, it seems to be more difficult to show an association between inflammation and progression to cirrhosis.

In our study, the level of the liver enzyme, AST, was the only factor independently associated with the extent of fibrosis. In HIV-infected patients, chronic elevation of AST and HCV infection have been previously described as independently associated with significant fibrosis [9]. When hepatitis is a mono-infection, AST has been correlated with sCD14 plasma levels, but was not associated with disease progression [9]. A previous study in HIV/HCV co-infected patients showed that heavy alcohol intake and increased AST levels were predictive of the severity of fibrosis [10].

In conclusion, in our series of HIV/HCV co-infected patients, sCD14 plasma level, the biomarker of monocyte activation, was not independently associated with the F3–F4 stage of liver fibrosis. Thus, we hypothesize that the higher levels of inflammation markers observed in HIV/HCV co-infected compared to HCV mono-infected patients may prevent such an association being observed in this population. Further studies that explore the possible roles of others biomarkers, for example the innate immune-activation marker, soluble CD163, may improve our understanding of the mechanisms of systemic immune activation.

Acknowledgments

We are indebted to the following for their assistance in data collection: E. Bouvet, S. Matheron, P. Yeni, S. Lariven, C. Rioux, M. Caseris, N. Dournon, H. Ferrand, M. Pichon, M. Ahouanto, E. Casalino, G. Castanedo, A. Dia, X. Duval, Z. Eid, S. Fegueux, V. Gregoire, F. Guiroy, S. Harent, C. Jestin, K. Jidar, M.A. Khuong, N. Landgraf, Y. Latorre, C. Leport, A. Lepretre, F. Lheriteau, P. Longuet, F. Michard, G. Morau, G. Pahlavan, E. Papot, B. Phung, M.H. Prevot, S. Puget, P. Ralaimazava, H. Rousselot, F. Louni, C. Godard, Z. Julia, M. Chansombat, G. Hamet.

Author Contributions

Contributed to this study concept: CC RL FBV DD YY. Performed the FibroScan® test: AG. Performed the immuno-analysis assays: LL. Performed the statistical analysis: KC. Contributed to the analysis and interpretation of the data: CC KC AG VJ SLG FD DD YY. Contributed to the writing of the manuscript: CC KC AG DD YY. Contributed to the critical reviewing of the manuscript: CC KC AG RL VJ SLG LL FD FBV DD YY.

References

1. Kalayjian RC, Machekano RN, Rizk N, Robbins GK, Gandhi RT, et al. (2010) Pretreatment levels of soluble cellular receptors and interleukin-6 are associated with HIV disease progression in subjects treated with highly active antiretroviral therapy. J Infect Dis 201: 1796–1805.

2. Sandler NG, Wand H, Roque A, Law M, Nason MC, et al. (2011) Plasma levels of soluble CD14 independently predict mortality in HIV infection. J Infect Dis 203: 780–790.

3. Marchetti G, Cozzi-Lepri A, Merlini E, Bellistrì GM, Castagna A, et al. (2011) Microbial translocation predicts disease progression of HIV-infected antiretro-viral-naive patients with high CD4+ cell count. AIDS 25: 1385–1394.

4. Sandler NG, Koh C, Roque A, Eccleston JL, Siegel RB, et al. (2011) Host response to translocated microbial products predicts outcomes of patients with HBV or HCV infection. Gastroenterology 141: 1220–1230.

5. Rodger AJ, Fox Z, Lundgren JD, Kuller LH, Boesecke C, et al. (2009) Activation and coagulation biomarkers are independent predictors of the development of opportunistic disease in patients with HIV infection. J Infect Dis 200: 973–983.

6. Boulware DR, Hullsiek KH, Puronen CE, Rupert A, Baker JV, et al. (2011) Higher levels of CRP, D-dimer, IL-6, and hyaluronic acid before initiation of antiretroviral therapy (ART) are associated with increased risk of AIDS or death. J Infect Dis 203: 1637–1646.

7. Thein HH, Yi Q, Dore GJ, Krahn MD (2008) Natural history of hepatitis C virus infection in HIV-infected individuals and the impact of HIV in the era of highly active antiretroviral therapy: a meta-analysis. AIDS 22: 1979–1991.

8. Macías J, von Wichmann M, Rivero A, Tellez F, Merino D, et al. (2010) Fast liver damage progression in HIV/HCV-co-infected patients in spite of effective HAART. [Abstract #659]. In: *Program and Abstract of the 17th Conference on Retroviruses and Opportunistic Infections;* 16–19 February 2010; San Francisco, USA.

9. Vermehren J, Vermehren A, Mueller A, Carlebach A, Lutz T, et al. (2012) Assessment of liver fibrosis and associated risk factors in HIV-infected individuals using transient elastography and serum biomarkers. BMC Gastroenterol 12: 27.

10. Cartón JA, Collazos J, de la Fuente B, García-Alcalde ML, Suarez-Zarracina T, et al. (2011) Factors associated with liver fibrosis in intravenous drug users coinfected with HIV and HCV. Antivir Ther 16: 27–35.

20

Up-Regulation of RACK1 by TGF-β1 Promotes Hepatic Fibrosis in Mice

Dongwei Jia[1], Fangfang Duan[2], Peike Peng[1], Linlin Sun[1], Xiaojuan Liu[1], Lan Wang[2], Weicheng Wu[1], Yuanyuan Ruan[1]*, Jianxin Gu[1,2]

1 Department of Biochemistry and Molecular Biology, Shanghai Medical College, Fudan University, Shanghai, P.R. China, 2 Institute of Biomedical Science, Fudan University, Shanghai, P.R. China

Abstract

Liver fibrosis represents the consequences of a sustained wound healing response to chronic liver injury, and activation of quiescent hepatic stellate cells (HSCs) into a myofibroblast-like phenotype is considered as the central event of liver fibrosis. RACK1, the receptor for activated C-kinase 1, is a classical scaffold protein implicated in numerous signaling pathways and cellular processes; however, the role of RACK1 in liver fibrosis is little defined. Herein, we report that RACK1 is up-regulated in activated HSCs in transforming growth factor beta 1 (TGF-β1)-dependent manner both *in vitro* and *in vivo*, and TGF-β1 stimulates the expression of RACK1 through NF-κB signaling. Moreover, RACK1 promotes TGF-β1 and platelet-derived growth factor (PDGF)-mediated activation of pro-fibrogenic pathways as well as the differentiation, proliferation and migration of HSCs. Depletion of RACK1 suppresses the progression of TAA-induced liver fibrosis *in vivo*. In addition, the expression of RACK1 in fibrogenic cells also positively correlates well with the stage of liver fibrosis in clinical cases. Our results suggest RACK1 as a downstream target gene of TGF-β1 involved in the modulation of liver fibrosis progression *in vitro* and *in vivo*, and propose a strategy to target RACK1 for liver fibrosis treatment.

Editor: Anna Alisi, Bambino Gesu' Children Hospital, Italy

Funding: This work was supported by the National Basic Research Program of China (973 Program) (2012CB822104), the State Key Project Specialized for Infectious Diseases of China (2012ZX10002-008, 2012ZX10002-012), the National High-tech R&D Program (863 Program) (2012AA020203), the Shanghai Leading Academic Discipline Project (B110), the National Natural Science Fund (31100977, 31170766, 31010103906, 31000348, 31000600, 31100586). The funders had no role in study design, data collection and analysis, decision to publish, or preparation of the manuscript.

Competing Interests: The authors have declared that no competing interests exist.

* E-mail: yuanyuanruan@fudan.edu.cn

Introduction

Liver fibrosis represents the consequences of a sustained wound healing response to various chronic liver injuries including viral, autoimmune, drug-induced, cholestatic and metabolic diseases [1]. In response to injury, HSCs undergo a well-characterized activation process during which they lose their characteristic vitamin A and lipid stores, and obtain a myofibroblastic phenotype [2]. This process is associated with the increased expression of contractile filaments such as α-smooth muscle actin (α-SMA) and production of extracellular matrix (ECM), and a large amount of production of pro-fibrogenic factors such as cytokines and reactive oxygen species (ROS) [3]. These cytokines, including interferons, interleukins, tumor necrosis factors (TNF), growth factors (e.g. TGF, PDGF) and chemokines, are released from hepatocytes, Kupffer cells, stellate cells, epithelial cells, endothelial cells and so on, and play critical roles in liver fibrosis through regulating hepatic inflammation, cell necrosis and apoptosis, and ECM production [4].

TGF-β is a cytokine/growth factor with immunosuppressive, anti-inflammatory, and pro-fibrotic properties. In the liver, TGF-β1 is the most abundant isoform, and is secreted by immune cells, epithelial cells and stellate cells. Bone marrow-derived and liver resident macrophages (Kupffer cells) are believed to be the major source of TGF-β1 in fibrotic liver, and the activated HSCs are also an important source of TGF-β1 in the liver [4,5,6]. During hepatic fibrogenesis, TGF-β1 plays a pivotal role in the progression of liver fibrosis by promoting the transdifferentiation and migration of HSCs [7,8]. It has been reported that activated HSCs, which are the principal cells to produce type I collagen in the fibrotic liver, contribute to the development of liver fibrosis through autocrine and paracrine loops of TGF-β1-stimulated collagen production [9]. Therefore, TGF-β1 is considered as a major factor in accelerating the progression of liver fibrosis. The classical Smads pathways (receptor-mediated Smads, Smad2/3), MAPKs as well as NF-κB signaling, have been reported to be implicated in the pro-fibrogenic effect of TGF-β1 [10,11,12]. In addition to TGF-β1, PDGF, mainly produced by Kupffer cells, is the most potent mitogen for HSCs and also upregulated in the fibrotic liver [13]. PDGF induces the activation of several signaling pathways such as MAPKs and AKT, which have been reported to involved in the modulation of HSCs proliferation and migration during the progression of liver fibrosis [14,15]

The receptor for activated C-kinase 1 (RACK1) is a member of the tryptophan-aspartate repeat (WD-repeat) family of proteins. RACK1 possesses the capacity for interaction with diverse proteins and plays important roles in a variety of physiological functions. The altered RACK1 expression has been identified in several kinds of human diseases, including brain developmental disorders, heart failure, muscle atrophy, breast cancer and pulmonary adenocarcinomas [16,17,18], and our previous research also indicates that RACK1 is frequently up-regulated in hepatocellular carcinoma and promotes its chemo-resistance and growth [19]. However, the role of RACK1 in liver fibrosis is little defined. In this study, we demonstrate that the expression of RACK1 is increased in activated HSC in TGF-β1 -dependent manner, and RACK1 promotes the initiation and progression of liver fibrosis by enhancing TGF-β1 and PDGF-induced differentiation, migration and proliferation of HSCs. Our results suggest RACK1 as a downstream target gene of TGF-β1 involved in the modulation of liver fibrogenesis, and propose a strategy to target RACK1 for liver fibrosis treatment.

Materials and Methods

Ethics Statement

The use of human tissue samples and clinical data was approved by the ethics committee of Fudan University. The individual in this manuscript has given written informed consent (as outlined in PLOS consent form) to publish these case details. Animal experiments were performed according to the criteria outlined in the Guide for the Care and Use of Laboratory Animals, prepared by the National Academy of Sciences and published by the National Institutes of Health, and also approved by the ethics committee of Fudan University. The surgery of liver perfusion was performed under sodium pentobarbital anesthesia, and all efforts were made to minimize suffering.

Mouse model of liver fibrosis

Wild-type and Tgfb1+/− mice of C57BL/6J background were used for inducing liver fibrosis. The wild-type C57BL/6J mice were obtained from SLAC Laboratory Animal Corp (Shanghai, China), and Tgfb1+/− mice were purchased from JACKSON laboratory. All mice were maintained at 25°C with a 12 h dark/light cycle. Liver fibrosis was induced by intraperitoneal injection of thioacetamide (TAA) (Sigma) at 0.2 mg/g body weight 3 times each week for 8 weeks. The control mice were received intraperitoneal injection of vehicle (distilled water). For the shRACK1 in vivo experiment, RACK1 shRNA lentiviral particles were delivered using the tail vein injection method [20]. Meanwhile, the mice were received TAA or vehicle treatment for 8 weeks. Samples of mouse livers were fixed in formaldehyde or immediately frozen in liquid nitrogen.

Patients and tissue samples

Forty-six liver biopsy samples were collected from patients with liver fibrosis at Zhongshan Hospital of Fudan University (Shanghai, China). The stage of liver fibrosis is according to previous report [21].

Primary cells and cell line

Primary hepatic stellate cells were isolated from mice using a modification of the methods of Geerts et al [22]. Briefly, the inferior vena cava was ligated and the portal vein was dissected. The liver was then perfused with Liver Perfusion Medium (GIBCO) followed by pronase E (Sigma Aldrich) and collagenase IV solution treatment. Digested liver tissue was filtered through nylon mesh and centrifugation to remove the parenchymal cells. The nonparenchymal supernatant was subjected to HSC separation by density gradient centrifugation. The purity was assessed by the autofluorescence of vitamin A droplets, and was between 90% and 95%. Primary hepatocytes were isolated by two-step collagenase perfusion [23]. Hepatocytes were filtered through 100 µM filter gaze, and then centrifuged to remove suspension. The HSC-T6 cell line was purchased from XiangYa Central

Experiment Laboratory (Changsha, Hunan province, China). All primary cells and cell line were cultured in Dulbecco's modified Eagle's medium (Sigma Aldrich, USA) supplemented with 10% fetal bovine serum (Gibco) at 37°C in a humidified atmosphere with 5% $CO2$.

Antibodies and reagents

Recombinant human TGF-β1 and mouse anti-TGF-β1 antibody were obtained from R&D system. SB203580 and SB431542 were purchased from CalBiochem. Rabbit anti-phospho-JNK, -JNK, -phospho-p38, -p38, -phospho-Smad2, -phospho-Smad3, -Smad2/3, -phospho-IKKα/β, -IKKα, -IKKβ, mouse anti-p65 antibodies and U0126 were purchased from Cell Signaling Technology. Rabbit anti-p50 antibody was obtained from BioVision and Santa Cruz Biotechnology. Rabbit anti-ERK1/2, -ERK, mouse anti-GAPDH, -phospho-I-κBα, -I-κBα, -RACK1, and goat anti-Col1A1 antibodies were obtained from Santa Cruz Biotechnology. Rabbit anti-RACK1 antibody was purchased from Abcam. Mouse anti-α-SMA antibody and PDTC were from Sigma Aldrich.

Plasmid construction, transfection and RNA interference

The NF-κB binding element of GNB2L1 promoter was subcloned into pGL3-Basic Vector. Transfection was performed using Lipo2000 (Invitrogen) according to manufacturer's instructions. The mouse RACK1 shRNA lentiviral particles were purchased from Santa Cruz Biotechnology.

Western-blot

Western-blot analysis was carried out according to our previous report [19].

Immunofluorenscence analysis

For immunofluorescence staining of RACK1 and α-SMA, 8 µm cryostat sections were fixed in ice-cold acetone for 10 min, blocked with 10% goat serum for 2 h at room temperature and incubated with antibodies for RACK1 and α-SMA overnight at 4°C. Immunofluorescence staining was examined using the confocal laser scanning microscopy (Leica Microsystems Heidelberg GmbH, Germany).

Histological analysis

For HE staining, the sections were stained with hematoxylin, rinsed with water, and stained with eosin, dehydrated and mounted. For Sirius red staining, sections were stained with Sirius red for 25 min, rinsed with 100% ethanol, dehydrated and mounted. For immunohistochemical staining, sections were soaked in 0.3% hydrogen peroxide, and incubated with primary antibody overnight at 4°C. All slides were processed using the peroxidase-antiperoxidase method (Dako, Hamburg, Germany).

For the scoring of RACK1 in clinical samples, double stained sections of RACK1 and α-SMA were interpreted under microscopic fields of 200 or 400-fold magnification. RACK1 scoring was based on a semi-quantitative method according to the intensity and percentage of staining in α-SMA positive cells, which was described previously [19]. The intensity of staining was scored on a scale of 0 to 3, in which 0 = negative staining, 1 = weakly positive staining, 2 = moderately positive staining, and 3 = strongly positive staining. The percentage of staining was estimated on a scale of 0 to 4, in which 0 = none, 1 = 1–25% positive staining in α-SMA positive cells. 2 = 26–50% positive staining; 3 = 51–75% positive staining; and 4 = 76–100% positive staining. The immunohistochemical score (IS) was calculated through multiplying the intensity score by the percentage score. Samples with IS between 0 and 1 were classified as Score 0, samples with IS between 2 and 4 were Score 1, samples with IS between 5 and 8 were Score 2, and samples with IS between 9 and 12 were Score 3. No samples from the 46 cases was grouped as Score 0. All of the sections were evaluated in a blinded manner without knowledge of the clinical and pathological parameters of the patients.

Real-time PCR analysis

Total RNA was extracted with TRIZOL (Invitrogen) according to manufacturer's instructions. Quality of the total RNA was detected by spectrophotometer (Pharmacia Biotech RNA/DNA Calculator). About 3 μg total RNA from each sample was used to perform reverse-transcribed by using RNA PCR Kit AMV (Takara). Real-time PCR was performed using SYBR Green Premix Ex Taq Ver. 3.0 (Takara) and detected by StepOne plus. The following primers were used: GAPDH Forward: GAGCGA-GACCCCACTAACAT; Reverse: TCTCCATGGTGGTGAA-GACA; RACK1 Forward: GGATCTCAATGAAGGCAAGC; Reverse: TTGCTGCTGGTGCTGATAAC

Luciferase activity assay

For luciferase activity assay, cell extracts were prepared and luciferase activities were detected according to the manufacture's instructions (Promega) using a Lumat LB9507 luminometer. All assays were performed in triplicate.

Chromatin immunoprecipitation assay (ChIP)

ChIP was performed using a commercial kit according to the manufacturer's instructions (Active Motif-ChIP-IT™ Express). Proteins cross-linked to DNA were immunoprecipitated with antibodies against p65, p50 or control IgG. The purified DNA was amplified by the promoter-specific primers. RACK1 Forward: ACTTGAGACCTACTCTCCCAG and Reverse: GGA-TAGCTCAGAGAGCCAAGC, and PCR products were separated by gel electrophoresis on 2% agarose gel and visualized.

Co-immunoprecipitation

Primary HSCs were treated with or without TGF-β1, washed with ice-cold phosphate-buffered saline (PBS) and solubilized with co-immunoprecipitation (co-IP) buffer. Cell lysates were rotated with relevant antibody and Co-IP was performed as before [19].

Migration assay

Migration assay was performed according to a previous report [8]. Briefly, the membranes with 8-μm pores were coated with type IV collagen on the upper side and with type I collagen on the lower side. Cells were added into the upper chamber. The number of infiltrating cells was counted from five visions and the experiments were repeated three times.

Cell proliferation assay

Cell proliferation was determined using Cell Counting Kit-8 (CCK-8) (Beyotime Inst. Biotech, China) according to manufacture's instructions. Briefly, cells were seeded in a 96-well plate and treated with or without PDGF, then incubated with WST-8 dye at 37°C. And the absorbance was determined at 450 nm using a Universal Microplate Reader (Bio-Tek Instrument Inc.). All assays were performed in triplicate.

Statistical analysis

Results were presented as mean ± S.D. Statistical analysis was performed using One-way ANOVA analysis. Statistical significance was determined at the level of $p < 0.05$.

Results

RACK1 is up-regulated in activated HSCs in vivo and in vitro

RACK1 is a classical scaffold protein ubiquitously expressed in the tissues of higher mammals and humans, and plays critical roles in the regulation of various signaling pathways and numerous aspects of cellular functions. To understand the role of RACK1 in the development of liver fibrosis, we examined the expression pattern of RACK1 in HSCs using the mouse model of TAA-induced liver fibrosis. As shown in Figure 1A and B, RACK1 expression was significantly up-regulated in activated HSCs after TAA treatment, but not in hepatocytes. Immunofluorescence analysis also revealed that the number of RACK1 and α-SMA (a marker for activated HSCs) double-positive cells was markedly increased in TAA-treated liver compared to vehicle control (Figure 1C). These results suggest that RACK1 is up-regulated in activated HSCs during the development of liver fibrosis in vivo.

It has been reported when cultured on plastic, freshly isolated quiescent HSCs undergo spontaneous fibrogenic activation to myofibroblast-like cells [24]. To further confirm whether RACK1 was up-regulated in activated HSCs, we next detected the expression profile of RACK1 in primary HSCs in vitro. With the progression of HSCs auto-differentiation, the protein and mRNA levels of RACK1 were coordinately increased (Figure 2A, left panel and 2B). Taken together, these results suggest that RACK1 expression is increased in activated HSCs in vivo and in vitro.

TGF-β1 is involved in the up-regulation of RACK1 in activated HSCs

Cytokines regulating the inflammatory response to injury play critical roles in the modulation of hepatic fibrogenesis, and TGF-β1 is considered as the most pro-fibrogenic cytokine and mediates the activation of HSCs and ECM production [25,26]. To explore whether TGF-β1 was required for HSCs activation, we next examined the expression of α-SMA and collagen in Tgfb1 heterozygous HSCs. As shown in Figure 2A, the up-regulation of α-SMA and collagen in Tgfb1 heterozygous HSCs was suppressed during the auto-differentiation in vitro. Moreover, TGF-β1-deficiency remarkably delayed the protrusions extending from the cell body as well as the recession of the vitamin A lipid droplet (Figure S1). These results suggest that TGF-β1 is required for auto-activation of HSCs in vitro.

To determine TGF-β1 is involved in the regulation of RACK1 expression, we also examined the expression profile of RACK1 in HSCs isolated from Tgfb1 heterozygous mice in vitro. As shown in Figure 2A and 2B, TGF-β1-deficiency impaired the up-regulation of RACK1 in primary HSCs during the auto-differentiation in vitro. Moreover, TGF-β1 neutralizing antibody efficiently inhibited the elevation of RACK1 protein and mRNA levels during the auto-activation of HSCs, suggesting that TGF-β1-induced RACK1 expression is in the autocrine manner (Figure 2C and D). We also examined the expression pattern of RACK1 in HSCs from Tgfb1 heterozygous mice in vivo. As shown in Figure 2E and F, the increase in RACK1 protein and mRNA levels upon TAA treatment was remarkably attenuated in Tgfb1 heterozygous HSCs in vivo, by comparing with that in wild-type HSCs. We next examined whether TGF-β1 treatment induced RACK1 expression in primary HSCs. As shown in Figure 2G and H,

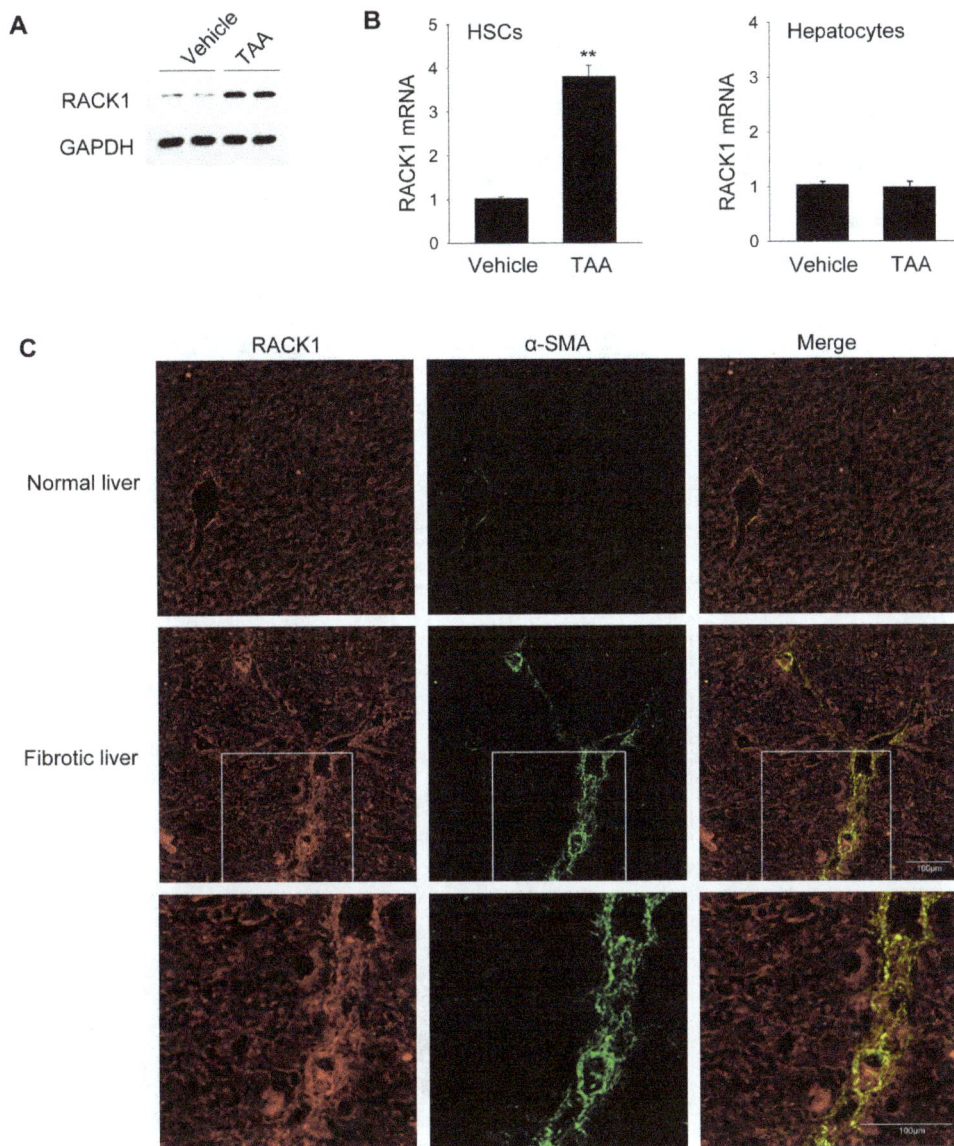

Figure 1. RACK1 is up-regulated in activated HSCs *in vivo*. The C57BL/6 mice were treated with vehicle or TAA for 8 weeks. (A) Freshly isolated HSCs from vehicle or TAA-treated mice were collected, and cell lysates were applied to western-blot analysis to detect RACK1 expression. (B) Freshly isolated HSCs or hepatocytes from vehicle or TAA-treated mice (n = 6) were applied to qRT-PCR analysis to assess RACK1 transcripts with GAPDH mRNA as the internal control. **, p<0.01. (C) Immunofluorescence staining against RACK1 (red) and α-SMA (green) was performed using frozen liver sections from vehicle or TAA-treated mice.

administration of recombinant TGF-β1 induced the elevation of RACK1 protein and mRNA levels both in dose-dependent manner. These data suggest that TGF-β1 is involved in regulation of RACK1 expression in HSCs *in vitro* and *in vivo*

TGF-β1 promotes the expression of RACK1 in NF-κB-dependent manner

To explore the underlying mechanism how TGF-β1 modulated the expression of RACK1, we first examined TGF-β1-mediated signaling pathways in primary HSCs. As shown in Figure 3A, treatment of TGF-β1 triggered the activation of JNK, ERK, p38 and Smad2/3 signaling. Moreover, TGF-β1 also induced the phosphorylation and degradation of IκBα, as well as the translocation of p65 and p50 NF-κB subunits into nucleus.

Previous reports have suggested that NF-κB and JNK pathways regulate RACK1 transcription and expression [24,27,28]. Therefore, we next determined whether NF-κB and/or JNK signaling mediated the up-regulation of RACK1 induced by TGF-β1. As shown in Figure 3B and C, treatment of PDTC, an inhibitor of NF-κB, but not the JNK inhibitor SP600125, suppressed TGF-β1-induced up-regulation of RACK1 both at the protein and mRNA levels. Moreover, inhibition of ERK, p38 and Smad2/3 signaling pathway showed little effect on TGF-β1-induced RACK1 expression.

To further confirm whether NF-κB was involved in TGF-β1-mediated RACK1 up-regulation, HSC-T6 cells were transfected with pGL3-Basic vector carrying NF-κB binding element of *GNB2L1* promoter, and luciferase gene reporter assay was carried out to examine the effect of TGF-β1 on the activity of the NF-κB

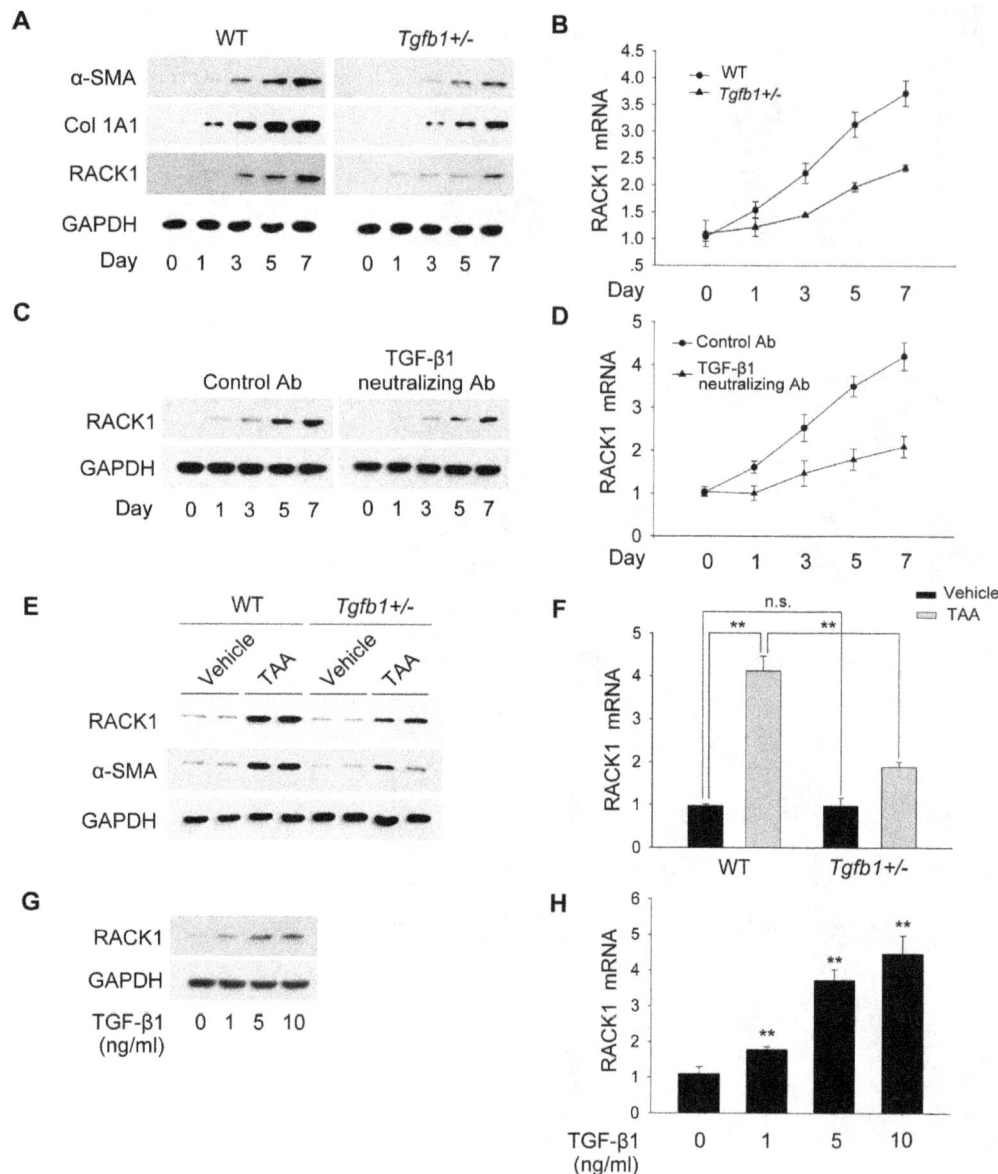

Figure 2. TGF-β1 is involved in the up-regulation of RACK1 in activated HSCs. (A, B) HSCs were isolated from wild-type or Tgfb1[+/−] mice, cultured for indicated time periods, and subjected to western blot (A) and qRT-PCR (B). (C, D) Freshly isolated HSCs were treated with neutralizing TGF-β1 antibody for indicated time periods, and subjected to western blot (C) and qRT-PCR (D) analysis. (E, F) Wild-type or Tgfb1[+/−] mice were treated with vehicle or TAA for 8 weeks. Freshly isolated HSCs were applied to western-blot and qRT-PCR analysis to detect relative RACK1 and α-SMA expression. (G, H) Freshly isolated HSCs after adherence were treated with TGF-β1 at varying concentrations for 48 h (G) or 6 h (H), harvested and subjected to western blot (G) and qRT-PCR (H) analysis to detect RACK1 expression. **, $p < 0.01$.

binding element. Results demonstrated that TGF-β1 treatment induced a remarkable increase in the luciferase activity in NF-κB-dependent manner (Figure 3D). ChIP assay also revealed that administration of TGF-β1 enhanced the binding of p65 and p50 NF-κB subunits to the promoter of GNB2L1 in HSCs, and PDTC attenuates the interaction between NF-κB subunits and GNB2L1 promoter (Figure 3E). These results imply that TGF-β1 promotes the expression of RACK1 in NF-κB-dependent manner.

RACK1 is involved in the regulation of TGF-β1-mediated signaling pathways in HSCs

Several reports have demonstrated that RACK1 interacts with the components of numerous signaling pathways [29,30,31], and

we next examined the effect of RACK1 on TGF-β1-induced pro-fibrogenic signaling in HSCs. As shown in Figure 4A and B, overexpression of RACK1 promoted TGF-β1-induced phosphorylation of JNK, ERK, Smad2/3 and IKKα/β as well as translocation of NF-κB subunits p65 and p50 into nucleus, while inhibition of RACK1 expression using specific shRNA attenuated TGF-β1-induced JNK, ERK, Smad2/3, IKKα/β and NF-κB activation (Figure 4C and D). However, RACK1 showed little effect on TGF-β1-induced p38 activation (Figure 4A–D).

RACK1 is a classical scaffold protein possessing the capacity for interaction with diverse proteins and regulation of multiple signaling pathways. To understand the role of RACK1 in TGF-β1-induced early signaling, we next examined the interaction between RACK1 and the early signaling components of TGF-β1

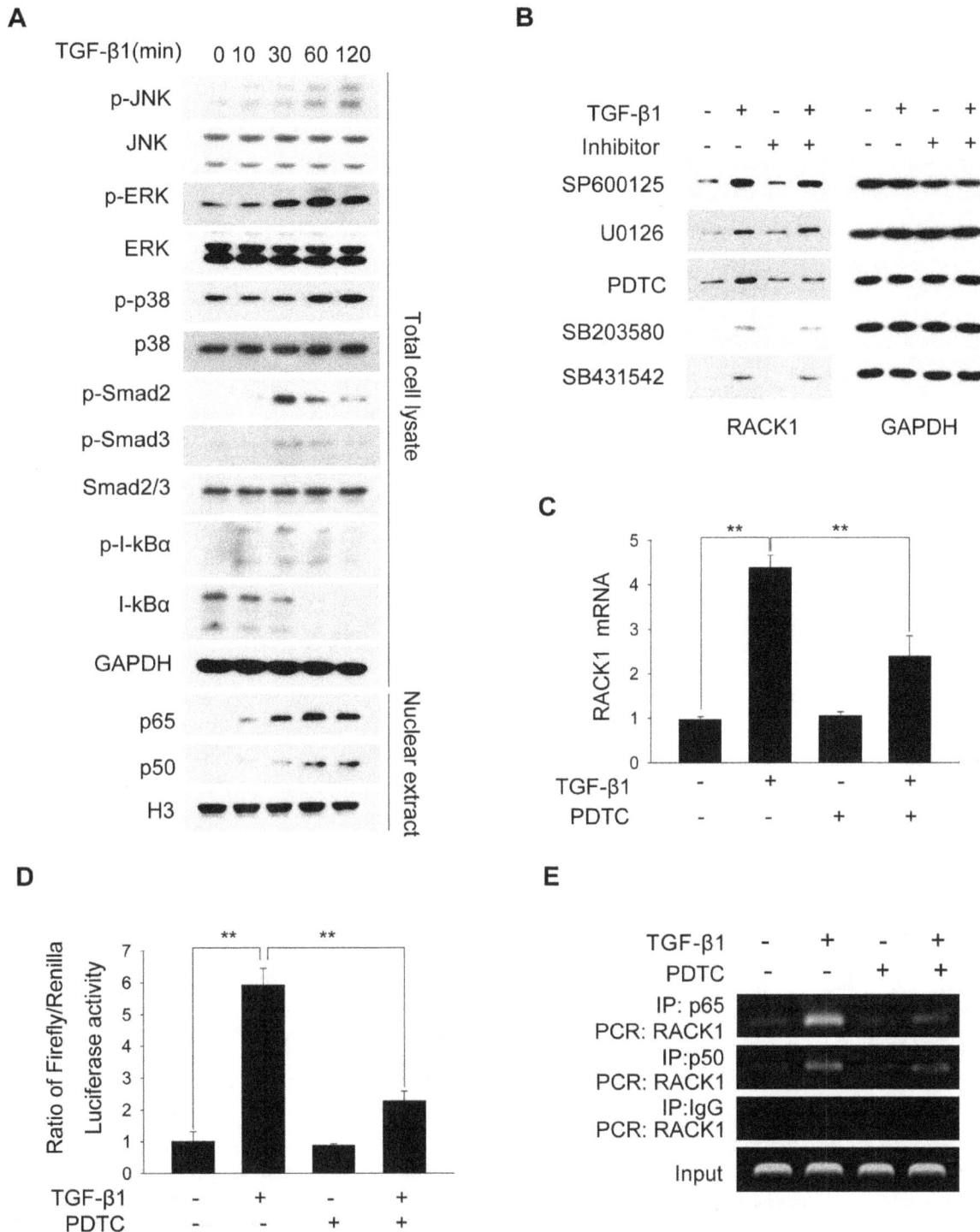

Figure 3. TGF-β1 promotes the expression of RACK1 in NF-κB-dependent manner. (A) Primary mouse HSCs were serum-starved for 6 h, and treated with TGF-β1 (10 ng/ml) for indicated times. Total cell lysates or nuclear extracts were subjected to western blot analysis. (B) Primary mouse HSCs were treated with TGF-β1 (10 ng/ml) for 48 h, along with vehicle, SP600125, U0126, PDTC, SB203580 or SB431542. (C) Primary mouse HSCs were stimulated with TGF-β1 for 6 h, along with or without PDTC, followed by qRT-PCR analysis. (D) The pGL3 vector carrying the NF-κB binding element of GNB2L1 promoter was transfected into HSC-T6 cells. 24 h later, cells were treated with TGF-β1 and/or PDTC for another 24 h for luciferase activity assay. (E) Primary mouse HSCs were treated with TGF-β1 and/or PDTC for 6 h, followed by ChIP assay. The data shown in (E) are representative of three independent experiments. **, p<0.01.

pathway. As shown in Figure 4E, RACK1 associated with JNK, ERK, Smad2/3 as well as IKKα/β, and their interactions were further enhanced upon TGF-β1 treatment. However, the inter-action between RACK1 and p38 was not detected. These results suggest that RACK1 functions as a critical scaffold protein in TGF-β1-induced early signaling.

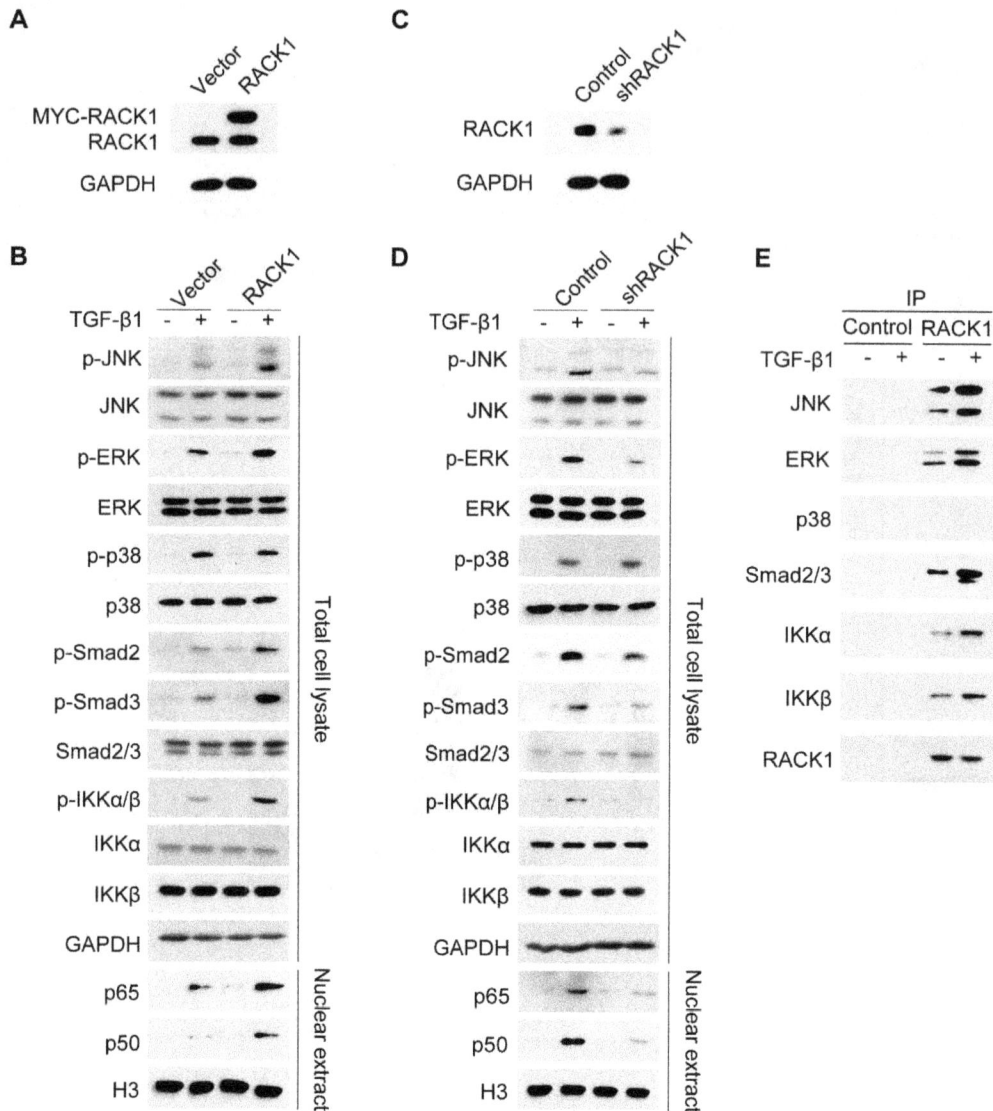

Figure 4. RACK1 is involved in the regulation of TGF-β1-mediated signaling pathways in HSCs. (A, B) Primary mouse HSCs were incubated with lentivirus expressing Myc-RACK1 or control for 96 h. Then cells were treated with TGF-β1 (10 ng/ml) and subjected to western blot analysis. (C, D) Primary mouse HSCs were incubated with lentiviral particles expressing shRNA targeting RACK1 or non-target control for 96 h. Then cells were treated with TGF-β1 (10 ng/ml) and subjected to western blot analysis. (E) Primary HSCs were treated with TGF-β1. Cell lysates were subjected to immuoprecipition with anti-RACK1 antibody, followed by western blot with related antibodies.

RACK1 is involved in the regulation of TGF-β1-mediated differentiation and migration of hepatic stellate cells

To understand whether RACK1 was involved in the regulation of HSCs activation, we first examined the effect of RACK1 on the morphological changes of HSCs during the auto-differentiation *in vitro*. As shown in Figure 5A, inhibition of RACK1 expression attenuated the spontaneous spreading of primary HSCs *in vitro*, suggesting that RACK1 is involved in the auto-differentiation of HSCs *in vitro*.

Since TGF-β1 is considered as the most potent pro-fibrogenic cytokine and mediates the HSCs activation and ECM production, we next examined the effect of RACK1 on TGF-β1-induced differentiation of HSCs. As shown in Figure 5B and C, overexpression of RACK1 promoted TGF-β1-induced up-regulation of α-SMA and collagen α1 type 1, while knock-down of RACK1 impaired the regulatory effect of TGF-β1 on α-SMA and

collagen expression. We also evaluated the role of RACK1 in TGF-β1-induced HSCs migration. Transwell assay revealed that overexpression of RACK1 promoted TGF-β1-induced HSCs migration from upper to the bottom wells of the chamber, while depletion of RACK1 by shRNA suppressed TGF-β1-mediated migration of HSCs (Figure 5D–G). Taken together, these results suggest that RACK1 is involved in the regulation of HSCs activation and migration induced by TGF-β1.

RACK1 is involved in the regulation of PDGF-mediated HSCs proliferation and migration

In addition to TGF-β1, PDGF also plays a critical role in liver fibrogenesis by stimulating the proliferation and migration of HSCs [32]. To understand whether RACK1 also enhanced the profibrogenic effect of PDGF, we first evaluated the role of RACK1 in PDGF-induced activation of profibrogenic signaling

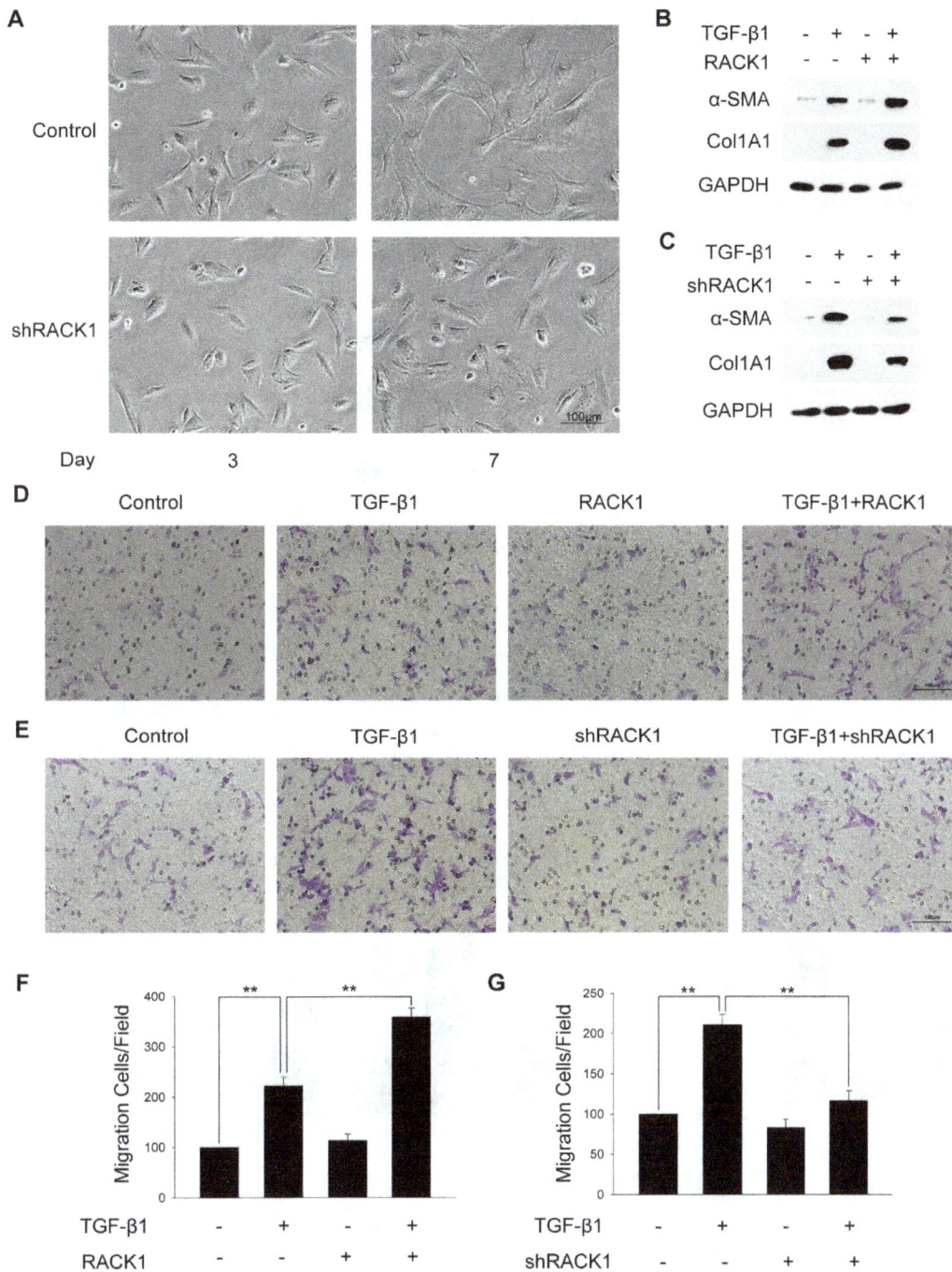

Figure 5. RACK1 is involved in the regulation of TGF-β1-mediated differentiation and migration of HSCs. (A) Fresh isolated primary mouse HSCs were incubated with lentiviral particles expressing shRNA targeting RACK1 or non-target control. The images were captured at the day of 3 and 7 after isolation. Scale bar, 100 μm. (B, C) 96 h after incubation with lentiviral particles, HSCs were stimulated with TGF-β1 (10 ng/ml) for 24 h, and expression of α-SMA and collagen α1 type 1 was analyzed. (D–G) Primary HSCs were incubated with lentivirus as indicated, and treated with or without TGF-β1, followed by transwell assay. In (D) and (E), images are representative of three independent experiments. In (F) and (G), the number of infiltrating cells was counted in five regions selected at random, and the experiments were repeated three times. **, p<0.01.

pathways. As shown in Figure 6A and B, overexpression of RACK1 promoted PDGF-induced phosphorylation of JNK, ERK, and AKT, while inhibition of RACK1 expression using specific shRNA attenuated PDGF-induced activation of JNK, ERK, and AKT.

We also examined the role of RACK1 in PDGF-induced proliferation and migration of HSCs. As shown in Figure 6C and

D, CCK8 assay revealed that overexpression of RACK1 promoted PDGF-induced HSCs proliferation, while depletion of RACK1 suppressed PDGF-mediated HSCs proliferation. Similar effect of RACK1 was also observed in PDGF-induced HSCs migration (Figure 6E and F). Taken together, these results suggest that RACK1 is involved in the regulation of the profibrogenic effect of PDGF.

A

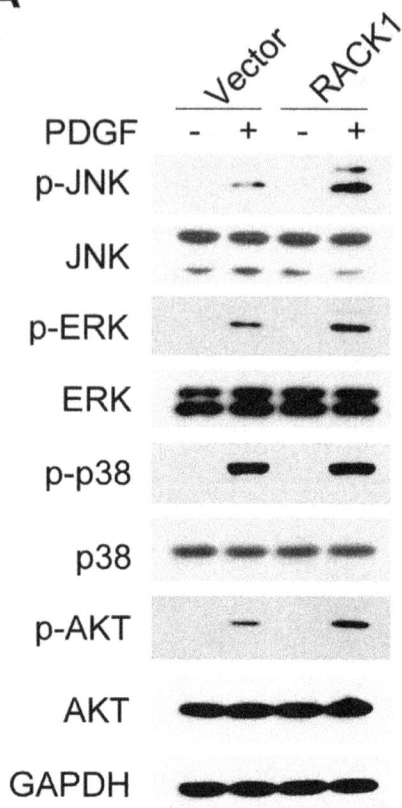

B

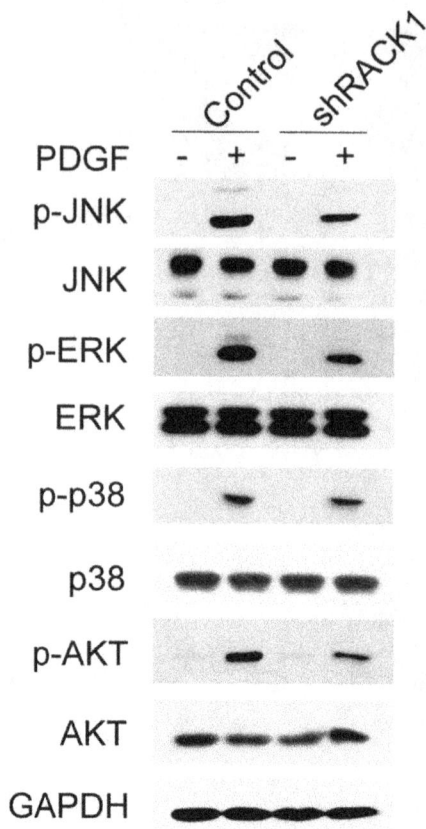

C

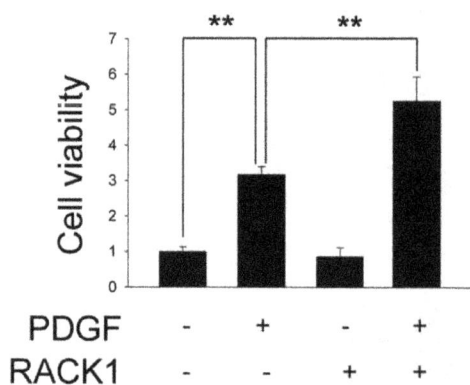

D

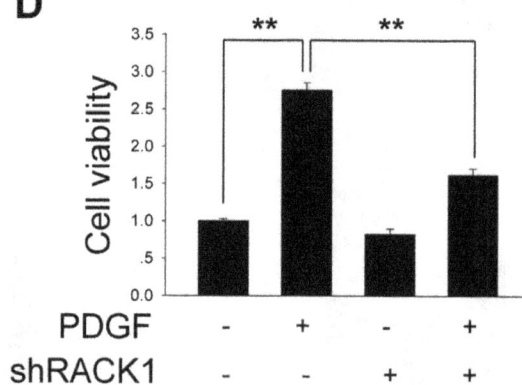

E

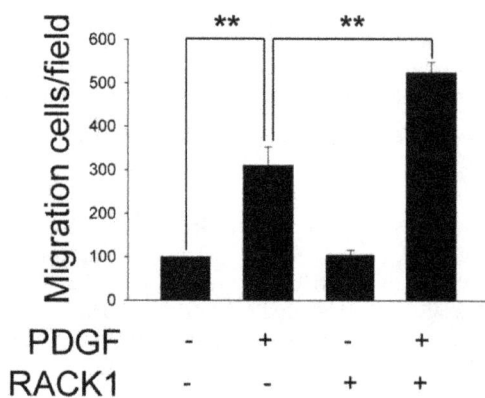

F

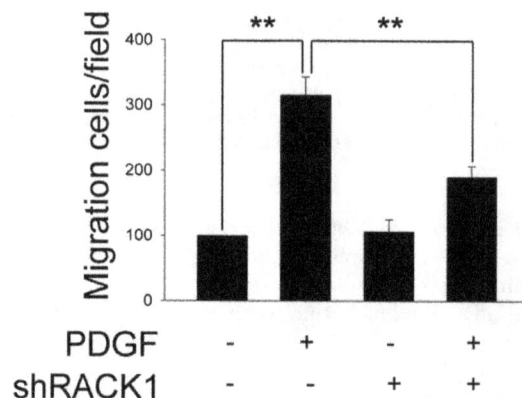

Figure 6. RACK1 is involved in the regulation of the pro-fibrogenic effects of PDGF. (A, B) Primary HSCs were incubated with lentivirus as indicated, starved for 6 h and treated with or without PDGF, followed by western blot analysis. (C, D) Primary HSCs were incubated with lentivirus as indicated, and treated with or without PDGF, followed by CCK8 assay. (E, F) Primary HSCs were treated as in (A, B), followed by migration assay. **, p<0.01.

RACK1 is involved in the regulation of TAA-induced liver fibrosis in mice

We next determined the role of RACK1 in TAA-induced liver fibrosis *in vivo*. Delivery of lentivirus carrying shRACK1 effectively suppressed the mRNA level of RACK1 both in HSCs and hepatocytes (Figure 7A and B). Moreover, western blot and histochemical staining also revealed that depletion of RACK1 remarkably attenuated TAA-induced up-regulation of α-SMA and collagen I in liver tissues (Figure 7C and D). Taken together, these results suggest that RACK1 is involved in the regulation of liver fibrogenesis *in vivo*.

RACK1 expression is positive relative to the stage of liver fibrosis

We next evaluated the expression of RACK1 in liver biopsy samples from patients with liver fibrosis. As shown in Figure 8A, the expression of RACK1 in fibrous septum is up-regulated, with the stage of liver fibrosis increases from F1 to F4. To further determine the role of RACK1 expression in fibrogenic cells, we also examined the correlation of RACK1 expression in fibrogenic cells with the fibrosis stage of clinical cases. As shown in Figure 8B, RACK1 expression in α-SMA+ cells positively correlated with the stage of liver fibrosis (F = 9.05, p<0.001). Taken together, these

results suggest that RACK1 may contribute to the progression of liver fibrosis in clinical cases.

Discussion

Liver fibrosis is the excessive accumulation of extracellular matrix proteins including collagen that occurs in most types of chronic liver diseases [13]. Advanced liver fibrosis results in cirrhosis, which is the most common non-neoplastic cause of death among hepatobiliary and digestive diseases, accounting for approximately 30000 deaths per year in the US [1]. In this study, we report that the expression of RACK1 is increased in activated HSCs in TGF-β1-dependent manner, and up-regulation of RACK1 induces TGF-β1 and PDGF-mediated pro-fibrogenic pathways as well as the differentiation, migration and proliferation of HSCs.

Activation of quiescent hepatic stellate cells (HSCs) into a myofibroblast-like phenotype is supposed to be the central event of liver fibrosis, and TGF-β1 is considered as a potent pro-fibrogenic cytokine responsible for HSC activation and migration. It has been reported that TGF-β1-deficient mice strongly attenuate the development of liver fibrosis, while overexpression of TGF-β1 in transgenic mice resulted in the acceleration of liver fibrosis progression [6]. TGF-β1 stimulates collagen gene transcription,

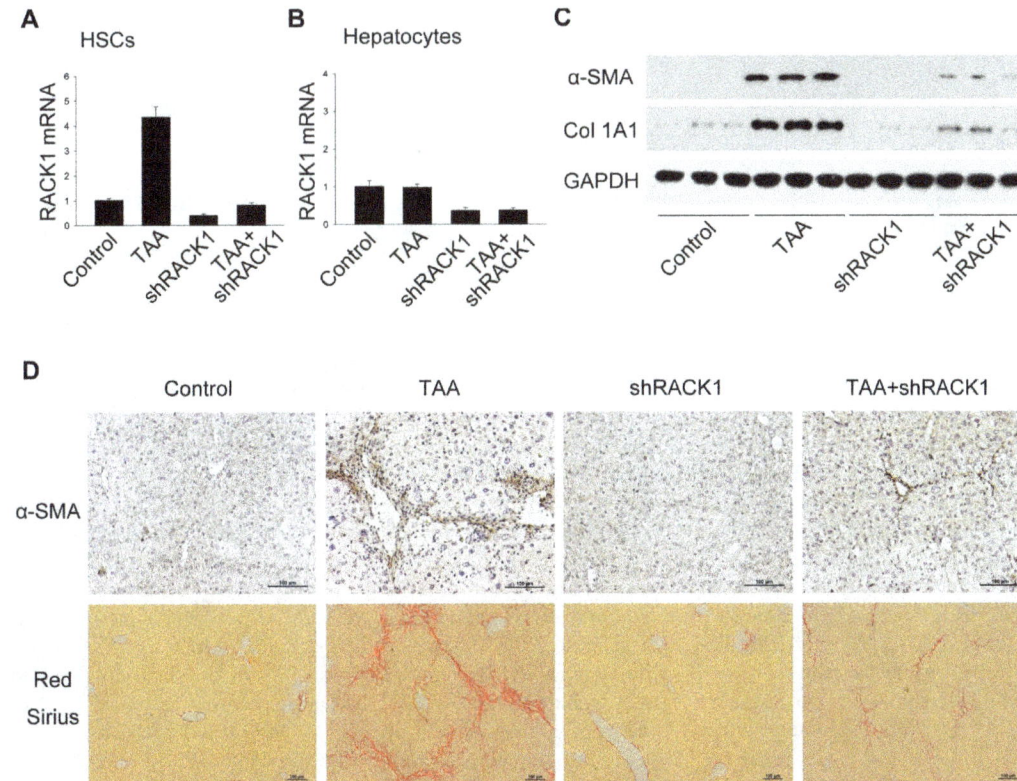

Figure 7. RACK1 is involved in the regulation of TAA-induced liver fibrosis in mice. Mice were treated with lentiviral particles expressing shRNA targeting RACK1 or non-target control, as well as TAA or vehicle control. (A, B) 8 weeks later, HSCs and hepatocytes were isolated and applied to qRT-PCR analysis to detect relative RACK1 expression. (C) Total protein lysates extracted from the livers were applied to western blot for α-SMA and collagen α1 type 1. (D) Liver sections were subjected to immunochemistry for α-SMA and Sirius Red staining. Scale bar, 100 μm.

A

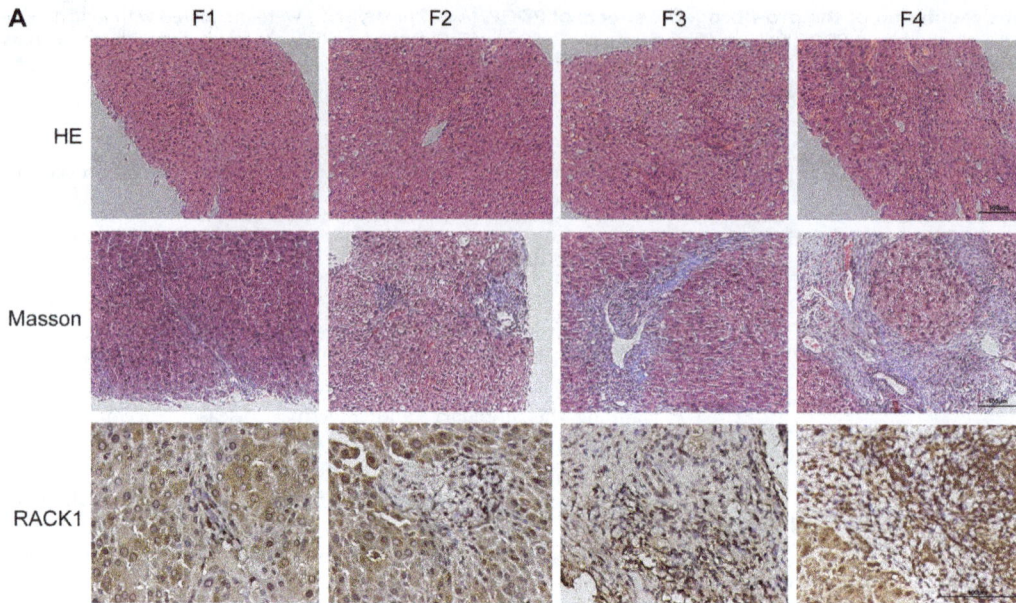

B

The correlation of RACK1 expression
in α-SMA⁺ cells with fibrosis stage in clinical cases

Score	Stage of liver fibrosis			
(RACK1)	F1	F2	F3	F4
1	6	3	0	0
2	4	7	3	1
3	2	4	7	9
Total	12	14	10	10

Note: One-way ANOVA analysis, F=9.05, p<0.001

Figure 8. RACK1 expression is positively relative to the stage of liver fibrosis. (A) The liver biopsy samples were collected from patients with different degrees of fibrosis, and applied to HE staining, Masson staining and immunohistochemistry analysis for RACK1. The images shown are representative of each group with different fibrotic stage. (B) The 46 cases were grouped according to the scoring of RACK1, and applied to One-way ANOVA analysis to detect the correlation of RACK1 expression in α-SMA+ cells with the stage of liver fibrosis.

suppresses MMPs expression and modulates the expression of integrins [33]. In our study, we also identified RACK1 as a novel downstream target of TGF-β1 in liver fibrosis through activating NF-κB. Though there have been reports that NF-κB and c-Jun might both modulate the transcription of RACK1 [27,28], our results indicated that TGF-β1 mediates the up-regulation of RACK1 in NF-κB-dependent and JNK-independent manners in HSCs, suggesting that the regulation of RACK1 transcription may vary in different types of cells (Figure 3). Moreover, in addition to TGF-β1, there are also several other fibrogenic and inflammatory cytokines that activate macrophages and HSCs, such as IL-6, IL-1β, TNF-α and PDGF. However, we found that administration of recombinant IL-6, IL-1β, TNF-α or PDGF showed little effect on RACK1 expression in HSCs, suggesting that the regulatory effect of TGF-β1 on RACK1 expression is specific in HSCs (data not shown).

RACK1 is a classical scaffold protein involved in the regulation of multiple signaling pathways and cellular functions. Though RACK1 has been reported to be implicated in the development of several kinds of diseases, the role of RACK1 in liver fibrosis is little understood. A previous research implied that RACK1 associated

with ADAM12 and promoted its translocation to membrane in PKC-dependent manner in HSCs, suggesting that RACK1 might contribute to the development of liver fibrosis [34]. In our study, we also found that RACK1 functioned as a potent regulator of TGF-β1 and PDGF signaling pathways, and promoted TGF-β1 and PDGF-mediated differentiation, proliferation and migration of HSCs, suggesting an essential role of RACK1 in the regulation of liver fibrogenesis. However, in addition to the HSCs differentiation into a myofibroblast-like phenotype, migration to the injured region and proliferation, there are several other aspects accelerating the initiation and progression of liver fibrosis, such as the survival of HSCs and the imbalance of ECM production and degradation. Since RACK1 has been reported to be involved in the regulation of cellular apoptosis and ADAM12 translation, it is likely that the up-regulation of RACK1 induced by TGF-β1 may contribute to liver fibrosis on other aspects.

Nowadays, mounting clinical evidences suggest that liver fibrosis can regress either by removing the cause of liver injury or treating the underlying diseases; however, there is no licensed anti-fibrotic therapies yet [35]. As the central event of liver fibrosis, activation of HSCs was investigated as the critical therapeutic target. It has been reported that in the animal model, removal of activated HSCs by apoptosis or reversal of hepatic myofibroblats to a quiescent state contributes to the regression of liver fibrosis [2,36]. Therefore, it is of great potential in developing new agents and strategies to regress liver fibrosis. Our data suggest RACK1 as a novel biomarker in the initiation and progression of liver fibrosis, and propose a strategy to target RACK1 as a potential adjuvant therapy for liver fibrosis treatment.

Supporting Information

Figure S1 TGF-β1 is required for the auto-activation of HSCs. Primary HSCs isolated from wild-type and *Tgfb1+/−* mice were cultured in DMEM supplemented with 10% fetal bovine serum. (A) The images showing the star shaped HSCs were captured at the day of 3 and 7 (scale bar = 100 μm). (B) The images showing vitamin A lipid droplet were captured at the day of 2, 5 and 8 (scale bar = 25 μm).

Acknowledgments

We would like to thank Prof. Xiaoling Wang (Shanghai University of Traditional Chinese Medicine) for the help in the isolation of primary hepatic cells. We thank Prof. Xizhong Shen and Dr. Jie Yin (Zhongshan Hospital of Fudan University) for the help in the collection of patient samples of liver biopsy.

Author Contributions

Conceived and designed the experiments: YYR DWJ. Performed the experiments: DWJ PKP FFD XJL. Analyzed the data: YYR DWJ LW WCW. Contributed reagents/materials/analysis tools: JXG LLS. Wrote the paper: DWJ YYR.

References

1. Friedman S (2003) Liver fibrosis ? from bench to bedside. Journal of Hepatology 38: 38–53.
2. Troeger JS, Mederacke I, Gwak GY, Dapito DH, Mu X, et al. (2012) Deactivation of hepatic stellate cells during liver fibrosis resolution in mice. Gastroenterology 143: 1073–1083 e1022.
3. Thomas P, Petrick AT, Toth CA, Fox ES, Elting JJ, et al. (1992) A peptide sequence on carcinoembryonic antigen binds to a 80 kD protein on Kupffer cells. Biochem Biophys Res Commun 188: 671–677.
4. Braunersreuther V, Viviani GL, Mach F, Montecucco F (2012) Role of cytokines and chemokines in non-alcoholic fatty liver disease. World J Gastroenterol 18: 727–735.
5. Sakata R, Ueno T, Nakamura T, Ueno H, Sata M (2004) Mechanical stretch induces TGF-beta synthesis in hepatic stellate cells. Eur J Clin Invest 34: 129–136.
6. Cong M, Iwaisako K, Jiang C, Kisseleva T (2012) Cell signals influencing hepatic fibrosis. Int J Hepatol 2012: 158547.
7. Gressner AM, Weiskirchen R (2006) Modern pathogenetic concepts of liver fibrosis suggest stellate cells and TGF-beta as major players and therapeutic targets. J Cell Mol Med 10: 76–99.
8. Yang C, Zeisberg M, Mosterman B, Sudhakar A, Yerramalla U, et al. (2003) Liver fibrosis: insights into migration of hepatic stellate cells in response to extracellular matrix and growth factors. Gastroenterology 124: 147–159.
9. Inagaki Y, Okazaki I (2007) Emerging insights into Transforming growth factor beta Smad signal in hepatic fibrogenesis. Gut 56: 284–292.
10. Kluwe J, Pradere JP, Gwak GY, Mencin A, De Minicis S, et al. (2010) Modulation of hepatic fibrosis by c-Jun-N-terminal kinase inhibition. Gastroenterology 138: 347–359.
11. Varela-Rey M, Montiel-Duarte C, Oses-Prieto JA, Lopez-Zabalza MJ, Jaffrezou JP, et al. (2002) p38 MAPK mediates the regulation of alpha1(I) procollagen mRNA levels by TNF-alpha and TGF-beta in a cell line of rat hepatic stellate cells(1). FEBS Lett 528: 133–138.
12. Luedde T, Schwabe RF (2011) NF-kappaB in the liver–linking injury, fibrosis and hepatocellular carcinoma. Nat Rev Gastroenterol Hepatol 8: 108–118.
13. Bataller R, Brenner DA (2005) Liver fibrosis. J Clin Invest 115: 209–218.
14. Marra F, Arrighi MC, Fazi M, Caligiuri A, Pinzani M, et al. (1999) Extracellular signal-regulated kinase activation differentially regulates platelet-derived growth factor's actions in hepatic stellate cells, and is induced by in vivo liver injury in the rat. Hepatology 30: 951–958.
15. Reif S, Lang A, Lindquist JN, Yata Y, Gabele E, et al. (2003) The role of focal adhesion kinase-phosphatidylinositol 3-kinase-akt signaling in hepatic stellate cell proliferation and type I collagen expression. J Biol Chem 278: 8083–8090.
16. Al-Reefy S, Osman H, Jiang W, Mokbel K (2010) Evidence for a pro-apoptotic function of RACK1 in human breast cancer. Oncogene 29: 5651; author reply 5652.
17. Nagashio R, Sato Y, Matsumoto T, Kageyama T, Satoh Y, et al. (2010) Expression of RACK1 is a novel biomarker in pulmonary adenocarcinomas. Lung Cancer 69: 54–59.
18. Adams DR, Ron D, Kiely PA (2011) RACK1, A multifaceted scaffolding protein: Structure and function. Cell Commun Signal 9: 22.
19. Ruan Y, Sun L, Hao Y, Wang L, Xu J, et al. (2012) Ribosomal RACK1 promotes chemoresistance and growth in human hepatocellular carcinoma. J Clin Invest 122: 2554–2566.
20. Deng L, Li G, Xi L, Yin A, Gao Y, et al. (2009) Hepatitis B virus inhibition in mice by lentiviral vector mediated short hairpin RNA. BMC Gastroenterol 9: 73.
21. Brunt EM (2000) Grading and staging the histopathological lesions of chronic hepatitis: the Knodell histology activity index and beyond. Hepatology 31: 241–246.
22. Geerts A, Eliasson C, Niki T, Wielant A, Vaeyens F, et al. (2001) Formation of normal desmin intermediate filaments in mouse hepatic stellate cells requires vimentin. Hepatology 33: 177–188.
23. Li WC, Ralphs KL, Tosh D (2010) Isolation and culture of adult mouse hepatocytes. Methods Mol Biol 633: 185–196.
24. Popov Y, Schuppan D (2009) Targeting liver fibrosis: strategies for development and validation of antifibrotic therapies. Hepatology 50: 1294–1306.
25. Barnes JL, Gorin Y (2011) Myofibroblast differentiation during fibrosis: role of NAD(P)H oxidases. Kidney Int 79: 944–956.
26. Friedman SL (1999) Cytokines and fibrogenesis. Semin Liver Dis 19: 129–140.
27. Choi DS, Young H, McMahon T, Wang D, Messing RO (2003) The mouse RACK1 gene is regulated by nuclear factor-kappa B and contributes to cell survival. Mol Pharmacol 64: 1541–1548.
28. Lopez-Bergami P, Huang C, Goydos JS, Yip D, Bar-Eli M, et al. (2007) Rewired ERK-JNK signaling pathways in melanoma. Cancer Cell 11: 447–460.
29. Ron D, Jiang Z, Yao L, Vagts A, Diamond I, et al. (1999) Coordinated movement of RACK1 with activated betaIIPKC. J Biol Chem 274: 27039–27046.
30. Yarwood SJ, Steele MR, Scotland G, Houslay MD, Bolger GB (1999) The RACK1 signaling scaffold protein selectively interacts with the cAMP-specific phosphodiesterase PDE4D5 isoform. J Biol Chem 274: 14909–14917.
31. Lopez-Bergami P, Habelhah H, Bhoumik A, Zhang W, Wang LH, et al. (2005) RACK1 mediates activation of JNK by protein kinase C [corrected]. Mol Cell 19: 309–320.
32. Bonner JC (2004) Regulation of PDGF and its receptors in fibrotic diseases. Cytokine Growth Factor Rev 15: 255–273.
33. Inagaki Y, Higashiyama R, Higashi K (2012) Novel anti-fibrotic modalities for liver fibrosis: molecular targeting and regenerative medicine in fibrosis therapy. J Gastroenterol Hepatol 27 Suppl 2: 85–88.
34. Bourd-Boittin K, Le Pabic H, Bonnier D, L'Helgoualc'h A, Theret N (2008) RACK1, a new ADAM12 interacting protein. Contribution to liver fibrogenesis. J Biol Chem 283: 26000–26009.
35. Ellis EL, Mann DA (2012) Clinical evidence for the regression of liver fibrosis. J Hepatol 56: 1171–1180.
36. Iredale JP, Benyon RC, Pickering J, McCullen M, Northrop M, et al. (1998) Mechanisms of spontaneous resolution of rat liver fibrosis. Hepatic stellate cell apoptosis and reduced hepatic expression of metalloproteinase inhibitors. J Clin Invest 102: 538–549.

21

Protection Effect of Kallistatin on Carbon Tetrachloride-Induced Liver Fibrosis in Rats via Antioxidative Stress

Xiaoping Huang, Xiao Wang, Yinghui Lv, Luli Xu, Junsheng Lin*, Yong Diao*

Institute of Molecular Medicine, Huaqiao University, Quanzhou, China

Abstract

Prolonged inflammation and oxidative stress are emerging as key causes of pathological wound healing and the development of liver fibrosis. We have investigated the effects of recombinant human kallistatin, produced in *Pichia. pastoris*, on preventing carbon tetrachloride (CCl_4)-induced liver fibrosis in rats. Daily administration of kallistatin prevented development of CCl_4-induced liver fibrosis, which was evidenced by histological study. In all kallistatin treated rats, activation of hepatic stellate cells (HSC) as assessed by s-smooth muscle actin staining was attenuated, TGF- β1 expression was inhibited, class I serum biomarkers associated with the process of fibrogenesis, such as hyaluronic acid, laminin, and procollagen III, were lowered, compared with that in the model control group. Furthermore, residual hepatic functional reserve was improved by kallistatin treatment. CCl_4 induced elevation of malondialdehyde level and reduced superoxide dismutase activity in the liver, while kallistatin reduced these oxidative parameters. We also investigated the effects of kallistatin on rat primary HSC and LX-2, the human HSC cell line. Kallistatin scavenged H_2O_2-induced ROS in the LX-2 cells, and suppressed the activation of primary HSC. These results suggest recombinant human kallistatin might be a promising drug candidate for therapeutic intervention of liver fibrosis.

Editor: David L. McCormick, IIT Research Institute, United States of America

Funding: This research is funded by National Natural Science Foundation of China (81271691, 81201183, 81270734); Program for International S&T Cooperation Projects of China (No. 2011DFG33320); Key Science & Technology Project of the Fujian Province in China (No. 2013N5007). The funders had no role in study design, data collection and analysis, decision to publish, or preparation of the manuscript.

Competing Interests: The authors have declared that no competing interests exist.

* E-mail: junshenglin@hqu.edu.cn (JL); diaoyong@hqu.edu.cn (YD)

Introduction

Advanced liver fibrosis resulting in cirrhosis, liver failure, portal hypertension and hepatocellular carcinoma (HCC) is one of the major causes of morbidity and mortality worldwide. The only curative treatment for liver cirrhosis is transplantation nowadays. But its wide application is restrained by the limitation of the donor organ availability and the recipient conditions. Research on molecular and cellular pathogenesis of hepatic fibrosis might contribute to provide a complementary approach of liver transplantation. The long-held dogma that liver fibrosis is irreversible and relentlessly progressive has been challenged by the increasing evidences that liver fibrosis is a highly dynamic process [1]. Progress in elucidation of the cellular and molecular mechanisms of hepatic fibrosis has brought us to a juncture where translation of these discoveries into treatments is nearing reality. Numerous clinical and experimental observations have demonstrated that prolonged inflammation and oxidative stress may cause pathological wound healing and the development of liver fibrosis [2]. Therefore, selectively target the detrimental effects of oxidant stress could be a strategy for antifibrotic therapy in the future.

Recent research has shown that kallistatin, a kind of plasma protein that belongs to the serine protease inhibitor family, is closely involved in cellular adaptation to oxidative stress, and the anti-inflammatory response. Kallistatin levels are reduced in the kidney and blood vessels under oxidative stress conditions; depletion of endogenous kallistatin with anti-kallistatin antibody exacerbates renal and cardiovascular oxidative stress and subsequence inflammation [3].

Adenovirus-mediated human SERPINA4 gene (coding kallistatin) delivery reduced the oxidative stress, and prevented salt-induced kidney injury, inflammation and fibrosis by inhibiting the expression levels of reactive oxygen species (ROS)-induced proinflammatory cytokines and transforming growth factor-beta1 (TGF-β1) [4]. Adenovirus-mediated human kallistatin gene delivery also suppressed arthritis by inhibiting inflammation in a rat model of arthritis [5]. Kallistatin gene transfer into rat hearts improved cardiac function and reduced ventricular remodeling, oxidative stress, cardiomyocyte apoptosis, and inflammatory cell accumulation after acute myocardial ischemia/reperfusion and chronic heart failure [6–8]. Collectively, these findings indicated that kallistatin may play an important role in the protection against oxidative stress-induced inflammatory responses and organ damage. In our previous study, human kallistatin gene therapy alleviated the carbon tetrachloride (CCl_4)-induced oxidative stress and inflammatory response, and reduced the liver damage in a mouse model [9]. However, fundamental difficulties remain associated with expression regulation of the transferred gene and viral vector-based immunogenicity.

Functional recombinant human kallistatin has been produced in our laboratory using a yeast expression system [10]. To determine whether the recombinant human kallistatin is beneficial in experimental liver fibrosis, rats were treated with the recombinant human kallistatin. It has been evidenced that the recombinant human kallistatin exhibited hepatoprotective and antifibrotic effects in CCl₄-induced liver fibrosis by daily intraperitoneal injection.

Materials and Methods

Reagents

Recombinant human kallistatin was expressed in *Pichia pastoris* strain GS115 and purified with a series of chromatographic steps, mainly Phenyl Superose and Heparin Sepharose FF chromatography. The rabbit anti-rat TGF-β1 polyclonal antibodies and rabbit anti-rat α-smooth muscle actin (α-SMA) monoclonal antibody were obtained from Biotechnology Development Co (Fuzhou, China). Kallistatin, hyaluronic acid (HA), procollagen III and laminin (LN) ELISA kits were purchased from R&D Systems (Minneapolis, America). Alanine aminotransferase (ALT), aspartate aminotransferaseam (AST), malondialdehyde (MDA) and superoxide dismutase (SOD) kits were purchased from the Biotechnology Research Institute (Nanjing, China). Hydrogen peroxide was purchased from Sigma. Molecular Probe dihydroethidium (DHE) was purchased from Invitrogen (New York, America). Hydrogen peroxide (H_2O_2) was prepared as described previously [11].

Rat models of liver fibrosis and treatment protocol

Male Sprague-Dawley (SD) rats (150–200 g) were obtained from the Experimental Center of Medical Scientific Academy of Fujian. Animal experiments were approved by Animal Ethics committee of Huaqiao University. The animals were cared for in accordance with protocols approved by the Animal Care and Use Committee of Huaqiao University. Animals were housed in a temperature-controlled environment (20–22°C) and 75±2% relatively humidity with a 12 h/12 h light/dark cycle, and acclimatized for one week before the experiment. A total of 40 rats were studied. The rats were divided into five groups, each group included 8 rats. All groups, excluding group 1, received a subcutaneous injection of 10 ml/kg carbon tetrachloride (CCl₄) dissolved in peanut oil (25%, v/v) twice a week for 7 weeks. Animals in group 1 were subcutaneously injected with the carrier vehicle peanut oil (10 ml/kg daily) only as a negative control and group 2 received CCl₄ delivered by the vehicle peanut oil as a model control. Group 3, 4 and 5 were injected intraperitoneally with kallistatin, at a dose of 2, 0.5 and 0.125 mg/kg daily, respectively, during the period of CCl₄ treatment.

At the end of the treatment, all animals were anesthetized with ketamine hydrochloride (30 mg/kg, *iv*) and then sacrificed. Blood samples were immediately collected into tubes and then centrifuged at 3000 g for 10 min at 4°C for serum preparation. Specimens were cut out from the liver and washed immediately with an ice-cold PBS to remove blood. A half of the each specimen was stored at −80°C for future analysis. The other half was fixed in a 10% formalin solution for histopathological analysis.

Biochemical analysis

The serum levels of AST, ALT and albumin were measured by the commercial colorimetric kits, according to the manufacturer's instructions. Serum hyaluronic acid, type III collagen and LN were determined by ELISA using commercially available kits according to the manufacturer's instructions.

Hydroxyproline assay

Liver hydroxyproline content was determined by the method reported by Iwaisako *et al* [12]. Hydroxyproline content was expressed as microgram of hydroxyproline per gram liver.

MDA and SOD assay

The extent of lipid peroxidation was estimated by measurement of MDA formation in the liver homogenates based on the reaction of MDA with thiobarbituric acid (TBA) [13]. Two molecules of chromogenic reagent (2-Thiobarbituric acid) react with one molecule of MDA to yield a stable chromophore. The assay was performed using a MDA kit followed the manufacturer instructions. Briefly, 200 μL TBA and antioxidants reagents from the kits were respectively added into a microcentrifuge tube containing a 100-μL aliquot of each of the liver homogenate and 100 μL of MDA standard solution, and then vortexed. The tubes was incubated at 95°C for 40 min and centrifuged at 4,000×g for 10 min. Then 300 μL of the supernatant from each of the tubes was transferred to a well of a microplate and the absorbance measured at 532 nm using a multi-detection microplate reader (Infinite 200, Tecan). The level of MDA is expressed as nmol MDA/mg homogenate protein. Protein concentration was determined according to Bradford method using bovine serum albumin as a standard.

Liver SOD activity was measured as previously described [14] with slight modification. Briefly, 0.1 mL of the liver homogenate was mixed with 1.5 mL of 20 mM Tris-HCl (containing 1 mM EDTA, pH 8.2), and then 0.1 mL of 15 mM pyrogallol was added. The activity was measured at 420 nm for 3 min and expressed as U/mg protein. One unit was determined as the amount of enzyme that inhibited the oxidation of pyrogallol by 50%.

Histopathology examinations

Specimens of the liver were fixed in 10% formaldehyde, processed using routine histology procedures, embedded in paraffin, cut in 5 μm sections and mounted on a slide. The samples were stained with hematoxylin and eosin (H&E) and Sirius red respectively. The content of collagen (stained light red on a pale yellow background) was quantified using the histogram module of Photoshop 8.0 software (Adobe).

Immunohistochemistry

To detect the immunohistochemical localization of α-SMA and TGF-β1, sections from formalin-fixed, paraffin-embedded specimens were deparaffinized and rehydrated in decreasing concentrations of ethylalcohol. All tissue sections were treated with fresh 3% hydrogen peroxide for 20 min, and then washed with PBS. The sections were sequentially incubated with 1% normal blocking serum for 30 min, with rabbit anti-rat α-SMA monoclonal antibody or the rabbit anti-rat TGF-β1 polyclonal antibodies incubate for 60 min, with appropriate HRP-conjugated goat anti-rabbit secondary antibody for 60 min and with DAB as a substrate. All the incubation steps were performed at room temperature and three washes with PBS were applied between the steps. Negative controls were obtained by omitting the primary antibodies. The sections, counterstained with haematoxylin, were then mounted and observed under light microscopy by a blinded pathologist.

Hepatic stellate cell culture and activation

Hepatic stellate cells (HSCs) were isolated from livers of male SD rats by the discontinuous density gradient centrifugation technique as previously described [11], cultured in DMEM supplemented with 10% fetal bovine serum and 100 U/mL penicillin, 100 μg/mL streptomycin in a dish coated with collagen, and maintained at 37°C in a 5% CO₂ incubator. The purity of the isolated HSCs was assessed through direct cell counting under a phase-contrast microscope by intrinsic vitamin A autofluorescence and by immunohistochemistry using a monoclonal antibody against desmin. Cell viability was examined by trypan blue dye exclusion. Both cell purity and viability were in higher than 90%.

To characterize the effect of kallistatin on HSCs activation, 1×10^4 primary HSCs were seeded in a 96-well-plate well with or without kallistatin in culture medium containing 10% FBS and incubated in 37°C. The media were changed every other day. Six days later, activated HSCs were identified with immunocyto-chemical analysis of rabbit anti-rat α-SMA monoclonal antibody.

Determination of intracellular Reactive Oxygen Species

Human HSC cell line (LX-2) is a widely used hepatic stellate cell in the fibrosis investigation [15,16]. The LX-2 cell line was purchased from BioHermes Inc (Jiangsu province, China). LX-2 were cultured in 96-well plates at a density of 1×10^4 cells/well for 24 h. Kallistatin at different final concentrations (2–50 μg/ml) was added and preincubated for 12 h. Then, the media were replaced with a serum-free medium with 1200 μM H_2O_2. Control cells were received a serum-free medium without H_2O_2. The cells were incubated for 6 h, and then with addition of 10 μM DHE for 30 min. Intracellular ROS contents were measured by quantifying conversion of DHE to fluorescent ethidium (ETH) [16]. ETH was excited at 535 nm, and emissions were monitored at 635 nm using a photoncounting photomultiplier.

Statistical analysis

Results were shown as mean±SD. Comparisons among groups were performed by one-way ANOVA, followed by Scheffe's test. The criterion for statistical significance was set at $p<0.05$ and highly significance at $p<0.01$.

Results

Kallistatin protected against CCl_4-induced liver injury

A rat hepatic fibrosis model with chronic CCl_4 injection was established, the degree of liver fibrosis was assessed by H&E and Sirius red staining (Figure 1A). Negative control (oil-injected without CCl_4) rats did not show any liver damage. Following CCl_4 administration, histological examination of the livers by H&E staining demonstrated a distorted architecture with extensive fibrosis combined with development of micronodules throughout the liver parenchyma. Liver injury was attenuated in the kallistatin-treated groups. Fibrillar collagen deposition as an indicator of liver fibrosis was determined by Sirius red staining. Repeated injection of CCl_4 induced bridging fibrosis. In contrast, by addition of kallistatin, the pathological progression was attenuated showing fewer and smaller fibrotic nodules. Quantification of Sirius red staining showed obvious increase in collagen accumulation in CCl_4-induced fibrotic rats compared with the negative control group, while combined administration of kallistatin resulted in a dose-response decrease in staining positive area (Figure 1B). These data supported that kallistatin administration was efficient in reducing pathological collagen deposition and structure damage in the CCl_4-induced rat hepatic fibrosis model.

The results were further confirmed by analysis of hydroxyproline content in liver. Fibrosis, which is the final result of prolonged liver injury, can be quantified by hydroxyproline analysis and expressed as liver collagen content. Hydroxylation of prolines stabilizes collagen, and increased hydroxyproline content is a marker of fibrosis [17]. The CCl_4-treated rats had significantly higher hepatic hydroxyproline content than the oil-injected control rats (Figure 2). Whereas, administration of kallistatin

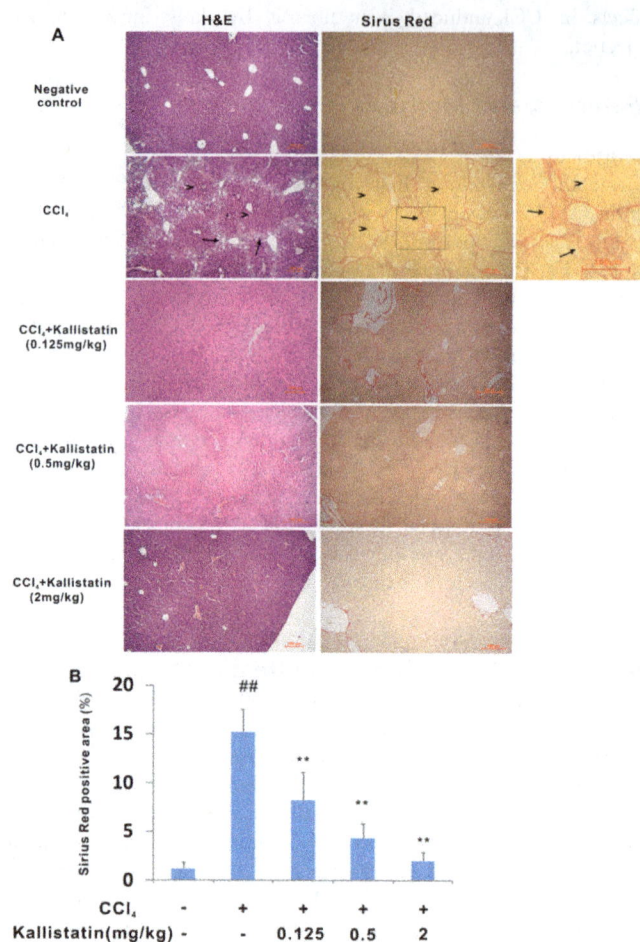

Figure 1. Kallistatin prevents CCl_4–induced injury to hepatic structure in rats. (A) Representative images of H&E or Sirius red stained sections (original magnifications ×40). Hyperplastic proliferation of hepatocytes in nodular formations (arrowheaded) surrounded by fibrotic septa (arrowed). Scale bars = 100 μm. (B) Collagen deposition was evaluated by Sirius red staining and quantitated by image analysis. Data are expressed as mean±SD (n = 8). ## $p<0.01$ vs. negative control; * $p<0.01$ vs. model control group.

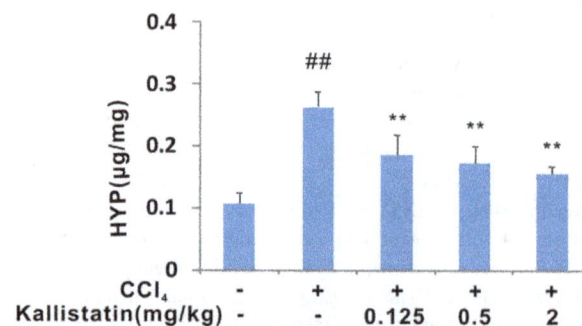

Figure 2. Effects of kallistatin on hepatic hydroxyproline content in CCl_4-induced liver fibrosis rats in a dose-dependent manner. The results are shown as the mean±SD (n = 8). ## $p<0.01$ vs. negative control; *$p<0.05$ vs. model control group; ** $p<0.01$ vs. model control group.

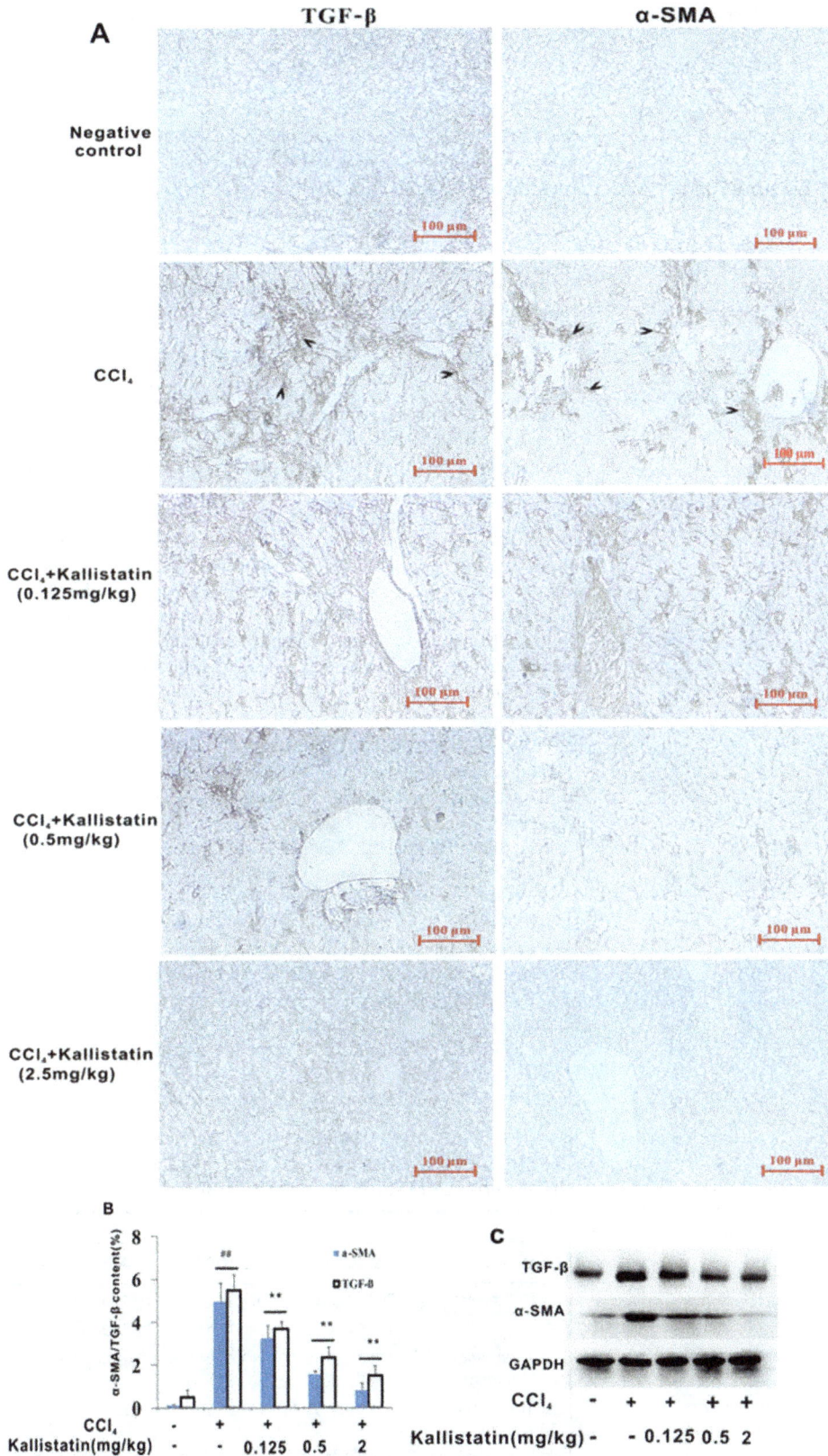

Figure 3. Kallistatin prevents CCl$_4$–induced liver fibrogenesis in rats. (A) Representative images of immunohistochemical staining for TGF-β1 (brown in color, arrowheaded) and α-SMA (brown in color, arrowheaded) are shown (original magnifications ×10) respectively. Expression of α-SMA around the periportal fibrotic band areas, central vein and fibrous septa were arrowed. Scale bars = 100 μm. (B) Deposition of α-SMA and TGF- β1 was quantitated by image analysis based on the immunohistochemistry results. Data are expressed as mean±SD (n = 8). ## $p < 0.01$ vs. negative control; ** $p < 0.01$ vs. model control group. (C) Immunoblotting analysis of α-SMA and TGF- β1 in livers from CCl$_4$ alone or plus kallistatin treated rats. Data from immunoblotting were confirmed, showing kallistatin-dependent abrogation of α-SMA and TGF-β1 expression. Immunoblotting and

immunohistochemistry results were consistent. Housekeeping proteins GAPDH are useful as loading controls for western blot and protein normalization.

reduced the hepatic hydroxyproline content in CCl_4-induced hepatic fibrosis rats in a dose-dependent manner (Figure 2).

Kallistatin protected the liver against CCl_4-induced fibrogenesis

Histological assessment of liver tissue has been the bedrock for diagnosis and staging of fibrosis. However, as a relatively static process of liver injury, fibrosis content alone is not enough to convey the information about the fibrogenic activity. Accordingly, tests that reflect fibrogenesis are important complements to the tests that assess only fibrosis content. As a marker of HSCs activation α-SMA is one of the sensitive indicators of the rate of fibrogenesis [2]. Although several potential non-HSC sources of

myofibroblast have been identified, the concept that major myofibroblasts in hepatic fibrosis can be recognized as activated HSCs is still generally accepted [2]. Our results showed that there were hardly any α-SMA positive cells in the negative control (Figure 3). In contrast, considerable expression of α-SMA was detected in the model control group, around the periportal fibrotic band areas, central vein and fibrous septa (Figure 3). Expression of α-SMA in all the CCl_4 plus kallistatin-treated groups showed a remarkable reduction, compared with the model control group, although higher than that in the negative control.

Pro-inflammatory cytokine TGF-β1 is a central regulator in chronic liver disease, contributing to all stages of disease progression, from initial liver injury through inflammation and fibrosis to cirrhosis and HCC. TGF-β1 is the most potent inducer of collagen I and other matrix constituents, and thus inhibiting its actions remain a major focus of antifibrotic efforts in liver. TGF-β1 expression was significantly increased in the liver sections in the model control group (Figure 3) comparing with the negative control. Expression levels of TGF-β1 in the CCl_4 plus kallistatin-treated groups were significantly lower than that in the fibrosis model control group, although higher than that in the negative control (Figure 3). These results indicated that kallistatin suppresses the CCl_4-induced fibrogenic activity related to down-regulation of TGF-β1.

Effect of kallistatin on class I serum biomarkers

Fibrosis accumulation is a dynamic process resulting from liver injury. The formation of an interstitial collagen-rich matrix represents a change in both the quality and quantity of the extracellular matrix (ECM). Class I serum biomarkers are associated with the process of fibrogenesis. Their presence in the serum is the result of the turnover of ECM. Several class I markers, such as HA, LN and procollagen III, represent attractive indicators to measure directly the fibrogenic process that leads to clinical complications [15]. CCl_4 treatment markedly stimulated HA, LN and procollagen III releasing in comparison with the control group ($p < 0.01$). The serum HA, LN and procollagen III levels in the three kallistatin groups were significantly lower than that in the model control group ($p < 0.01$–0.05) in a dose-dependent manner (Figure 4). These data further demonstrated

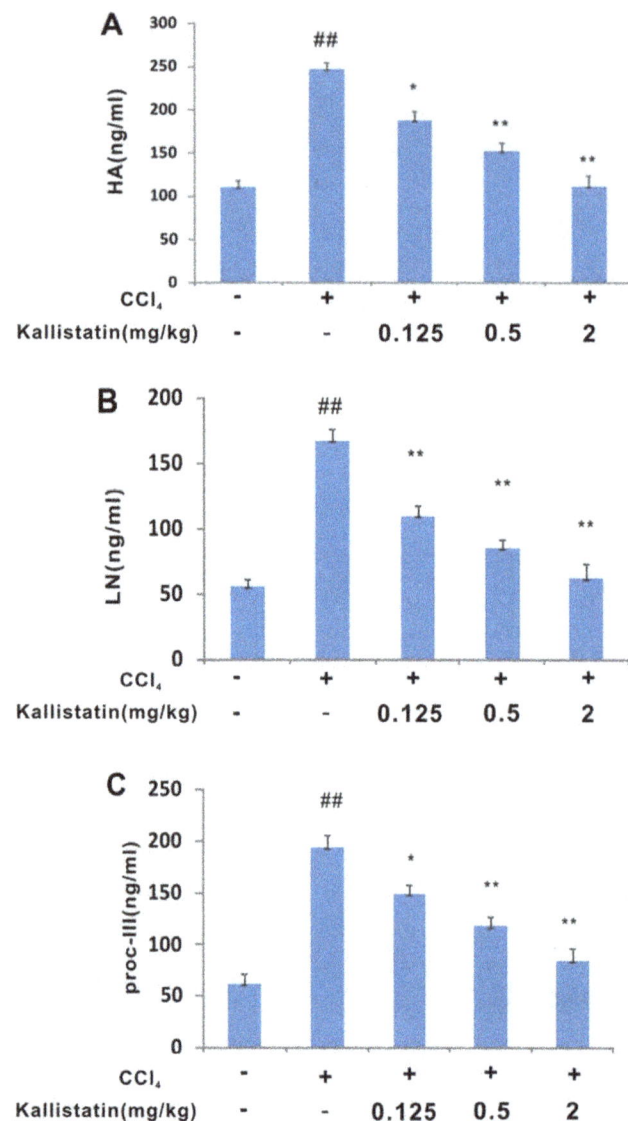

Figure 4. Kallistatin prevents CCl_4–induced increase of serum HA (A), LN (B) and procollagen III (C) levels in rats. The results are shown as the mean±SD (n = 8). ## $p < 0.01$ vs. negative control; *$p < 0.05$ vs. model control group; ** $p < 0.01$ vs. model control group.

Table 1. Effects of kallistatin on serum AST, ALT and Albumin in CCl_4-induced liver fibrosis rats (n = 8).

Treatment	AST(U/L)	ALT(U/L)	Albumin(g/L)
negative control	78.99±2.63	66.29±5.29	45.50±3.20
CCl_4	177.43±4.11##	140.77±15.27##	25.3±2.50##
CCl_4+kallistatin (0.125 mg/kg)	114.07±5.88**	102.86±17.04**	29.38±2.10*
CCl_4+kallistatin (0.5 mg/kg)	101.25±4.53**	92.65±10.25**	35.68±4.35**
CCl_4+kallistatin (2 mg/ kg)	85.77±3.51**	81.23±5.99**	42.51±3.090**

The results are showed as mean±SD.
##$p < 0.01$ vs. negative control;
*$p < 0.05$ vs. model control;
**$p < 0.01$ vs. model control.

Table 2. Effects of kallistatin on MDA and SOD in CCl₄-induced liver fibrosis rats (n = 8).

Treatment	MDA(nmol/mg)	SOD(nU/mg)
negative control	0.48±0.14	37.13±3.70
CCl₄	0.95±0.09##	22.66±2.66##
CCl₄+kallistatin (0.125 mg/kg)	0.72±0.10*	27.45±3.48**
CCl₄+kallistatin (0.5 mg/kg)	0.59±0.08**	30.56±4.56**
CCl₄+kallistatin (2 mg/kg)	0.48±0.07**	33.39±3.32**

The results are showed as the mean±SD (n = 8).
##$p < 0.01$ vs. negative control;
*$p < 0.05$ vs. model control group;
**$p < 0.01$ vs. model control group.

the efficacy of kallistatin on preventing liver from fibrogenesis.

Effect of kallistatin on functional reserve of rat liver

Assessment of residual hepatic functional reserve is indispensable for stratifying the severity of liver fibrosis and cirrhosis. No single marker is entirely reliable for predicting residual function, since hepatocytes possess a wide array of different functions. Tests of this type provide more information than simple hepatic histologic features about the progression of liver fibrosis, irrespective of the etiology. Hepatic capacity of protein synthesis is regarded as an important aspect of the hepatic functional reserve [14]. Serum albumin levels are commonly used as an important marker. The administration of CCl₄ caused severe liver damage characterized by significant decreases ($p < 0.01$) in serum albumin, compared with the control group (Table 1). Serum albumin levels in the three kallistatin groups increased significantly, compared to the model control group. There was an obvious dose-respond relationship on the liver function recovery among kallistatin treatment groups.

We also measured the serum AST and ALT levels to determine the degree of residual hepatic functional reserve in the rats (Table 1). Consistent with the albumin data, significantly lower levels of the serum AST and ALT were resulted from the addition of kallistatin compared to the fibrosis model group.

Kallistatin protected from liver oxidative stress

Oxidative stress is known to play a critical role in CCl₄-induced liver damage and fibrosis formation. MDA is one of the end products from lipid peroxidation, and can be used as a marker of oxidative stress to assess lipid peroxidation. On the other hand, SOD and catalase are important antioxidant enzymes that function as endogenous free radical scavengers. Our data showed that the MDA level was significantly higher in liver homogenates of CCl₄-intoxicated rats compared with the negative control group (Table 2). Treatment with kallistatin significantly reduced the MDA levels. Conversely, the levers of SOD were significantly increased in the livers of rats in the fibrosis groups treated with kallistatin (Table 2), compared with the fibrosis model group. These data suggest that kallistatin increases SOD activity and suppresses oxidative stress in the liver.

Kallistatin scavenged H₂O₂ -induced ROS in vitro

H₂O₂ is widely used to make oxidative stress model *in vitro*. After H₂O₂ exposure, oxidative stress results from increased intracellular ROS production and decreased ROS scavenging. To explore the mechanism of the protective effect of kallistatin on oxidative stress-induced damage in LX-2 cells, we examined the effect of kallistatin on intracellular ROS production. To determine whether kallistatin prevents H₂O₂-induced ROS generation, the concentration of intracellular ROS was evaluated by the changes in ETH fluorescence intensity. H₂O₂ exposure caused an apparent increase in ROS levels compared to control group, whereas pretreatment with kallistatin resulted in reduced ROS levels dose-dependently (Figure 5).

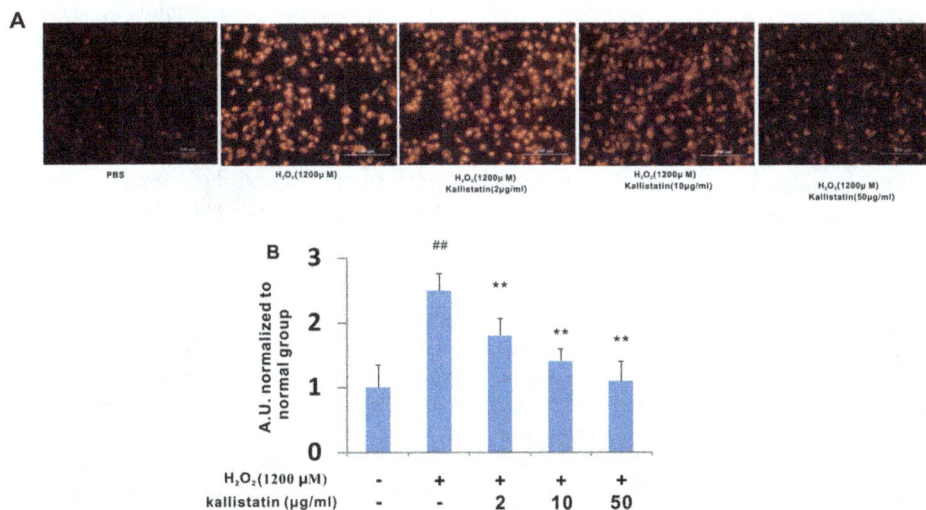

Figure 5. Effect of kallistatin on intracellular ROS levels after H₂O₂ exposure in LX-2. Cells were treated without or with kallistatin (2 μg/ml, 10 μg/ml and 50 μg/ml, respectively) prior to H₂O₂ challenge. ROS levels were measured using fluorescent probe DCFH-DA from the cells. (A) Representative images of ROS levels. Scale bars = 100 μm. (B) Intensity arbitrary units (A.U.) reflecting the relative value of intracellular ROS levels. Each value represents the mean±SD of triplicates. ## $p < 0.01$ vs. normal; **$p < 0.01$ vs. H₂O₂ alone.

A α-SMA

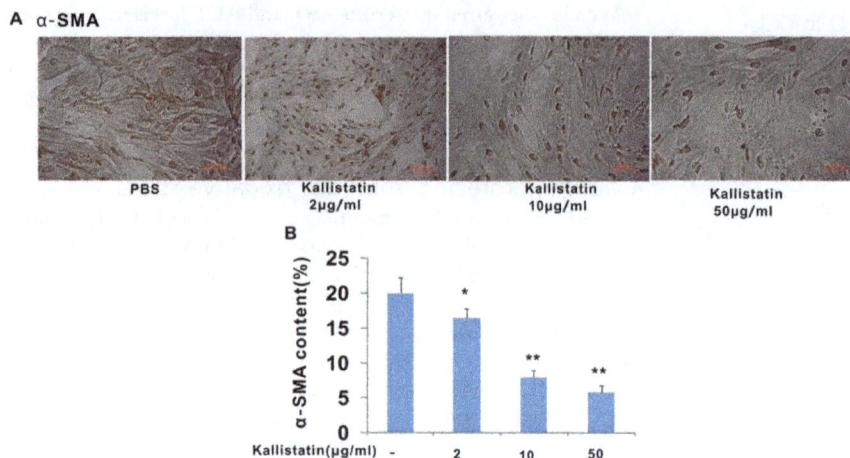

Figure 6. Kallistatin suppressed the expression of α-SMA, the marker of activated HSCs. (**A**) Cultured HSCs on days 6 were fixed in 4% paraformaldehyde and subjected to immunocytochemistry analysis of α-SMA (brown colored). Scale bars = 100 μm. (**B**) Deposition of α-SMA and TGF-β1 was quantitated by image analysis based on the immunohistochemistry results. Data are expressed as mean±SD (n = 8)*$p<0.05$ vs. PBS group; ** $p<0.01$ vs. PBS group.

Kallistatin suppressed the activation of primary cultured HSCs

To find whether kallistatin can inhibit HSCs activation, we performed *in vitro* studies in primary cultures of HSCs. Generally, isolated primary HSCs undergo autonomous activation when cultured in plastic dishes, and the activation is associated with the expression of α-SMA. The expression levels of α-SMA were demonstrated with immunocytochemistry analysis. Our data showed that α-SMA was expressed and uniformly distributed in the cytoplasm (Figure 6). The activated HSCs exhibited a stretched morphology with developed stress fibers, which consisted of α-SMA. Kallistatin suppressed α-SMA expression in HSCs dose-dependently.

Discussion

Chronic liver diseases constitute a global challenge. Current medical treatments for these diseases have achieved limited efficacy. All chronic liver diseases can lead to hepatic fibrosis and eventually liver failure. It is in high demand to find new medicines for the treatment of liver diseases and control of fibrogenesis [18,19].

Kallistatin is a pleiotropic cytokine which has anti-inflammatory and anti-oxidant properties, and may hold therapeutic promise in prevention of various diseases, including cardiometabolic disorders [20], vascular injury [3,8], arthritis [5,21,22], cancer [5,23–25], kidney fibrosis [4], cardiac hypertrophy and fibrosis [6]. Studies of kallistatin gene delivery have shown significantly alleviated the CCl$_4$-induced oxidative stress and inflammatory response, and reduced the liver damage in mouse models [9].

All the *in vivo* experiments with the efficacy of kallistatin on fibrosis were based on kallistatin gene delivery methods [4,6,9]. The safety concern on gene delivery vectors slows down the successful translation to the clinic. On the other hand, the recombinant human proteins sector still represents a significant and growing proportion of the overall pharmaceutical market. The recombinant kallistatin contains 100% human sequence. To our knowledge, the present study has for the first time shown the hepatoprotective effect of recombinant kallistatin protein on CCl$_4$-induced hepatic fibrosis in rats.

HSCs have been recognized as the main matrix-producing cells in the process of liver fibrosis. The identification of HSCs has been a key development in understanding the process of liver fibrosis. Activation of HSCs is the dominant event in hepatic fibrogenesis, which is characterized by the transformation of quiescent cells into proliferative, fibrogenic, and contractile myofibroblasts. The expression level of α-SMA is a sensitive indicator of the fibrogenic myofibroblasts. We have found that the recombinant human kallistatin effectively inhibited the myofibroblast-like activation of isolated rat HSCs and reduced the expression of α-SMA in vitro. We have tested the hypothesis that the suppression of myofibroblast-like transformation and activation of HSCs upon kallistatin treatment may help alleviate CCl$_4$-induced liver fibrosis in vivo. Indeed, the *in vivo* data showed that CCl$_4$-induced liver injury and collagen deposition in the experimental groups were accompanied by high expressions of TGF-β1, indicating that the TGF-β1 active HSCs classic pathway is active. Damaged resident liver cells triggered a profibrogenic response that stimulates TGF-β1 expression, and converts latent TGF-β1 into the active form, which provokes early HSCs activation. The recombinant human kallistatin was administered at the initial stage of hepatic fibrosis, and continued on a period of 7-week, so that an adequate biological effect could be exhibited. The recombinant human kallistatin treatment significantly reduced the expression levels of TGF-β1 and α-SMA in liver along with the progress of fibrogenesis in the rat model, indicating that the recombinant kallistatin had an inhibitory effect on hepatic fibrosis (Figure 1), at least partly via down regulation of the expressions of TGF-β1 and suppression of HSCs activation (Figure 3).

Since persistent inflammation and oxidative stress always precede and accompany with liver fibrosis, drugs that inhibit the inflammatory cascade and ROS generation typically have antifibrotic effects. Recent findings have indicated that kallistatin may play an important role in the protection against oxidative stress-induced inflammatory responses and organ damage. In a highly reproducible rat resistant hepatocyte model, kallistatin was not detectable or at very low levels in nodule tissue compared with normal liver by proteomics study [26]. A significantly reduced kallistatin level was seen in plasma samples from patients with chronic, severe liver disease [27], suggesting that kallistatin is produced mostly in the liver and can be consumed during inflammation in the liver. The results of the present study demonstrated that cells pretreated with kallistatin decreased the formation of ROS products after exposure to H_2O_2 (Figure 5), which supported the idea that kallistatin protected cells from oxidative stress-induced cytotoxicity by its antioxidant property. SOD is considered to be the most relevant enzyme involved in detoxification of H_2O_2 and protection of hepatocytes from oxidative stress. The inhibited activities of SOD induced by CCl_4 *in vivo* were attenuated by kallistatin. The results obtained here provide strong evidence that kallistatin attenuated ROS formation, and exerted a protective effect against CCl_4-induced liver injury.

Chronic liver disease results in hepatic fibrosis and cirrhosis. Complications of cirrhosis include ascites, portal hypertension, encephalopathy, liver failure, and high risk of HCC. Despite no drug has yet clinically available as an effective antifibrotic agent, the progress in the research on cellular and molecular biology of the liver fibrosis and cirrhosis has provided an opportunity to develop antifibrotic therapies. The findings reported here suggest kallistatin is effective to reduce inflammation and immune response, and to attenuate ROS induced by CCl_4 injection. Further investigation toward treating patients with chronic liver diseases should be promoted.

Author Contributions

Conceived and designed the experiments: XH YD. Performed the experiments: XH XW LX. Analyzed the data: YL JL. Contributed reagents/materials/analysis tools: JL. Wrote the paper: XH YD.

References

1. Pellicoro A, Ramachandran P, Iredale JP (2012) Reversibility of liver fibrosis. Fibrogenesis Tissue Repair 5 Suppl 1: S26.
2. Friedman SL (2010) Evolving challenges in hepatic fibrosis. Nat Rev Gastroenterol Hepatol 7: 425–436.
3. Liu Y, Bledsoe G, Hagiwara M, Shen B, Chao L, et al. (2012) Depletion of endogenous kallistatin exacerbates renal and cardiovascular oxidative stress, inflammation, and organ remodeling. Am J Physiol Renal Physiol 303: F1230–1238.
4. Shen B, Hagiwara M, Yao YY, Chao L, Chao J (2008) Salutary effect of kallistatin in salt-induced renal injury, inflammation, and fibrosis via antioxidative stress. Hypertension 51: 1358–1365.
5. Wang CR, Chen SY, Wu CL, Liu MF, Jin YT, et al. (2005) Prophylactic adenovirus-mediated human kallistatin gene therapy suppresses rat arthritis by inhibiting angiogenesis and inflammation. Arthritis Rheum 52: 1319–1324.
6. Gao L, Yin H, S. Smith R J, Chao L, Chao J (2008) Role of kallistatin in prevention of cardiac remodeling after chronic myocardial infarction. Lab Invest 88: 1157–1166.
7. Chao J, Yin H, Yao YY, Shen B, Smith RS, Jr., et al. (2006) Novel role of kallistatin in protection against myocardial ischemia-reperfusion injury by preventing apoptosis and inflammation. Hum Gene Ther 17: 1201–1213.
8. Yin H, Gao L, Shen B, Chao L, Chao J (2010) Kallistatin inhibits vascular inflammation by antagonizing tumor necrosis factor-alpha-induced nuclear factor kappaB activation. Hypertension 56: 260–267.
9. Diao Y, Zhao XF, Lin JS, Wang QZ, Xu RA (2011) Protection of the liver against CCl_4-induced injury by intramuscular electrotransfer of a kallistatin-encoding plasmid. World J Gastroenterol 17: 111–117.
10. Huang X, Wang X, Dong H, Zhao X, Li Z, et al. (2010) High level expression of recombinant human kallistatin in Pichia pastoris and its bioactivity. Chin J Biotech 26: 249–255.
11. Xu R, Harrison PM, Chen M, Li L, Tsui TY, et al. (2006) Cytoglobin overexpression protects against damage-induced fibrosis. Mol Ther 13: 1093–1100.
12. Iwaisako K, Haimerl M, Paik YH, Taura K, Kodama Y, et al. (2012) Protection from liver fibrosis by a peroxisome proliferator-activated receptor delta agonist. Proc Natl Acad Sci U S A 109: E1369–1376.
13. Kim HJ, Yu MH, Lee IS (2008) Inhibitory effects of methanol extract of plum (Prunus salicina L., cv. 'Soldam') fruits against benzo(alpha)pyrene-induced toxicity in mice. Food Chem Toxicol 46: 3407–3413.
14. Shaker ME, Salem HA, Shiha GE, Ibrahim TM (2011) Nilotinib counteracts thioacetamide-induced hepatic oxidative stress and attenuates liver fibrosis progression. Fundam Clin Pharmacol 25: 248–257.
15. Itoh A, Isoda K, Kondoh M, Kawase M, Watari A, et al. (2010) Hepatoprotective effect of syringic acid and vanillic acid on CCl4-induced liver injury. Biol Pharm Bull 33: 983–987.
16. Guillaume M, Rodriguez-Vilarrupla A, Gracia-Sancho J, Rosado E, Mancini A, et al. (2013) Recombinant human manganese superoxide dismutase reduces liver fibrosis and portal pressure in CCl4-cirrhotic rats. J Hepatol 58: 240–246.
17. Valva P, Casciato P, Diaz Carrasco JM, Gadano A, Galdame O, et al. (2011) The role of serum biomarkers in predicting fibrosis progression in pediatric and adult hepatitis C virus chronic infection. PLoS One 6: e23218.
18. Kisseleva T, Brenner DA (2011) Anti-fibrogenic strategies and the regression of fibrosis. Best Pract Res Clin Gastroenterol 25: 305–317.
19. Cohen-Naftaly M, Friedman SL (2011) Current status of novel antifibrotic therapies in patients with chronic liver disease. Therap Adv Gastroenterol 4: 391–417.
20. Zhu H, Chao J, Kotak I, Guo D, Parikh SJ, et al. (2012) Plasma kallistatin is associated with adiposity and cardiometabolic risk in apparently healthy African American adolescents. Metabolism.
21. Hsieh J-L, Shen P-C, Shiau A-L, Jou I-M, Lee C-H, et al. (2009) Adenovirus-mediated kallistatin gene transfer ameliorates disease progression in a rat model of osteoarthritis induced by anterior cruciate ligament transection. Hum Gene Ther 20: 147–158.
22. Wang CR, Chen SY, Shiau AL, Wu CL, Jou IM, et al. (2007) Upregulation of kallistatin expression in rheumatoid joints. J Rheumatol 34: 2171–2176.
23. Miao RQ, Chen V, Chao L, Chao J (2003) Structural elements of kallistatin required for inhibition of angiogenesis. Am J Physiol Cell Physiol 284: C1604–1613.
24. Miao RQ, Agata J, Chao L, Chao J (2002) Kallistatin is a new inhibitor of angiogenesis and tumor growth. Blood 100: 3245–3252.
25. Diao Y, Ma J, Xiao WD, Luo J, Li XY, et al. (2007) Inhibition of angiogenesis and HCT-116 xenograft tumor growth in mice by kallistatin. World J Gastroenterol 13: 4615–4619.
26. Luo Q, Siconolfi-Baez L, Annamaneni P, Bielawski MT, Novikoff PM, et al. (2007) Altered protein expression at early-stage rat hepatic neoplasia. American Journal of Physiology-Gastrointestinal and Liver Physiology 292: G1272–G1282.
27. Chao J, Schmaier A, Chen LM, Yang Z, Chao L (1996) Kallistatin, a novel human tissue kallikrein inhibitor: levels in body fluids, blood cells, and tissues in health and disease. J Lab Clin Med 127: 612–620.

Permissions

The contributors of this book come from diverse backgrounds, making this book a truly international effort. This book will bring forth new frontiers with its revolutionizing research information and detailed analysis of the nascent developments around the world.

We would like to thank all the contributing authors for lending their expertise to make the book truly unique. They have played a crucial role in the development of this book. Without their invaluable contributions this book wouldn't have been possible. They have made vital efforts to compile up to date information on the varied aspects of this subject to make this book a valuable addition to the collection of many professionals and students.

This book was conceptualized with the vision of imparting up-to-date information and advanced data in this field. To ensure the same, a matchless editorial board was set up. Every individual on the board went through rigorous rounds of assessment to prove their worth. After which they invested a large part of their time researching and compiling the most relevant data for our readers.

The editorial board has been involved in producing this book since its inception. They have spent rigorous hours researching and exploring the diverse topics which have resulted in the successful publishing of this book. They have passed on their knowledge of decades through this book. To expedite this challenging task, the publisher supported the team at every step. A small team of assistant editors was also appointed to further simplify the editing procedure and attain best results for the readers.

Apart from the editorial board, the designing team has also invested a significant amount of their time in understanding the subject and creating the most relevant covers. They scrutinized every image to scout for the most suitable representation of the subject and create an appropriate cover for the book.

The publishing team has been an ardent support to the editorial, designing and production team. Their endless efforts to recruit the best for this project, has resulted in the accomplishment of this book. They are a veteran in the field of academics and their pool of knowledge is as vast as their experience in printing. Their expertise and guidance has proved useful at every step. Their uncompromising quality standards have made this book an exceptional effort. Their encouragement from time to time has been an inspiration for everyone.

The publisher and the editorial board hope that this book will prove to be a valuable piece of knowledge for researchers, students, practitioners and scholars across the globe.

List of Contributors

Lei Zhan, Mingzhe Yu, Cheng Huang, Xiaoming Meng, Taotao Ma, Lei Zhang and Jun Li
School of Pharmacy, Anhui Medical University, Hefei, China
Institute for Liver Diseases of Anhui Medical University (AMU), Hefei, China

Yang Song
School of Pharmacy, Anhui Medical University, Hefei, China
Institute for Liver Diseases of Anhui Medical University (AMU), Hefei, China
The First Affiliated Hospital of Anhui Medical University, Hefei, China

Jun Liu, Alex N. Eischeid and Xian-Ming Chen
Department of Medical Microbiology and Immunology, Creighton University School of Medicine, Omaha, Nebraska, United States of America

Hongtao Zhang, Xing Wang, Ning Xia, Desheng Wang and Kefeng Dou
Department of Hepatobiliary Surgery, Xijing Hospital, The Fourth Military Medical University, Xi'an, China

Jiandong Yang
Department of Hepatobiliary Surgery, Xijing Hospital, The Fourth Military Medical University, Xi'an, China
Department of Biochemistry and Molecular Biology, State Key Laboratory of Cancer Biology, The Fourth Military Medical University, Xi'an, China

Lin Wu, Xinping Liu, Libo Yao and Yan Li
Department of Biochemistry and Molecular Biology, State Key Laboratory of Cancer Biology, The Fourth Military Medical University, Xi'an, China

Jin Zheng
Department of Traditional Chinese and Western Medicine of Oncology, Tangdu Hospital, The Fourth Military Medical University, Xi'an, China

Ming Shi
Department of Neurology, Xijing Hospital, The Fourth Military Medical University, Xi'an, China

Brandon J. Auerbach
Infectious Diseases Institute, College of Health Sciences, Makerere University, Kampala, Uganda
Harvard Medical School, Boston, Massachusetts, United States of America

Steven J. Reynolds
Division of Intramural Research, National Institute of Allergy and Infectious Diseases, National Institutes of Health, Bethesda, Maryland, United States of America
Division of Infectious Diseases, Department of Medicine, School of Medicine, Johns Hopkins University, Baltimore, Maryland, United States of America

Collins Kukunda-Byobona
Department of Botany, Makerere University, Kampala, Uganda

Gregory D. Kirk
Department of Epidemiology, Bloomberg School of Public Health, Johns Hopkins University, Baltimore, Maryland, United States of America

Florence Abravanel, Stéphanie Raymond and Jacques Izopet
INSERM, U1043, Centre de Physiopathologie de Toulouse Purpan, Toulouse, France
CHU Toulouse Purpan, Laboratoire de Virologie, Institut Fédératif de Biologie de Purpan, France

Elodie Pambrun, Maria Winnock and François Dabis
INSERM, U897 and ISPED, Université Victor Segalen, Bordeaux, France

Philippe Bonnard
Service des Maladies Infectieuses et Tropicales, Hôpital Tenon, AP-HP, Paris, France

Philippe Sogni
Unité d'Hépatologie, Hôpital Cochin, AP-HP, Paris, France
Université Paris Descartes, Paris, France

Dominique Salmon-Ceron
Université Paris Descartes, Paris, France
Service des Maladies Infectieuses et Tropicales, Hôpital Cochin, AP-HP, Paris, France

Pascale Trimoulet
CHU Pellegrin, Laboratoire de virologie, Bordeaux, France
CNRS, UMR 5234, Microbiologie fondamentale et pathogénicité, Universite´ Bordeaux Segalen, Bordeaux, France

Yoshiki Murakami and Fumihiko Matsuda
Center for Genomic Medicine, Kyoto University Graduate School of Medicine, Kyoto, Japan

Hidenori Toyoda
Department of Gastroenterology, Ogaki Municipal Hospital, Ogaki, Japan

Masami Tanaka and Masahiko Kuroda
Department of Molecular Pathology, Tokyo Medical University, Tokyo, Japan

Yoshinori Harada
Department of Pathology and Cell Regulation, Kyoto Prefectural University of Medicine, Kyoto, Japan

Atsushi Tajima
Department of Molecular Life Science, Tokai University School of Medicine, Isehara, Japan

Nobuyoshi Kosaka and Takahiro Ochiya
Division of Molecular and Cellular Medicine, National Cancer Center Research Institute, Tokyo, Japan

Kunitada Shimotohno
Research Institute, Chiba Institute of Technology, Narashino, Japan

Jinxia Liu, Xin Cheng, Zhengrong Guo, Zihua Wang, Dong Li, Fubiao Kang, Haijun Li,

Baosheng Li and Dianxing Sun
The Liver Diseases Diagnosis and Treatment Center of PLA, Bethune International Peace Hospital, Shijiazhuang, People's Republic of China

Zhichen Cao
Department of Traditional Chinese Medicine and Liver Disease, The Third Affiliated Hospital of Hebei Medical University, Shijiazhuang, People's Republic of China

Michael Nassal
University Hospital Freiburg, Internal Medicine II/ Molecular Biology, Freiburg, Germany

Patricia Sancho, Jèssica Mainez and Eva Crosas-Molist
Biological Clues of the Invasive and Metastatic Phenotype Group, Bellvitge Biomedical Research Institute (IDIBELL), L'Hospitalet, Barcelona, Spain

Isabel Fabregat
Biological Clues of the Invasive and Metastatic Phenotype Group, Bellvitge Biomedical Research Institute (IDIBELL), L'Hospitalet, Barcelona, Spain
Department of Physiological Sciences II, University of Barcelona, Barcelona, Spain

César Roncero
Departamento de Bioquímica y Biología Molecular II, Facultad de Farmacia, Universidad Complutense and Instituto de Investigacio'n Sanitaria del Hospital Clı'nico San Carlos (IdISSC), Madrid, Spain

Conrado M. Fernández-Rodriguez
Service of Gastroenterology, Hospital Universitario Fundación Alcorcón and Universidad Rey Juan Carlos, Alcorcón, Madrid, Spain

Fernando Pinedo
Unit of Pathology, Hospital Universitario Fundacio'n Alcorcón, Alcorcón, Madrid, Spain

Heidemarie Huber and Wolfgang Mikulits
Department of Medicine I, Division: Institute of Cancer Research, Medical University of Vienna, Vienna, Austria

Robert Eferl
Department of Medicine I, Division: Institute of Cancer Research, Medical University of Vienna, Vienna, Austria
Ludwig Boltzmann Institute for Cancer Research (LBI-CR), Vienna, Austria

Catalina Atorrasagasti, Estanislao Peixoto, Néstor Kippes, Mariana Malvicini, Flavia Piccioni, Esteban J. Fiore and Juan Bayo
Gene Therapy Laboratory, School of Medicine, Austral University. Derqui-Pilar, Buenos Aires, Argentina

Jorge B. Aquino, Laura Alaniz, Mariana Garcia and Guillermo Mazzolini
Gene Therapy Laboratory, School of Medicine, Austral University. Derqui-Pilar, Buenos Aires, Argentina, CONICET (Consejo Nacional de Investigaciones Científicas y Técnicas), Buenos Aires, Argentina

Ramón Bataller
Department of Medicine and Nutrition, University of North Carolina, Chapel Hill, North Carolina, United States of America

Elizabeth Guruceaga and Fernando Corrales
Centro de Investigación Médica Aplicada, Universidad de Navarra, Pamplona, España

Osvaldo Podhajcer
Gene Therapy Laboratory, Fundación Instituto Leloir, Buenos Aires, Argentina
CONICET (Consejo Nacional de Investigaciones Cientı'ficas y Técnicas), Buenos Aires, Argentina

Li-xia Tang, Rui-hua He, Guang Yang and Jia-ju Tan
Institute of Medical Research, The First People's Hospital of Foshan, Foshan, Guangdong, China

Li Zhou
Department of Medicine, West China Hospital of Sichuan University, Chengdu, China

Xiao-ming Meng, Xiao Ru Huang and Hui Yao Lan
Li Ka Shing Institute of Health Sciences and Department of Medicine and Therapeutics, The Chinese University of Hong Kong, Hong Kong, China

Henning W. Zimmermann, Sebastian Seidler, Jens J. W. Tischendorf, Tom Luedde, Christian Trautwein and Frank Tacke
Department of Medicine III, University Hospital Aachen, Aachen, Germany

Jacob Nattermann
Department of Medicine I, University of Bonn, Bonn, Germany

Nikolaus Gassler
Institute of Pathology, University Hospital Aachen, Aachen, Germany

Claus Hellerbrand
Department of Medicine I, University of Regensburg, Regensburg, Germany

Alma Zernecke
Institute for Molecular Cardiovascular Research, University Hospital Aachen, Aachen, Germany

Ralf Weiskirchen
Institute of Clinical Chemistry and Pathobiochemistry, University Hospital Aachen, Aachen, Germany

Chuanshan Zhang, Xufa Wei, Guodong Lv, Xiaomei Lu, Hao Wen and Renyong Lin
State Key Lab Incubation Base of Xinjiang Major Diseases Research (2010DS890294) and Xinjiang Key Laboratory of Echinococcosis, First Affiliated Hospital of Xinjiang Medical University, Urumqi, Xinjiang, China

Junhua Wang
State Key Lab Incubation Base of Xinjiang Major Diseases Research (2010DS890294) and Xinjiang Key Laboratory of Echinococcosis, First Affiliated Hospital of Xinjiang Medical University, Urumqi, Xinjiang, China
Department of Nuclear Medicine, University of Franche-Comté and Jean Minjoz University Hospital, Besançon, Franche- Comté, France

Oleg Blagosklonov
Department of Nuclear Medicine, University of Franche-Comté and Jean Minjoz University Hospital, Besançon, Franche- Comté, France
WHO-Collaborating Centre for the Prevention and Treatment of Human Echinococcosis, University of Franche-Comté and University Hospital, Besanc,on, Franche-Comté, France

Georges Mantion and Dominique A. Vuitton
WHO-Collaborating Centre for the Prevention and Treatment of Human Echinococcosis, University of Franche-Comté and University Hospital, Besanc,on, Franche-Comté, France

Ursula Manuelpillai, Vijesh Vaghjiani and Jing-Yang Tee
Center for Reproduction and Development, Monash Institute of Medical Research, Monash University, Melbourne, Australia

James Chan
Center for Inflammatory Diseases, Monash University, Melbourne, Australia

Dinushka Lourensz, Jorge Tchongue, Alexander Hodge and William Sievert
Center for Inflammatory Diseases, Monash University, Melbourne, Australia
Gastroenterology and Hepatology Unit, Southern Health, Melbourne, Australia

Derek Lacey
University of Melbourne, Arthritis and Inflammation Research Centre, Royal Melbourne Hospital, Melbourne, Australia

Padma Murthi
Department of Obstetrics and Gynecology, University of Melbourne, Melbourne, Australia
Pregnancy Research Center, Department of Perinatal Medicine, Royal Women's Hospital, Melbourne, Australia

Morten Asser Karsdal, Quoc Hai Trieu Nguyen and Diana Julie Leeming
Nordic Bioscience A/S, Herlev, Denmark

Sanne Skovgård Veidal and Efstathios Vassiliadis
Nordic Bioscience A/S, Herlev, Denmark
Faculty of Health Science, University of Southern Denmark, Odense, Denmark

Arkadiusz Nawrocki and Martin Røssel Larsen
Faculty of Health Science, University of Southern Denmark, Odense, Denmark

Yunyun Luo and Qinlong Zheng
Nordic Bioscience Beijing, Beijing, China

Per Hägglund
Department of Systems Biology, Technical University of Denmark, Kgs. Lyngby, Denmark

Ben Vainer
Department of Pathology, Rigshospitalet, Copenhagen University Hospital, Copenhagen, Denmark

Si-Wen Chen, Ben-Yan Wu, Shi-Ping Xu, Li Yan, Yuan Gong, Jun-Bao Wen and Dao-Hong Wu
Department of Gastroenterology, NanLou Clinic, General Hospital of PLA, Beijing, China,

Ke-Xing Fan
International Joint Cancer Institute, The Second Military Medical University, Shanghai, China

Gang Tan, Shangha Pan, Xuesong Dong, Xian Jiang, Haiquan Qiao and Hongchi Jiang
Department of General Surgery, The Hepatosplenic Surgery Center, The First Affiliated Hospital of Harbin Medical University, Harbin, China

Xueying Sun
Department of General Surgery, The Hepatosplenic Surgery Center, The First Affiliated Hospital of Harbin Medical University, Harbin, China
Department of Molecular Medicine and Pathology, Faculty of Medical and Health Sciences, The University of Auckland, Auckland, New Zealand

Kai Kang and Mingyan Zhao
Department of ICU, The First Affiliated Hospital of Harbin Medical University, Harbin, China

Jie Li
Department of Hepatobiliary Surgery, Affiliated Qianfoshan Hospital of Shandong University, Jinan, China

Jagat R. Kanwar
Laboratory of Immunology and Molecular Biomedical Research, Centre for Biotechnology and Interdisciplinary Biosciences, Institute for Technology and Research Innovation, Deakin University, Geelong, Victoria, Australia

Yuping Wang and Hongmei Jiang
Department of Clinical Microbiology and Immunology, Affiliated Hospital of Guiyang Medical College, Guiyang, Guizhou Province, China

Mingliang Cheng and Baofang Zhang
Department of Infectious Diseases, Affiliated Hospital of Guiyang Medical College, Guiyang, Guizhou Province, China

Fei Nie
Guizhou Academy of Sciences, Guiyang, Guizhou Province, China

Ruchi Bansal and Jai Prakash
Department of Controlled Drug Delivery (Targeted Therapeutics), MIRA Institute for Biomedical Technology and Technical Medicine, University of Twente, Enschede, The Netherlands
Department of Pharmacokinetics, Toxicology and Targeting, University of Groningen, Groningen, The Netherlands

Marieke De Ruiter and Klaas Poelstra
Department of Pharmacokinetics, Toxicology and Targeting, University of Groningen, Groningen, The Netherlands

Charlotte Charpentier, Lucile Larrouy, Florence Damond, Françoise Brun-Vézinet and Diane Descamps
Laboratoire de Virologie, Assistance Publique-Hôpitaux de Paris (AP-HP), Groupe Hospitalier Bichat-Claude Bernard, HUPNVS, Université Paris Diderot, Paris 7, PRES Sorbonne Paris Cité , EA4409, Paris, France

Karen Champenois
Inserm ATIP-Avenir: "Modélisation, Aide à la Décision, et Coût-Efficacitéen Maladies Infectieuses", Lille, France

Anne Gervais, Roland Landman, Véronique Joly, Sylvie Le Gac and Yazdan Yazdanpanah
Service des Maladies Infectieuses et Tropicales, AP-HP, Groupe Hospitalier Bichat-Claude Bernard, HUPNVS, Université Paris Diderot, Paris 7, PRES Sorbonne Paris Cité, EA4409, Paris, France

Dongwei Jia, Peike Peng, Linlin Sun, Xiaojuan Liu, Weicheng Wu and Yuanyuan Ruan
Department of Biochemistry and Molecular Biology, Shanghai Medical College, Fudan University, Shanghai, P.R. China

Jianxin Gu
Department of Biochemistry and Molecular Biology, Shanghai Medical College, Fudan University, Shanghai, P.R. China
Institute of Biomedical Science, Fudan University, Shanghai, P.R. China

Fangfang Duan and Lan Wang
Institute of Biomedical Science, Fudan University, Shanghai, P.R. China

Xiaoping Huang, Xiao Wang, Yinghui Lv, Luli Xu, Junsheng Lin and Yong Diao
Institute of Molecular Medicine, Huaqiao University, Quanzhou, China

Index

www.ingramcontent.com/pod-product-compliance
Lightning Source LLC
Chambersburg PA
CBHW080518200326
41458CB00012B/4250